1 MONTH OF
FREE
READING

at

www.ForgottenBooks.com

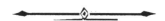

By purchasing this book you are eligible for one month membership to ForgottenBooks.com, giving you unlimited access to our entire collection of over 1,000,000 titles via our web site and mobile apps.

To claim your free month visit:
www.forgottenbooks.com/free785375

ISBN 978-0-483-50767-8
PIBN 10785375

This book is a reproduction of an important historical work. Forgotten Books uses
state-of-the-art technology to digitally reconstruct the work, preserving the original format
whilst repairing imperfections present in the aged copy. In rare cases, an imperfection in
the original, such as a blemish or missing page, may be replicated in our edition. We do,
however, repair the vast majority of imperfections successfully; any imperfections that
remain are intentionally left to preserve the state of such historical works.

THE
MONTREAL MEDICAL JOURNAL.

A Monthly Record of Medical and Surgical Science.

EDITED BY

GEORGE ROSS, A.M., M.D.,

Professor of Practice of Medicine, McGill University; Physician to the Montreal General Hospital.

T. G. RODDICK, M.D.,

Professor of Clinical Surgery, McGill University; Surgeon to the Montreal General Hospital, etc.

AND

JAMES STEWART, M.D.,

Professor of Materia Medica and Therapeutics, McGill University.

VOL. XVIII.

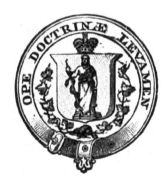

Montreal :

PRINTED & PUBLISHED BY THE GAZETTE PRINTING COMPANY.

1890.

a.

INDEX TO VOL. XVIII.

LIST OF CONTRIBUTORS TO VOL. XVIII.

ALLOWAY, T. JOHNSON, M.D.

BIANCHI, PROF.

BLACKADER, A. D., M.D.

BULLER, F., M.D.

CAMERON, J. C., M.D.

CAMPBELL, JNO., M.D.

CORBIN, F. G., M.D.

DAREY, J. H., M.D.

EDGAR, C. J., M.D.

EVANS, ED., M.D.

GARDNER, WM., M.D.

GIBNEY, V. P., M.D.

GRANT, SIR JAMES, M.D.

HOLMES, T. K., M.D.

IRWIN, J. L., M.D.

JOHNSTON, WYATT, M.D.

KENNEDY, G. A., M.D.

LANG, M. W., M.D.

MAJOR, G. W., M.D.

MacDONNELL, R. L., M.D.

PRAEGER, E. A., M.R.C.S.E.

ROSS, G. T., M.D.

SHEPHERD, F. J., M.D.

SMALL, H. B., M.D.

STEWART, JAS., M.D.

STIRLING, J. W., M.D.

WHITTAKER, J. T., M.D.

WRIGHT, A. H., M.D.

WRIGHT, H. P., M.D.

THE

MONTREAL MEDICAL JOURNAL.

| VOL. XVIII. | JULY, 1889. | No. 1. |

Original Communications.

ABSTRACT OF A CLINICAL LECTURE

DELIVERED AT THE MONTREAL GENERAL HOSPITAL, JUNE 18TH.

BY T. JOHNSON-ALLOWAY, M.D.,

The first case I bring before you to-day, gentlemen, is one of recto-vaginal fistula:

R. H., aged 32, married six years; two pregnancies at full term; youngest child two years of age. Complains of pain in back and iliac regions, a burning sensation in vagina, and escape of gas by that passage.

The opening is situated in the lower third of the vagina, or just anterior to the sphincter ani muscle. As I pass my index finger into the rectum and turn the point of it up-wards, you see it passes through an opening in the septum, into the vaginal tube. By this manœuvre we obtain a fair esti-mation both of the size of the opening and the strength of the sphincter; also what has been left of that muscle after so grave an injury. The recto-vaginal septum may be perforated by a fistula in any part, but the site corresponds in quite a typical manner to the mode of its occurrence.

In the lowermost part of the septum are found those fistulæ which are left over after incomplete cure of total perineal rup-tures, or after perforation of foreign bodies which have stuck fast in the rectum. Somewhat higher, from, say, 2 to 5 cm. above the anus, are found those fistulæ produced by pressure. necrosis during difficult labor, and they generally correspond

1

to the position of the bony exit of the pelvis—the point of the sacrum, or coccyx.

The upper peritoneal portión of the septum is the site of perforations resulting from encapsulated exudations in Douglas's pouch bursting through rectum into the vagina, or the rupturing of an extra-uterine pregnancy through both tubes.

The case before us belongs to the first class I describe; that is, the abnormal communication is due to necrosis of the soft parts as a result of long-continued pressure of the head during her first labor. The size of these pressure-necroses fistulæ varies very much ; this one is about the average, being about 2 cm. in its longest diameter, which is in the direction of the long axis of the vagina. The mucous membrane of the posterior wall of the rectum protrudes through the opening into the vagina, and, as you see, carries with it a rolling border of the mucous membrane of the anterior rectal wall as well.

The opening, you will also see, is not in the centre of the passage—in fact it rarely is ; it is situated to the right of the posterior columna rugarum, which sometimes overlaps it as a valve. The nature of such a blemish as this involves the loss of the most important function of the rectum. The patient cannot prevent gases and liquids passing from the bowel into the vagina, and thus renders her life most miserable. Our object, therefore, is to restore the recto-vaginal septum by operative means. And operative treatment is indicated in cases except those resulting from cancerous ulceration. The best time to operate is about six to eight weeks after labor.

I do not intend here to relate to you all of the different methods of repairing such an injury ; time would not permit ; but will demonstrate the method I intend to adopt in the present case by means of this little model of potter's clay. Previous to repairing recto-vaginal fistulæ and ruptured perinea, by Tait's flap-splitting, it was thought necessary always to divide the sphincter and whatever remained of the perineum right up to the fistulous opening, and undoubtedly it was the proper method to pursue.

I do not think in this case, however, it will be necessary to do more than forcibly stretch the sphincter so as to paralyze it for a short time while union is going on. After having done this I split the recto-vaginal septum with this obtuse-angled scissors until I have reached quite an inch above the upper portion of the fistula. I now pass silk-worm gut sutures in such a manner as to draw down that portion of the split anterior rectal wall above the fistula, over it, and thereby seal it. At the same time the sides of the perineum are drawn together with the sutures. After having thus demonstrated to you the operation on this model, I will perform it on the patient which has just been brought in anæsthetized. I would say, however, that complicating the recto-vaginal fistula, this patient has an old bilateral laceration of the cervix, which I will first repair by means of Emmet's trachelorrhaphy, occupying but a few moments.

In performing these flap-splitting operations you will often find large dilated veins running across the surface of cleavage. It is best to cut them through completely, as, if left and are afterwards transfixed by the needle, may give rise to a troublesome hæmatoma in the wound. This patient's bowels will be, from to-morrow, kept very loose by saline purgatives, and the sutures removed on the ninth or tenth day. Rest in bed, however, will be enforced for another week.*

The next case, gentlemen, is an exceedingly interesting one. Her history is as follows :

M. L., aged 48, married twenty-eight years ; thirteen children, youngest five years of age. Frequent and painful micturition, dysmenorrhœa, and profuse menstruation.

In brief, the conditions here are bilateral laceration of cervix, enormous hypertrophy of posterior segment of cervix, ectropion and cystic disease. The uterus is lying in the well of the pelvis, in the third degree of retroversion ; easily replaceable, though enlarged and hard—old-standing chronic metritis. The perineum is destroyed down to the sphincter and the vaginal walls prolapsed. We have, considering all these conditions, a

---

* Perfect union, with complete closure of fistula, was found on tenth day after operation.

very bad state of affairs, though, fortunately, easily remedied.
As regards treatment, we will do well to consider the various
conditions *seriatim.* There is first to attract our attention the
cervical laceration, which, from the extreme ectropion and hyper-
trophic disease, will not admit so well of Emmet's trachelorrhaphy as of Schrœder's supra-vaginal hysterectomy. Then
we have to deal with the lacerated perineum and an injured pelvic
floor. Tait's flap-splitting method will be most suitable here.
Finally, we have to deal with the still prolapsed and retroverted
uterus, and the two operations that I have spoken of will in no
wise give this woman, with more than ordinary intra-abdominal
pressure, relief. In order, therefore, to obtain a good result for
her, we will have to perform Alexander's operation—that of
shortening the round ligaments. By this latter procedure we
draw the uterus, ovaries, and broad ligament-folds well
forward, and we do away entirely with the injurious effects of
intra-abdominal pressure, by changing the direction of its force
from the anterior to the posterior face of the uterus and broad
ligaments. Therefore, after the round ligaments have been
shortened, the whole intra-abdominal pressure will have been
directed behind the uterus, into the posterior half of the pelvic
cavity, and will tend, if anything, to support the uterus and broad
ligament.

We have now completed Schrœder's operation on the cervix
and Tait's on the perineum, and my house surgeon tells me that
we have absorbed twenty minutes in so doing; we will therefore
have ample time to go on with Alexander's operation.

The field of operation, you see, is treated, as regards preparatory toilet, in the same way as for a laparotomy.

I stand on the opposite side of the patient to that on which
I make the incision.

First find the spine of the pubis, and cut down upon it with
one stroke of the knife, continuing the incision upward and outwards about half an inch to the inside of Poupart's ligament to
the extent of one and a half to two inches in length. On finding the ring and separating slightly its pillars, the round ligament will rise up to the surface, covered with a mass of fat

which appears to me to be an off-set from the subperitoneal fat,
as it is exactly like it in appearance. This, gentlemen, is the
structure we are in search of. You will always know it by its
white, pearly, glistening appearance, about the thickness of two
ordinary lucifer matches placed side by side, and capable of
being gradually drawn out of the opening by slight traction
with the fingers. We have now drawn out about four inches of
the ligament, and you will notice that it becomes gradually
thicker and more pink in color as it approaches the uterus.
Five or six silk-worm gut sutures are now passed, taking in the
wound thickness, half the ligament, and the pillars of the opening. A small drain made of a few strands of silk-worm gut is
placed in the lower angle of each wound, the slack of the ligament cut and torn away from its distal attachment, and the wound
dressed with sublimated gauze, etc. The drain will be removed
on the third day, the sutures on the fourteenth, and the patient
retained in hospital for four weeks.

REMARKS ON ANTISEPTIC EYE-SURGERY.

By F. Buller, M. D.,
Professor of Ophthalmology McGill University; Ophthalmic Surgeon to the
Montreal General Hospital.

(Read before the Ontario Medical Association, Toronto, June 6, 1889.)

Shortly after " Listerism " began to be recognized as a
substantial improvement in the art of surgery ophthalmologists commenced to seek for means of applying similar
methods in ophthalmic surgery. Unfortunately the great
principal of Listerism, which is absolute cleanliness, was for a
long time over-shadowed by the elaborate and ever changing
details of its application. I well remember at that time hearing the subject of antiseptic eye-surgery discussed by several
leading ophthalmologists of that period. The general opinion
seemed to be that the anatomical and physical conditions of
the eye were such as to render the methods of Lister wholly
inapplicable in ophthalmic practice. So soon, however, as the
great principle on which all antiseptic surgery is founded
came to be generally recognized ophthalmologists the world
over commenced to pay more strict attention to cleansing
measures, both in operative cases and in all affections of the

eye attended with unhealthy secretion. They soon found, too, that some of the so-called germicidal substances could be applied in efficient strength to the eyelids and conjunctiva not only without danger but with palpable advantage in the presence of certain morbid conditions. Such drugs as boracic acid, carbolic acid, and solutions of perchloride of mercury were used on account of their reputed germicidal properties, not only in purulent affections of the cornea and conjunctiva, but as a preventive of suppuration in all major operations on the eye.

Antiseptic eye surgery in its widest sense includes— 1st, the treatment of all inflammatory affections of the eye of a presumably septic character or in which the tissues or secretions or both contain micro-organisms supposed to be active agents in the inflammatory process. 2nd. The use of antiseptic precautions before, during and after operations on the eye for the purpose of preventing suppurative inflammatory action. I do not intend to speak of the first-class of cases except to state in a general way that I am fully convinced by my own experience in the treatment of this class of eye diseases that many eyes can be saved by strict attention and the free use of antiseptic remedies that would perish if left to nature, or such routine treatment as the text-books of a few years ago contain.

Everyone who has had much experience in operating on the eye must have observed that suppurative and ulcerative complications nearly always occur if they are going to take place at all, within a comparatively short time after the operative interference. In operations which involve penetrating wounds of the eyeball, such as the extraction of cataract, the formation of pus is sometimes noticed within a few hours after the operation, and I may say as far as my own observation goes, I believe this complication seldom, if ever, occurs later than twenty-four hours after the operation.

Another striking fact is the promptness with which union of the cut surfaces takes place when the eye is in a healthy condition. This, too, is, as a rule, a matter of only a few hours. In addition to this we have the unquestionable and no less important fact that the more recent the wound the more favourable are the conditions for septic action.

It follows from these observations that if we can in any way manage to keep the eye free from septic influences for the space of twenty-four hours, we carry it safely through the most dangerous period. This at least is true, if, as most of us now believe, suppuration can be shown to depend on septic influences, and especially so if the septic influence is from without, as it undoubtedly is in nearly every instance.

The only possible way of proving the actual value of antiseptic eye surgery is that of comparing results obtained under this system with those obtained when no special precautions are used. The comparison would be most complete if made on a large scale by the same operator with all other circumstances unaltered. For obvious reasons these conditions can never be entirely fulfilled. We can, however, institute a comparison between the antiseptic and the older methods, with other conditions approximately the same, and in this way conclusions may be drawn which will give us a fairly accurate idea of the relative value of the two methods.

Operations for the removal of cataract afford the greatest scope for making such comparisons, and for this reason I will give a *résumé* of the cataract operations which I have performed during the past two years, that is from May, 1887, to May, 1889. The number, though not very large, is, nevertheless, perhaps sufficient to justify this attempt to illustrate the subject of my paper. During the period just mentioned I have removed ninety cataracts by the various methods of extraction now in vogue.

The great majority of these were senile cataracts and the operation usually employed was the one known as sclero-corneal extraction with iridectomy. There are, however, in the series, cataracts of almost every variety, such as congenital, lamellar, traumatic, and soft cataract in early adult life of unknown origin. I do not think the value of the antiseptic method is materially modified by introducing these into the series because I am fully persuaded disastrous results are relatively quite as frequent in operations for the removal of these as in the more common senile cataract.

I will not give details as to the exact amount of vision attained in each case for the reason that many of them were hospital patients and most of these were discharged from the

hospital without an accurate record of vision having been
made. Moreover the records of visual acuteness commonly
given in the statistics of cataract operations are seldom of
much practical value because they do not by any means
represent the final results. It often happens that an eye,
which at the time of the patient's dismissal appears most
unpromising, ultimately turns out very satisfactorily, and
vice versa.

Vision of $\frac{1}{10}$ or $\frac{1}{5}$ after a successful operation may often
be vastly improved and perhaps brought up to the normal by
a secondary operation, and as a rule illiterate persons are
satisfied with imperfect vision and do not return for any
secondary operation. I may here state that in private
practice I do not consider any cataract operation satisfactory,
if the eye is otherwise healthy, unless the patient ultimately
gets sufficiently good vision to admit of reading ordinary
print. But in making up statistics of cataract operations I
would, if classifying according to visual results, divide into
four classes :—

    1.—Good result $V => \frac{1}{10}$.
    2.—Satisfactory result $V = \frac{1}{10} - \frac{1}{15}$.
    3.—Unsatisfactory result, $V = \frac{1}{15} - \frac{1}{100}$.
    4.—Bad result, $V =< \frac{1}{100}$.

As in the present instance I am not giving a precise statement of the visual results I shall classify as follows :

1. *Good result.*—All cases in which no complication
occurred likely to prevent the eye from attaining its maximum
vision. For instance, a senile cataract is removed, no
complications of any kind result from the operation. The
fundus oculi is subsequently seen perfectly by the ophthalmoscope in all its details. Yet V. only $\frac{1}{40}$. There is found to
be a central chorio-retinitis of old standing, accounting for the
defective vision.

2. *Satisfactory result.*—All cases in which complications
occurred after the operation, and fairly attributable to it,
which would obviously prevent the eye from attaining its
maximum vision but without greatly impairing its usefulness.

3. *Unsatisfactory results.*—All cases in which serious complications arose in consequence of the operation and caused
diminution of vision, but not such as to prevent the patient
from seeing sufficiently well to get about.

4. *Bad result or failure.*—All cases in which complications occurred of so serious a nature as to prevent the patient from regaining sufficient vision to see his way about.

On this basis then how does it stand with the ninety cases now under consideration? I find there are 76 good results, or 84.4 per cent.; 12 satisfactory results or 13.3 per cent.; 2 unsatisfactory results or 2.2 per cent., and no failures. Most of these operations were done under the influence of cocaine, and I think this has had something to do with results being better than were usually obtained before the days of cocaine, for there is no doubt operations on the eye are now performed with much greater deliberation and precision than was the case where no anæsthetic, or such anæsthetics as ether or chloroform were used; and there is, moreover, no doubt but that the patient's general condition is much more favorable after cocaine anæsthesia than it used to be after the profound disturbance so often seen in consequence of the administration of a general anæsthetic.

In my own experience I have never had so long a series of cataract operations without loss of one eye as the one now presented, and I am quite inclined to attribute this unusual success to the strict use of antiseptic precautions rather than to increased skill in operating or any other collateral circumstance. Compared with the cataract statistics of other ophthalmic surgeons as we find them in current literature of a few years ago, my results are certainly more favorable as it is not uncommon to find the failures amounting to five and even ten per cent.

I will not go into details of the ninety cases just referred to, but at the same time I cannot refrain from calling attention to the remarkable absence of suppurative inflammation in the whole series.

In only one instance there was a slight yellowish infiltration of the vitreous humor which had the appearance of a suppurative process, and when the patient disappeared from observation vision was reduced to qualitative perception of light. The eye in question was beginning to clear up and about six months after the woman returned wrote to say that she could not see very well.

The two worst results were in both eyes of one same patient.

a debilitated hard-working man, of intemperate habits, with thin flaccid corneæ. There was an interval of six months between the two operations and in both the course of events was the same. For three or four days all appeared to be well, then, for no obvious reason an insidious iritis set in, resulting in nearly complete occlusion of the pupil. Subsequently an iridotomy gave vision $=\frac{12}{200}$ with one eye, and with the other vision was $\frac{10}{200}$ without further interference.

In these operations I prepare the patient in the following manner :

Fifteen or twenty minutes before the operation one drop of a four per cent. solution of cocaine is instilled into the eye. Immediately before the operation the patient's face and eyelids are thoroughly cleansed with soap and water and then with solution of perchloride of mercury 1–5000, and the eye is also flushed with the same. Then another drop of cocaine is instilled and the eye again flushed with solution of the perchloride, 1–10,000, and the same solution is used during the operation as much as may be necessary.

I always wash each instrument to be used, with alcohol immediately before and after the operation. After the operation a thin layer of cotton soaked in the 1–10,000 solution is laid on the lids and over this a light compressure bandage applied in the usual way. I have not found any injurious effects from the perchloride used in this way unless it were once perhaps a little transient opacity of the cornea and twice a slight eczema of the lids which disappeared in a few days.

Among other ophthalmic operations for which antiseptic precautions are essential to success I would especially mention the operation of inserting an artificial vitreous, and also plastic operations involving both skin and conjunctiva of lower lids, in which latter the conjunctival secretion is particularly prone to contaminate the wound and prevent union by first intention.

CASE IN PRACTICE—TETANUS INFANTUM.

By Ed. Evans, M.D., LaCrosse, Wisconsin.

Infant, five days old, lies on back, with eyes closed, mouth slightly open, tongue pressed against teeth and interspace filled with frothy saliva; face contracted, and of a muddy, yellowish hue; slight cyanosis of lips; respirations are fast and very irregular (62 per minute); the head is held straight; the neck is stiff, so that the body can be lifted from the bed by placing the hand behind the head. The eyes are examined with difficulty; they are slightly rotated upwards; pupils are equal and normal in size. The arms are pressed to sides, the forearms flexed on chest, and the hands clenched, the thumbs in the palm. There is spasm of the diaphragm, irregular in intensity and rhythm. The abdominal muscles are somewhat rigid. The umbilicus is moist and slightly red, but not inflamed-looking, and no sign of pus. The thighs are flexed on trunk; the legs and feet are also flexed, as are the toes. There is no jaundice of the trunk or limbs. Pulse 150, heart steady and regular; temperature 101.5°F. There is persistent rigidity of all the muscles, paroxysmally intensified. Attempts at passing the finger into the mouth, stirring the limbs, or moving the clothes causes firm closure of the mouth, jerking of the muscles of the face and limbs, and a paroxysmal increase of the rigidity, during which the respirations become more impeded and the cyanosis is increased. Examination of the head reveals nothing abnormal.

The first symptoms were noticed about twelve hours before, when the child refused to nurse and was cross and fretful. It gradually grew worse, and in a short time the jaw became rigid and respirations impeded. It had the first "spasm" about six hours after illness was first noticed. During the night it grew rapidly worse and had opisthotonos twice. The nurse treated it for "spasms" with hot bath, etc.

It was an easy labor; the child was remarkably robust and fat. The bowels were regular and it passed urine all right. (She was attended by a midwife.) As it was impossible to give anything by the mouth, I gave gr. ii chloral hyd. by enema, to be repeated, and ordered perfect quiet.

The child died four hours later, apparently from exhaustion. The muscles relaxed a few minutes before death. Duration, seventeen hours. The slight jaundice I noticed in face rapidly increased till it spread over head and trunk before death, being very marked in face, but little, if any, in limbs. An hour after death the body was quite warm and rigor mortis very marked. An autopsy was refused. The child belonged to healthy parents. The sanitary conditions about good. It had not been exposed to cold in any way. There did not seem to be any intestinal irritation up to the time of the attack, and after I first saw the child the bowels moved twice, the stools being normal in color and consistency. The jaundice which appeared so rapidly was scarcely noticeable when I saw the child five hours before death. The nurse remarked on the very rapid emaciation during its short illness.

I might mention incidentally that a few months ago two horses died in the vicinity of idiopathic tetanus, and a few days previous to this case a gentleman of the city died of traumatic tetanus.

Retrospect Department.

REPORT ON THE PROGRESS OF OPHTHALMOLOGY.

BY FRANK BULLER, M.D.,
Professor of Ophthalmology, McGill University.

G. Martin of Bordeaux has labored assiduously to prove that migrain is an arthritic disease which only appears in cases of partial contraction of the ciliary muscle. He has found astigmatism present in nearly all cases of migraine, often marked by a partial contraction of the ciliary muscle. Very low degrees of astigmatism suffice to set up faulty action in the ciliary muscles and thus cause migraine In the majority of cases, the astigmatism amounted to less than one dioptry. The prolonged use of atropine was often necessary to discover the actual degree of astigmatism, the spasmodic action yielding only after several weeks of atropinization. Before the use of the drug both eyes might appear to be astigmatic, but afterwards the static astigmatism would commonly be found in one eye only ; to overcome this, the irregular contraction of the ciliary muscle had induced an apparent astigmatism in the other eye. When only one eye is affected the hemicrania is confined to that side.

The development of migraine, according to this authority, depends on three factors:

1. A constitutional anomaly, arthritis.
2. Partial contraction of the ciliary muscle.
3. Upon accidental causes varying with each case.

Martin bases his views upon a long series of clinical cases given in detail, and concludes from them as follows: " Our theory of astigmatism as the cause of migraine ophthalmique therefore rests upon a number of proofs. First, upon the constancy of astigmatic contraction; secondly, upon the confinement of the unilateral migraine to the side of this contraction; and, finally, on the good effect of cylindrical glasses."

[Our experience of the use of atropine in correcting errors of refraction would lead us to believe that in this country comparatively few patients would submit to the long course of atropine that Martin has found essential.—F.B.]

Causes of Myopia.—Risley has found several instances of originally hyperopic eyes eventually becoming myopic. He refers this remarkable change to the presence of astigmatism. It may here be stated that Sattler's views regarding the influence of astigmatism in causing myopia have not generally been accepted.

The real cause of the development of axial myopia is as yet by no means settled, notwithstanding the many theories advanced in explanation thereof. One of the latest of these theories is that propounded by Weiss of Tübingen, whose anatomical investigations as to the cause of myopia led him to believe that the optic nerve is not exposed to any strain by the movements of the eyes when the piece extending from the anterior end of the optic canal to the insertion at the globe is long, but that such strain results when this portion of the nerve is short. This strain accounts for the tissue changes at the extreme end of the optic nerve. When, however, the growth of the body has ceased, the influence of this strain as a cause of myopia ceases.

Purulent Ophthalmia.—Aldfield (Prevention of Contagious Diseases of the Eye during the first week of life, *Berliner Klin. Woch.*, No. 14, 1888) recommends "irrigation of the vagina with solution of corrosive sublimate during parturition, and as soon as the child's head appears he washes the face and eyes with ordinary water and then covers the child's face with a folded cloth so that the vaginal discharges cannot come in contact with the child's eyes." [This procedure is not likely to be generally adopted, and in view of the very small percentage of new-born infants that suffer from ophthalmia neonatorum, even when no special precautions are taken in the way of prevention, it would hardly seem to be necessary. If, however, the accoucheur has any reason to suspect venereal disease in the parturient woman, some such precautionary measures should on no account be neglected, and would doubtless often save the infant from a dangerous disease of the eyes.—F.B.]

In the treatment of acute purulent ophthalmia, Hoor recommends, in the early stages of the disease, ice compresses to the lids and frequent washing of the conjunctiva with a solution of permanganate of potash. In the treatment of this disease the condition of the cornea must be carefully watched; if ulceration appears cold compresses are contra-indicated. Frequent cleansing of the conjunctival sac with warm, unirritating antiseptic solutions is, however, essential. Mules treats blenorrhoic conjunctivitis by washing the everted lids and brushing them with alcohol; he also washes them with corrosive sublimate 1×2000. Whatever may be the choice of remedies in the treatment of purulent ophthalmia, the chief element of success lies in scrupulous cleanliness and thoroughness in the application of the antiseptic selected. The treatment should never be left to uninstructed attendants.

Granular Ophthalmia.—The operative treatment of granular ophthalmia (trachoma) seems to be growing in favor. Peunow favors scraping out the granulations with a sharp spoon. When they form a fold he excises this before scraping out the remaining granulations. When they cannot all be scraped out on account of marked infiltration (*trachoma diffusum*), he presses out the remainder with the fingers or the forceps. In this manner Peunow treated 180 patients, whom he divides into three groups. The first (43 patients) comprises those cases in which the trachoma-granules had developed upon the sound or only slightly hyperæmic conjunctiva. The results were excellent. The treatment lasted from ten to thirty days ; the spoon was used from one to three days. All were completely cured ; no relapses thus far, though some were treated more than a year ago. In the second group (102 patients), trachoma with marked hyperæmia and swelling of the conjunctiva and muco-purulent discharge. Length of treatment, fifteen to sixty days ; the spoon was used from two to five days. Fifty patients were completely cured : in thirty-two there was thickening of the palpebral conjunctiva, while in the remainder there was thickening and unevenness of the conjunctiva generally ; in three some granulations remained, as they lay deep in the tissues and could not therefore be perfectly scraped out. Third group (35 patients), trachoma with scars of the conjunctiva and corneal complications ; length of treatment two months and more. In some cases there remained unevenness and pannus, which yielded to jequirity.

Staderini has made a careful study of the trachomatous process, and has uniformly discovered the presence of germs, which he calls the trachomacoccus, closely resembling the gonococcus, but much smaller. Introduced beneath the conjunctiva it produces trachoma, especially in poorly nourished animals. This author has always found the specific coccus in groups of three to nine, abundant in the protoplasm of the lymph cells of trachoma, rarely in the fibrous tissue of the granules, or in the connective tissue of the conjunctiva. As regards treatment, he recommends daily brushing with sublimate solution 1 to 500, together with the instillation twice daily of a solution of the same, 1 to 2000. When there is much discharge, nitrate of silver may be used alternately with the sublimate. Creoline has been found to act beneficially in the treatment of granular ophthalmia ; a one or two per cent. solution is said to possess powerful antiseptic properties without causing any lasting irritation. It may be used as an instillation several times daily ; stronger solutions may also be applied to the everted lids, but the excess should be washed off before replacing the lids.

Ectropion.—For senile ectropion of the lower lid, Boucheron recommends excision of the tarsus, which is performed through the conjunctiva. A strip of tarsus 1 mm. wide is allowed to remain. In total ectropion he excises the whole tarsus with the exception of this strip, but in partial ectropion he only removes a portion of it.

Trichiasis.—For the relief of trichiasis, Van Milligan divides the edges of the lid longitudinally between the lashes and the meibomian glands, thus making a wound 3 to 4 mm. wide, becoming narrowed at each extremity, into which he transplants a corresponding strip of mucous membrane from the lips, keeping it in position with a bandage. [This operation, if successful, would have the advantage of giving a perfectly smooth surface to the edge of the lid, which is more than can be claimed for those operations in which a portion of integument from the upper lid is similarly transplanted either with or without pedicle.—F.B.]

Diagnosis of Lachrymal Fistula.—J. Scheff, in an article on the differential diagnosis of fistula of the cheek and gums below the inner canthus, and lachrymal fistula, states that the former is never situated exactly at the infra-orbital margin, but below it, and can be probed only downward and backwards.

Disease of Lachrymal Sac.—The pernicious effect on the eye of secretions retained in the lachrymal sac in cases of chronic ducryocystitis has long been recognized. In order to study the effect of the bacteria of the lachrymal sac upon the conjunctiva and lac-sac, Widmark introduced the lachrymal secretion from three patients into the eyes of healthy persons seven times in all. With the exception of slight lachrymation and injection lasting only a few hours, no change was noticed. He therefore thinks that the bacteria are harmless when the conjunctiva and lachrymal sac are healthy, and assumes that an obstruction to the flow of tears may perhaps be the cause. In this connection it must be observed that in chronic dacryocystitis the conjunctiva is constantly exposed to the unhealthy secretion, which in the experiments gave rise to only transient irritation. Under these circumstances the chronic conjunctivitis and tendency to suppurative disease of the cornea is sufficiently obvious. Widmark has also made cultures in cases of serpiginous ulcers of the cornea, and has found streptococcus pyogenes and micrococcus. In 25 cases of blephoradenitis examined, he always found the streptococcus pyogenes. When gelatine containing bacteria is introduced into a pocket-like wound of the conjunctiva, a pustule is the result; and when a culture emulsion of staphylococcus pyogenes is injected under the conjunctiva, a local infiltration with catarrh of the conjunctiva ensues. The author thinks that the phlyctenula conjunctivitis and blephoradenitis are due to infection, the same micro-organisms being the cause in both.

Ocular Muscles.—The correction of faults in the muscular functions of the eyes is a subject which has in the past few years received a great deal of attention and excited much discussion among ophthalmologists. The nomenclature as well as the principles advanced and advocated by Dr. Geo. T. Stevens are fully accepted by some and almost entirely rejected by others. There seems, however, to be a growing conviction that many cases of asthenopia and headache can be satisfactorily treated by graduated tenotomy of the ocular muscles, where a surplus of power in certain muscles is found associated with deficiency of power in their opponents. In a paper read before the last meeting of the American Ophthalmological Society by Dr. Webster of New York, and entitled " Some Tenotomies for the Correction of Heterophoria, with Results," he arrived at the following conclusions :—

1. No person should have tenotomy performed simply and solely because he is the subject of heterophoria ; that is, unless some annoying symptom, local or general, is present that *may* be due to the want of harmony in the action of his ocular muscles. There must be a reason for the operation in addition to the existence of the condition to be corrected.

2. Very slight degrees of heterophoria may and should be

2

ed where troublesome symptoms exist which may be due
too great use of nervous force in co-ordinating the eyes.
t is well that all other means that afford any prospect of
hould be tried before resorting to a tenotomy, although
) should be lost by unnecessary or dilatory treatment.

enotomies for the correction of heterophoria should always
ormed under cocaine, so that the effect of the operation
) accurately measured and properly limited.

n judiciously selected cases, where the operation is prop-
rformed, the average results will be quite as satisfactory
results of most other surgical operations.

eter had operated on four patients who were epileptics.
ilepsy was not cured in any case, though the fits were
arily suspended in one case. In another case the fits
vorably modified, though the epilepsy was organic. In
case there was temporary improvement, but later the
was worse than ever. In the fourth case the fits had
ispended for over six months, and the operation was done
)r the relief of asthenopia than for epilepsy, and with
)od result. He further says : "There can be no objection
)ring the proper balance of the ocular muscles, when it
in lost, in cases of epilepsy and chorea, but, judging from
sonal experience, it does not cure either disease. Aside
ie cure of the disease, however, enough good results in
ig asthenopic symptoms to justify the procedure."

or two hysterical cases were operated upon at Dr. E. C.
's suggestion with surprisingly good results. One gentle-
civil and mining engineer from the west, had come to
guin with a diagnosis of "incurable spinal disease." Dr.
found spinal irritation of extreme degree. He had been
1 for business "by semi-periodical paroxysms of excruci-
pain, in which he made contortions (semi-involuntary),
had been termed convulsions." Webster says : "I found
one of these attacks when I went to his room prepared
ate on one of his interni. I sat with him over an hour,
which the agony, the plaintive cries, and the apparent
sions continued without remission, the patient constantly

writhing in the most intense pain, until Dr. Seguin arrived, and we gave him chloroform and divided the tendon. From that time to the present, so far as I can learn, he has had but one attack, and that a very mild one, and after sufficient psychical abuse to account for a recurrence."

The majority of cases operated upon and relieved were cases of headache, varying in degree, character and location.

A lengthy discussion followed the reading of this paper. Referring to the case of the engineer just cited, Dr. Seguin said : " The man, it seems to me, was subject largely to delusional, nervous suffering, and the question will arise, whether the operation did not do good partly by " suggestion," as well as it may have helped in a psychical way."

Another case was one in which all the muscles of the eyeball were remarkably feeble, and in which dizziness, attacks of a fainting nature, and confusion of mind were the chief nervous symptoms. In this case all efforts at correction proved unavailing. That was one of the cases which brings up the question strongly in the mind of the neurologist, whether the condition of the eye muscles might not be the result of neurosis and the general condition of the patient. This patient was anæmic and had a feeble heart. Seguin is inclined to the opinion that in many cases unsuccessfully treated by tenotomy of the ocular muscles, the failure is due to faults in the general condition rather than to asthenia of one or more of the ocular muscles, and although not over-sanguine as to the results to be obtained in many nervous cases from tenotomies, he intends to prosecute further enquiries in this direction. He defines his position as neutral between the extravagant claim that neuroses are curable by tenotomies and the adaptation of spectacles, and the position which assumes that these means are useless.

Dr. Henry D. Noyes objects to such expressions as exophoria, orthophoria, etc., " because they tend to lump things together and mislead as to the real state of muscular equilibrium." The objection is hardly a valid one, because the complete clinical record which must be made in every case of known muscular fault before remedial measures can be adopted shows not only the faulty tendency, but also the relative power of all muscles whose actions can be measured with prismatic glasses. Dr. Noyes believes that insufficiencies of the external recti are by far the preponderating troubles to be dealt with, and endeavors, when at all practicable, to relieve the difficulty by the use of prisms rather than by tenotomy. He would not operate at all unless fully satisfied that there was a considerable excess of muscular power in some one direction so that he could interfere with an over-strong muscle for the benefit of a weak one. He is convinced that a large proportion of cases of defective muscular action are mainly due to nerve exhaustion and not to pure muscular error, that the symptoms on the part of the muscles are developed in consequence of nerve exhaustion, and they are not suitable cases for tenotomy. The same conclusions have been arrived at by others who have had much experience in dealing with this class of cases.

Sexual Organs and their Relation to Eye Disease.— Mr. Henry Power, in a lengthy paper (*Trans. of the Ophth. Society of the United Kingdom,* Vol. VIII.), sums up as follows : In males, the excessive excitement of the sexual organs in youth occasions various subjective symptoms in one or both eyes—as muscæ, photopsiæ, asthenopia, and loss of accommodation, together with blepharospasm, and, at a later period, possibly retinitis, retinal hemorrhages, and white atrophy. That in young women, the epoch of the installation of menstruation may be attended with conjunctivitis, both phlyctenular and follicular, and ulcers of the cornea, with special disposition to the development of keratitis consequent on constitutional taint. That amenorrhœa, especially if suddenly induced, may be followed by hemorrhage into the anterior chamber or into the vitreous, iritis, irido-choroiditis, optic neuritis, and white atrophy of the optic disc. That dysmenorrhœa may be accompanied by conjunctivitis, keratitis, episcleritis, as well as by inflammation of the uveal tract. That the menopause is often accompanied by effusion into the vitreous, and by a disposition to glaucoma, by paresis or paralysis of the ocular muscles. That pregnancy is often attended during the early months with asthenopia, and towards the close with albuminuric retinitis with its consequences (hemorrhages and white patches on the retina); and that if delivery is attended with copious hemorrhage, loss or great impairment of vision, with white discs, may occur. That in the puerperal state we may meet with embolism, which is sometimes of a septic character, and may rapidly lead to loss of the eye. And, finally, that in lactation—if we may be allowed to include that process in the consideration of the sexual organs—we find asthenopia, great tendency to suppuration of the cornea on slight scratches, and lachrymal diseases to be of common occurrence.

The Prognosis as to Life in Renal Retinitis.—Mr. Simeon Snell (*Trans. Oph. Soc. of the United Kingdom*, Vol. VII) relates eight cases bearing on this subject, only one of which lived longer than one year after the retinal disease first came under notice. Mr. Snell remarks: " The prognosis of the retinal lesion is truly that of the renal disease, and does not think that English writers insist sufficiently on the point that in certainly the majority of cases the presence of the retinal changes betokens such a grave condition that the period of existence is limited. In the renal retinitis of pregnancy the prognosis, however, is by no means so serious, partial or complete recovery commonly taking place under these circumstances."

QUARTERLY RETROSPECT OF GYNÆCOLOGY.

PREPARED BY T. JOHNSON-ALLOWAY, M.D.,
Instructor in Gynæcology, McGill University; Assistant Surgeon to the Montreal General Hospital; Gynæcologist to the Montreal Dispensary.

The Perineum ; its Anatomy, Physiology and Methods of Restoration after Injury, by HENRY O. MARCY, M.D., &c., Boston.—A voluminous and profusely illustrated paper appearing in the January number of the *Amer. Journal of Obstetrics* by Dr. Marcy is well worth careful study. It is, however, altogether too exhaustive and minute in detail to make an abstract notice of with justice. Dr. Marcy says in conclusion: " My method differs from others in the following particulars :

1. The dissection of the posterior third of the vagina, not its mucous membrane, from its vulvar attachment, carried as deemed necessary into the recto-vaginal space, and the retention of the flap.

2. In rectocele with prolapse, the closure of the deep layers of post-vaginal fascia by a continuous buried animal suture, taken either in single or double stitch.

3. In lifting forward the vagina from its vulvar attachment, the retracted transverse perineal muscles with their connections can be reached and closed also by a deep-buried suture, making in this way a true restoration of the pelvic floor.

4. Coapting all superficial surfaces by a buried animal suture, applied in a blind, continuous stitch from side to side, covering the same when dry with iodoform-collodion.

5. The application of lateral supports, pins external to the sutures as a splint to hold the parts in complete apposition without strain.

6. In complete ruptures, the lateral dissection, the joining of the rectal and vaginal edges with buried sutures, and then finishing the operation as in incomplete ruptures."

In the above, taken with the diagrams, we have the gist of Dr. Marcy's exhaustive paper ; and although the author states that his method differs from those of others, we cannot admit the statement to be exactly correct. The operation described by Dr. Marcy as original is simply Tait's " flap-splitting" method as applied to the lacerated perineum. The addition of deep-buried sutures, as a method, belongs to Werth, and we think the application of supporting pins a superfluity, entailing much suffering to the patient during convalescence. As regards the animal sutures used by Dr. Marcy, whether from kangeroo or other animal, no man can prove them to be absolutely aseptic unless they have been previously boiled, and as silk-worm gut will best undergo this process, it should be chosen before all others. We would also draw Dr. Marcy's attention to the fact that few men now even think of applying more than *one* perineal suture in performing the primary operation.

Psychoses and Gynæcological Operations. (CHARLES W. FILLEBROWN, M.D.)—The appearance of psychosis after operations upon the female genitals has only lately been observed by operators. The causative relation of the operation is by no means clear, and the analysis of cases only renders the association as cause and result more and more difficult to comprehend. Naturally we look first for some evidence of predisposition, either in the family history or in the history of the patient. In some cases we certainly do find a predisposition, but in others the psychosis is attributable only to the operation. We cannot overlook the possibility of the co-existence of organic cerebral disease, or the occurrence of embolism or hemorrhage ; and, again, in cases where the patient has suffered great losses, or where a long, painful illness previous to the operation has weakened the nervous system, as well as the whole constitution. We must attach some etiological importance to this general condition.

Prof. Werth of Kiel, who read a paper upon this subject before the Gynæcological Congress of Halle last May, reported six cases of psychosis following operations. In 32 total extirpations of the uterus two cases occurred ; in 160 ovariotomies, two cases ; in 36 oöphorectomies, two cases. In five cases the mental disorder assumed the form of melancholia, and in one mania. In two cases the disorder made its appearance five and eight days respectively after the operation ; in two cases after two or three weeks ; and in the two remaining cases the disturbance developed after discharge. Of these six cases, three recovered—one after fifteen days, one after four months, and one after eight months.

In the discussion which followed this paper, Sänger of Leipsig considered the psychosis in these cases latent, and the operation the exciting cause. He was of opinion that careful inquiry into the family history or that of the patient would probably show some evidence of predisposition ; further, that the presence of psychical symptoms should not alter the treatment indicated by the local condition. Martin said that the gynæcology played no particular part in the causation of psychosis. He claimed that it was seen after other surgical operations in both men and women.

The author concludes with the following :—

1. Gynæcological operations can produce psychosis in patients free from hereditary predisposition.

2. Where there exists no predisposition, the mental derange-

ment is transitory and the prognosis is good. In predisposed patients the prognosis is unfavorable.

3. Mental disturbance appearing later than four months after the operation is probably independent of the latter.

4. The development of psychosis is probably limited to those cases in which the convalescence from the operation did not run a normal course.

5. The existence of a predisposition to psychosis in a patient ought not to deter the gynæcologist from carrying out the treatment indicated by the physical condition.

6. In cases of really insane patients, operations should only be performed when the physical condition endangers life or renders it insupportable."

Dr. Shepherd of Montreal recently published a paper on this subject, giving cases of psychosis following operations in men. There seems to be some relationship between these cases of psychosis following surgical operations and the cases of so-called puerperal insanity. It is well recognized by all observers how little is understood concerning the etiological nature of this form of insanity, and it would appear that the puerperal traumatism or process had the same relation to " puerperal insanity" that the gynæcological operations had to the psychosis following.

Dr. Hirst reports six cases of puerperal insanity occurring within the period of eighteen months.—(*American Journal of Obstetrics*, Feb. 1889.)

Surgical Treatment of Retroversion of the Uterus with Adhesions, with New Method of Shortening the Round Ligaments. W. GILL WYLIE, M.D. (*Amer. Jour. Obstet.*, May 1889.)— Dr. Wylie's method consists in opening the abdominal cavity, catching up the round ligaments with forceps about midway between the cornu of the uterus and the pubic bone, then forming a loup with the ligament and tying this loup with three ligatures so as to considerably shorten the length of the ligament. He says : " Given ten cases of retroversion with adhesions which have been subjected to what I may call the preparatory treatment with rest, boroglyceride cotton pledgets, and etherization to reach an approximate diagnosis and to enable me to exclude those cases of endometritis and enlargement with retroversion simulating fixation by adhesions, it will be found, on opening the abdomen, that nine out of the ten cases are in reality cases of salpingitis complicated by retroversion and usually chronic endometritis ; that in the majority the adhesions which fix the uterus are mainly in the broad ligaments, these ligaments being rolled back over the ovaries in such a way as to displace the fundus backward.   The peritoneum covering the fundus may have adhesions binding the uterus backward, but as a rule the fundus is comparatively free, the fixation being chiefly caused by the change in the broad ligament.   In about one out of the ten cases the tubes and ovaries are free, or are only slightly affected by adhesions, the adhesions not being sufficient to close the fimbriated extremities of the tubes, and the ovaries not at all or only slightly fixed by adhesions ; while the fundus of the uterus is fixed by adhesions binding it to the posterior wall of the pelvis, to the rectum, etc.   It is evident that the exudations in this case were not due to the extension of the uterine disease from the uterus out through the tube to the peritoneum, but that the endometritis had been accompanied by such a severe metritis as to cause inflammation and exudation on the peritoneum covering the uterus, and resulted in adhesions and fixation to the tissues in direct continuity with the walls of the uterus.   Now I know that by careful treatment, notwithstanding these adhesions, some of these cases can be cured by local treatment without resorting to either laparotomy or forcible means of breaking up the adhesions ; but in many cases all such treatment fails, either from the difficulty of getting the patients to submit to the treatment or the obstinacy of the endometritis, and the only way to ever reach a certain diagnosis after failure of local treatment is to open the abdomen.   I maintain that laparatomy is in such cases safer than the old plan of *attempting* to break up the adhesions, either with or without ether, by means of a repositor or by any forcible means applied through the vagina."

We cannot see where Dr. Wylie's method has advantage over the operation known as hysterorrhaphy—that of attaching the

fundus of the uterus to the anterior abdominal wall by means of
sutures passed through the broad ligaments, close to the entrance
of the Fallopian tubes, including part of the round ligaments,
and then through the peritoneum and subperitoneal tissue of the
anterior abdominal wall.   The procedure of Dr. Wylie is, however, a departure, and deserves notice, but whether it will
become an advance or not in operative surgery, time will decide.

Two Cases of Primary Epithelioma of the Vulva and Vagina.
PAUL F. MUNDÉ, M.D.—Dr. Mundé gives the following short
report of this rare disease :

" While a number of cases of primary malignant disease of
the external genital organs of the female and of the vagina are
on record, they are still sufficiently rare to justify reporting and
illustration.   This is particularly true of the vagina, of which
location Kuester collected only twenty-two cases, to which
Olshausen added two.   I myself have seen two cases, the one
here reported, and one two years ago in a girl of 24, where a
freely bleeding and secreting growth of the size of an almond
projected from the posterior vaginal pouch.   I excised it as
deeply as I dared without opening Douglas's pouch, but it soon
returned and I again excised it, this time opening the peritoneal
cavity.   I closed the wound at once with catgut, and the patient,
although confined to her bed for some time by a cellulitis and
pelvic abscess, eventually made a good recovery and remained
well.   The microscope showed the growth to be a true epithelioma.   Epithelioma is more common on the vaginal walls than
medullary infiltration.   The posterior wall is most frequently
affected.   Only in the early stage, when complete extirpation
is possible, can a cure be expected.   Schroeder has dissected
off the entire vaginal wall down to the rectum and united the
edges of the wound, including the rectal wall, and drained.
Out of three cases one died of sepsis ; the second recovered,
and two and one-half months thereafter there was no recurrence ;
the third was still too recent when reported to admit of a conclusion as to the ultimate result.   When a radical cure is impossible, the sharp curette, thermo-cautery, or some styptic,
with subsequent dressing with iodoform and tannin powder, is

all that can be done to make the patient comfortable. Carcinoma of the vulva occurs about once in thirty-five to forty cases of cancer of the female sexual organs. Epithelioma is by far the most frequent variety, and remains local a long while, not infecting the inguinal glands until quite late. When it involves only the labia or mons veneris, it can usually be radically removed without difficulty; but when it has spread to the urethra, as in the case here reported, it may be necessary to remove more or less of that canal to reach sound tissue, and contraction of the urethra, or, if the neck of the bladder has been injured, incontinence of urine, may ensue. In the matter of diagnosis, only occasionally is it necessary to differentiate between epithelioma and lupus. The microscope will easily settle the question.

"I. EPITHELIOMA OF VAGINA.—Mrs. E., 54 years, no children, consulted me on January 26th, 1889, for an ulceration of the right labium majus, which had developed during the past six months. I diagnosed it an epithelioma and advised immediate extirpation. The inguinal glands were not involved. On January 30th I excised the whole mass with the knife, finding it necessary to remove all of the urethra outside of the pubic bones. The wound was stitched together with catgut suture and united by first intention, except the lower portion, which closed by granulation. The patient was discharged cured on February 25th, and, so far as I know, remains well. The microscope showed the disease to be epithelioma without a doubt.

"II. PRIMARY EPITHELIOMA OF THE VAGINA.—A. V. was admitted to Mt. Sinai Hospital on January 27th. She had been treated for a vaginal discharge for six months. I found a friable, spongy, easily bleeding mass of the size of an orange growing from the posterior wall of the vagina, not involving the cervix, and extending to about one inch from the vaginal orifice. Its character was readily apparent. On January 30th I removed it with the constricteur wire, scraped the wound smooth, and cauterized it thoroughly with the thermo-cautery. The patient was discharged on February 12th. On April 11th she presented herself at the Polyclinic with a mass as large as and much more offensive than the one removed two months before. She had become cachectic, and nothing could be done for her but to alleviate her discomfort and prolong her life for a time." —(*Amer. Jour. Obstet.*, May 1889.)

Foreign Bodies in the Bladder.— Dr. Ellison, of Canisted, N.Y., reports in the February number of the *American Journal of Obstetrics* a remarkable case, where a thread spool had been passed by a young girl (aged 12) into her vagina and from there ulcerated gradually into her bladder. It took over one year to do this, and was found lying in the bladder imbedded in a phosphatic calculus. This case is interesting in proving the sexual precocity of the patient, and also that so large and clumsy an instrument as a spool could be introduced past the vulva of so young a girl. The foreign body was removed by section of the vesico-vaginal septum.

Indications for Vaginal Hysterectomy in Cancer of the Cervix. C. THEIM.—(*Trans. German Gyn. Society.*)—Most authors were agreed that in carcinoma total extirpation must not be done when the parametria and the other adnexa are clearly infiltrated with cancer ; that the result was too unsatisfactory, and out of proportion to the gravity of the operation. Fritsch has defined his standpoint in the sentence, " to perform hopeless operations is an inhuman sport." But we may assume, for the honor of German gynæcologists, that they have operated only quite exceptionally in such cases. At all events, inhuman reasons cannot be alleged in the cases of men like B. Schultze and Brennecke, both of whom, but especially the latter, are well known to have pleaded for confining the indications for total extirpation in carcinoma within the limits of technical possibility. Olshausen has demonstrated that in Berlin relatively more operable cases of carcinoma come under treatment than in Halle. This fact is most noteworthy. In Berlin, with its large number of prominent gynæcologists, every woman knows where to apply, when, for instance, she suffers from atypical uterine hemorrhages ; hence inoperable cases are relatively few. In Halle, the conditions are less favorable, and as for Jena and Breslau, Schultze and Fritsch complain of the alarmingly large percentage of inoperable cases. In small country towns the prospects are deplorable. In the first place, the women bear the hemorrhages for months without complaining to anybody ; then they ask older women, who, of course, assure them that it is the change of life ; then a midwife who professes some knowledge of gynæcology is consulted ; and finally the family physician is asked to prescribe something for the hemorrhage, and if he, as is unfortunately the case at times, complies without making an examination, more months pass before the woman comes to the operator, usually when it is too late. When in such terrible cases total extirpation is performed, not with the hope of affording the woman radical cure, but as the safest and best palliative relief, it truly cannot be considered an inhuman measure. The very large number of other palliatives in so-called inoperable cases of carcinoma proves, as does the multiplicity of infallible remedies in diphtheria, that there is no panacea against these diseases, and that in a long series of cases all together are of no use. In carcinoma, before a satisfactory point is reached with any of the palliative measures—for instance, cauterization with concentrated chloride of zinc—so long a time elapses that the relatives do not leave the patient in the institution until its conclusion, especially when they are informed that actual operation has not been done. So long as irrigation and tamponing of the cancerous cavity with disinfectants can be done according to rule with the aid of the speculum, the women are fairly comfortable ; but whenever, after discharge from the institution, this manipulation is left to the patient, or to the equally unskilled midwife, the old misery recommences. Many sloughing cases of carcinoma constitute a *noli me tangere*, even for the usual palliative measures. As soon as they are touched, proliferation and sloughing become excessive. After total extirpation we generally attain, in from three to five weeks, a cicatrization which frequently becomes so firm that in relapses there is no longer any ulceration, but only a formation of tumors in the cicatrix. The women then die of secondary carcinoma of internal organs, or of general cancerous cachexia, and frequently are spared to the last that most horrible of all symptoms—sloughing. If, after certain palliative measures, isolated instances of improvement of prolonged duration, or even apparently complete cure have been attained, this proves, in the author's opinion, only that such cases were not inoperable and would have had an all the more favorable issue after total extirpation. Two years ago the author performed a total extirpation on a woman, although the left parametrium was immovably infiltrated and the patient had been refused operation four months before in some out-of-town gynæcological clinic. This woman is still alive and enjoys good health. Even should she still suffer a relapse, the speaker would count the case among the best results from all his total extirpations, because a similar effect is, unfortunately, not always to be reported after operations undertaken with apparently good prognosis. But should she remain permanently cured, this would prove that we are not always able to distinguish old inflammatory parametric thickenings from cancerous infiltrations. Then it would be safest for a woman to try the total extirpation at all hazards. The speaker will continue to do this operation, even in so-called inoperable cases, whenever it appears to him technically feasible, and he hopes that many others will do the same, particularly where the operation appears comparatively simple.—(*Amer. Jour. Obstet.*, Feb. 1889.)

Suppurative Disease of the Uterine Appendages. H. J. BOLDT, N.Y.—There has been recently quite a revolution and there is now marked difference of opinion concerning the justifiability of surgical interference in diseases of the uterine adnexa. It is true that very many women have been deprived of their ovaries or tubes without having been benefited ; in fact, not a few feel worse than they did previously. Many a patient, if she presented herself to the same surgeon to-day, would not be subjected to the knife at all, or the operation in some cases would be done differently. As some have gone to extremes in operating, others, again, are going to extremes in the opposite direction, instead of keeping the medium and selecting the cases for operation with greater care. Diseases of the uterine appendages may be roughly divided into three groups—1st, those in which an operation is unjustifiable ; 2nd, where it is wise to watch the patient and keep her under constant treatment to see what benefit may be derived and then decide upon the course to be pursued ; 3rd, those cases where delay is not only unadvisable but dangerous. A remark may not be out of place here with regard to cases occurring in private practice, especially among our better class of patients, namely, that in such cases there is altogether too much hesitancy on our part to interfere with the knife. It is very true that many cases of acute salpingitis recover without operative interference ; but even if they do get over the acute attack, what is the condition of such patients in the future ? Do not the majority remain invalids from pelvic disease ? It cannot be too strongly urged that we open the abdomen in every case of *active* pyo-salpingitis, from whatever cause it may arise, except under positive contra-indications, to be noticed below, or when the tubal trouble is complicated with another disease which in itself will destroy life in a *short* time, as advanced phthisis, carcinoma, etc. The question arises : Can we *always* make the diagnosis of pyo-salpingitis ? This, of course, must be answered negatively ; yet, from personal obser-vation, often corroborated by subsequent operation, I say that it can be done in most cases, and I think that a careful observer, experienced in this line of work, will not often fail. The con-ditions which we must differentiate are usually hydro- and hæmato-salpinx ; if, however, the tube or tubes are much dis-tended, ovarian and parovarian cysts must also be considered. The history of the case is of the greatest importance in the dif-ferential diagnosis. There are many operators who consider it unjustifiable to operate for hydro- and hæmato-salpinx, yet as it is unfortunately impossible for one to always make the positive diagnosis before operation, I still adhere to the opinion expressed in a paper read three or four years ago before the physicians of the German Poliklinik, where I held that even cases of hydro-salpinx should be operated upon if they give rise to serious morbid symptoms, which cannot be alleviated by other treat-ment, because even the simplest and most inert fluid may become purulent after any inflammatory condition set up in the walls of the tube, or from the extension of an endometritis.

I desire to lay particular stress on the fact that, when we have
reason to suspect suppurating disease in activity, without evidence of free communication between such diseased tube and
the uterus, the abdomen ought to be opened ; even though our
diagnosis prove erroneous, not much harm is done to the patient,
except that she is deprived of her liberty for a period of three
to four weeks, to allow comparatively firm healing of the abdominal wound ; besides this there is only the restriction of diet
for from ten to fourteen days. The danger of an exploratory
incision by a careful and experienced surgeon is almost nothing.
If our diagnosis is correct, as it should usually be, what immense
advantages are gained by the patient : in the first place, it rids
her of the pains which in the majority of cases accompany this
condition (pyo-salpingitis), although one must not look for the
cessation of the old pains immediately after operation ; sometimes a number of months or even one or two years may pass
before the full benefit is felt—changing her from an invalid to
a healthy being. Secondly, the danger from rupture of the
diseased tube is removed—an accident almost necessarily fatal,
unless with immediate operation, the risks of which are far
greater at that time than if done earlier. In fact, if done prior
to such accident, the danger is very slight. Although a prominent German operator's mortality from salpingo-oöphorectomies
is very great (over twelve per cent.), we must bear in mind that
his cases were extremely unfavorable, having waited very long
before determining on operation. It is against this too long
waiting that I would protest. Why let a patient suffer when
we have from history, examination and observation satisfied ourselves almost with positiveness that she is suffering from a disease
not amenable to ordinary treatment ? I call to mind a patient
who was referred to me, and whom an esteemed colleague
examined for me, because another very prominent gynæcologist
had advised the patient against operation. The poor woman
was such a great sufferer that I declined any further attempt
at ordinary treatment ; the gentleman who had referred her to
me, several other physicians, and myself having tried it for
some time without obtaining the slightest benefit. I operated,

and proved the justifiability and correctness of our diagnosis—
pyo-salpingitis dating from abortion. The patient is now fully
restored, a picture of health. When we have opened the abdomen for a suspected pyo-salpingitis, and find that such is not
present, but that we have an hydro- or hæmato-salpinx to deal
with, shall we close the wound, leaving the tubes intra-abdominal
in this condition in which we find them, because some say that
it is wrong to do a laparatomy for such disease ? I say *no* most
emphatically, provided I satisfied myself that the tube in question is at some point *firmly* occluded as the result of adhesive
inflammation. No matter what the contained fluid may be, the
tube ought to be unhesitatingly removed, for it is certainly of
no further use to the patient, and only jeopardizes her health, if
not her life. By what right should we allow such appendages
to remain ? On the ground and with the belief that the blood
or serum, whichever the tube may contain, will be absorbed,
which may be possible ; but does that restore the patency of the
occluded tube ? Or, if we aspirate the fluid from the tube, may
it not refill ? If we leave it alone, we run the risks previously
mentioned in such conditions ; these chances must all be taken.
No one will venture to say that such an organ, once firmly
occluded from the results of adhesive inflammation, can ever
again become permeable ; compare the old pleuritic adhesions
which are found daily in autopsies—can such pleuræ, after having become firmly adherent to the chest-walls, detach themselves ? The condition of an occluded Fallopian tube is pathologically similar. The question will now naturally be asked,
How may we recognize whether a tube is so firmly occluded as
to require removal, and when can we with probable safety for
the patient leave it undisturbed ? The answer is quite simple ;
the appendage is taken in the left hand, and with the thumb and
forefinger of the right hand it is gently manipulated or stroked
towards the uterine opening of the tube, care being taken not
to handle too roughly lest it rupture ; whether the contained
fluid be diminished or not will decide the permeability of the
tube, and also the further procedure. I have on my record but
two instances in which I regret t at I interfered, both occurring

in the beginning of my work of abdominal surgery. The first was a case of catarrhal salpingitis, with frequent occurrences of local peritonitis. The adhesions in this case were very extensive, and had it not been for the kind assistance of two experienced abdominal surgeons, who were also good enough to examine the patient previously and then advised operation, I should doubtless have abstained from completing the operation. This patient died of general peritonitis on the sixth day. In the second case, the same condition called for operation, with equally extensive and dense adhesions, the patient dying on the third day from septic peritonitis. With my present views, I think it very doubtful that I would be induced to remove the appendages at all in such cases, especially if the patients were near the menopause. —*Amer. Jour. Obstet.*, March 1889.

Extra-Uterine Foetation ; Abdominal Section Eight Months after Death of Foetus ; Recovery.—DR. CULLINGWORTH reported this case to the Obstetrical Society of London, Dec. 5th, 1888. The patient was 27 years old ; her last confinement happened five years ago. In April, 1887, she menstruated for the last time. In July she quickened and continued to enlarge and feel the movements of the foetus till December, when she suffered for an hour with labor-pains. Then the movements ceased, and the abdomen decreased in size. Seven months later she was admitted into hospital. An abdominal tumor lay behind the uterus, an eight months foetus was found in a sac composed of the left Fallopian tube and broad ligament. The liquor amnii and umbilical cord had disappeared. The placenta lay in front and was removed without hemorrhage. The foetus was firmly adherent to the sac-wall. A portion of the sac was removed, the remainder being stitched to the abdominal wound and drained. The sac closed in well ; a small piece near the incision sloughed. The patient made an uninterrupted and aseptic recovery, the temperature during convalescence never exceeding 100.4°.

Intestinal Occlusion after Ovariotomy. W. HIRSCH. (*Arch. f. Gyn.*, xxxii, 2.)—According to Hirsch, occlusion could take place in three different ways : First of all, it may be of direct origin ; the gut is included in cicatricial tissue. Secondly, it may be of indirect origin, the occlusion occurs here independently of the wound-surfaces, which heal without implicating the gut; but the irritation attending the operative procedure and that of the antiseptic fluids used in irrigating the abdominal cavity induce an aseptic peritonitis; the adhesive bands resulting inclose the intestines in the omentum and hinder peristalsis. Any external agency, such as blows or pressure upon the abdominal walls or the impaction of fæces, may then determine occlusion. He reckons as in the third class all cases of occlusion not dependent upon inflammation. The accident is purely mechanical, as kinking, catching of the gut between the pedicle and abdominal wall, or between the pedicle and the pelvic wall. A mixture of all these causes is frequently concerned in the etiology. In cases of the first two classifications the occurrence takes place only after the lapse of some time; the patients die of occlusion after the wound has healed, and time for convalescence to set in has arrived. The purely mechanical occlusion occurs shortly after the operation, ere the process of healing is completed. An acute and chronic form of occlusion may nevertheless be observed after ovariotomy. Observations were too limited to determine what part previous pathological processes in the intestines play in the production of obstruction, but this factor is theoretically very probable. In one thousand ovariotomies, eleven deaths were due to this trouble according to Spencer Wells. The time of occurrence varies, generally developing shortly after operation; instances are recorded where the first symptoms showed themselves years afterwards. The symptoms are those usually associated with this affection. In some of Hirsch's cases the pulse and temperature remained normal throughout. The diagnosis is so difficult as to make secondary laparatomy a procedure extremely hazardous. It had been done once in the fourteen cases reported by H. with successful result to the patient. The diagnosis approaches nearest certainty only where there is distinct stercoraceous vomit and the bowels remain confined. All other symptoms are those attending an ordinary peritonitis. Diagnosis is also easier in cases where the trouble supervenes some time after the operation. The occlusion occurs most frequently at the abdominal wound. In occlusion of the small intestine the symptoms are the more violent; Jaffé's test for indican in the urine will also show an increase of that substance where the trouble is in the small, while it remains unaltered when the occlusion occurs in the large intestine. The prognosis is extremely unfavorable. Of H.'s fourteen cases all but one, upon whom secondary laparatomy had been performed, died. A number of authorities are quoted to show the advantages of various prophylactic measures. If occlusion has once set in, choice must be made between two operations—laparatomy or colotomy. The choice depends upon the degree of certainty with which the site of the occlusion is located, and whether the procedure will guarantee against a recurrence of the strangulation. If the site be positively known, and there are slight prospects of reducing the occlusion, and if the latter be in the colon or rectum, an artificial anus must be established. Success depends essentially upon a timely operation. In those cases where, by reason of great debility or unwillingness of the patient to appreciate the necessity for operating, repeated washing out of the stomach with Hebe's apparatus may be resorted to, leading to moderate success; in some cases it may possibly produce spontaneous correction of the evil; three cases of ileus were cured by this procedure by Kussmaul, and other cases are reported which were relieved to a considerable extent. A case is reported in which a patient suffering from great tympanites was held head downward on the sixth day, when a great quantity of gas was suddenly expelled from the anus. Medication consisted of the administration of narcotics, principally excessive doses of opium. A detailed history of fourteen cases of the malady under consideration is presented by the author, illustrating various phases of occlusion; in one case the latter being apparently due to the pressure from large masses of fat in the mesentery.—*Amer. Jour. Obstet.*, March 1889.

Oöphorectomy in Australia. T. CHAMBERS, M.D. (*Brit. Med. Jour.*, May 25th, 1889.)—Dr. Chambers, in his presidential address at Sydney, N.S.W., made some very remarkable statements. First he spoke of Oöphorectomy in cases of OVARIAN

PROLAPSE, and reported the following case : A patient, aged 25, and married two years, came under his care. When five months married and four months pregnant she was thrown from a carriage and fell on the lower part of her back ; much shock and hystero-epileptic fits followed, with abortion within a week. The fits recurred at every period, and also at every attempt at sexual intercourse. At the end of nine months, hystero-epileptic attacks took place spontaneously between the periods, at gradually lessening intervals, and finally they occurred weekly. On examination, which proved very painful and nearly caused recurrence of the fits, both ovaries were found prolapsed and fixed by adhesions in Douglas's pouch. After grave deliberation it was decided to operate. On September 23rd, 1886, Dr. Chambers removed both ovaries and tubes, which were bound down by old adhesions in the recto-vaginal pouch. The ovaries were studded with cysts of various sizes, and the tubes were enlarged and filled with a sanguineous fluid. The attacks at once ceased, the patient made an excellent recovery, and is now in good health. Dr. Chambers then discussed Oöphorectomy for MENSTRUAL OR OVARIAN EPILEPSY. He believed that epilepsy was associated with menstruation and ovulation, and depended wholly upon deranged function of the sexual organs. He quoted a case in point with recovery after operation. He then spoke of Oöphorectomy in cases of UTERINE FIBROID, and related cases. In cases of CHRONIC OVARITIS the operation should be performed. Dr. Chambers next turned to cases of CONGENITAL ABSENCE OF THE UTERUS AND VAGINA, where the ovaries as well as the external genitalia remain well developed. He cites a case of a married, well-formed woman, complete in all except uterus and vagina, where attempted intercourse brought on " inward convulsions." Dr. Chambers removed both ovaries, one of which was large and cystic. Some months later this patient wrote to say that she had no more suffering, and that intercourse was not only possible but quite satisfactory. Dr. Chambers gives the following remarkable table of results :—

Diseases.	Number of Operations.	Cured.	Greatly Relieved.	Died.
Ovarian prolapse	11	10	1	—
Menstrual epilepsy	6	4	2	—
Uterine fibroids	10	9	1	—
Chronic ovaritis.............	11	9	1	1
Congenital absence of uterus and vagina............	4	4	—	—
Salpingitis with fluid in tubes	8	8	—	—
	50	44	5	1

Nearly all of Dr. Chambers' cases had had "fits" of some kind, and were cured by the operation. But the most remarkable statement of all is that congenital absence of the uterus and vagina with well developed ovaries is much more common than generally supposed. This statement we do not think correct. Müller of Berne says* : "If under this designation we mean complete absence of every trace of this organ in the pelvic cavity, the anomaly is an extremely rare one. It has been found with extensive general malformations, acephalia, cardiac monstrocities, and others which render life impossible, but the absence of rudiments of the womb at all events is extremely rare." So that as Dr. Chambers has met with four cases of congenital absence of the uterus and vagina, he himself must be " Munchausen " or the women of Australia somewhat of a risky matrimonial investment. We also notice that Dr. Chambers has not had occasion to resort to drainage in any of his fifty cases, which is certainly remarkable, especially so considering that he has had only two per cent. mortality, lower than Tait himself.

Uses of Curette. (A. F. CURRIER, M.D., in *Gaillard's Medical Journal.*)—Congestive and inflammatory conditions of the tubes or ovaries may be associated with copious uterine hemorrhage. Unless the process extends to the uterine mucous membrane curetting will do no good. As a matter of fact, the uterine mucous membrane is first involved in a very large number of cases, especially in those in which the disease has an infectious origin. Curetting for such cases may serve a very

---

* Cycl. Obstet. and Gyn.

useful palliative purpose. Uterine congestion and hemorrhage may attend disease of the pelvic peritoneum and cellular tissue. That this disease occurs in more or fewer cases irrespective of disease in the tubes and ovaries cannot be doubted, though to what extent is still an unsettled question. The great mass of clinical evidence which has been accumulating in the last few years certainly proves that disease of these organs is the principal factor in pelvic disorders far more frequently than would have been admitted ten or even five years ago. In the acute forms of this disease curetting should be performed, but in the chronic, degenerated condition of the mucous membrane which frequently results from them curetting will be efficient. Uterine displacements, especially posterior ones, are frequently attended by hemorrhage, and this is apt to be unusually troublesome during the menstrual epoch. The most rational explanation for such bleeding seems to me to be the stasis which must exist in the venous system of the pelvis, at least in many of the cases. This is one of many facts which puts greater importance upon uterine displacements than is now the fashion in many quarters. A continuation of this condition of course implies hypernutrition of the uterine mucous membrane, and curetting becomes a means for at least temporary relief. The radical cure must come from a restoration to the normal mechanical conditions, except in the few cases in which the pelvic apparatus and its dependencies all apparently adjust themselves to the situation which is forced upon them. I do not recall any instance of this kind in which atrophy and sterility have not resulted from a failure to restore the normal conditions to the circulation. The most violent uterine hemorrhage may occur from uterine polypi, and retention of fragments of placenta and decidua. For the first of these a cure will come after the cause has been removed ; for the second the curette will act with a promptness and efficiency which can be equalled by nothing else. To summarize, it may be stated that if uterine hemorrhage accompanies degeneration, infiltration, hyperplasia, or chronic inflammatory changes of the mucous membrane, there is no treatment which offers such satisfactory results as careful and thorough curetting, performed under anæs-

thesia and with antiseptic regulations, and followed immediately
by the application of an astringent or caustic antiseptic solution
—such as tincture of iodine, carbolic acid, or nitrate of silver
(60 grains to the ounce).   Mucus and muco-purulent discharges
from the uterus, especially in connection with chronic catarrhal
inflammation of the glandular system of the cervical mucous
membrane, are also readily checked by the use of the curette.
This operation is so simple and usually so painless that it seems
strange that it is not more generally adopted.   It is with me
almost a daily operation, and one from which I never have seen
harm result.   Like all other operations, it should be done antiseptically, and preferably within a week after the cessation of
the menstrual flow, as the normal pelvic congestion has then
subsided.   It is far more satisfactory than simply swabbing
away the discharges with cotton, drawing them out with a syringe,
or covering them with a layer of iodine or other astringent.   An
antiseptic astringent should be applied to the curetted surface,
both to prevent toxic absorption and to supplement the work of
the curette.

Purgative Effects of Glycerine.—DR. F. F. MILREFF, in
Novosti Terapii, details his experience concerning the use of
small glycerine enemata and suppositories in habitual constipa-
tions of various kinds.   The main results of his observations
may be condensed as follows :

1. In those cases where accumulation of fæcal masses takes
place in the lower portions of the large bowel, a rectal injection
of one or two drachms of pure glycerine in an adult, and of one-
half to one drachm in a child, is invariably followed by stools
occurring in two or three minutes.

2. The fæcal masses do not show any signs of liquefaction or
even softening ; still, owing to lubricant properties of the drug,
the act of defecation proves to be fairly easy and comfortable.

3. The enemata do not give rise to the slightest painful or
unpleasant sensations about the rectum.   Neither do any phenomena of rectal irritation supervene, even on a prolonged
employment of the injections.

4. The purgative effects of glycerine should be attributed to

its stimulating action on the nervous and muscular apparatus of the large bowel, which action is probably determined by the drug greedily extracting water from the intestinal mucous membranes with its nerve-fibres.   The desiccation irritates the latter, and thus exacts a reflex contraction of the intestinal muscular coat. The hypothesis finds a strong support in the fact that any dilution of glycerine with water markedly weakens its purgative action, and that the more in proportion the larger is the amount of water added.

5. Glycerine enemata are especially indicated (*a*) in the constipation of pregnancy, where ordinary water enemata are inconvenient on account of their considerable bulk, which causes discomfort to the woman; and (*b*) in infantile constipation caused by unduly prolonged feeding on milk alone, and associated with fæcal accumulations in, and consecutive distension of, the sigmoid bowel.   In cases of the kind, glycerine enemata are very useful on account of their energetic action in the intestinal muscles, and convenient because of their small bulk.

6. As to glycerine suppositories (containing half a drachm of the drug each), they are said to act well (in five minutes or so) only in such cases where no pure glycerine enemata were previously employed, otherwise they remain inactive.   Hence he commences the glycerine treatment of constipation with suppositories (a piece at bedtime), and passes to enemata as soon as the former cease to secure the desirable result.

7. As regards the apparatus for the enemata, any special contrivances are superfluous.   He uses for the purpose an India-rubber urethral syringe with a piece of thick walled elastic tube on the nozzle.

Dr. Grewcock, in *London Med. Recorder*, says he "found out quite accidentally a novel method of applying glycerine," which is "equally efficacious with the clyster. . . . If a piece of cotton wool alone, the size of a nut, is well saturated with glycerine, and inserted as a suppository, in a short time a copious motion is produced."

Laparotomy for Tubal Disease—Re-operation fourteen days after for symptoms of Peritonitis and Intestinal Obstruction. (DR. E. S. STEVENSON *in So. African Med. Jour.*)—Mrs. L., aged 38, V-para, one miscarriage, has been suffering for fourteen years. She was under treatment in London for constant pelvic pains more than twelve years ago, and since that time has been continually ailing ; she cannot lie or sit down without great pains, and has excruciating pains when her bowels are open. Six months ago she became seriously ill with severe pelvic pains and hemorrhage, which has continued ever since. Two months ago she was again laid up with the same symptoms. I found her suffering from disease of the right appendages, and advised operation, to which she readily consented. On Dec. 28th, 1888, I operated. On opening the peritoneal cavity I found the right tube much enlarged and adherent to the uterus and surrounding parts. On trying to separate the tube it burst, and its contents, a clot the size of a small orange and dark blood, escaped into the cavity. On drawing out the parts, I found the tube split longitudinally in its whole length and the fimbriated extremity torn. This part was found closely adherent to a coil of intestines, its fimbriæ spread out, covering a spot the size of a five-shilling piece, and firmly adherent. Great care was required to remove this, and free oozing took place. The right ovary, which was cystic, burst on being pulled out, and was also removed. The left annexures were also removed. The cavity was well irrigated with hot water, and, on account of oozing, a glass drainage-tube inserted. The patient recovered rapidly, and on the tenth day she felt all right. The wound was well healed, and all the pains which she had suffered constantly from previous to the operation had left her. On the eleventh day the patient committed an indiscretion, and soon after felt worse, with vomiting, constipation, severe griping pains, tympanitis, pulse quick and hard, tongue dry, and general tenderness over the abdominal walls. The vomiting became very urgent, and on the fourteenth day after the operation Mrs. L. appeared to be sinking. Feeling sure that I had to deal with peritonitis and intestinal obstruction, I concluded to reopen the abdomen. The wound was healed all through. At first it was found impossible to map the parts, there being a general glueing of parts together. Fortunately the adhesions were recent and easily parted. The intestines were engorged and dilated, especially in the pelvic cavity, and there several soft fibrinous bands had to be torn. The large omentum, instead of floating on the surface of the intestines, was twisted like a loose rope, and dipped into the abdominal cavity down to the back. The whole of it was glued to coils of intestines, and was at its extremity firmly attached to a coil deep down. This adhesion required considerable force to free it. The whole part of the twisted omentum was ligatured and removed, and the cavity freely irrigated with a 1 in 3000 solution of corrosive sublimate, and a drainage-tube left in. Six hours after the operation the bowels were moved by an enema of turpentine and hot water, and a long rectal tube frequently passed in to allow the escape of flatus. Immediately after the operation all symptoms of obstruction and peritonitis left her, and she soon got over the shock of a second operation. The bowels were kept open daily by turpentine enemata. I must mention that after the first operation the same course was pursued, with the exhibition of salines, and the rectal tube was freely used. This intestinal obstruction was due to the omental adhesions. The firm, deep-seated adhesion was, I have no doubt, attached to the intestinal wall whereon the tube had been glued, and which at first accounted for the unbearable pain the patient felt when the bowels were relieved. This case demonstrates the rapidity of formation of inflammatory bands in peritonitis and how easily intestinal obstruction can take place after laparatomy. The patient is now up and about, feeling well and strong.

Pelvic Peritonitis ; Forced Dilatation and Curetting. (DR. WALTON.)—The lesions of the endometrium constitute an important factor in the etiology of diseases of the Fallopian tubes, peritoneum, ovaries and parametrium, though it does not follow that this is the only way by which the inflammatory element is transmitted from the uterus to the neighboring organs. Septic infection, after having been located in the endometrium, is propagated principally by the lymphatic vessels. Pelvic cellulitis, phlegmasia alba dolens, and the great majority of puerperal accidents are caused by the absorption of septic germs. Contagion is acquired rapidly on account of the existence of traumatic lesions caused by parturition or abortion. While the so-

called puerperal septicæmia can be transmitted directly by the
uterine parenchyma, the lymphatics, or the veins, the same condition is not propagated apart from the puerperal condition.
Catarrhal inflammation and gonorrhœal infection have a tendency
to invade the uterine mucous membrane. After having produced
the lesions of the womb, there is extension to the tubes, salpingitis being first produced and then perimetritis. The initiatory
agent of inflammations of the mucous membrane is always a
microbe. This micrococcus, located in the folds of the mucous
membrane, gives rise to symptoms of endometrial inflammation,
which indicate active treatment for their relief. To cure this
inflammation and avoid subsequent pelvic peritonitis, dilatation,
curetting and antiseptic precautions are indicated. The following conclusions result from the author's experience :

1. In non-exudative pelvic peritonitis the pain, which is the
principal symptom, may be relieved by dilatation.

2. In the exudative variety forcible dilatation by facilitating
the return circulation may check the progress of peritoneal infarctions and assist the absorption of exudates.

3. In circumuterine or pelvic abscesses, which are usually
nothing more than cysts of the tubes, it is possible, by dilating
the womb, to evacuate the cysts by way of the uterine canal.

4. In cases of puerperal septicæmia the septic symptoms will
disappear under this treatment. No other is so efficient for the
disinfection of the cavity of the uterus and disposing of the products of infection.

5. Reflex symptoms, such as vomiting, are immediately
relieved by forcible dilatation.

Hysteropexia for Prolapse of the Uterus.—DR. M. POLAILLON
reports a case of prolapse of the uterus of long standing, in which
he had performed hysteropexia, or abdominal fixation of the
uterus. The patient was a woman aged 50, eight years past
the menopause, in whom prolapse caused violent lumbar pain
and dysuria. The prolapse was complicated with cystocele.
On opening the abdomen he experienced the greatest difficulty
in bringing up the uterus, which was studded all over with small
fibroids. He passed several sutures through it, and fixed it to

the abdominal parietes. The operation was carried out with the strictest antiseptic precautions, but the day following the operation the patient complained of abdominal pain, and was sick. A week later she succumbed to peritonitis. At the autopsy no sign of union could be seen in the abdominal wound, and the sutures maintaining the uterus in apposition with the abdominal wall had given way. The peritoneum was the seat of a general inflammation. He attributes his want of success to the absorption of the catgut sutures, which he will discard in any future operation in favor of metal or silk. M. Terrier, however, has performed the operation five times with catgut sutures without their having given way.

The relation of the above case is an instance of the thoughtless, pedantic things some surgeons will at times do. That a surgeon will perform hysterorrhaphy using catgut ligatures is beyond all comprehension. Here we want a ligature of strength, of long duration, and absolutely aseptic ; the very opposite of all these characters we have in catgut. It is being almost entirely discarded by Montreal surgeons ; in strength it is unreliable, and it is absolutely impossible to make it any more aseptic than a sponge-tent—neither can be boiled. These two characteristics make it dangerous as a ligature, and it should be used no more.

Elytritis and Blenorrhœal Endometritis. (DR. FRITSCH.)— Make a mixture containing equal parts of chloride of zinc and water ; twenty grammes of this mixture are combined with a litre of water ; this is heated to a temperature of 30°R., and is used by irrigation in the treatment of blennorrhœal vaginitis and endometritis twice daily, being continued during the menstrual period. About ten irrigations are usually required. If the disease has extended to the cervical canal, the mucous membrane of the uterus, and the tubes, the discharge will soon recur. In such cases the uterine cavity should be cauterized with concentrated solution of chloride of zinc, and a pencil of iodoform should be introduced at suitable intervals within the cavity. Bandl's method of treatment is the following : The speculum having been introduced, a fenestrated canula is passed within the cervical canal as far as the os internum ; then a 10 per cent. solution of sulphate of copper is passed within the canula, the latter being rotated so that all portions of the mucous membrane shall receive the copper solution through the fenestra. After the canula has remained in position a few minutes, it is to be removed and a tampon introduced within the cervix.   Such applications should be made every three or four days, irrigations of a very weak solution of sulphate of zinc being used during the intervals.

During Dr. Macan's inaugural address as president of the British Gynæcological Society for the present year, he drew attention to the rapid strides in importance the bimanual method of making pelvic examinations was obtaining.   And in discussing the subject, he gave the following account of uterine massage as introduced by Thure Brandt of Stockholm some twenty years ago, and practiced in the treatment of pelvic inflammation with adhesions.   Brandt not being a medical man, the method was not taken up by the profession until quite recently.   Bandl of Vienna lately gave it a trial, and through him it has gained some popularity with the profession.   The method is practised as follows :

" The treatment itself consists of two parts, the first being the elevation of the uterus.   To carry this out the aid of a skilled assistant is necessary, whose duty it is with one hand to elevate the uterus from the vagina, and to keep it in a state of anteflexion, while his other hand is laid on the abdomen exactly over the uterus.   The latter hand indicates to the operator the exact position of the fundus.   Standing now at the foot of the couch or sofa on which the patient is lying, the operator lays his two hands, strongly supinated, flat on the abdomen, the fingers being pointed towards the pubes, and grasps the fundus between them, its position, as already said, being indicated by the hand of the assistant that is on the abdomen, while the fingers of the other hand of the assistant, which are in the vagina, prevent the fundus being pushed out of reach of the hands of the operator. Having firmly grasped the uterus, the operator raises it steadily upwards in the abdomen, in the axis of the pelvis, watching the face of the patient the whole time. This is necessary, as the slightest expression of pain is an indication to desist or to go more slowly. In this way the uterus can be elevated as much over its normal level as it had formerly been prolapsed. When the uterus has been elevated as far as is possible it is allowed to slip gently from between the hands, and sinks slowly in the abdomen. The duty of the assistant is now to receive the uterus as it descends on his finger which has remained in the vagina, and to keep it in a condition of anteflexion. This movement of elevation is repeated two or three times at each sitting, a few minutes' interval being allowed between each, during which time the assistant massages the fundus in order to arouse it to contraction and thereby lessen its bulk. The second movement now follows and consists of forcible separation and forcible closure of the knees. To carry it out the patient should be placed in the recumbent position, and closing the knees and thighs should elevate the sacrum from the couch, so that the body rests on the elbows and feet only. While in this position the operator forcibly separates the knees, the patient resisting as much as possible. This is repeated about three times. The contrary movement is now practised, the patient lying with the knees widely separated, and the operator bringing them forcibly together. This is also repeated three times, and closes the sitting. The patient now turns over gently on the face and remains in that position for from five to ten minutes. It is well, when it is possible, for the patient to remain in the recumbent position for the first few days of the treatment, but this is not essential. The treatment is repeated daily till the cure is effected, the time required varying greatly, but being usually from four to eight weeks."

Reviews and Notices of Books.

The Physiology of the Domestic Animals. A Text-Book for Veterinary and Medical Students and Practitioners. By ROBERT MEADE SMITH, A.M., M.D., Professor of Comparative Physiology in the University of Pennsylvania. Philadelphia and London : F. A. Davis, publisher.

That there was an urgent need for a work on the physiology of the domestic animals for the use of students of veterinary medicine few acquainted with the facts of the case will deny. Professor Smith had a rare opportunity such as occurs to few men in a lifetime now-a-days, viz., that of supplying a new and really needed thing ; and, we regret to say, we believe he has in large measure missed the mark. Students of human medicine do not require such a work ; but few practitioners, we fear, make much use of works of physiology of any kind, and the real *desideratum* was a work for undergraduate students as we actually find them in the schools of veterinary medicine on this continent. When it is remembered that in by far the larger proportion of such institutions the students spend but two years on the whole course of study, it becomes perfectly plain that their physiology must be prepared for them in at most but a moderate compass. But this book is a ponderous volume of 920 closely packed pages. How the class of students we refer to can be expected to read, understand and inwardly digest this huge mass passes our comprehension. We think it most unfortunate that Dr. Smith has seen fit to add another to the list of books that are too large for those for whom they are professedly written. It is a great and growing evil, and if this crowding of the mind continues, Who shall say what the result may be ?

The general conception of the work is good, but has been much marred in the execution by lack of balance. We find more than three hundred pages devoted to " Food and Digestion," and but seventy to the " Circulation of the Blood." It is true that for the veterinarian the former subjects are of great, perhaps of paramount importance, so much have they to do with explaining actual disease ; but will any one assert that they are more than four times as important as is the " Circulation of the Blood" for example ?   Then, that a subject so important for comparative physiology as " Reproduction " should be dealt with in twenty pages greatly surprises us.

Discussion of chemical and physical principles largely in the abstract at the very beginning of a work, and apart from the actual subjects (chapters) in which their application is obvious, though not without precedent, has always seemed to us to be contrary to some of the well established principles of teaching as founded on the laws of our mental constitution.   In practice it does not work well; it increases the difficulties of the student's already rugged path and tends to intellectual nausea and dyspepsia.   The book is a good compilation of the physiology of the domestic animals as known.   The author claims for it no originality, though we are sorry he did not lessen the bulk of his work, and if he did not make it in any high sense original, at least impart some degree of his own individuality to it.   The teeming press of to-day sadly lacks books with individuality.

But though we have felt called upon to criticise this work upon its merits, we nevertheless feel that Professor Smith has done good service, if not for the undergraduates, at least for the practitioners of veterinary medicine.   Those who will read may now learn in their own language enough of physiology as it is known to make the practice of their profession an intelligent study and not a rule of thumb routine.   Though too lengthy in comparison with other chapters, those on " Food and Digestion" are excellent ; so is that on " Locomotion," as was to be expected from the original work done on this subject by Mr. Muybridge at the University of Pennsylvania.   The illustrations are abundant, wisely chosen and sufficiently well executed. It is to be remembered that the author's task was a new one and the difficulties great.   With Prof. Smith we also lament that in comparative physiology the harvest is plentiful, but the laborers few ; and such, we fear, must be the case till medical men perceive more clearly the true relations of the study of their great profession.   Nevertheless, progress is now rapid, and the whole of medicine has before it a new, broader and better way.

The great question with regard to this work seems to be : Is the profession of veterinary medicine the richer by it ? Unquestionably it is. It was a needed book. We should have preferred it different in many respects, but accept it thankfully notwithstanding.

The Cerebral Palsies of Children. A Clinical Study
From the Infirmary for Nervous Diseases, Philadelphia. By WILLIAM OSLER, M.D., Fellow of the Royal College of Physicians, London. London: H. K. Lewis, 136 Gower Street, 1889.

This very valuable contribution to practical medicine is founded on the observations of no less than 151 cases of cerebral paralysis, an amount of material which far exceeds in amount any previously analyzed. In 120 of the 151 cases, the paralysis was hemiplegic in distribution, in twenty cases the hemiplegia was bilateral, and in the remaining eleven cases the paralysis was paraplegic. Out of the total of 120 cases of hemiplegia, the disease made its appearance in ninety-six before the end of the third year, fifteen of the ninety-six being congenital. It is important to note that in nine of these cases the child was delivered with the forceps. " In six of the cases the child is said to have been injured by the forceps, and in all the paralysis was either noticed at once or a few months afterwards without definite onset." In sixteen of the 120 cases there is a history of the palsy coming soon after an attack of one of the eruptive fevers. From these histories it appears probable that exceptionally convulsions may give rise to a cerebral hemorrhage which leads to a permanent cerebral palsy.

The second chapter deals with the symptoms and morbid anatomy of cerebral palsy of children (hemiplegic type). The author groups the lesions under three headings: 1. Embolism, thrombosis and hemorrhage. 2. Atrophy and sclerosis. 3. Porencephalus. It is pointed out that our knowledge of the pathological conditions underlying infantile hemiplegia is very defective. This is owing mainly to the fact that the great majority of post mortems have been made years after the onset of the disease, and when all trace of the primitive lesion has disappeared.

Chapters three and four are devoted to blilateral spastic hemiplegia and spastic paraplegia respectively. The final chapter deals with the pathology and treatment of the different forms of paralysis. Dr. Osler is of the opinion that hemorrhage is the cause in only a very small percentage of the cases. In those cases of palsy coming on at birth there is strong evidence that meningeal hemorrhage is frequently the cause, while a fœtal meningo-encephalitis is probably the cause in a few of the cases.

In speaking of infantile hemiplegia coming on during the first two or three years of life, Dr. Osler says that we are called upon to explain " the mode of origin of sclerosis and porencephalus, the conditions present in the great majority of cases. A certain number of cases of infantile hemiplegia are due to hemorrhage, to embolism and aneurism, a few to tumor, as glioma or chronic tubercle; but, as we have seen, these form a fractional part. We require to know the pathological process lying at the basis of the convulsive attacks with coma, which come suddenly, or after a slight febrile movement, frequently succeed an infectious disease and leave a hemiplegia with too often its disastrous consequences—epilepsy and imbecility. In a large proportion of the cases the disease is such a clinical unit, with symptoms as marked and definite as those of infantile spinal paralysis, that we might expect a corresponding uniformity in the anatomical lesion. Unfortunately we are, so far as I can ascertain, entirely without information upon the state of the brains of children dying during or shortly after the attack; and the question resolves into an explanation of the conditions most commonly met with years after the onset, viz.: sclerosis and porencephalus."

The author then discusses fully the more important views advanced to explain the origin of these changes and tabulates his conclusions as follows: Infantile homiplegia is probably the result of a variety of different processes, of which the most important are: 1. Hemorrhage, occurring during violent convulsions or during a paroxysm of whooping cough. 2. Post-febrile processes: (a) embolic; (b) endo- and peri-arterial changes, and (c) encephalitis. 3. Thrombosis of the cerebral veins.

We have only been able to point out a few of the more important points dealt with in this important monograph. It represents a vast amount of clinical and literary work and reflects the greatest credit on its author.

Society Proceedings.

MEDICO-CHIRURGICAL SOCIETY OF MONTREAL.

Stated Meeting, March 22nd, 1889.

WM. GARDNER, M.D., PRESIDENT, IN THE CHAIR.

Radical Cure of Hernia. — DR. SHEPHERD exhibited a patient on whom he had operated a year ago. The man, a blacksmith by trade, was 45 years of age, of intemperate habits, and very stout. He had had a swelling in the left groin since boyhood, which always disappeared on lying down. It gradually increased in size and entered the scrotum. It now could only with difficulty be reduced. Two years before had received a severe blow on the scrotum with a bar of iron; from this time the tumor rapidly increased in size and became irreducible. Latterly the tumor had become so large and troublesome that he could not do his work, and with difficulty could wear large-sized trousers. The tumor in the scrotum was larger than a good-sized foot-ball. He was sent into hospital and kept in bed some time. Operation for the radical cure of the hernia was advised, and the man having consented, the operation was performed on April 26th, 1888. An incision some eight inches long was made over the tumor and the sac reached. The sac was found to be very thin, and was with difficulty partially dissected out. Failing to reduce the hernia the sac was opened. The sac contained all the large intestines with the exception of the cæcum and rectum, and nearly all the small, besides a large mass of omentum. Several pounds of omentum were removed after ligature, and then an endeavor made to return the bowels. This was not easily accomplished, the abdominal cavity appearing too small to contain them. After manipulating the intestines for a considerable time without making much impression on the quantity outside the abdomen, the man was suspended by the feet. This enabled Dr. Shepherd to reduce the small intestines first, then the large. The whole time occupied was nearly two hours. It was found that, in reducing the large intestines, when pushing them in a certain direction failed to diminish the quantity, as soon as they were pushed in the opposite direction they slipped in easily. When all the intestines were returned the abdomen was as tight as a drum, and it seemed as if it would not have been possible to introduce an inch more of bowel. Having taken so much time in reducing the hernia, Dr. Shepherd decided that it was better to sacrifice the testicle of that side, and so complete the operation as soon as possible. The sac was cut off and the ends of the ligature passed through the abdominal walls, as suggested by Mr. Barker of London, one through each pillar of the internal ring and then tied together; the canal, which, of course, was of large size, was then closed by two silk sutures which were passed through the conjoined tendon and Poupart's ligament, and the external wound closed with continuous silk suture. The patient was in fairly good condition after the operation, and quickly rallied. Next day there was some pain and tympanites. Small doses of salts were given frequently and the bowels freely moved. The recovery of the patient was uninterrupted and without special incident. He remained in bed some six weeks after operation, when he was discharged with a sinus still unhealed at the point of drainage. After a few weeks more he returned to his work, at which he has been constantly engaged ever since. There has not been the slightest return of the hernia, but the fistulous opening has never completely closed, and some few days ago Dr. Shepherd removed one of the silk sutures from it.

.Dr. Shepherd stated that he brought this case before the Society because of the special interest taken at the present time in this subject. The operation performed was a formidable one, and relieved the man from a very disagreeable tumor which had seriously interfered with his occupation. The sacrifice of the testicle he did not regret, as he was convinced that in these large herniæ, cure could be more readily accomplished if the spermatic cord were cut, as the stump helped to close the internal opening. The fistulous opening, he thought, was no doubt due to the silk sutures. One had already come away, and when the other was discharged he had no doubt the fistula would heal.

DR. BELL congratulated Dr. Shepherd on the satisfactory result obtained in a very unpromising case. He thought the fistulous opening might be caused by the continuous escape of peritoneal fluid. He had seen a similar case in Dr. Fenwick's practice and two cases of women operated on for femoral hernia; fistulæ remained for months. These, however, were completely cured by rest in bed. In the case of the women, he found that fistulæ only persisted when patient assumed a semi-erect position. He removed a silk suture from a sutured patella four months after operation. He formerly believed that the silk he used in suturing the intestines of dogs was absorbed, but now he thinks that after union the sutures are passed per rectum.

DR. TRENHOLME said that the case illustrated the advantage of hempen over silk sutures, as numerous observations show that hempen sutures are entirely absorbed. He has always advocated the advantage of using sutures of shoemaker's thread. He asked if Dr. Shepherd had failed to reduce the intestines would he have resected a portion to reduce the bulk?

DR. GARDNER asked why fistulæ should persist after hernial operations when they do not do so after abdominal section for ovariotomy, etc. He said that post-mortem examinations had shown that silk ligatures disappear from the pedicles after ovariotomies if the silk has been properly prepared.

DR. SHEPHERD, in reply, said that he believed the fistula to be due to the presence of a suture, because he had already removed two out of the three used in the operation.

Ligature of the Common Carotid.—DR. SUTHERLAND intro-duced the patient, a girl of 24, on whom he had performed ligature of the common carotid for arterio-venous aneurism. She was brought to the Montreal General Hospital on Sept. 3, 1888, having been accidentally shot in the neck by an ordinary parlor rifle carrying a bullet the size of a pea. The bullet entered the neck midway between the symphysis and angle of the lower jaw on the left side, passed across the neck, and was found under the skin two inches below the right mastoid process, behind the sterno-mastoid. The right side of the neck was swollen, and a distinct pulsation and thrill was felt on placing the hand over the upper carotid triangle. With the stethoscope a distinct bruit could be heard. The thrill and pulsation of the tumor gave one the idea that the affection was an arterio-venous aneurism. The pulsation was arrested by compressing the common carotid on the neck. The patient was kept quiet for a few days, and the tumor and pulsation increasing, it was decided to throw a ligature around the right common carotid and then search for the wounded vessel. This was done, but failing to find the vessel, which appeared to be deep (probably the internal carotid), Dr. Sutherland determined temporarily to occlude the carotid by ligating it over a piece of drainage-tube after the manner suggested by Mr. Lewis of London, and await results. The patient did well for several days, but the ligature loosening, the pulsation in the aneurism returned, so the patient was again placed under ether and the carotid tied in its continuity above the omohyoid. The patient did well, the wound healing by first intention, except at the point where the bone drain had been. After three weeks she was discharged from hospital with the swelling in the neck much decreased and with the aneurism cured. The fistulous opening remained until January 12th, when the ligature came away, and then the opening rapidly closed. The patient is at present perfectly well.

Dr. Sutherland stated that with regard to the tying of the ligature over the rubber tube outside, it was a practice he would not repeat. Although it had the advantage of accustoming the brain to a lessened supply of blood, yet he considered that the retarded flow of blood in the main vessel might lead to a thrombus being formed in some of its anastomotic branches, and so interfere afterward with the nutrition of the part. He preferred ligature of the carotid to temporary compression, as the former was much more certain and not more dangerous.

Cyst of the Broad Ligament.—DR. WM. GARDNER exhibited a thin-walled cyst, of the size of a goose-egg, removed from a married woman of 25. The origin appeared to be from some structure of the broad ligament other than the parovarium. The contents were thin and faintly colored. The ovary was healthy and not involved. The symptoms were pelvic pain and disturbance of the bladder.

Membranous Cast of the Uterus.—DR. ALLEN exhibited a complete membranous cast of the uterus and gave the following history : Mrs. P., aged 26, married, had always enjoyed good health ; menstruation had been irregular, giving rise to no special pain. One month after marriage, before leaving England, suffered from an attack which she says came on with abdominal pains, which lasted a few days, being followed by loss of something, but what I was unable to find out. Amenorrhœa followed from that date to the present attack. On 21st July, while walking on the mountain, was taken with severe abdominal pains and slight sickness, compelling her to return home at once and go to bed, where she remained ever since. The pains were greatly relieved by heat to abdomen and warm drink for a time. During the night of the 22nd they again returned, were very severe and bearing down in character, followed by loss of some blood towards morning. I was called in on the morning of the 23rd and found patient in bed, restless, slight flush of cheeks, temperature 99.5°, pulse 100 (regular), and bearing down pains, less severe than they were some time before according to her account. On examination, cervix soft and slightly dilated, membrane protruding into vagina, covered with some coagula. With the aid of Syms' speculum, with patient in Syms' position, membrane could be seen to be only slightly held in cervix, being removed by index finger without any force. Uterus contracted well and was entirely empty ; no trace of a fœtus could be found. Irrigated vagina once with warm Condy's fluid (very weak), keeping her in bed on light diet for a few days. Slight amount of blood lost during the first twenty-four hours, after which pulse and temperature became normal, remaining so. Three weeks later, when seen, felt well, after which date I lost sight of her, so am unable to give the subsequent history, which I regret very much. The membrane, on further examination, proved to be a complete cast of uterus, very thin in some parts.

Dr. LAPTHORN SMITH regarded the case as one of severe membranous dysmenorrhœa.

A Case of Urœmia.—Dr. FINLEY exhibited a pair of hypertrophied and cystic kidneys about three times their proper size. The fibrous tissue was largely increased. The heart from the same case showed the left ventricle largely hypertrophied and dilated. Dr. Finley said he was not able to find any reference to cases of cardiac hypertrophy from cystic disease of the kidney.

Dr. SPRINGLE stated that the patient was a man of about 53 years old, who had been taken suddenly ill in the morning; he was brought to the hospital in a moribund condition the same afternoon, and died in about ten minutes.

Esbach's Method of Determining Proteids in the Urine.—Dr. RUTTAN exhibited and explained Esbach's method of determining proteids in the urine, and showed how it might easily be applied to ascertain the relative proportion of serum-albumin and serum-globulin in urine. He expressed surprise that this method, though over two years old, was not used more by physicians, as it was extremely easy of application and occupied little or no time. It was time that the unscientific and misleading statements which appear in the journals regarding the quantitative relation of albumin in urine were replaced by more accurate and reliable observations. Such statements as 30 or 40 per cent. by volume of albumin conveyed no information whatever as to the actual quantity of proteids, not even of the relative proportion from one observation to the next. Dr. Ruttan said that it was obvious that the volume of precipitated albumin depended on whether precipitated in flakes or in granules, and this, again, depends on the time it is boiled and the amount and nature of acid used. Again, the specific gravity of the urine, the time elapsing before the observation is made, etc., all should be constant and should be stated before it is possible, by the old method, to convey even an approximate idea of the actual amount in the sample of urine. Esbach's method, though not absolutely accurate, is more nearly so than any other chemical method, and has the advantage of giving the actual proportion

of albumin by weight in any given sample of urine. Dr. Ruttan
also referred to Dr. Grainger Stewart's observations on the significance of the relative proportion of serum-albumin and globulin in urine. These observations, though few in number, go to
show that the globulin, if in excess or present alone, is significant of functional albuminuria.

A Method of Detecting Traces of Albumin.—DR. RUTTAN
demonstrated a modification of Heller's test for albumin. Instead of floating the urine on the acid in a wine-glass, as Heller
recommends, he proposed to warm both urine and acid in separate test tubes, then fill a pipette with the warm acid, and, with
the end closed by the finger, introduce it to the bottom of the
tube containing the urine, then by withdrawing the finger the
acid will flow out and float up the urine. A sharply defined
line of opacity at the junction of the two fluids indicates the
presence of albumin. The advantage claimed for this modification of Heller's test is that the reaction is more sharply defined
than in Heller's test, when but traces of albumin are present,
and that in the warm urine the acid urates are not precipitated
by the acid, so the only opacity that can occur at the line of
contact is one due to coagulated albumin. Dr. Ruttan emphasized the necessity of filtering all samples of urine not perfectly
bright before testing for albumin.

Modification of the Urinometer.—DR. RUTTAN also exhibited
Squibb's urinometer, which consists of urine tube with flutings
and a float with doubly conical bulb. The flutings prevent the
float from adhering to the sides of the urine tube, thus lessening
one of the errors inseparable from this method of taking specific
gravity. This instrument is particularly useful for ascertaining
slight differences in specific gravity, as when the sugar in urine
is estimated by Sir William Roberts' method.

Stated Meeting, April 5th, 1889.

WM. GARDNER, M.D., PRESIDENT, IN THE CHAIR.

Dr. E. P. Williams was elected a member of the Society.

Nævus of the Face.—DR. W. R. SUTHERLAND exhibited a
very marked case of nævus in a man of 60 years. It had existed

for twenty years ; formerly it was flat, but now the tumor was pedunculated in places and everywhere raised above the level of the skin. Dr. Sutherland remarked that in such extreme cases in an old man surgical interference would avail but little.

Dr. Buller could not see why even such a case as the one exhibited could not be cured by electrolysis. Nævi of the orbit are controlled and frequently entirely eradicated by electrolysis. In one case, however, optic neuritis set in after, and the eye was lost.

Dr. Hingston agreed with Dr. Sutherland that interference in the case of a man of the age of the patient was uncalled for. In his practice he used the thermo-cautery in extreme cases like the one shown after removing the peduncles with the knife. The effect of the cautery is to substitute a white scar for the unsightly red blemish. In earlier stages of the affection, especially in young persons, he scarifies with razor or scalpel with close parallel cuts so as to deprive the spot of its circulation. He could recall one case in which he completely removed by this method a nævus covering the whole shoulder of a young girl.

Dr. Lapthorn Smith believed that since the hæmostatic effect of the positive pole has been understood, the electric method was the best for the treatment of such cases.

Dilated Fallopian Tube with attached Ovary.—Dr. Armstrong exhibited a dilated Fallopian tube which was removed from a married woman aged 37. She had had repeated attacks of severe abdominal pain, with tenderness on pressure and elevation of temperature. The operation was performed on the 24th of March. A chart was handed round, which showed that the temperature never rose above normal. The right ovary was displaced downwards behind the uterus and there held by inflammatory adhesions. Both tubes were more or less attached by the same method.

Dr. Gardner said that the specimen illustrated well the danger of trying to diagnose by digital manipulation the exact condition before operation, as such a tube filled with pus might easily be ruptured, especially if the examination be made while the patient is under ether. His experience fully corroborates Dr. Lawson Tait's statement that if both ovaries be not removed, as Dr. Armstrong did in this case, a second abdominal section is, as a rule, necessary to remove the other ovary.

DR. HINGSTON was present at the operation, and fully agreed as to the necessity of immediate operation. He was opposed to all such operations when not absolutely warranted by the symptoms.

DR. TRENHOLME said he had seen the case before operation, but owing to the attachment of the ovary to the right cornua of the uterus was not able to make a satisfactory diagnosis.

Clot from the Internal Saphenous Vein.—DR. ARMSTRONG also exhibited a blood-clot having a circumference of three inches which he removed from the internal saphenous vein, just opposite the knee-joint. The vein was completely occluded on the proximal and distal side. It caused the woman a good deal of annoyance from becoming painful and inflamed, and its size exposed it to frequent injury.

Note on Shortness of the Umbilical Cord as a cause of Dystocia.—DR. LAPTHORN SMITH then read the following paper :—

The following remarks have been suggested to me by my having noticed at two labors occurring on the same day, a very long and a very short cord, which I now show you. The longer one measured when fresh just fifty inches, while the shorter one measured less than twelve. The only trouble which the short cord case gave me was that the placenta was retained for half an hour, which I attribute to the fact that whenever the cord is is pulled upon either by the accoucheur or by such an accident as its being too short, irregular contractions are set up in the middle or lower segments of the uterus, thereby causing more or less a condition known as hour-glass contraction. The labor, the patient's third one, was remarkably rapid, occupying in all only two or three hours, and was terminated naturally with the exception that I introduced my hand within the os in order to remove the placenta. The long cord, strange to say, caused more trouble, for after leaving the head on the perineum for several hours, the patient being a primipara, I applied the forceps, and as soon as the head was delivered I felt for a possible turn of the cord around the child's neck and found one. While undoing this, by slipping it over the child's head, I found that there were two other turns which I also unwound. By this time the child was quite black and the cord was pulseless. I practised artificial respiration for nearly half an hour before it breathed well.

Both of these conditions are recognized as offering considerable danger to both mother and child. Shortness of the cord, either absolute or owing to its being wound around the child's neck, may retard labor while the head is at the superior strait, while it is in the cavity of the basin, or while it is passing the inferior strait. And even after the head has passed, according to Cazeaux, it may arrest the progress of the shoulders. The latter author cites a case of his own in which delivery was terminated two hours after the expulsion of the head only after section of the cord had been resorted to, the foetus being dead. Dalmotte relates a similar observation.

Labor will generally terminate itself spontaneously, however, in one of three ways : Either the uterus will be forced down by the expulsive efforts of the mother, so as to bring the placenta near enough to the vulva to allow the delivery of the child ; or the cord may be ruptured ; or the placenta may be torn off. In a case observed by Malgouyre the latter accident happened and the placenta was expelled simultaneously with the foetus. In a case reported by Rigby the cord was ruptured two inches from the navel. In a case occurring in the practice of a *confrère* in the country, in which labor had been going on furiously for several hours without any progress, and in which he intervened with the forceps, the cord was so short that on the extraction of the child he was horrified to see it followed outside of the body by the placenta with the inverted uterus adherent. In spite of every effort and precaution he was unable to replace it, and the patient died.

In my opinion most, if not all, cases of inversion are due to tractions on the cord either owing to its being too short or to its being wound around the child's neck, or to the tractions of the

too hasty accoucheur.   I cannot admit that inversion can take
place from any kind of normal or abnormal uterine contractions.
Not only does shortness of the cord, either absolute or by being
wound around the child's neck, increase the pains of the mother
and retard the delivery of the fœtus, besides contributing largely
towards producing inversion, but it is very hazardous for the
child.   According to Mayer, out of 3,587 confinements the
cord was wound around the child's neck in 685 cases. Of these
121 were born asphyxiated.   Of these latter 72 were restored
by appropriate measures while 42 died.

Although the two cords I have shown you are respectively
much longer and shorter than the average, they are by no means
the longest or shortest on record.   Baudeloque has reported a
case in which the cord measured nearly 59 inches in length,
and which was wound around the child's neck seven times ;
while Schneider relates a case in which the cord measured 118
inches and was wound six times round the child's neck.   The
shortest recorded was less than four inches long.

Discussion.—DR. WM. GARDNER said he had little or no experience with acute inversion of the uterus. He certainly could
not agree with Dr. Smith that all cases were due to injudicious
traction on the cord ; many undoubtedly are, but chronic cases
often arise from a depression in the uterine walls, from a tumor
or local weakness.   This depression increases until inversion,
more or less complete, results.

DR. GIRDWOOD referred to a case of inversion three days after
delivery, where the uterus projected out of the vulva when the
patient sat up.

Fritz Bozeman Return-Flow Catheter. — DR. LAPTHORN
SMITH exhibited this valuable instrument, and pointed out its
value for irrigating the uterus after manipulation of the uterus
and cervical canal.   He also stated that by this instrument the
danger, which he contended was no imaginary one, of forcing
fluids into the peritoneal cavity through open Fallopian tubes
was avoided.   The instrument is so constructed that constriction
of the internal os will not prevent the return flow, and it possesses
as well the advantage of being easily taken apart and cleaned.

DR. TRENHOLME did not believe in curetting the decidua after miscarriage, but if considerable quantity remain, the only safe plan is to remove it.

DR. ALLOWAY also agreed that curetting was not advisable except where there is considerable retention. He was inclined to doubt the patency of Fallopian tubes in endometritis. The passage of a sound through the uterine wall is a more common accident than is usually supposed.

DR. ARMSTRONG said that in his experience there is less danger of sepsis after miscarriages than of hemorrhage. The latter is often very difficult to control.

DR. SMITH, in reply, stated that Dr. Wallace of Liverpool had demonstrated to his satisfaction the patency of the Fallopian tubes in endometritis. He also did not believe in curetting after miscarriages, but preferred the use of the catheter exhibited.

Drain Sore-Throat.—DR. J. C. CAMERON read a short paper on this subject, in which he showed that when a number of cases of sore throat broke out in the same family, and when it was of a marked adynamic character and accompanied with a rash somewhat resembling scarlet fever, there was usually good grounds for suspecting the drainage of the house. He then gave the details of ten cases of sore throat which occurred in one family. Suspecting the drainage, it was examined and a defect in the ventilation of the soil-pipe was discovered. In six of these cases both severe tonsillitis and ulceration almost diphtheritic in character were present.

DR. BLACKADER said that in his practice about the same time he had twelve cases of tonsillitis followed by an erythematous rash in families residing in the same district. The rash was especially marked on hands and neck. The temperature reached 101° to 102°, and headache with pain in the back were symptoms common to all. The sore throat in the adults was diphtheritic in character; in the children it was severe and scarlatiniform. The only possible cause common to all the cases was the milk supply. This, however, on investigation, showed nothing to indicate that infection proceeded from this source. He could not trace the cases to bad drainage, but he did not have the drains inspected by a sanitary engineer, as he certainly would do should he have a similar experience.

DR. WILKINS thought many of these cases were due to changes in temperature. All practitioners about that time had a number of such cases.

DR. Ross pointed out that in the early stages scarlatina was very difficult to diagnose. A rash accompanied or preceded by sore-throat, such as Dr. Blackader described, should always be treated as scarlet fever.

DR. MILLS had no doubt but that sore throat is frequently caused by open drains.

DR. PROUDFOOT thought that the question of contagion is often lost sight of in these cases.

DR. SPENDLOVE said he was able to trace six cases of tonsillitis with rash to a broken soil-pipe. A separation of two inches was found at one of the joints.

MR. FLEMING, Sanitary Engineer, was introduced by the President, and said he had numerous experiences of cases of sore throat clearly traceable to defective drainage. In one family no fewer than eleven were ill. Here he found sewage gas blowing into all the rooms, and the worst case was the one most exposed to the gas. Wherever the ventilating shaft of the drain passes through the house, any opening will cause a draught from the pipe into the rooms. He found upwards of 75 per cent. of the best houses in Montreal had defective house drains.

DR. CAMERON, in reply, made a strong appeal on behalf of the Montreal Sanitary Protection Association, of which Mr. Fleming is the engineer.

The Late R. P. Howard, M.D.—The following resolution of regret was proposed by Dr. W. Hingston, seconded by Dr. G. Fenwick, and as a mark of respect was passed by a silent standing vote :—

Resolved,—That this Society record its profound regret at the death of Dr. R. P. Howard, one of its most distinguished members and more than once its president, whose brilliant professional career was fairly earned by his untiring application to study, by his unflagging zeal in the discharge of his duties, and by the most delicate observance of the amenities of social and professional life.

Stated Meeting, April 19th, 1889.

WM. GARDNER, M.D., PRESIDENT, IN THE CHAIR.

Angina Pectoris : Occlusion of Coronary Artery.—DR. LAFLEUR presented the heart of a patient who had suffered from angina pectoris. The left ventricle was much dilated, and there was extensive fatty and fibroid degeneration of the myocardium. The coronary arteries were much thickened from atheromatous changes, and the interventricular branch of the left artery was completely occluded, near its origin, by a firm, calcified thrombus. Fine anastomoses with branches of the other vessels were traced out. The degenerative changes of the myocardium were most marked in the neighborhood of the occluded vessel.

DR. BELL stated that he had amputated the leg of this patient, and during convalescence he had been attacked by gangrene of the stump, severe pain coming on suddenly at night, and death occurring from exhaustion.

DR. ROSS, who had seen the patient for his thoracic symptoms, described his first attack of angina as coming on in bed, with excessive pain, anxiety and distress. The only physical signs were those of enfeeblement of the heart sounds. He regarded cases in which the attacks took place when at rest as much more serious than the more common ones, in which pain occurred during exertion.

DR. F. W. CAMPBELL referred to a case of angina and sudden death, with advanced disease of coronary arteries.

Cancer of Liver ; Metastasis involving Fifth Cranial Nerve.—DR. LAFLEUR exhibited a liver affected with encephaloid cancer. The organ was enormously enlarged, weighing over ten pounds. The cancerous nodules were scattered through the organ, the largest being about an inch and a half in diameter, were soft, fluctuating, and not umbilicated. The centres of the larger ones were softened and broken down to a fluid detritus. There was no primary growth in the stomach or elsewhere. A small secondary tumor was present involving the fifth cranial nerve of the left side. Microscopic examination showed a typical encephaloid cancer.

5

DR. WILKINS stated that in addition to the emaciation, enlargement of the liver, and jaundice, the patient had suffered from
severe shooting pains in the course of the trigeminus, which was
explained by the growth involving the nerve.   Briefly, the history of the case is as follows : Patient, a soldier, aged 48, who
drank freely, was jaundiced for twelve months some years ago.
Admitted to the hospital, March 25th, with great pain in epigastrium and general weakness ; face of an earthy, cachetic appearance.   The epigastric region was full and tender ; dullness over
all the upper abdominal region and in right nipple line for eight
inches from the fifth rib, and in the axillary line it reached the
crest of the ilium.   A hard, rounded, tender mass with nodules
could be felt across the abdomen two and a half inches below
the navel.   The patient could not sleep without morphia, the
abdomen became distended and tympanitic, failed rapidly, and
died April 12th.

Subdiaphragmatic Abscess; Gangrene of the Extremities.—
DR. FINLEY exhibited the organs.   A large abscess cavity,
bounded below by the liver, above by the lung, and communicating freely by an opening in the diaphragm.   The liver, which
was pushed down three and a half inches below costal border,
presented a shallow, saucer-shaped excavation surface, three
inches in diameter, and lined by pyogenic membrane.   The lung
bounding the abscess was firm and carnified, and showed early
interstitial changes microscopically.   Old adhesions closed the
pleural sac over its lower two-thirds.   A large bronchus opened
directly into the cavity.   The spleen was large, soft and pulpy ;
the other organs normal.   Moist gangrene was present in right
leg almost as high as knee, also in both upper extremities. Dissection of the vessels of the lower limb showed the arteries, as
far as the bifurcation of the popliteal, to be normal, but the
popliteal vein was blocked by a partially organized thrombus.
The origin of the abscess was probably subdiaphragmatic.   Abscess of the liver could be excluded by the anatomical conditions
in addition to its rarity.   Localized basal empyema usually presents greater pleural thickening and often small pockets of pus,
and very seldom caused perforation of the diaphragm.

DR. STEWART gave the following history of the case :—

L. R., aged 39, carter, was admitted into hospital Jan. 30th, 1889, complaining of an incessant and distressing cough with copious and occasionally blood-stained expectoration, also pain in right side in taking a long breath, and dyspnœa, which occasionally amounted to orthopnœa. Patient has been irregular in his habits and often severely exposed himself during periods of intemperance. No history of syphilis. Family history negative. Present illness began four weeks ago by pains in right shoulder and chest; had a chill followed by severe catching pain in right side, with hacking cough and a sense of oppression across chest. During last ten days expectoration has become muco-purulent, copious, and occasionally blood-stained; has lost strength rapidly and dyspnœa has increased; pulse 80, full and compressible; temperature $100\frac{1}{2}°$; respirations 24, shallow, restrained, and catching in character; constant cough and anxious expression.

Physical Examination.—Slight deficiency of expansion of right side; vocal and respiratory fremitus slightly diminished; dullness in front, on right side, from second rib to base and throughout axilla, and from eighth rib to base behind; breath sounds over dull area diminished and proceeding towards the base, almost extinct at apex; breathing harsh; sputum copious, purulent and blood-tinged. Examination of sputum showed red blood-cells, small amount of elastic tissue, no tubercle bacilli.

Feb. 4th.—Is spitting up large amount of frothy red blood, sometimes one pint per diem. Severe pain below right nipple. Sputum contains large amount of elastic tissue. 10th—Still copious hemorrhage, which is becoming more profuse. 20th— fine moist sounds heard at base of right lung; breath sounds more distinct. 23rd—Sputum less copious, but chiefly composed of bright red blood; dullness diminished to third rib in front, less marked. 27th—Patient becoming weaker

sputum lessened and not so much blood; signs nipple. —Complains of great pain in morning, also in right parts; temperature

105.2° ; pulse imperceptible at wrists ; brachial artery felt feebly beating ; neither tibial arteries can be felt ; pain on pressure in popliteal space on right side. 16th—Complains of coldness and numbness of hand and leg mentioned ; temperature 100° ; sputa less copious ; great pain in leg and arm. 18th— Parts are becoming livid and cold, and this condition is extending up leg and arm, as also is seat of pain ; sensation in fingers and toes nearly gone ; no pulse in radial or tibial arteries ; perspires profusely at times ; complains of pain in right wrist coming on suddenly ; left hand livid and cold. 20th—Complains of severe pain in left foot (instep) ; gangrene extending in other parts. 23rd—Complete stasis of blood in both hands and feet ; is failing rapidly and suffering great pain. 28th—Gangrene still extending, is half-way up right leg and above right wrist-joint ; blebs appearing ; suffering great pain ; very weak and delirious at times.

April 10th.—Patient died to-day, gangrene having extended over two-thirds of left arm, nearly to knee of right leg, and over other foot and hand.

DR. Ross had seen the patient in the earlier part of his illness. Hæmoptysis had then been the most prominent symptom.

DR. LAFLEUR suggested that the gangrene was due to capillary thrombi of micro-organisms.

Old Encysted Trichina.—DR. FINLEY exhibited the larynx of a woman aged 45, in the muscles of which trichinæ were imbedded. The trichinæ were found in moderate numbers in the muscles of the tongue and larynx, but were not observed elsewhere. They were distinctly visible to the naked eye as fine yellowish particles. There was fatty degeneration of the heart and cirrhosis of liver and kidneys, attributed to chronic alcoholism.

DR. WILKINS stated that the woman had been brought to the hospital a couple of days before death with convulsions, and died of uræmia, a noticeable feature of the case being the slow pulse, which was only 40 per minute. Albumen and tube casts were present. Trichinosis had, of course, not been suspected.

Chronic Alcoholism—Cirrhosis of Liver and Kidneys ; Gastric Ulcer ; Death from Hæmatemesis.—DR. FINLEY exhibited for Dr. Wilkins the stomach of a patient who had died of hæmatemesis. The organ presented a small ulcer, with sharply-cut edges, one-third of an inch in diameter, on the posterior wall, near the middle of the lesser curvature. A small, open-mouthed artery is present in the centre of the ulcer, into which a small probe is readily passed. The stomach contained a small amount of blood, and there was a large quantity of more or less altered blood in the small and large intestines. The liver was fatty and cirrhotic, about normal in size. The kidneys were small and cirrhotic. The spleen was atrophied, and the heart showed fatty infiltration and degeneration.

DR. WILKINS stated that the patient, a female aged 40, had been brought to hospital the day before her death. She was too ill to give an account of herself. Severe hæmatemesis began forty-eight hours before death, and was looked upon as probably due to ulcer. The patient was known to have been a hard drinker, and to this the changes in the kidneys, liver and heart were probably due.

Selections.

Some Observations on Œdema, WITH TWO CASES OF IRREGULAR ŒDEMA COMPLICATING MALARIA.—

Different names are applied to œdemas of different location and extent, but for all practical purposes I may say that the following list embraces substantially all the different varieties of œdema : 1. Œdema due to portal obstruction, or liver œdema. 2. Œdema due to cardiac disease, heart œdema. 3. Œdema due to renal disease, or kidney œdema. 4. Essential œdema of Wagner.

Œdemas from other causes worthy of mention, though their causative relation is disputed, are, those from exposure to cold and damp, the sudden suppression of an habitual discharge, the rapid cure of a cutaneous disease and extreme anæmia and debility. The four last named are considered to induce œdema by exciting congestion in internal organs from the afflux of blood to them, on its being driven from the surface, and in this way disturbing the renal as well as other functions; or in consequence of abnormal states of the blood and tissues. It is doubtful, however, if either of them can of itself actually occasion œdema, It is very likely indeed that many or all of them exist at the same time and contribute each its part to the production of the undesired result. After some remarks on the first three varieties, Dr. Keefe continues: I would now draw your attention to the essential œdema of Wagner. This is more frequently found in children than adults, and generally occupies the entire surface of the body. Although we do not know its etiology it is thought that cutaneous, vascular and blood changes and cardiac asthenia are among the most frequent causes. Heredity also seems to be a factor in its production, the father or mother having been rachitic, while in other cases a brother or sister has been subject to general œdema. "Neither autopsies nor experiments on animals have served to explain the genesis of this disease. It is considered doubtful if the vaso-motor or trophic nerves have any part whatever in its production." The generalized œdema accompanying febrile disease is also a kind as to the cause of which we are entirely ignorant, though there are many speculations in this regard. I will relate briefly two cases of irregular œdema occurring in my practice as a complication of malarial disease.

Case 1. Single female, domestic, aged 24, extremely restless, chill, nausea and vomiting; left hand and wrist greatly swollen, pitting on pressure, as were both ankles also; temperature 104½°, pulse 110, pain in head, back and limbs; had been told she had dropsy, which greatly frightened her. Urinary examination proved negative, as did physical examination of chest and abdomen. I accordingly gave quinine in anti-periodic doses, and was pleased to find a ready response. There was no return of the paroxysm and she returned to her work in a few days. In about six weeks I was again called and found her in a similar condition. Quinine gave, a second time, a prompt cure.

Case 2. Married female, Swede, aged 38, had lived in a malarious district, and had several tertian attacks. Called to see her for œdema under eyes, and in right wrist and arm; later, painful chilly feelings in back, headache and weakness in limbs. Quinine with iron and arsenic removed all symptoms.

While I do not pretend to be able to explain how malarial

poison acts on the organism to produce such exudations, I would suggest that it is due to the poison of the disease acting on the nerve centres, just as I have explained regarding urea in kidney diseases, and through the sympathetic ganglia paralyzing the vaso-motor nerves, thereby dilating the arterioles and thus causing an afflux of blood to one part. In other words it causes an inco-ordination on the part of the vaso-motor nervous system. This superabundance of blood, the veins of the part find it more than usually difficult to return to the circulatory centre, in consequence of the congestion existing in nearly all the important viscera and consequent pressure on and narrowing of the lumen of the veins and lymphatics passing into and through them. For these reasons stasis and transudation are encouraged and produced. The points of interest, as it seems to me, in these cases are: the importance of keeping in mind the possibility of malarial disease as a causative factor in irregular œdema; its speedy yielding to anti-malarial treatment; and the advisability of resorting to such treatment in doubtful cases.—
Dr. D. E. Keefe in Bost. Med. and Surg. Jour., May 16.

Diseases of the Circulatory Organs—

PROGNOSIS IN HEART AFFECTIONS.—At the meeting of the Verein fur innere Medicin on April 1st, 1889, Dr. Leyden discussed the prognosis of diseases of the heart. After some preliminary observations on the general importance of prognois, the speaker went on to say that the advance in our present knowledge was due to the emancipation of observers from purely physical methods which were assuredly not undervalued, but on which formerly reliance had been too exclusively placed. The clinical method now in vogue took into account, in addition to physical diagnostic measures, all other local and general symptoms, and had thus acquired a broader standpoint. Until a short time ago the prognosis of heart disease had been extremely bad. A more hopeful outlook had for the first time been taken quite recently. Experience had shown that many sufferers from heart disease lived in fairly comfortable ease. A gloomy prognosis appeared to be confirmed by the fact that persons with diseased heart often died suddenly. Closer examination, however—especially by English physicians—had shown that in the majority of chronic heart affections, sudden death was rare, except in the case of inadequacy of aortic valves, and true angina pectoris (of Heberden). In both of those, although the patient is not safe any day, his life may be prolonged for years. In relation to aortic insufficiency, Dr. Leyden had

had a very large experience, both in hospital and private practice. In other kinds of valvular inadequacy sudden death was comparatively rare; in mitral incompetence it occurred in about two per cent. of the cases, that is to say, so seldom that the practitioner might leave this unfortunate termination out of account. Further observations on prognosis might be grouped under three heads: (1) with reference to general disposition and circumstances of life; (2) with special groups of cardiac affections; (3) with reference to particular physical and physiologico-pathological symptoms. In connection with the first of these, the age must first be considered. Young children bear heart disease very badly. In adolescence and early adult life the prognosis is better. This depends on the fact that at that age those forms of cardiac affection chiefly occur in which the prognosis is relatively favorable. At more advanced periods of life, heart diseases are for the most part associated with arterio-sclerosis. This often became developed at a very early stage. Arterio-sclerosis had always a progressive tendency; this progressive character might, however, be very gradual. Compensative changes were easily brought about in more mature years. But precisely because of this progressive tendency, those forms of valvular insufficiency presented an unfavorable prognosis. The second general etiological factor was the sex. The prognosis was on the whole better in the female than in the male sex. If this was less clearly the case in hospital than in private practice, that was due to the fact that women of the lower classes led a life exposed to the same hard work, the same mental disturbances, and partly the same excesses as men. In women of the upper classes these etiological factors were wanting. Arterio-sclerosis was, moreover, less frequent in the female sex, and even in families in which it was hereditary it affected the female members to a less extent. The female character was better adapted to bear troubles. Finally, experience proved that in women mitral incompetence, in which the prognosis was good, was more frequent than aortic insufficiency. A third factor was to be found in the patient's circumstances and manner of life. Hard bodily labour was the most dangerous enemy to sufferers from cardiac disease. Even mental emotion often aggravated the condition. The less disturbed by worry the patient's life was, the more care he took of himself, the better was the prognosis; therefore patients in better and easier circum-stances bore heart affections better than persons less fortunately situated. A further point was connected with possibility of treatment and the re-action of 'A - ' to medicines, of which digitalis was the m' right use of that drug was one of the in medicine.

THE

Montreal Medical Journal.

| VOL. XVIII. | JULY, 1889. | No. 1. |

DIABETES MELLITUS FOLLOWING EXTIRPATION OF THE PANCREAS.

Mering and Minkowski (*Centralblatt f. Klin. Med.*) have found that extirpation of the pancreas in the dog is invariably followed by diabetes mellitus. Sugar appears in the urine shortly after the operation and is constantly to be found till the death of the animal, which usually occurs some weeks after. In addition to the sugar in the urine, the other well known symptoms of the disease also make their appearance; polyuria, excessive thirst and emaciation in spite of abundant nourishment. The urine was also found to contain acetone, the blood sugar was also found to be increased in quantity. The normal glycogen of the liver and muscles was found absent in a dog that had been operated on four weeks previously and after being fed with a rich nitrogenous diet. As care was taken not to wound the solar ganglion during the operations, the authors conclude that the diabetes was due to the extirpation of the pancreas.

LEPROSY IN ENGLAND.

Within the last few months great alarm has been expressed lest leprosy should secure a footing in England and become a prevailing disease. There is no doubt that it is spreading in India and those of our colonies which are situated in tropical climates. But in spite of the alarmists it is not present in England to any extent, especially when we take into consideration the fact that so much oriental traffic centres in that country. Altogether there are supposed to be not more than twenty lepers in England, and two of them were exhibited lately at the Epidemiological Society. A discussion ensued on the increase of the malady in India, and the necessity for strict segregation. Several speakers pointed to the danger of leprosy becoming common in this country unless precautions were taken to limit the risk of contagion. They all agreed that there was no curative treatment. Legislation to compel lepers to enter asylums was demanded by some medical men present, whilst others, including the chairman, Dr. Thorne Thorne, advocated a Government enquiry upon the subject.

HOSPITAL FOR THE TREATMENT OF THE DISEASES OF THE GREAT TOE.

In the course of a very able address given at the Mansion House, London, on the 20th ult, in aid of the Hospital Sunday Fund, Sir Andrew Clark alluded to the growth of special hospitals as one of the causes of the falling off in the revenues of the general hospitals and dealt heavy blows at the founders of special institutions and those who had been induced to contribute to their support. To use his own words "Then there is another reason, and that is the foundation and maintenance of improper hospitals which divert funds in a direction in which they ought not to be employed and rob the great hospitals of the support which they ought to receive. A doctor who cannot get on in the ordinary way takes to studying the great toe, and he discovers something about it that has never been discovered before. In the course of his studies he ascertains that the diseases of the organ are not only supremely important in themselves but that they have the most intimate relation to all the other serious diseases of the body. He also invents a wonderful instrument whereby he can look into the great toe and see what is threatening and prevent all those terrible things which happen in the organ and affect the whole system. He goes to his friends, shows them his instrument and tells them of his discoveries. They then club together and establish a hospital for the treatment of the diseases of the great toe. The hospital is manned by his friends who, having joined in the venture, must make it a success. They soon get patients who are convinced of the vast importance of the great toe; marvellous cures are expected and all sorts of frightful diseases are prevented.

Then they have an annual meeting; they have a chairman who sets forth bashfully, in the presence of the great physician, the diseases of the great toe, the wonderful things that had been done, the great service which has been rendered by the hospital, the terrible prejudice it has had to encounter, the determination that this great institution shall be liberally supported notwithstanding the prejudices of the medical profession and of those who herd along with them."

CHANGES IN THE CURRICULUM OF THE ONTARIO MEDICAL COUNCIL.

We are pleased to hear that the Ontario Medical Council have determined to make one summer session compulsory. This is a much needed change in the interests of the student. Another change instituted is the attendance on a course of fifty demonstrations on medical and surgical anatomy during the final year. Such a course will no doubt be an aid to many students in working for their examinations in the final subjects, but on the other hand it will seriously interfere with what should be the real work of the year—clinical work. We have also noticed that the Council in future will require two six months' courses on medical jurisprudence. This is the only change made in the requirements of attendance on didatic lectures. It is a most unfortunate change in many ways. The previous requirements of two three months' courses on this subject were, in the opinion of many, well able to judge entirely too much. There can, we think, be no two opinions on the unadvisability of doubling what was previously a burden. The Council as yet do not require any attendance on lectures on general pathology, a subject of very much greater importance than jurisprudence.

THE ONTARIO MEDICAL ASSOCIATION.

The recent meeting of the Ontario Medical Association in Toronto was the most successful that this body has as yet held. The attendance was good, and many excellent papers were read. The discussions were keen and interesting. The address of the president, Dr. Henderson of Kingston, dealt in a very able manner with many of the questions that are specially attracting the attention of the pro-

profession in this Canada of ours. The following officers were appointed for the ensuing year: President, Dr. J. Algernon Temple; first vice-president, Dr. Landy, of Preston; second vice-president, Dr. G. Shaw, of Hamilton; third vice-president, K. N. Fenwick, Kingston; fourth vice-president, Dr. Hanley, Waubaushene; general secretary, Dr. D. G. Wishart, Toronto; treasurer, Dr. Barrick, Toronto; assistant secretary, Dr. W. P. Caven, Toronto.

AMERICAN MEDICAL ASSOCIATION.

The fortieth annual meeting of the American Medical Association, recently held in Newport, was, especially in a scientific aspect, one of the most successful meetings that this important bodies has ever held. The address of the President, Dr. Dawson, of Cincinnati, dealt mainly with questions affecting medical education. The address on Medicine, delivered by Provost Pepper, of the University of Pennsylvania, was mainly a sketch of the life work of Benjamin Rush. Prof. W. H. Welch, of Baltimore, delivered an exceedingly able address on State Medicine. We hope in an early issue to publish this address. Our distinguished countryman, Sir Jas. Grant, of Ottawa, ably represented the profession in Canada.

COLLEGE OF PHYSICIANS AND SURGEONS OF THE PROVINCE OF QUEBEC.

At the triennial meeting of the College of Physicians and Surgeons of the Province of Quebec held at Laval University, Quebec, on July 10th, the President, Dr. Hingston, presiding. The Treasurer, Dr. Lachapelle, submitted his financial statement, showing that the total receipts of the College from 1st July, 1886, to 1st July, 1889, had been $16,013.03 and that, after paying all expenses, there remained a balance on hand of $4,672.64, together with five shares of the Bank of Montreal.

The thanks of the College were unanimously voted to the Treasurer for the able manner in which he had discharged his duties during the last nine years, and the meeting then proceeded to the election of forty new governors for the next three years, with the following result:

City of Quebec.—R. F. Rinfret, L. Larue, C. T. Parke, A. G. Belleau, A. A. Watters and E. A. de St. George.

District of Quebec.—P. M. Guay, Come Rinfret, R. Fiset, L. H. Labrecque, L. T. Rousseau, P. E. Grandbois and A. Moiresset.

District of Three Rivers.—Hon. J. J. Ross, E. C. P. Chevre. fils and F. Trudel.

City of Montreal.—T. A. Rodger and J. M. Beausoleil.

District of Montreal.—Hon. Dr. Paquet, P. Laberge, J. O. Mousseau, J. H. L. St. Germain, J. Lippe, H. A. Mignault, Hon. Dr. Marcil, Jules Prevost and J. B. Gibson.

District of St. Francis.—Drs. J. F. Austin, F. Pare and T. Larue.

The new Board met immediately, when the President, Dr. Hingston, presented his report, which was unanimously adopted. The representatives of the universities were then named as follows :

McGill.—Drs. Craik and Geo. Ross.

Montreal School of Medicine, etc.—Drs. Hingston and Desjardins.

Laval, Quebec.—Drs. Lemieux and Simard.

Bishops.—Drs. Campbell and Perrigo.

Laval, Montreal.—Drs. Rottot and Dagenais.

The election of officers resulted as follows:

President, Hon. Dr. J. J. Ross; Vice-Presidents, Drs. R. F. Rinfret and Gibson; Treasurer, Dr. Dagenais; Secretaries, Drs. Campbell and Belleau; Registrar, Dr. L. Larue.

Professors Laflamme, Verrault, Howe and Petry were chosen as preliminary examiners.

The following were named assessors :—

Laval, Quebec.—Drs. Sewell and Gameau.

Laval, Montreal.—Drs. Marcel and Gibson.

McGill.—Drs. Austin and P. E. Mignault.

Victoria.—Drs. Angus Macdonnell and O. Raymond.

Bishops.—Drs. H. A. Mignault and Rodger.

Thanks were then voted to the retiring President, Dr. Hingston, and the other outgoing officers, and the meeting adjourned to the 25th of September next.

————

—THE fifteenth annual meeting of the Bathurst and Rideau Medical Association was held in Arnprior on July 3rd last, Dr. Cranston, of Arnprior, president, in the chair. The following officers were appointed for the ensuing year: President, J. G. Cranston, of Arnprior; vice-presidents, Dr. R. W. Powell, of Ottawa, and Dr. Burns, of Almonte; secretary,

H. B. Small, of Ottawa; treasurer, Dr. Hill, of Ottawa; executive committee, Dr. Horsey, Rogers and Sir James Grant for the City of Ottawa; and Drs. Dickson, Lynch, Armstrong, Mann, Allan and Grant for the rural districts. It was decided to hold the next meeting in the City of Ottawa in January, 1890.

Obituary.

DR. JAS. B. HUNTER OF NEW YORK.

Death has again cut into the ranks of the leaders of medical thought of this city. This time the victim was James Bracebridge Hunter, who, although a native of New York State, in which he had lived the major part of his life, always felt a warm filial feeling for Canada—the scene of the happy days of his boyhood. His family continued residing in Toronto and there his remains were taken for burial. Dr. Hunter died on June 10th, at the age of fifty-two years, after an illness of twenty-six weeks, having suffered from acute rheumatism complicated with endo- and pericarditis.

He was a medical student in Cincinnati at the time that the civil war broke out in 1861, when he entered the army as a volunteer and was soon promoted to the rank of first lieutenant and adjutant. Later on he passed the Army Medical Board Examination and was assigned to the 60th Indiana Regiment as asssistant surgeon. In this capacity he saw active service under Grant at Vicksburg and at other points. On the termination of the war he came to this city and continued the study of medicine at the College of Physicians and Surgeons, where he was graduated in 1866. He then went to London and attended Moorfields Hospital with a view of becoming an oculist. On his return here he became associated with Dr. T. G. Thomas in hospital and college work and this circumstance determined his efforts and energies into the paths of gynæcology. He was appointed house surgeon to the Woman's Hospital in this city in 1867, assistant surgeon in 1871. In 1878 he was elected attending surgeon—a post which he occupied until his death. He was one of the early members of the New York Polyclinic, holding the chair of Gynæcology, and was visiting surgeon to the Cancer Hospital, of which he was one of the founders.

From 1872 to 1880 he was connected with the *New York Medical Journal*, first as assistant then as chief editor, and exhibited the same thoroughness, earnestness and good common sense in this position as in all that he filled. Dr. Hunter's career in this city is a forcible illustration of what patience, industry and perserverence will accomplish even in the face of great odds. Naturally reserved, modest, unostentatious, with no family connections, with a face and manner which repelled rather than attracted at first sight, he was the last person of whom one would predict a brilliant career in this vast metropolis where the competition is so keen and great. And yet for at least the past decade he was reckoned among the leading gynæcologists of the day and had a very large and profitable *clientile*. There were a few more brilliant operators, but there were none more cool, more neat and more skillful than he. As a diagnostician there were few his equal. As a teacher he was conscientious, clear and practical. Those who have reason to know him best speak very highly of the goodness of his heart, of his loyal friendships and of his almost morbid sensitiveness lest his acts of charity should become known to the world. Of him it might be truly said " he gave with the right hand and the left hand did not know it." His heart beat warmly for all in distress and in physical suffering. To those of his colleagues who served with him he was kindness in itself and full of consideration. It is deplorable that such an active and useful life should be cut off just in its prime, at a time when the thorny paths that beset it were beginning to be left behind, when the summit of the mountain was about to be reached, and when the vision was gaining in width and in height, for there can be no doubt that had he lived for another decade he would have enriched medical science to a considerable degree. Even in this immense aggregation of human beings, where one soul is like a drop in the ocean, his loss will be felt by the profession and by the community for some time to come.   H. N. V.

New York, 1 July, 1889.

THE LATE DR. WOOLDRIDGE OF GUY'S HOSPITAL.—Guy's Hospital has been singularly unfortunate within the last few years in that it has suffered the loss of so many of the members of the medical staff. Moxon, Fagge, Carrington and

Mahomed, all men of mark, all in their prime, and in the very thick of professional life, followed each other very rapidly to the grave. The last English mail brings news of the death of another assistant physician of Guy's, Dr. Leonard Charles Wooldridge. The nature of the fatal illness seems to have been obscure. The onset was acute and death unexpectedly sudden. The autopsy showed congestion and ecchymosis of the stomach and duodenum, with follicular ulceration of the colon. There was slight but undoubted dilatation of both ventricles of the heart. It would appear that the morbid state of the stomach and colon produced in his exhausted condition a cardiac dilatation, which proved fatal from syncope. Dr. Wooldridge was the son-in-law of Sir Edward Sieveking.

Medical Items.

—THE following is the list of officers of the Ontario Medical Council for the current year: President, Dr. Cranston, Arnprior; vice-president, Dr. Crawford; treasurer, Dr. W. T. Aikins; solicitor, B. B. Osler; registrar, R. A. Pyne.

—We beg to draw attention to Dr. Holford Walker's change of advertisement in this issue, announcing that his new hospital in Toronto is now open for the reception of patients. The doctor has taken a wise course to confine himself to the speciality of Diseases of Women and Abdominal Surgery, and as such is the pioneer specialist in that department of the profession in Toronto or in fact in Ontario. We understand his Hospital is a model one in every respect, and worthy of the support of the profession throughout Ontario.

TREATMENT EOR CATARRHAL AFFECTIONS OF THE THROAT.— Dr. G. B. Hope of New York, attending surgeon Metropolitan Throat Hospital, and Professor Diseases of the Throat, University of Vermont, says: " For a long time I have been employing Horsford's Acid Phosphate as a constitutional treatment for catarrhal affections of the throat. I consider it to be among the very best tonic excitants of the vocal organs, and particularly applicable in relieving the fatigue and huskiness of voice incident to those who pursue a professional career of actor or vocalist, and far preferable to the various forms of wines now so generally recommended for this purpose. I have seen no other allusion to its employment in this direction, which I believe you are perfectly safe in recommending both from a theoretical and practical point of view.

THE

MONTREAL MEDICAL JOURNAL.

| VOL. XVIII. | AUGUST, 1889. | No. 2. |

Original Communications.

ON THE PROGRESS OF MEDICAL SCIENCE DURING THE PAST HALF CENTURY.

BY SIR JAMES GRANT, M.D., K.C.M.G., OF OTTAWA.

An Address delivered at the Fortieth Annual Meeting of the American Medical Association, at Newport, R.I., June 27th, 1889.

Mr. President and Gentlemen :—I beg to return to you my sincere thanks for the invitation extended by a committee of this Association to be present at this meeting of the medical profession of the United States, and it is an additional source of gratification that I am asked to a seat on this platform. I am reminded of the fact that when the Marquis of Lorne was Governor of Canada, the Royal Society was invited to lunch at the Government House. When the health of the President of the United States was proposed, a sentiment which we Canadians fully appreciate, and which we are delighted to honor next to that of our glorious Queen Victoria, Mark Twain was asked to respond. He thanked His Excellency for the compliment, and was proud to be the recipient of the distinction, but regretted that being unprepared he was unable to respond. I feel very much in the same position on being called upon to speak to this large body before me. For fully twenty-five years I have been in the habit of attending the meetings of your Association at various points, and it is to me a source of pride and gratitude to be able to note the progress of that profession to which I have. the honor to belong. This is an exceedingly important epoch in the history of our profession. You have just celebrated your

6

one hundredth anniversary, which marks the progress of this great country. In entering the hall to-day, the observation dropped from a bystander that the insane doctors were meeting here. It struck me as somewhat peculiar, inasmuch as I was not aware of the fact that this meeting could appropriate that idea. It was soon cleared up, as I learned that that branch of the profession met here. Let me for a short time draw your attention to the remarkable advance in the several departments of the profession which has been made within the past century.

It was in 1835 that Gardner Hill, of Lincoln Lunatic Asylum, announced the treatment of insanity by non-restraint. Prior to that time the poor lunatic was subject to be confined in the corner of a cell with chains round his neck, his arms manacled, and pendulous clubs attached to his feet in order to prevent locomotion. His food was served to him as it would be to an ordinary quadruped, and in fact the whole treatment of the insane in those days was most irrational in its character. Much credit is due to Pinel in Paris, Tuke of York, and Charlesworth in the city of Lincoln asylum, in which the grand final experimenting of entire freedom of the insane was carried out.

We find here that in the great institutions of this country for the treatment of the insane every indication of progressive development as to the principles of treatment in cases of mental aberration have been carried into operation most successfully. You have undoubtedly great workers in the subject of psychological investigations. When in Edinburgh some years ago, Dr. Tuke, the author of that admirable work on " Insanity," remarked to me that by far the best journal on psychological medicine was that published by the late Dr. Jewell of Chicago. The investigations of the late Dr. Gray of Utica are well known, doubtless, to every member of the Association. The subject of cerebral pathology attracted his closest attention, and his demonstrations by the large microscopic sections of the brain which he was enabled to make did much to convey an accurate idea of cerebral structure under very diverse circumstances. Strange to say that some of the most violent forms of insanity ever under the microscope have not been traced to anything like change of structure. Such, also, was the impression conveyed to me by Tuke of Edinburgh. These, of course, may be looked upon as irregular cases, as usually insanity rarely takes place without some definable reason in the great nervous centre. Under these circumstances, is not the trite and laconic observation of *Punch* brought home to us with more than ordinary force : " What is matter ? never mind ; and what is mind ? that's the matter." Pursuing this subject still further, the investigations of our physiologists within the past quarter of a century have certainly accomplished much as regards our knowledge of the nervous system. Disturbed cerebral centres frequently telegraph their normal condition to the peripheral surface, producing an abnormal condition of facial expression. By a process of careful analytical induction, such men as Ferrier of London, Hamilton and Seguin of New York, and Hammond of Washington, have been enabled to take stock of the changes and define the region of the disturbed centres. This embraces the great recent advances in the subject of cerebral localization, and is the very key to the advances in cranial surgery undertaken by such men as Horsley of London, Macewen of Glasgow, and Seguin and Weir of New York.

In looking around me on this platform, I am extremely grateful to find present one of the ex-Presidents of this Association, Dr. Bowditch of Boston, whose name is so closely associated with the subject of pleuritic effusion, and who worked so vigorously to convey his accurate impressions as regards the treatment of that important thoracic disease. Not alone have his observations been confined to the chest, but in the domain of preventive medicine he has also been one of the pioneers. It has been well said that " an ounce of prevention is better than a pound of cure," and notwithstanding the fact that the members of the medical profession, in the advocacy of sanitary science, are curtailing effectively the means of their ordinary livelihood, still their philanthropic efforts are never stayed where they can be of advantage to the public at large. The great public institutions of to-day give evidence of the principles of sanitary science. Life is made comfortable even for the most dejected criminal. The hospitals give evidences of thorough ventilation and ample supply of light, and all the modern improvements for sewage and water supply, very important factors in the treatment of the sick. The articles of diet are being carefelly investigated. Milk is now known to be a prolific source both of scarlet fever and diphtheria, and in early life being a common source of diet, how necessary are the investigations of the sanitarian. Less than half a century ago Farr of London gave a great impulse to the progress of sanitary science by the introduction of tabulated statistics as to the life and death rate. In the various medical institutions in this country, as well as in Canada, the subject of sanitary science is receiving the most careful consideration, and very justly so, inasmuch as it pertains most closely to the welfare of society at large.

Let me draw your attention for a few moments to a great gymnasium of the human system, of which we have evidence in the surgery of the abdominal cavity. This country has reason to feel proud of what has been accomplished in this department. The name of Ephraim McDowell of Kentucky with you, as with ourselves, is a household word. He possessed the skill, the forethought and the knowledge which enabled him to undertake the first ovariotomy. Following rapidly ln his path came Dunlop of Ohio and Kimball of Lowell, Mass., the latter of whom maintains the vigor of youth although considerably over his seventieth year. These men constitute an intellectual tripod, if I may so term it, in the domain of abdominal surgery. Before me I see a gentleman whose name I cannot refrain from giving expression to— Dr. Senn of Chicago—who has accomplished so much with reference to the lesions of the intestinal canal. His name will undoubtedly become a household word amongst the members of our profession. While adverting thus personally to what your men have achieved, I feel confident you will join with me in recognizing the admirable achievements in the same line of thought brought about by such men as Sir Spencer Wells, Drs. Thornton, Bantock, Lawson Tait, and Keith of Edinburgh. Almost every organ in this cavity has been operated on successfully, and the achievements mark beyond a doubt the progress of surgery during the latter half of this century.

There is another department concerning which I desire to allude briefly, namely, that of therapeutics. Medicines are now no longer, we hope, administered empirically; the why and wherefore are being inquired into most carefully. How the remedial agents act directly or indirectly on the blood and tissues is the subject of much physiological research. Here comes in a question of the slowing of the heart's action by digitalis and the reduction of febrile states of the system by antipyretics. Much credit is due to the pharmaceutical associations of this country for the elegance of the preparations placed before the profession, so much so that the old British pharmacopœia must undergo considerable modification. There is also a marked advance in dietetics, embracing peptonoids and very digestive materials introduced to tone and assist digestive function. Cod liver oil and its emulsion also occupy an important place as therapeutic adjuncts. And in addition, the triturates so recently introduced are doubtless valuable as means of medicinal administration.

On my way from Boston yesterday I was gratified to read the instructive address of the Hon. Chauncey Depew to the legal profession, in which he referred to the representation of this country. Of the thirty-two presidents, eighteen were members of the legal profession, and during the past one hundred years, in eighty-two of that period the presidential chair has been occupied by legal lights of this country. The bearing of this subject is extremely important, inasmuch as the medical profession is concerned. In the Commons of Canada there are at least fifteen or twenty medical men, and in the Senate also quite a number of members of the medical profession. In the Local Provincial Parliaments our profession is ably represented. Thus we have been enabled to guide and direct public opinion towards the important question of medical education. I listened with pleasure to the report of your committee on this subject, recommending the introduction of a higher standard in this country, both as to preliminary education and subsequent academic study. Having been upwards of twenty-two years consecutively in the Medical Council of Ontario, I have had opportunities of observing the importance of this question. The Local Parliament of Ontario passed a bill for the formation of a Council, giving it the power to appoint examiners in medicine, irrespective of the teaching bodies, and thus guard the portals of entrance into the medical profession. Prior to this time the entrance of homœopathists and eclectics into the profession was very considerable, but now that matters have been placed on a uniform basis of examination, except in special subjects such as homœopathy and eclectic materia medica, we find that this elevated standard has improved very materially the entire status of our profession ; in fact, to-day there are very few graduating homœopathists or eclectics compared to the regular profession, greatly brought about by the introduction of the elevated standard of medical education.

In the great medical centres of this country we cannot fail to miss many of the old landmarks, men like Dunglison, Gross and Pancoast, of Philadephia ; Parker, Buck, Marion Sims, Flint, Hamilton and Van Buren, of New York ; White, of Buffalo ; Brainard and Jewell, of Chicago. These men gave a force, a character and an impulse to the profession recognized throughout the civilized world. Younger men are following rapidly into the path of distinction, and have achieved more than an ordinary celebrity, such as Thomas and Emmet, of New York ; Storer of Boston, and Goodell of Philadelphia ; particularly in the diseases of women. I am pleased to observe here so many younger members of the profession. To attend these meetings is a duty they owe not only to themselves but to the communities in which they are laboring. Here we receive, as it were, a bird's eye view of the progress of our profession in every department, and the very intellectual friction produces a tonic influence which sends every member of this Association home with renewed vigor in that profession we delight to honor. A young Western physician, recently visiting Paris, remarked to his professor if he knew So-and-So in the medical profession ; the reply was that he did not. " What has he written ?" was the question asked. The young physician answered, " He has not written anything so far as I know, but he has a very large practice." To the younger members of the medical profession I would say, in order to achieve a lasting reputation, record your facts, note carefully bedside observations, and do not be in a hurry in drawing sudden conclusions.   Thus you will be enabled to contribute your mite to the journalism of this country, and support a most commendable department of literature which guards over the best interests of our profession.

To the profession in Canada permit me to say that I consider ourselves one people.   Placed as we are on either side of an imaginary Chinese wall, we speak the same language, we enjoy the same literature, we take our inspirations from the same fountains of science in all that pertains to the best interests of our profession, and I will say, in as far as the unity of that profession is concerned, that the beautiful sentiment expressed by Her Majesty the Queen on the completion of the Atlantic cable applies equally well to our profession : " What God hath joined together let no man put asunder."

In conclusion, let me again return you my warmest thanks for the kind reception I have received and the delight I have experienced in the presence of your great historian, Bancroft, and many other old friends I see around me still in the vigor of life.   Let us then work on to do honor to our profession, to alleviate the sufferings of humanity, and in that profession to perform the important responsibilities assigned to our respective charges.   And I feel I cannot do better than express the lines so beautifully written by your gifted poet who now slumbers amidst the illustrious dead of this great Republic :

> " Let us then be up and doing,
> With a heart for any fate ;
> Still achieving, still pursuing,
> Learn to labor and to wait."

ABSTRACT OF A CLINICAL LECTURE

DELIVERED AT THE MONTREAL GENERAL HOSPITAL, JULY 18TH.

BY T. JOHNSON-ALLOWAY, M.D.,

The first case upon which I intend to operate to-day was admitted into hospital July 1st, and has the following history:

Aged 21 years; married four years ago. Two pregnancies; the first terminated at the eighth month of gestation, the other at the third month. Ever since this miscarriage, which took place two years ago, she has complained of the following symptoms: severe pain in left lumbar region, back and hypogastrium; a bearing-down feeling constantly present; dysmenorrhœa; frequent micturition; leucorrhœal discharge; dyspareunia and painful defecation. She has lost her health generally, and is quite unable to do ordinary housework.

On examination, I find she has the small, delicate, though proportionately-formed pelvis so characteristic of the poorly-fed French-Canadian race. The perineum is intact, and will not require attention. There is bilateral laceration of the cervix uteri, with ectropion and extensive glandular hypertrophy. The uterus is enlarged, hard, tender, and retroverted to the third degree. It is mobile, and easily replaced to its normal position, showing that if we can only adopt some method of treatment which will keep it permanently in the forward position, we will in all probability relieve our patient of her suffering.

Before we touch upon the subject of treatment, however, it would be well to ask ourselves how so grave a pathological condition of the uterus could occur in so young a woman. If we look back we will see that she was married at 17 and became immediately pregnant. Now at this age the pelvic organs have not sufficiently matured to be capable of carrying out the functions of pregnancy and parturition without suffering injury to themselves in making the attempt. In this case the uterus with difficulty fulfilled its functions until the eighth month of gestation, when, unable to do so any longer, it expelled the contents. The cervix, not being properly prepared for such an event, gave way instead of dilating, giving rise to one of the most serious might be explained by the suggestion that in the case of acute rheumatism in the female sex the presence of a simultaneous gonorrhœa was less frequently enquired for. Gluzinski argues that it must not be supposed that these complications were analogous to orchitis or cystitis set up by extension of the inflammatory process *per continuitatem* or *per contiguitatem.* He gives the following explanation. The synovia of joints affected with gonorrhœal rheumatism has been repeatedly examined for micro-organisms. Some, who believe they have discovered a specific microbe, consider the rheumatism to be a direct result of the gonorrhœa. Others who have failed to find gonococci or other pyogenic micro-organisms in the synovial fluid, regard this affection as a secondary one, due to the penetration of pyogenic micro-organisms owing to a lesion in the urethral mucous membrane. This hypothesis was confirmed by a case published by Weichelbaum where gonorrhœa was complicated with endocarditis and cardiac failure and the streptococcus pyogenes was proved to be present in the vegetations on the valves. Dr. Gluzinski said that complications did not always occur in so acute a form as the endocarditis ulcerosa or pericarditis acuta. In eight cases which he had observed these complications were of a mild character. The patients complained of "stitch" in the left chest and palpitations of the heart. There was accelerated and increased action of the heart, and frequently also a slight pericardial râle. In spite of the most careful examination no other affection could be detected but gonorrhœa. These cases mostly ran a rapid and mild course and might very easily be overlooked. They deserved the greatest attention, however, as endocardial murmurs and cardiac failure came on in two of these cases. In the majority, rheumatism was either quite missed or came on after the cardiac affection had set in. In all the patients there was gonorrhœa of long standing. Gluzinski concluded that just as acute affections of the heart occurred in acute gonorrhœa, mild diseases of the serous membrane of the heart could also supervene in the course of chronic gonorrhœa.

ENTERIC FEVER.

Ehrlich's Diagnostic Sign.—Dr. Howard Taylor, of the

woman is pregnant ; now steps in the laceration to " kill all her joy." As the uterine cavity expands, the organ assumes a spherical shape, with a short, flattened cervix attached to its lower segment ; the cervical canal is practically effaced, and the internal os is immediately continuous with the vaginal tube. Here the parts which should be protected and kept at rest are exposed to friction and injury. The result is that the internal os gradually opens, a slight hemorrhage takes place, uterine contraction sets in, and the ovum is expelled. As a result of the same factors, pregnancy rapidly takes place again, followed again by abortion, and so on until a vicious circle has been established, which will continue until the laceration has been repaired and other concomitant conditions remedied.

Returning now to the case before us, it is evident that we must first begin by repairing the lacerations of the cervix, which I will do according to Emmet's method ; I will then elevate the uterus and broad ligaments by shortening the round ligaments. I have now repaired the cervix, using silk-worm gut (salmon size) as sutures (three on each side). From the dorso-gluteal position we will extend the patient flat upon her back as if for a laparotomy, and take up the round ligaments according to the method explained in a previous lecture.

The next case to be brought in is one of some interest. She is an extremely emaciated woman of 38 years of age ; married eight years. Six months after marriage she had a miscarriage at the third month of gestation. There was retention of the decidua, accompanied with severe hemorrhage which lasted for some days. She was confined to her bed for six weeks with severe pain and a continuous bloody discharge of a fœtid character. Rigors and other evidence of recurring attacks of sepsis took place from time to time during the following three months. She lost flesh gradually, and became finally a confirmed invalid, unable to leave her bedroom. This state of things continued for three years after marriage, when she consulted me. I found one of her most distressing symptoms was constant vomiting ; she could not retain the smallest quantity of food, which resulted in the extreme emaciation at present so noticeable a feature of her disease. There were also severe dysmenorrhœa and menorrhagia ; constant pain in the back, hypogastrium and right iliac region.

On making a vaginal examination I found the uterus sharply anteflexed, not enlarged appreciably, but very tender during pressure of the bimanual method. The whole pelvic floor was somewhat limited as regards mobility, with a bulky mass fixed in the region of the right lateral pouch. This mass was very sensitive to the touch, causing the patient to cry out and exhibit a tendency to faint. The ovary on the left side could be defined, and seemed slightly enlarged, but there was no fixity of parts on this side, the ovary could be moved freely about during the bimanual and was not very tender to pressure. The cervix was bilaterally lacerated and lips everted ; extensive glandular hypertrophy of the everted mucous membrane. A glairy, tenacious discharge occupied the cervical canal, and the inflamed cervical surface bled freely on being touched. Consistent with above symptoms and pathological condition nothing could be done beyond confining the patient to bed on hot-water douches and the iodine and glycerine treatment. This course was faithfully carried out for three months. At the end of that time the pelvic floor became more mobile ; the tenderness to a great extent had disappeared, the inflamed erosion showed a tendency to heal, and the patient was in a sufficiently improved condition to permit of the cervical laceration being repaired without danger. This operation was accordingly done and all went well. For some months she appeared to have derived benefit from the trachelorrhaphy, but eventually·all her old troubles relapsed, especially the inability to retain food. She became an attendant at the out-clinic, but did not improve. Every now and then a sharp onset of severe abdominal pain with some fever and constant retching would recur. These attacks would necessitate her confinement to bed for a week or more at a time, causing her to become morose and careless about life. Two weeks ago she called on me in this state of mind, and I took the opportunity of suggesting the removal of the appendages, which I considered the seat of disease. She and her husband readily consented, and now I propose to do that operation by laparotomy. The incision I make is about two inches in length. The left ovary is enlarged, and being free from adhesions is delivered with ease and after the application of a silk ligature is removed. The right ovary is adherent to adjacent parts by old inflammatory remnants, which I have carefully separated with my fingers, and the ovary is now delivered and removed in the same manner as the left. The abdominal cavity is now carefully cleansed, and as there is no colored fluid of consequence found in Douglas's pouch, the wound is closed by four silkworm-gut sutures and dressed with cotton wool, a single layer of sublimated gauze intervening. This dressing will not be disturbed until the ninth day, when the sutures will be removed.*

Retrospect Department.

QUARTERLY RETROSPECT OF MEDICINE.

By R. L. MacDonnell, M.D.,

Professor of Clinical Medicine, McGill University ; Physician to Montreal General Hospital.

Heart Complications in Gonorrhœa.

Gluzinski, in a recent number of the *Przeglad Lekarski*, gives some details with respect to circulatory diseases depending on gonorrhœa.† Complications connected with the serous membranes of the internal organs, such as that of the heart, were unknown until recently. Brande (1854) published two cases of endocarditis and pericarditis respectively in connection with gonorrhœal rheumatism. Sigmund (1858) observed two cases of pericarditis in women. Gluzinski has collected thirty-one cases. The following conclusions might be derived from these observations : 1. Pericarditis as well as endocarditis might supervene in the course of gonorrhœa. 2. These may develop after gonorrhœal rheumatism, but also without the presence of such an affection. 3. The complaint often assumes the character of a severe infectious disease, as in endocarditis ulcerosa, runs an acute course, and sometimes gives rise to failure of the heart. The fact that of the thirty-two cases published, in only two were the patients women

---

* Sutures removed ; primary union ; no pain nor vomiting since operation, first time for years ; expresses desire for food.

† Vienna correspondence of the *British Medical Journal.*

might be explained by the suggestion that in the case of acute rheumatism in the female sex the presence of a simultaneous gonorrhœa was less frequently enquired for. Gluzinski argues that it must not be supposed that these complications were analogous to orchitis or cystitis set up by extension of the inflammatory process *per continuitatem* or *per contiguitatem*. He gives the following explanation. The synovia of joints affected with gonorrhœal rheumatism has been repeatedly examined for micro-organisms. Some, who believe they have discovered a specific microbe, consider the rheumatism to be a direct result of the gonorrhœa. Others who have failed to find gonococci or other pyogenic micro-organisms in the synovial fluid, regard this affection as a secondary one, due to the penetration of pyogenic micro-organisms owing to a lesion in the urethral mucous membrane. This hypothesis was confirmed by a case published by Weichelbaum where gonorrhœa was complicated with endocarditis and cardiac failure and the streptococcus pyogenes was proved to be present in the vegetations on the valves. Dr. Gluzinski said that complications did not always occur in so acute a form as the endocarditis ulcerosa or pericarditis acuta. In eight cases which he had observed these complications were of a mild character. The patients complained of "stitch" in the left chest and palpitations of the heart. There was accelerated and increased action of the heart, and frequently also a slight pericardial râle. In spite of the most careful examination no other affection could be detected but gonorrhœa. These cases mostly ran a rapid and mild course and might very easily be overlooked. They deserved the greatest attention, however, as endocardial murmurs and cardiac failure came on in two of these cases. In the majority, rheumatism was either quite missed or came on after the cardiac affection had set in. In all the patients there was gonorrhœa of long standing. Gluzinski concluded that just as acute affections of the heart occurred in acute gonorrhœa, mild diseases of the serous membrane of the heart could also supervene in the course of chronic gonorrhœa.

ENTERIC FEVER.

Ehrlich's Diagnostic Sign.—Dr. Howard Taylor, of the

London Hospital, discusses the value of this sign in a recent (May 4th) number of the *Lancet*. Several years ago Ehrlich first drew the attention of the profession to the importance of a certain condition of the urine to be found, he claimed, in enteric fever and not in any other disease. In 1882 he announced the fact that such urine gives a re-action—with one of the aniline derivatives—different from that of normal urine, and from the re-action of the urine of patients suffering from other diseases.

His test solutions are as follows : A, a saturated solution of sulphanilic acid in dilute (1 in 20) hydrochloric acid ; B, a five per cent. solution of sodic nitrite in distilled water. Both of these solutions must be fresh, especially the latter, which cannot be depended upon for more than a week at a time at the longest. When they are mixed, of course, a solution of sulphanilic acid containing free nitrous acid is produced, which is the actual test of solution, but on account of the extreme instability of the latter the two solutions must be mixed fresh at each testing. In using the test, about twenty-five parts of A are added to one of B. Mix with this an equal bulk of the urine to be examined, and render alkaline with strong ammonia.

With healthy urine, the only change which ordinarily occurs is a mere deepening of its colour to a cherry or a vinegar brown. In conditions of pyrexia other than typhoid fever the color also deepens, but still remains merely brown, although usually it becomes of a darker tint than the average color given by normal urines. But in typhoid fever the color rapidly turns red, the exact tint it acquires varying from the yellowish red of bichromate of potassium solution, though ruby red to a rich port wine color. On shaking the test tube a froth is produced which has usually a delicate pink color that is very characteristic.

Now as to the limitations of the test. Dr. Taylor says that (1) it is not always given until the latter end of the first week ; (2) after the morning temperature has once reached normal during the intermittent stage (usually in the fourth week) it may—though it frequently does not—cease to be given. " Still, so far as my experience has gone * * * the re-action is present during the greater part of the febrile period *in every case.* It is this which constitutes the great value of the test."

Unfortunately in exceptional cases the test is given in other diseases. Dr. Taylor has found occasionally, even in healthy urines, the development of a slightly reddish color, but this is *very* rare and the redness is hardly ever well marked, indeed, he has never seen the deep rich crimson which is given in so many cases of enteric fever.

Several cases of Bright's disease, both acute and chronic, gave this "typhoid re-action." It is more frequent in albuminous urines. But with this exception it is extremely rarely given in the urine of non febrile patients. "Thus, out of a large number of cases of valvular disease of the heart it only occurred in one out of six cases, and in two cases of diabetes mellitus and one of diabetes insipidus which had been repeatedly tested, the re-action has not been given on any occasion.

Of the febrile diseases it seems to be especially common in measles. In acute general tuberculosis, which most simulates enteric fever, it has been found absent in all the cases examined. In acute and advanced chronic phthisis the re-action has been found, but in ordinary cases it has not been found. In the cases of lobar and of lobular pneumonia which have been examined, none of the urines have turned red; but other observers have found the re-action in some cases of the former disease. In only two of a large number of cases of acute rheumatism has the re-action been present.

The absence of the re-action is practicably proof positive that the case is not one of enteric fever (provided that the disease has lasted six days or more and that the temperature has not yet fallen to normal.) Its presence suggests, but does not prove, that the case is one of typhoid; the probability being greater the deeper the tint produced.

URÆMIA.

Treatment of Chronic Uræmia by Morphine.—At the Medical Society of London (April 8th, 1889) Dr. Stephen Mackenzie read a paper on this subject. Three cases were reported. *Case* 1—A women aged thirty-eight. Diffuse chronic nephritis of some years standing; anasarca; ascites; breathlessness;

urine one-half to two-thirds albumen; heart hypertrophied; double papillo-retinitis. Treatment for renal symptoms at first afforded great benefit, and in about six weeks she was free from dropsy and breathlessness and able to leave her bed. One evening there was a sudden attack of intense dyspnœa (fifty respirations to the minute); heart's action weak (150-200 per minute); cyanosis; clammy sweat; intense mental excitement. Nitrite of amyl, alcohol, ammonia and ether were administered without any relief and then one-sixth of a grain of morphine was injected hypodermically. In a few minutes the dyspnœa was less urgent, in twenty minutes the patient was able to lie down and on the following morning was in her usual condition. Several subsequent attacks, after intervals of complete freedom from dyspnœa were treated in a similar manner after the failure of other remedies. Morphine hypodermically and internally never failed to afford relief, and at no time were toxic effects induced. The patient died three months and a half later of symptoms of chronic Bright's disease.

Case 2—Woman aged twenty-eight; granular kidneys of four years' standing. Considerable anasarca, about one-third albumen in the urine; hypertrophy of the left ventricle; mitral incompetency, double papillo-retinitis; much breathlessness; headache. After decided improvement for a time she suffered from severe headache, nausea, breathlessness, irregular action of the heart and great sleeplessness. Chloral, bromides, nitro-glycerine, and inhalations of oil of juniper were used without effect or with but little effect. Ten minims of solution of hydrochlorate of morphine were then administered, with rapid alleviation of all the symptoms. It was repeated on many subsequent occasions with equal benefit and with no drawbacks. The patient died of the combined effects of a carbuncle and the renal disease about two months after the treatment was employed. Ten minim doses of solution of morphine always promptly relieved distressing symptoms; five minim doses were not sufficient.

The principles of the treatment of uræmia were declared to be three: 1, the elimination of the poison; 2, the counteraction of the poisons; 3, the prevention of the absorption and the retention of further poisons. Morphine is valuable in fulfilling the second indication, as it frees the bloodvessels from the spasm induced by the poison in the blood.   The indiscriminate use of morphine was not recommended and in the light of the asserted susceptibility of patients with disease of the kidneys to the toxic effects of opium, it would be given with eyes open to its possible danger.

CIRRHOSIS OF THE LIVER.

Cirrhosis of the Liver Causing Hemorrhage into the Pelvis.— At the Hunterian Society (March 28th, 1889) Dr. Pitt showed a specimon of extensive hemorrhage into the pelvis associated with cirrhosis of the liver.   Small hemorrhages are common but extensive hemorrhages are rare.   The blood was effused freely into the left broad ligament, slightly into the right and formed a large tumor over four pounds in weight, surrounding the bladder by a blood clot one inch and a half thick, compressing it and causing retention of urine probably from pressure on the ureters for the last twenty-four hours of life. The blood extended into the submucous tissue of the bladder, it also spread through the inguinal canal up on to the abdomen, chiefly on the left side, as far as the ribs and nipple forming a layer one inch thick and three inches wide. The liver was a typical hobnail cirrhosis. The kidneys were healthy except for some seaming. The specimen was taken from a woman aged thirty-eight, admitted with œdema, pyrexia and cough, who became increasingly drowsy and died.

Non-alcoholic Cirrhosis.—Dr. Goodhart, at a meeting of the Pathological Society, of London (April 16th, 1889) described a case of cirrhosis of the liver occurring in a female aged twenty-one.   There was absolutely no history of alcoholism or syphilis.   Two years before her death she had married and three months later had a miscarriage which was followed by septic poisoning.   Later she developed jaundice and ascites and vomited large quantities of blood.   The post mortem examination revealed an ordinary case of cirrhosis with enlarged spleen.   He suggested that the cause was plugging of the portal vein from the septic process with secondary shrinking of the liver and fibrotic change.   In the ensuing discussion Dr. Moore related in detail a case of hæmatemesis which was associated with the presence of a firm cord-like

7

clot in the portal vein, the liver was firm but not cirrhotic.
Dr. Crooke referred to the effects of specific febrile disease on
the livers of young children; he had many times met with
interstitial hepatitis after scarlet fever, and this might lead to
a contraction like that which occurred in the kidney. The
President (Dr. W. H. Dickinson) had known severe cases of
cirrhosis fatal under two years of age, and many such cases
had followed measles and scarlet fever.

The Curability of Interstitial Hepatitis.—Professor Semmola*, of Naples, protests against the exaggerated
importance attached to the anatomical basis of disease. The
error is common of associating the post mortem changes of
the last and probably incurable stage with the symptoms of
an earlier and possibly curable stage. He regards the
atrophic stage as seen in the dead house as the dregs of the
disease, and as far as therapeusis goes he refers merely to the
early condition when the liver is large and the new tissue has
not become hard, contracted and fibrous. Semmola has long
ago (1869) suggested the possibility of the curability of
interstitial hepatitis, and at the International Medical
Congress at Amsterdam in 1879 he brought forward a series
of cases in support of his views. Millard (*Progrès Médical*)
has advocated the same proposition and has also published a
series of cases in which a cure has taken place.

Semmola, in his recent cases, does not appear to have
drawn a line between those due to malarial and those of
alcoholic and syphilitic origin. It is possible that the former
may be more readily curable than the latter. It would also
appear that sufficient account is not given to the establishment of a collateral circulation and to the consequent disappearance of ascites and other symptoms, the interstitial
hepatitis remaining unaltered. The principle of Semmola's
treatment is the rigid restriction to a milk diet. More solid
dietary, and especially meat, increases the hepatic irritation
and exaggerates the disease.

GRAVES' DISEASE.

The Connection of Graves' Disease with Nasal Symptoms.—
This subject, it will be remembered, came under discussion at

---

*Le Progresso Medico, January 15th, 1889.   From the *London Medical Recorder*.

the Medico-Chirurgical Society of Montreal last November.*
On the 12th April last Mr. Felix Semon read an important
paper on a case of Unilateral Incomplete Graves' Disease
after removal of nasal polypi, at a meeting of the Clinical
Society of London. The patient was exhibited. As an introduction three cases were cited. These were recently observed
by Hopmann, of Cologne, Hack, of Freiburg, and B. Frankel,
of Berlin, and in all three cases intra-nasal operations undertaken for the relief of nasal obstruction had very unexpectedly
led to the diminution or even disappearance of the symptoms
of Graves' Disease, from which the patients in question had
concomitantly suffered. Mr. Stoker, of London, has reported
two cases in which intra nasal operations had caused diminution or disappearance of goitres, though in his cases no other
symptoms of Graves' Disease had been present. That in these
cases the changes in the domain of the sympathetic were
actually due to the intra nasal operations, and that the
diminution of exopthalmos and of goitre corresponded to the
side which had been operated upon. Dr. Semon now
regretted having to bring forward a case illustrating the
possibility that the changes occasionally brought about by
intra nasal operations in the domain of the sympathetic might
be other than favorable ones. In his case operations undertaken by means of the galvano-caustic loop for the removal of
multiple recurrent mucous polypi of the nose had suddenly
caused exopthalmos of the patient's right eye, occurring
within a day or two of the operations. The presence of
Graefe's and Stellwag's symptom plainly showed that the
exopthalmos was of the nature of Graves' disease, but there
was neither enlargement of the thyroid gland nor increased
frequency of the pulse rate. Not the least remarkable fact in
connection with this case was that whilst the intra-nasal
operations had produced one neurotic symptom (the
exopthalmos), they had cured the patient of another, viz.,
asthma, from which he had begun to suffer shortly after the
appearance of the nasal polypi. Should further operations be
undertaken ? Mr. Brudenell Carter felt inclined to regard
the alleged connection as a mere coincidence. A case had
come under his notice of a young lady aged sixteen whose left

*Montreal Medical Journal, Vol. VII, No. 8.

eye suddenly appeared wide open.   On careful examination it
was found that there was little or no real protrusion of the
globe beyond what was produced by the downward pressure
of a displaced eyelid.   An operation on the lid relieved the
symptom which he did not regard as belonging to Graves'
disease, and he thought that probably a similar operation
would give relief in Mr. Semon's case.   Dr. Semon in reply
thought that coincidence was rendered extremely improbable
by the fact that at least five cases were on record in which
exopthalmos had been associated with affection of the nose.
In these cases the symptoms had developed shortly after a
nasal operation and always on the same side as the latter.

The Relation of Exophthalmic Goitre to Tabes Dorsalis.—
Barié reports* the history of a patient who presented many
symptoms—on the one part those of tabes, lightning pains,
Romberg's sign, absent patellar reflex, plantar anæsthesia,
inco-ordination of movement, vertigo, gastric crises; on the
other, the signs of Graves' disease, exopthalmos, tachycardia,
hypertrophy of the heart, enlargement of the thyroid gland.
He concludes that these concurrent phenomena are the expression of a pathological complexus with its seat in the bulbo-
protuberantial centre.   He admits that goitre may be a symptom not of the actual condition of tabes but of its early stages,
that it is of the nature of a simple congestive hyperæmia which
is likely to be improved by a course of ergot with faradization.

Seven cases, all in females are reported by Loffroy.†   All
had tachycardia, six had ocular protrusion, two had thyroid
tumor.   He is not in accord with the views of Barié but
believes that one may see in the same patient the two
diseases side by side, but he recognizes the fact that ataxia
may give rise to tachycardia and possibly to a slight degree
of protrusion of the eye.

The Pathology of Exophthalmic Goitre.—Observation has
taught us that in all probability the pathological changes are
to be found in the nervous system, and for many years it was
supposed that the cervical sympathetic was the seat of the
disease, but experience showed that this view was not based on
fact.   The sympathetic was often found diseased when there

---

* Soc. méd des hop., 14th décembre, 1888.
† Revue des Science Medicales, 15th April, 1889.

was no exopthalmic goitre, and as many times was found normal in structure when the three cardinal symptoms were most highly marked. In the *British Medical Journal* (March 30th, 1888), Dr. White, of Guy's Hospital, publishes a case where very suggestive changes were found in the floor of the fourth ventricle.

The patient, a woman æt 31, had two attacks of "ulceration of bowels" two years previously. Mother died at 21 of rheumatic fever. The symptoms of Graves' disease were well marked; palpitations, goitre; slight exophthalmos with Graefe's sign; normal optic disks; pulse, 150. In spite of treatment diarrhœa, jaundice and pneumonia on the right side set in, and the patient soon died.

At the autopsy the following were the more important observations made: Normal amount of fat in orbits; cervical glands slightly enlarged; thymus easily recognized, but not enlarged; thyroid extremely enlarged uniformly; confluent lobular pneumonia. Heart, 11 oz.; no fatty change. Stomach large, and small intestines all intensely congested, with swelling of the mucous membrane: solitary follicles more prominent than usual. Liver, kidney and supra-renal capsules normal; mesenteric glands swollen, injected. The capillaries of the brain were everywhere full, especially on the floor of the fourth ventricle.

A series of sections was made extending from the lowest part of the medulla to the corpora quadrigemina. At the level of the lower part of the olivary nucleus there was just under the posterior surface of the medulla, evidence of slight inflammation, shown by engorgement of the vessels, blood being present in their sheaths, and by a few wandering cells in the posterior median nucleus on each side. The next few sections were healthy, but those near the nucleus of the sixth nerve showed considerable changes. Just under the posterior surface of the medulla, from the middle line to the restiform bodies, which were slightly involved, were numerous hæmorrhages. The area occupied by these did not extend deeply, so that, except for a slight inplication of the sixth nucleus on one side, the nerve cells had escaped injury. The fibres of the facial nerve, which approach the surface here were free. The hæmorrhages seemed almost *entirely limited to* the posterior

superficial part of the reticular formation, but there were two
or three small deeper ones. Though most marked at this level,
they existed in all sections up to the lower part of the aqueduct of Sylvius where, however, only one or two were seen.
They always occupied the posterior part of the reticular
formation. The hæmorrhages were not old, but had not
occurred immediately before death. The cervical sympathetic
cord was quite healthy. In the superior cervical ganglia the
nerve cells were healthy, the sections were full of leucocytes.

The hæmorrhages were visible to the naked eye, and none
of those present had ever seen them so marked in the medulla.
Dr. White supposes that these hæmorrhages occurred as a
result of the pneumonic fever from which the patient suffered.
He infers that since hæmorrhages would naturally take place
in that part of the central nervous system which was rendered
weak by local disease-changes, they indicate the seat of the
pathological processes which underlie the various symptoms
of exophthalmic goitre.

INFECTIOUS JAUNDICE.

Some notes of this interesting condition, by some writers
described as Weil's disease, have appeared in the *Retrospect of
Medicine* of this JOURNAL. Several cases have been observed
in Montreal within the last few months. The patients were
children, and the prominent symptoms were jaundice and fever.
Infection was probable, as some of the children in the neighborhood was similarly attacked. The whole subject is attracting considerable interest in Europe, and many clinical observers are paying attention to it. Fränkel, in the course of an
article "On the Study of the so-called Weil's Disease,"*
relates the history of a case in which symptoms resembling
decidedly those of Weil's disease, came on as the result of an
external wound which had taken on a slightly erysipelatous
action. The symptoms soon declined, and the patient became
free from fever and felt almost well, except that he suffered
from great lassitude. After some eleven days he experienced
a slight relapse with moderate elevation of temperature and
an increase in the enlargement of the liver and of the spleen.
This observation induced Fränkel to make a careful critical

---

* Schmidt's Jahrbücher der Gesammten Medicin, 15 Mai, 1889.

Cardiac Crises in Tabes Dorsalis.—Groedel (*Deut. Med. Woch.*, No. 20, 1888) describes three cases of tabes in which attacks of angina pectoris were present. The symptoms were similar to those described by Vulpian and Leyden. I. A Hamburg merchant, æt 49, who had suffered for one year from shooting pains in the lower extremities, was aroused in the middle of the night by a tightening pain about the chest with dyspnoea. The medical man who was summoned diagnosed tabes. No physical signs of organic heart lesion were discovered. The patient was sent to Nanheim where, after some unusual fatigue at an excursion, there occurred another attack of angina with pallor of the face, dyspnœa, and smallness of the pulse. No cardiac lesion. In the following year there were several less severe attacks, while the ataxia gradually increased. II. An American, aged 50, for some years a tabetic. For several months past, without any assignable cause, attacks of angina pectoris. II. A third case is mentioned, but it is not as characteristic as the two others since the patient has also chronic nephritis with cardiac hypertrophy to a slight degree.

ADDISON'S DISEASE.

Contributions to the Pathological Anatomy of Addison's Disease.—Kahlden reports two observations of autopsies made in two cases of this disease, The patients were aged respectively 54 and 70 years.* In both cases the suprarenals presented at their centres caseous masses, in which the anatomical structure of the glands was lost, and in which a considerable number of tubercle bacilli were present. The semilunar ganglia were the seat of remarkable changes; the ganglionic cells, as well as their nuclei and their protoplasm were transformed into pigmentary granulations : the greater number of blood vessels here had undergone hyaline degeneration with an infiltration of the adventitia with rounded cells, at the same time that the splanchnic nerves showed a thickening of the lamellar sheath. There were hemorrhages more or less abundant in the periphery of the ganglia. These lesions were not equally manifested on either side. The author is of opinion that these anatomical modifications of the semilunar ganglia can explain partly the symptoms of the disease, although one is

---

* *Archiv für Pathol. Anat. u Physiol.*, Band cxiv., Heft 1.

not justified in concluding from two cases that the alteration in the semilunar ganglia is sufficient to account for all the symptoms which belong to Addison's disease.

As for the pigment of the skin it was altogether accumulated in the layers of the rete Malpighi, though it could be traced to the horny layer. The most external layers of the outer epithelial sheath of the hairy follicle were to a similar extent filled with pigmentary granulations. These are not formed in the epithelial cells themselves ; they take their origin in the derma, whence the migratory cells transport them into the epidermis. Each epithelial cellule receives its pigment from several migratory cellules at a time. These latter are found arranged in the papillæ of the derma on each side of the blood-vessel going there, and seem to be loading themselves in order to carry the pigment which is formed by alteration of the blood to the epithelial cells. This origin of the pigment is the more probable, since nowhere was there any trace of hemorrhages, and since the lesions of the coats of the vessels were insignificant and of secondary origin.

QUARTERLY REPORT ON DISEASES OF CHILDREN.

By A. D. BLACKADER, B.A., M.D.,

Instructor in Diseases of Children, McGill University ; Assistant Physician, Montreal General Hospital.

WHOOPING COUGH : ITS NATURE AND TREATMENT—SUMMER DIARRHŒA : PREVIOUS LESIONS ; INTESTINAL IRRIGATION —FUNCTIONAL MURMURS OF HEART IN EARLY LIFE— POSITION OF APEX BEAT.

During the past few years the exact contagion of whooping cough has been the subject of much research. In 1870 Letzerich found in the sputa of whooping-cough patients round and oval spores, which at a later stage in their development gave place to certain fungi, which, introduced into the trachea of tracheotomized rabbits, were followed in eight days by laryngo-bronchitis with attacks of convulsive cough and increased secretion from the nasal fossæ. In 1876 Tschäunner repeated these experiments and produced a modified whooping-cough in his own person. Two years subsequently Birsch-Hirschfeld went carefully over the same ground, but failed to confirm their conclusions. In

1883 Benger described a new bacillus, which he declared was not found in any other affection of the respiratory system, but his work has never been verified. In 1886 Afanassieff made a very thorough investigation of the micro-organisms found in the sputa of those suffering from the disease. His facilities were good, for his own children, four of whom had the whooping-cough, were the patients. "The bacilli which he obtained, and which he considered characteristic of whooping-cough, were circular or oval, of a pale cinnamon color, and from 0.2 to 2.2 millimetres in length. They appear in from four to fifteen days after the first manifestation of the disease, and may sometimes be found for a period of four months. Inoculations made with the greatest care in rabbits and puppies produced a disease closely resembling human whooping-cough. Semtchenko has confirmed these results of Afanassieff, and concludes that the bacilli are specific, that they may appear as early as the fourth day of the disease, that they multiply in the organism until the disease reaches its height, that they disappear while the paroxysmal cough still persists, and become more numerous if broncho-pneumonia supervenes." (*Rev. des Malad. de l'Enfance*, May 1888.) Since then, Schwenker (*Lancet*, Jan. 7, '88) and Wenat (*Medical News*, June 2, '88) have both confirmed Afanassieff's discovery.

As regards treatment, there is still much diversity of opinion. It would appear as if different epidemics vary much in the way they yield to the several medicines. Good reports continue to reach us in regard to the value of antipyrin in checking both the frequency of the attacks and their violence, and when given in the doses originally recommended by Sonnenberger, viz., as many centigrammes per day as the infant is months old, or as many decigrammes as the child is years old, administered in three or four divided doses during the twenty-four hours, I have never seen any ill results occur. The best results are obtained when the treatment with antipyrin is begun at the first appearance of the disease. Like everything else, it sometimes fails, and in such cases, considering the ill effects sometimes produced by prolonged administration of the drug, it would not appear advisable to push its further use. In a recent number of the

Archiv f. Kinderheilk, t. x, fasc. vi, Dr. O. Mugdan reports the results which have been obtained under several modes of treat. ment at Baginsky's clinic in Berlin.   (1) *Resorcin*—Moncorvo was the first who employed this drug in whooping-cough.   He painted the pharynx and larynx with a solution of resorcin, com. mencing at first with one of a strength of 1 to 2 per cent., in. creasing it afterwards gradually to 8 per cent.   At Baginsky's clinic it was administered internally without any appreciable beneficial result.   Since the researches of Afanassieff, it is ad. mitted that the special bacillus of this disease, instead of fixing itself exclusively on the laryngeal mucous membrane, invades all the respiratory tract, and particularly the mucous membranes of the bronchi, of the trachea and of the nasal fossæ.   Consider. ing these facts, inhalation practised with a strong solution of resorcin might perhaps give more appreciable result.   (2) *Co. caine*—Painting the mucous membrane of the pharynx and after. wards of the larynx with a solution of cocaine, 5 to 10 per cent., has been highly extolled by Prior.   In the patients subjected to this mode of treatment at Baginsky's clinic the number and in. tensity of the fits of coughing have been favorably modified in the majority of the cases, but, nevertheless, the writer is of the opinion that this mode of treatment should not be employed except in grave cases which do not yield to other medication, on account of the resistance which many children make to its employment, and on account of the frequency of symptoms of intoxication.   (3) *Antipyrin*—The results obtained from the use of this drug, in the few cases in which it was tried at this clinic, were disappointing.   Dr. Mugdan says of it : " In the seven patients thus treated, neither the number nor the intensity of the fits of coughing underwent any modification ; while it is to be remembered that this drug is far from being inoffensive, and accidents of intoxication have been already reported on all sides."   (4) *Insufflation*—Michael, considering pertussis as a nervous reflex provoked by the specific irritation of the poison of the bacillus in the nasal and pharyngeal mucous mem. branes, used insufflations into the nasal fossæ, at first of boric acid and quinine, then, later, exclusively of benzoic acid.   The results obtained by him were very satisfactory. Since then, Bachem, Hagenbach, Stœrk and Lublinski have also acknowledged the good results obtained by this means of medication. Gesser alone found no appreciable result from these insufflations. In Baginsky's clinic, of 25 children subjected to methodical insufflation of benzoic acid, 17 presented a marked amelioration from the first insufflation. A cure was generally obtained in the space of one to three weeks.

Jacobi still strongly advocates the use of belladonna in this affection, and writes as follows (*Arch Pœdiatrics*, July, '89) : " The prevention of whooping-cough, which is a specific and contagious disease, is certainly not easy, as contagion may take place very suddenly, especially during the first or second stages of the disease. . . . Isolation is an absolute necessity, difficult though it be. In one point isolation is more effective in this than in other contagious diseases, namely, that the disease does not appear to be carried by persons not affected. As regards treatment, the air must be kept pure, uniform, and moderately warm. No draught of wind must be permitted. Utensils must be kept clean and be disinfected. The mucous membranes must be kept in, or restored to, a healthy condition, particularly those of the mouth and respiratory organs. Thus no injudicious exposure must be allowed. The digestive organs have to be watched, the stomach must not be full at any time ; the food must be digestible and the bowels kept regular. An important indication is that of treating a catarrhal or inflamed mucous membrane. It is quite possible that only such a mucous membrane is capable of admitting the contagion of whooping-cough, as it does that of other infectious disease—for instance, diphtheria. Besides, by attending to the mucous membranes in time, the occurrence of serious complications, such as pneumonia, may be prevented. Catarrh of the mouth and pharynx ought to be treated with doses of potassium chlorate of from half a grain to a grain in a teaspoonful of water every hour. Expectorants may be used, but all those which have a depressing effect must be avoided, particularly antimonials. . . . Cases exhibiting a severe degree of pharyngitis and laryngeal hyperæmia, par-

. . . ong time from chronic
. . . to well, as far as the
use of the tincture of
. . . over the twenty-four
. . . of from one to three
. . . sorted to by many. . . .
. . . the difficulty encountered
. . . and for the confidence of
. . . submission of his wards.
. . . and externally by a number
. . . first recommended by Let-
. . . drug with the power of re-
. . . Binz, however, attributes
. . . He gives as many decigrammes
. . . a child of four years would take
. . . He expects to find an improve-
. . . days, the attacks by that time
. . . severe. When it cannot be
. . . in suppositories or by injec-
. . . particularly Forchheimer who has
. . . been benefited by the administration
. . . in which either convulsions have
. . . attacks, or in which the interruptions of
. . . cerebral hemorrhage or convulsions
. . . of chloroform, or, according to
. . . recommended. In the case of a very young
. . . chloroform once every hour for every
. . . course of a number of days in succession
. . . apparently beneficial result. . . . Of all
. . . whooping-cough, I prize belladonna
. . . returned to it after having discon-
. . . trying one after the other of the
. . . during these thirty years. As
. . . ress in the *American Medi-*
. . . belladonna is the most power-
. . . scarcely remember a single
. . . years past proved unsuccess-

ful in shortening the duration of the process. The effect is
generally not a sudden one. Many cases in which belladonna
is given from the first commencement will become worse for a
short while, then remain at their height for some days or a week,
and gradually improve in both the character and frequency of
the attack. In others the effect is perceptible from the outset
of its administration. From fear of ill effects it is generally
given in doses entirely too small, and which cannot but prove
unsatisfactory. . . . To obtain a cure in whooping-cough the
remedy must be given in a dose sufficient to produce erythema
or at least a flushed condition of the face and, as it were, a
feverish appearance after every dose. If not obtained at first,
the dose is to be gradually increased until this result is
obtained. Some of the old authors recommended the administration of belladonna to such an extent as to produce the
first symptoms of poisoning ; but others insisted on this practice being dangerous and wholly objectionable. I, for my
part, soon found that those children suffering from whooping-
cough who exhibited general erythema from an apparent overdose recovered soon, while others in whom no such symptoms
were observed remained sick for a long time, and continued experience has proved that the occurrence of this symptom is
necessary for the full remedial effect. Vogel also speaks highly
of the effect of belladonna, taking the dilatation of the pupils as
a guide. This effect is rather late in appearing in children, and
is not required ; indeed it may become quite uncomfortable.
Evans, in the *Glasgow Medical Journal* (1880), recommended
the administration of a large dose first, to be followed by smaller
ones afterwards. Very young infants may take proportionately
large doses ; I do not remember a single case in which less
than half a grain of the extract was taken in the course of
twenty-four hours. The tincture of belladonna is a convenient
remedy, inasmuch as the dose can be readily and gradually increased. A baby of two years may take daily doses, the
first of which may be six drops. If the flush be perceptible
within twenty or thirty minutes, that is the dose ; if not, the
the number of drops must be increased to obtain the effect.

receive early and intelligent treatment, best obtained by ensuring proper digestion, which implies proper feeding, with especial care to avoid over-feeding.

In a very excellent lecture on the treatment of enterocolitis in infants, Dr. E. P. Davis (*Med. News*, July 6, '89) says :— Should the case go on to well marked intestinal catarrh with enteritis, a more decided policy must be adopted. An effort should at once be made to remove the irritating ingesta from the intestines, to prevent the growth of bacteria, and to feed and support the patient in every possible way. An intestinal antiseptic is indicated, and from experience calomel seems best fitted for an early stage of the disease. In one-tenth or one-twentieth grain doses with soda or milk sugar, it may be given every hour or half hour until the stools show a free secretion of bile. For the first six or eight hours food should be replaced by teaspoonfuls of whiskey and boiled water, or Jacobi's mixture of white of egg and whiskey and water, care being taken that fluid in *small* quantities is taken very freely. Temperature may be reduced by the warm or hot bath, and a cold cloth upon the head. A spice plaster upon the abdomen may often be used to advantage. If pain and restlessness with fever are not controlled by the bath, antipyrin in one-half grain doses may replace opium to advantage. If the antiseptic action of nature's intestinal antiseptic, the bile, with the calomel, are not sufficient to check the growth and invasion of bacteria, intestinal irrigation should be promptly undertaken, before prostration supervenes. A soft catheter (No. 11), a connecting glass tube and fountain syringe are needed. The fluid may be boiled water made alkaline by sodium bicarbonate, thymol 1 to 1000, or sodium salicylate 20 gr. to 20 ounces of water. The infant is to be laid across the lap of the nurse, who receives it on its abdomen upon a rubber sheet gathered into a pail below. The oiled catheter is introduced by the right hand and pushed gently into the bowel. As it advances it is held by the thumb and finger of the left hand placed against the child's nates, while the right rotates it ; if a decided obstruction presents, it is slightly withdrawn and then advanced. It may be introduced six or eight inches without difficulty.   The fountain syringe should be held from two to three feet above the patient and the fluid allowed to flow freely.   Its temperature should be from 90° to 110° ; if the child is in collapse, a hot irrigation is a decided stimulant.   The quantity of fluid used may vary from twenty ounces to double that amount.   In collapse after the fluid returns clear, several ounces of hot water, or water containing a little whiskey, may be introduced into the bowel for absorption with decided advantage.   While the introduction of the catheter may be resented, the passage of the fluid is a positive comfort ; and it is not an unusual occurrence for infants to fall asleep on the nurse's lap while receiving the irrigation, and sleep for an hour or two, the temperature at the same time falling considerably.   The irrigation may be employed twice daily without injury to the patient, and even oftener in urgent cases.

Functional Murmurs of the Heart during Childhood.—M. Hochsinger, in a paper (*Rev. Mens. des Mal. de l'Enf.*, Jan., 1889), states that the inorganic *bruit de souffle* of the heart is absent during childhood until the second half of the fourth year of life.   The fact is surprising, as the circumstances which habitually call forth these sounds in adults are met with in early childhood with much greater frequency and more marked intensity.   The writer states that he has examined several hundred children under three years of age with the view of determining the question as to the presence or absence of these sounds.   He did not find them present in a single case, although there were evidences of extreme anæmia in several of the cases ; in all, the heart sounds were clear, sharp, and well defined.   Of twenty-four very anæmic children who had passed the third year, only eight presented evidences of the bruit.   Of twenty-nine who had suffered from attacks of scarlatina, diphtheria, pneumonia, phthisis, etc., in four cases only could a systolic murmur be heard at the level of the valves, and the youngest of these was

Position of Apex Beat during Childhood.—In a paper (*Rev. Mens. des Mal. de l'Enfance*, Nov. '88) M. Storck gives us the result of careful examinations made upon upwards of three hundred children between the ages of one month and fifteen years to determine, as far as possible, the position of the apex beat and præcordial dulness during infancy and childhood. The following are his conclusions :—(1) It is frequently impossible, during the first year of life, to determine with precision the exact point at which the apex of the heart strikes the chest-wall. (2) In most cases the apex of the heart is located on or outside the mammillary line until after the twelfth year. (3) The apex of the heart is never found within this line until the age of two years. It is very rarely found within it until the seventh year. (4) During the first four years the apex beat is almost always found in the fourth intercostal space. With regard to percussion, there are great differences of opinion. The author's investigations led him to recognize during childhood three degrees of præcordial dulness—the first corresponding, as a rule, to the first year of life, the second to the sixth year, and the third to the twelfth year.

Reviews and Notices of Books.

Diabetes : its Cause and Permanent Cure from the standpoint of experience and scientific investigation. By EMIL SCHNEE, M.D., Consulting Physician at Carlsbad, &c. Translated by A. L. TAFEL, A.M., Ph.D. London : H. K. Lewis.

In reading over this book one is very forcibly reminded of Benvenuto Cellini's interesting autobiography, in which, noted for his vanity, he by no means under-estimates his skill as an artist nor his prowess as a soldier. Schnée's work is composed of about two hundred small pages, and contains " everything of importance that has thus far been written about diabetes " ; so says the author. His view, " based on experience," attributes diabetes to a luetic (*i.e.*, venereal) constitution, consequently the curative method proposed by him " is able to effect a lasting cure of diabetes, which fact borders on the miraculous," more especially seeing that the disease results in " organic destruction which no physician thus far has been able to heal." The author has no doubt as to the cause of diabetes, inasmuch as " it manifests itself only in persons who are hereditarily predisposed for it." The author further writes with italics : " *Herein lies the great mystery, never before discovered by anyone, of the cause of diabetes, and here, according to my conviction, hereditary lues on the part of one of the parents, grandparents or great-grandparents of the patient has to be taken into consideration. A transmission of lues through vaccination also is not excluded.*" This fact discovered by him " lets a flow of light into the chaotic darkness of diabetes. A new epoch in the therapeutics of diabetes has no doubt been inaugurated with this discovery." Chapter IX is headed with large capitals : " The so-called cures of diabetes that have hitherto been made are illusions." Thank God that chaotic period passed away in 1881, the time of Dr. Schnée's discovery. Now the rational practitioner, if he will only follow Dr. Schnée's method—that is, not to omit the methods heretofore generally adopted—to practice massage with a preparation of mercury ; the use of moderate intercourse so that there may be a " regular circulation of the juices" ; ventilating the lungs by drawing deep breaths ; an intelligent care of the skin, " *the use of hot Carlsbad waters, regulated for individual cases, which is of especial value, as one of the factors in this my therapeutical system.*"

His " entire secret consists in restoring the equilibrium," which, from the rather indefinite suggestions advised by the writer, would be best attained by the unfortunate victim of this malady going to Carlsbad, consulting Dr. Schnée, and, under his instructions, drinking and using its waters and drugs prescribed by him.

We cannot refrain from making use of quotations in reviewing this interesting and instructive book. It is interesting in revealing the fact that on the other side of the Atlantic there yet remain some whose talents might be a successful investment for the proprietor of " safe cure" or other similar merchandizable material in editing or preparing advertisements ; it is instructive, because it really contains much useful information that would be valuable to anyone desirous of being posted on the literature of the disease referred to. Any one interested in the subject of the work will certainly read it with mixed pleasure.

Elements of Histology. By E. KLEIN, M.D., F.R.S. Philadelphia: Lea Brothers & Co.

The subject of histology, both normal and pathological, has become such an important one that the physician or surgeon who is not well posted in it cannot be considered quite up to the times. Herein is one subject in which the young graduate has the decided advantage of his older *confrère*—even no further back than twelve or fifteen years. Diagnosis is now frequently made by the use of the microscope : indeed that instrument cannot be dispensed with. Of course, to be able to recognise diseased structures implies the knowledge of the appearance of healthy tissues, hence the necessity of a good text-book on normal histology. Klein's book is, without doubt, the best modern book in the English language ; other good books exist, some of them translations, but anyone having the *last* edition of Klein will be able to post himself to date. It is a common saying that the medical practitioner is always a student. We would suggest to the practitioner of over twelve or fifteen years standing to borrow a few slides from a first or second year student, and, with the use of a microscope and these slides, to peruse Klein's book, and in it he will find three hundred and fifty-seven pages, every one of which will only serve to convince him more and more of his ignorance of the subject and of the truly progressive nature of the *science* of medicine. We have no hesitation in recommending this book highly to both students and practitioners.

Synopsis of Human Anatomy. By J. K. YOUNG, M.D. Philadelphia: F. A. Davis. 1889.

This is another of those numerous " aids " for the busy practitioner and student. It is a mere compilation which any student could make for himself, and contains nothing new either in arrangement or matter. It is merely a "cram-book" on anatomy, the sort made use of by lazy students for examination purposes, and one which would not help them in any practical examination on the subject. Anatomy should be chiefly learned in the dissecting-room, and such works as the one under review can teach but little that is of use. We cannot recommend this work (which is good enough of its kind) to students or practitioners, when so many good text-books on anatomy can be so easily procured.

Electricity in the Diseases of Women. By G. BRETTON MASSEY, M.D. Philadelphia: F. A. Davis, publisher. 1889.

This little work is probably the only one written at the present day upon this subject worth perusing—those of Apostoli and Engelmann being, of course, excepted. There is one special virtue in connection with it—it is written by a specialist in nervous diseases and their treatment by electricity. The author begins with a short treatise on the general physics of electricity, the various kinds of batteries and necessary instruments to complete an outfit for the treatment of uterine disease. The author then goes very fully into Apostoli's methods, including the use of the galvanic and the faradic currents, their distinctive difference and relative application. The treatment of fibroid tumors is next taken up. Cases are cited in full, and the usual ending in such cases is adopted— "still under treatment." The treatment by electricity of uterine hemorrhage comes next. Then the treatment of endometritis, subinvolution, uterine hyperplasia, and pelvic indurations; of pelvic pain, dysmenorrhœa with stenosis, extra-uterine pregnancy, etc., etc.

A more thorough and useful little book to those interested in the electrical treatment of disease we do not think can be obtained, and we heartily recommend it.

Transactions of the American Ophthalmological Society. Twenty-fourth annual meeting, New London, Conn., 1888. Hartford : Published by the Society.

The transactions of this society's last annual meeting is full of interesting material, although nothing very new was communicated. The society and the medical world in general

have to lament the loss of some of the leading men in this
branch, viz.: Dr. C. R. Agnew and Dr. Loring—men whose
able work lives after them.   Also Dr. Joseph Aub, of
Cincinnati.   Dr. Swan Burnett presents an interesting
analysis of the refraction of 576 human corncæ by means of
Javal and Schiotz Ophthalmometer, which is well worthy of
study and reflection.   Dr. Sutphen, of Newark, reports
three operations of puncture of the retina for detachment in a
patient. Dr. Sutphen at first tried profuse diaphoresis and
rest in bed without any success. Puncture was then made of
the right eye, vision being only perception of light.   No
return of detachment had occurred up to seven months later.
Vision was $\frac{15}{100}$ with $-\frac{1}{20} = \frac{15}{40}$. In the left eye the result
was negative.   Detachment returned after first operation,
when it was repeated, but a short time after detachment
again appeared.

Dr. Edward Jackson, of Philadelphia, exhibited a new form
of cataract knife, being a combination of the Graefe and
Beers' forms.   The advantages are: The puncture and
counterpuncture are as perfectly under control as with the
Graefe knife. The flap may always be completed with one
forward thrust. The escape of the aqueous can be largely
prevented until the incision is nearly completed.   The
counterpressure of the back of the knife balances the pressure
of the cutting edge and aids in fixation.

Dr. Tansley, of New York, exhibited a lachrymal syringe,
canaliculus compressor, and a new form of lachrymal probe.

The proceedings of the Ophthalmological Branch of the
International Congress at Washington are also embodied in
the transactions. These include a very interesting series of
cases of tenotomies for heterophoria, by Dr. David Webster.

Society Proceedings.

MEDICO–CHIRURGICAL SOCIETY OF MONTREAL.

Stated Meeting, May 3rd, 1889.

WM. GARDNER, M.D., PRESIDENT, IN THE CHAIR.

Dr. M. C. McGannon was elected a member of the Society.

Cystic Ovarian Tumor.—DR. WM. GARDNER showed a large ovarian tumor, the interest of which lay in the fact that it was composed of two very large cysts containing papillomatous growths and a small dermoid cyst containing a bunch of hair and one tooth. From the hilum of this ovary there also hung a thin-walled cyst of the size of a large orange. It had a thin separate pedicle. This tumor was removed from a married woman of 57 years of age.

In answer to DR. SMITH, DR. GARDNER said that the prognosis was favorable, but not cloudless.

DR. HINGSTON agreed that tapping papillomatous cysts was unwise, inasmuch as it led to the spreading of the disease to the peritoneum. He referred to a case in which he began an operation for removal of an ovarian cyst, but on opening the abdomen he found both tumor and peritoneum covered with papillomata. He emptied the cyst, but did not attempt to remove it. The woman got better and lived for seven or eight years.

Pharyngeal Fibroid.—DR HINGSTON exhibited a large pharyngeal fibroid and said that the subject of it was a strong, able-bodied young man, full of life and vigor. The tumor, which was of a very solid character, had formed in the respiratory tract. It had pushed forward into the nostril, where a prolongation was visible at the alæ of the nose. It had dilated the nostril considerably, till it had given a frog-like expression to the countenance. There was a profuse discharge from the nostril and occasionally bleeding. Within a month the growth had projected into the throat about half an inch below the uvula. The soft palate was rendered tense, and the hard palate was arched downwards and forwards. Nasal respiration was impossible, and there was considerable dysphagia. On passing the little

finger, well oiled, into the left nostril, there was found to be
perfect freedom of its walls, but the longer index made out a
broad and extremely firm attachment. With the right index
behind the soft and hard palates, and working upwards, an
equally broad and firm attachment was recognized, reaching
from the extremity of the right finger behind the palate to the
point of the left index in the nostril. The attachments were
certainly to the basilar process of the occipital bone and the
body of the atlas, and seemingly also to the body of the sphenoid.
The growth was entirely subperiosteal, and, as is usual in such
cases, the periosteum was much thickened. The ligamentous
structures between the bones rendered the attachments more or
less uneven. The tumor was removed by the slow and painful
(to operator also) method of enucleating by the two index fingers.
With the left index in the left nostril, and the right behind the
soft and hard palates, working steadily downwards and backwards from above and upwards from below, the fingers ultimately
met and separation was effected. During the operation the
patient, with a gag between his teeth, was seated in a firm, stiff-
backed chair during the operation, and was kept fairly steady
by a couple of students. A thick, strong string, which was
entrusted to an assistant, was passed through the tumor behind
the palate. No chloroform was administered. The hemorrhage
was alarming, and more than once during the operation partial
syncope occurred. Blood passed in large quantities from the
right nostril and in streams from the mouth, while a large quantity was swallowed and afterwards vomited. The patient made
a good recovery. Dr. Hingston stated that the operation would
have been impossible in one less robust. The operation, which
lasted an hour and forty minutes, was too long and too severe
to be borne without an anæsthetic by any but the strongest;
and anæsthesia without tracheotomy would be inadvisable; and
the amount of blood lost was too great for any but the full-
blooded to withstand.

*Carbolic Acid Poisoning; Parenchymatous Degeneration of
Kidneys.*—DR. FINLEY presented the kidneys of a woman aged
40, a case of carbolic acid poisoning. The organs were of

natural size ; capsules non-adherent ; cortex pale and pyramids somewhat injected. Microscopically the cells of the cortex showed marked parenchymatous degeneration and a few slight interstitial infiltrations of leucocytes, together with a few small hemorrhages. The heart muscle was soft and pale, and the fibres showed fatty degeneration. The other organs were healthy. Judging from the absence of gastro-intestinal irritation, it was probable that the poison had been taken in a dilute form. Dr. Finley stated that the patient, an intemperate woman, had swallowed an unknown quantity of carbolic acid, and died forty-eight hours afterwards. The urine was smoky, contained albumen and a large quantity of granular and hyaline casts, also renal epithelium.

Tracheotomy vs. Intubation.—DR. ARMSTRONG then read a paper on this subject,which appeared in full in the June number of the JOURNAL.

Discussion.—DR. BELL said he had had no experience with intubation, but a great deal with tracheotomy. He would be glad if intubation would replace tracheotomy, as the latter is the most unsatisfactory of operations, but he could not help thinking it never would. On examination of statistics, those of tracheotomy are better than those of intubation, as quoted by Dr. Armstrong. Trousseau claims 30 per cent. of successful operations. Among the German operators 33 per cent. is attainable ; others report from 25 to 33 per cent. of successful cases. Northrup's statistics show less than 30 per cent. Statistics, however, are of slight value, as the conditions under which the operation is performed vary greatly. It is generally supposed that an early operation is better than a late one. He has seen very many cases where physicians agreed that the child could not live more than a few hours ; tracheotomy was not allowed, yet recovery took place. He had come to the conclusion that relief should be left to nature till the child could live no longer, then resort to operation. In his experience early operation tended to cause extension of the membrane down the trachea. He believed the relief of the future for such cases would be an aseptic operation requiring no tube or other foreign substance in the larynx.   He did not think Dr. Armstrong had laid stress enough on the effect of the intubation tube on the larynx causing ulceration and subsequent stenosis.   On the whole, the results of intubation had been to him disappointing.

DR. WILKINS said that he thought cases were rare where tracheotomy was done where the child would have recovered without. Cases where the constitutional symptoms of the disease were marked, such as enlarged glands, high temperature, etc., neither tracheotomy nor intubation would avail.   Where the symptoms were only those of obstruction, operative procedure was always called for.

DR. MAJOR said it was difficult to compare cases, as intubation was allowed where tracheotomy would not be thought of. He had performed intubation twenty-seven times, with ten complete recoveries.   Five cases were absolutely hopeless from complications of the disease. Feeding the patient is always difficult.   He had had six cases of foreign-body pneumonia after intubation from entrance of food into the air passages. He now uses a No. 4 catheter, with tube and funnel, and feeds the child himself by passing the tube down the œsophagus. A nurse cannot be trusted to pass the tube.

DR. HINGSTON said that no question in surgery would be more difficult to decide by statistics than this.   To arrive at a satisfactory conclusion as to which was the better operation, we would require operators of equal skill operating at the same period of the disease in similar cases. He only operates reluctantly and as a last resource ; hence his results have not been brilliant. Many times he has been urged to operate where the child has recovered without it. He has had but little experience with intubation.

DR. McCONNELL said that four of the cases quoted by Dr. Armstrong occurred in his practice ; of these, two were successful.   The only advantage of either operation was to overcome obstruction in the air passages. Neither could have any effect on diphtheria as a disease.   During intubation he applied antiseptics to the throat by means of an atomizer. He thought the administration of medicine in these cases unnecessary.

F. W. CAMPBELL thought that the balance of evidence in favor of intubation. It certainly had the great advantage of allowing the air to enter the lungs warm and moist, thus preventing congestion.

J. APTHORN SMITH said that under the most favorable circumstances, the experiences of the London hospitals for children went to prove that tracheotomy is a very dangerous operation. He firmly believed intubation would entirely replace tracheotomy.

Stated Meeting, May 17th, 1889.

WM. GARDNER, M.D., PRESIDENT, IN THE CHAIR.

... of the Cornea treated by evisceration of eyeball and introduction of a glass globe in the Sclerotic.—DR. BULLER introduced to the Society a boy, 8 years old, who received an injury to his right eye from a stick thrown at him by a playmate. He related the following history :—

The patient was brought to me on April 19th ; the injury inflicted eight days previously. I found the eye shrunken and beginning to present the appearances characteristic of traumatic cyclitis. There were two fresh scars from recent wounds in both upper and lower lids. The wound of the eyeball extended vertically through the entire cornea and for a short distance into the sclerotic, both above and below. The cornea presented the appearance of two small turbid cornea separated by a shallow groove. Perception of light was lost, there was no conjunctivitis, and the deeper structures had evidently not undergone any active inflammatory changes. The shrunken eyeball was quite soft and slightly tender to the touch. The condition was such as would evidently involve considerable risk to the other eye from sympathetic ophthalmia. The case was one which demanded some mode of treatment calculated to obviate this danger. I do not approve of removing the eyeball in children on account of the faulty development of orbit and conjunctiva which such an operation involves in young people, and the operation by neurectomy would have, at best, left a very imperfect eyeball. The child being perfectly healthy, with no tendency to suppurative inflammation, I determined to try the operation recently devised by Mr. Mules of Manchester; that is, the insertion of a globe into the cavity of the sclerotic. The operation was done under rigid antiseptic precautions. The cornea was removed entirely with so much of the sclerotic above and below as to give the opening the shape and direction of a vertical ellipse. All the contents of the globe were carefully scraped out with a sharp scoop and the bleeding from the inner scleral surface arrested by packing with aseptic sponges. All bleeding had ceased in about fifteen minutes, and the smallest sized glass globe was inserted. This globe was perfectly smooth and rather more than half an inch in diameter. I selected the smaller size in order to avoid all danger of undue tension when the lips of the scleral wound were united in a vertical direction by three silk sutures. The conjunctival aperture was then united horizontally, also by three silk sutures. After carefully cleansing the eye again with solution of hydrarg. perchlor. 1 to 5000, I dusted fine iodoform powder into the conjunctival sac and covered the lids with absorbent cotton likewise freely dusted with iodoform, this being retained in place by a tolerably firm compressive bandage over both eyes. This dressing was allowed to remain undisturbed for forty-eight hours. When removed I found the eyelids and orbital tissues considerably swollen and tender; both swelling and tenderness completely subsided in a few days under the constant application of cold aseptic compresses, and the case, as you perceive, has done remarkably well. Two days ago I inserted an artificial eye, which presents a very satisfactory appearance. There is no sinking of the upper lid, and the movements of the artificial eye are apparently almost normal. He is only permitted to wear the eye for a short time each day as yet. The sutures in the sclerotic are hidden from view, and create no irritation. The result is far more satisfactory than could have been attained by enucleation or by optico-ciliary neurectomy, and it seems probable that all danger of sympathetic ophthalmia has been removed.

Hodgkin's Disease.—DR. STEWART exhibited a case of Hodgkin's disease. The patient, a powerfully-built man, 22 years of age, first noticed enlargement of the glands in the left side of the neck ten months previously. The glands have steadily continued to increase in size, until now there is a very extensive infiltration of the glands on both sides of the neck and axilla. There is no appreciable enlargement of any other group of superficial lymphatic glands. Both liver and spleen are normal in size. The patient is slightly anæmic. There is, however, no change in the absolute number of either the red or white blood cells, neither can any change in the size or shape of the red cells be determined. For the past six weeks he has been taking Fowler's solution in considerable doses, but without any benefit.

Neoplasm of Stomach.—DR. FINLEY exhibited for Dr. Stewart the organs of a patient with a malignant growth at the pylorus. On either side of the valve the gastric walls were uniformly infiltrated and a third of an inch thick. The mucosa was not ulcerated, and although the opening at the pylorus was only half an inch in diameter, there was no dilatation of the stomach. The pyloric growth was continuous with a nodule projecting into the hepatic flexure of the colon, causing puckering and moderate contraction of the lumen of the bowel. Microscopically, there was inflammatory infiltration of the mucosa with much hyperplasia of the submucous and muscular layers. No cancerous elements had been found after examining a large number of specimens from different parts of the growth. The liver and heart were considerably atrophied, but no metastases were present. The absence of hemorrhage was explained by vomiting always coming on after meals. The growth was doubtless of a malignant nature, as the cancerous elements are at times occluded by the fibrous elements of the growth.

DR. STEWART stated that the patient, a woman aged 46, had been subject to severe and frequent vomiting since June last; also had pain, but no hemorrhage. Moderate and progressive emaciation had accompanied the affection. A tumor was felt in the epigastrium, but no dilatation of the stomach. A diagnosis of pyloric cancer had been made.

Abnormal Subclavian Artery and the Right Pulmonary Veins emptying into the Superior Cava.—DR. SHEPHERD exhibited a specimen obtained from the dissecting-room showing the right subclavian artery arising from the descending arch and passing upwards betweeen the trachea and œsophagus to reach its normal position in the neck. It was given off from the descending aorta and opposite the third dorsal vertebra. The right vertebral artery arose from the right carotid and the left from the aorta between the left carotid and left subclavian. The right recurrent laryngeal nerve did not hook around the right subclavian, but formed a loop in close relation with the right vertebral, which represented, no doubt, the shortened fourth arch. This anomaly is somewhat uncommon, but is easily explained by reference to the development of the aorta. It is an example of a persistent right aortic root, and in this case the fourth right arch, which usually forms the subclavian, does not develop but atrophies. This explains the fact of the right recurrent nerve not hooking round the subclavian; both fifth and fourth arches disappear, so the nerve passes directly to its place of supply. In this case the vertebral was given off at the place where the subclavian usually begins, and really represented the remains of the fourth arch. The sympathetic of the right side was somewhat pulled down by the right subclavian. In the same subject on the right side there was only one large pulmonary vein, and it emptied itself into the vena azygos major instead of the left auricle of the heart. The combined vein was of large size, and entered the superior vena cava by hooking round the root of the right lung. In the same subject the renal arteries were multiple, and there were several muscular anomalies of no special rarity. The conformation of the teeth was peculiar ; the intermaxillary bone appeared to be not fully developed, and the teeth of the upper jaw proper overlapped on each side the incisors. Patient was a woman, aged 30, who died of phthisis in the General Hospital.

Adenoma.—DR. MAJOR read a paper on adenoid growths of the naso-pharyngeal cavity, and described his method of operating in the recumbent position, by means of which blood is prevented from entering the larynx. He places the patient on the back, with a pillow under the shoulders and the head well thrown back so as to make the naso-pharynx the most dependent part. He generally employs curettes of various patterns, and when the vegetations occur high up on the roof he uses his adenomatome. He considered that in diphtheria the presence of adenoid vegetations was a source of aggravation and danger. He believed that nocturnal enuresis was somewhat common in children suffering from extensive adenoid growths. Dr. Major had operated on 186 cases under ether, but had no record of cases done without anæsthetics.

Sublingual Sebaceous Cyst.—DR. SHEPHERD reported the case. The patient was a girl aged 19, who first noticed a swelling beneath the tongue three years ago. This interfered somewhat with articulation and mastication. A year ago the swelling projected into the submaxillary region, and when seen at the hospital was about the size of a small orange. The girl had been several times insane and once after an anæsthetic, so Dr. Shepherd decided to open the cyst under cocaine and not attempt to dissect out. An incision was first made into the cyst beneath the tongue and some fluid evacuated ; then a pair of dressing forceps was pushed down through the cyst and made to project beneath the chin, with the intention of passing a drainage-tube through. An incision was here made and the forceps presented, covered with a thick cyst-wall ; this was seized, the incision enlarged, and with occasional touches of the knife the cyst was drawn out entire through the opening beneath the chin. It contained sebaceous matter of a putty-like consistency. Dr. Shepherd remarked that these cysts were congenital, and, as a rule, grew slowly, so that they caused no inconvenience until about the age of 18 to 20. They are somewhat rare; but are described in most works on surgery. Sir William Ferguson gives a graphic account of the difficulties of their removal in his System of Practical Surgery.

DR. BELL stated that he had met with but two dermoids in unusual situations ; one occurred in the mammary gland and oved from a man's back.

red if Dr. Shepherd had any difficulty in all. In his experience with dermoids about the orbit he had found great difficulty in removing them without rupture and escape of the contents, which then necessitated a very careful dissection, as their walls, when occurring in this region, are extremely delicate.

Selections.

ABSTRACT OF THE HARVEIAN LECTURES ON THE RHEUMATIC STATE IN CHILDHOOD AND EARLY LIFE.

By W. B. CHEADLE, M.D.

The various Manifestations of the Rheumatic state as exemplified in Childhood and Early Life is the subject of the Harveian Lectures delivered this year by Dr. W. B. Cheadle. To reproduce such a lecture even in abstract would require more space than the columns of this journal would allow, so fully and exhaustively is the subject dealt with. The special points brought forward will be here briefly touched upon.

Rheumatism must not be regarded as a mere affection of the joints. The rheumatic virus which produces the articular affection produces in like manner inflammation of the fibrous tissue of the pericardium, endocardium and pleura and that of fasciæ and tendons. It affects fibrous tissue not of joints alone but of these other structures, moreover it affects mucous membrane and skin and disturbs nervous centres. Arthritis must then be regarded as being only one of many rheumatic phenomena. In childhood, the articular affection has not become the chief feature, but is usually slight and subordinate, and, indeed, may be absent altogether from a seizure undoubtedly rheumatic in its nature. The joint tissues are less susceptible, the other fibrous tissues more so. Subcutaneous nodules which are so frequent and significant in early life practically disappear with the advent of puberty; and chorea, so common in connexion with the rheumatism of childhood, disappears as full maturity is reached. Endocarditis and pericarditis are more frequent in children, i.e., they tend to decline as age advances. In the rheumatism of early life arthritis is at its minimum, endocarditis, pericarditis, chorea and subcutaneous nodules at their maximum. As life advances the joint phenomenon becomes more prominent, constant and typical of the disease and reaches its maximum ;

while the other phenomena decline and tend to die out. The various phases of rheumatism must be regarded not as complications or sequelæ but as direct manifestations of rheumatic activity.

Another point of distinction between the rheumatism of childhood and that of later life is the tendency of the various phases to arise independently and apart from each other. The series of rheumatic events is often spread out, scattered over a period of months or years, so that the history of a rheumatism may be a history of childhood. (Cases are cited where the various phases have appeared at intervals through childhood).

The incidence of the disease upon the two sexes.—Taking males and females of all ages together, articular rheumatism is somewhat more common in the former. Up to the age of twenty the balance is the other way. Further, this preponderance of females over males is not uniform at all periods of this first twenty years, but shows a remarkable variation which is of considerable significance. In the first five years of life boys preponderate, viz.: 5–1. At the next quinquennial period between five and ten years, they become nearly equal, viz.: 15 boys to 14 girls. At the next period eleven to fifteen years of age inclusive, comes a remarkable change. The proportion is suddenly and decisively reversed. Girls suffer from articular rheumatism in great preponderance, viz. : 47 girls to 25 boys. After fifteen there is another change; the greater liability of girls gradually declines up to twenty, so that at the close of this period males again preponderate. The greater proclivity of females which has been noted up to twenty years of age is then in reality, chiefly due to their extraordinary liability to the disease during this particular period of from eleven to fifteen. A strong confirmation of this special susceptibility of young girls to rheumatic arthritis is afforded by the fact that the rule holds with regard to scarlatinal rheumatism. The greater liability of girls to rheumatic arthritis during this report (10–15) corresponds with a similar liability to endocarditis and chorea.

Family predisposition.—The tendency to rheumatism is transmitted as strongly as the tendency to gout. This is more striking than in the case of adults, partly perhaps for

9

the reason that the constitutional tendency existing is usually in activity before maturity—if it is there it comes out in childhood; and partly, perhaps, because of the greater ease with which the history of relatives is obtained in the case of children.

The consideration of various phases in detail.—The articular affection is usually comparatively slight and may even be absent altogether. It is, however, nearly always present at some period of the rheumatic efflorescence. Often when medical advice is sought the ailment passes for nothing but a slight feverish attack. Such cases are constantly described as " low fever." The profuse sweatings, the intensely and sour smelling perspiration, are rarely seen, the rarity being in inverse proportion to age. Sudamina and miliary eruptions are rarely seen in children. The pyrexia is slight, and this is the more remarkable, because, as a rule, it rises readily in children. The slight arthritis of childhood often assumes a misleading aspect, and it is sometimes difficult to distinguish it from other ailments involving pain and tenderness of parts. This recognition is of immense importance, since a deadly endocarditis or pericarditis may be insidiously developing concurrently.

Other conditions are often mistaken for articular rheumatism. Essential paralysis in its early stage, when there is great hyperæsthesia, is one of them. But in essential paralysis there is extreme flaccidity of muscle, the limb falling limp and loose, drooping of the toes, and the fact that the tenderness in general is not confined to joints and tendons. Later the disappearance of faradic contractility and tendon reflex would be decisive.

Syphilitic disease of the ends of the long bones is sometimes mistaken for rheumatism. In this there are tenderness and swelling from accompanying periostitis, and there may be even some arthritis, the limbs being kept perfectly motionless from pain on movement. It may be distinguished by the presence of other signs of congential syphilis, and by the history possibly; but the age at which it occurs, viz.: in the first few months after birth, is almost diagnostic. Rheumatic arthritis is almost, if not quite, unknown in early infancy. In infantile scurvy—scurvy-rickets—the swellings are usually limited to the shafts of the long bones, although Dr. Cheadle has once seen a periosteal swelling on the malar bone and swelling and tenderness of the joints. Such, however, are rare exceptions. Other diagnostic points are the existence of spongy gums, subcutaneous hemorrhages and albuminuria. And then infantile scurvy is limited to the bottle-feeding period, i. e. when articular rheumatism is almost unknown.

Anæmia.—The effect of rheumatism in producing anæmia is more remarkable in children than in adults. The presence of the rheumatic poison appears to be inimical to the red corpuscles or their hæmatin. The rheumatic poison is not so rapidly destructive of red blood as that of diphtheria, which causes marked blanching in a few days; but still its effect is decided and unmistakeable. The presence of valvular disease and pericarditis aggravates this tendency, and it is accompanied by progressive emaciation.

Tonsillitis.—Tonsillitis should be ranked as one of the rheumatic series. It occurs frequently in direct and immediate association with articular rheumatism and some pathological connexion cannot be doubted. (Trousseau and Fowler). According to the statistics of the Collective Investigation Committee the association was present in 24.12 per cent. It is not always the rule that the tonsillitis ushers in the articular affection. Tonsillitis may occur at any period of the rheumatic series, although most often it comes first—immediately preceding arthritis. It is probable that tonsillitis may occur as a solitary expression of the rheumatic state and in many cases it arises in rheumatic subjects quite apart from the articular manifestation. Dr. Cheadle has seen recently three examples of its occurrence with chorea and in all these the chorea occurred in a child who had articular rheumatism at another period. " But, of its connexion with endocarditis or pericarditis apart from arthritis I have no certain knowledge."

The decision whether a given case of tonsillitis not immediately associated with articular rheumatism is of rheumatic nature must be based upon a comprehensive survey of the patient's life history and family predisposition as well as of the accompanying symptoms.

Erythema Exudativum.—The *connexion is* more clear in

children than in adults, and is of common occurrence. Of twenty-seven patients with rheumatic nodules eight had erythema papulatum or marginatum, one urticaria and one purpura *i. e.* ten out of twenty-seven cases and these in close association with the evolution of the nodules (Barlow and Warner). It appears in various forms—erythema margina-tum, erythema papulatum, erythema nodosum and urticaria, the first named being the most common. The erythema may occur at any point in the rheumatic series, but it is usually at any rate associated with the development of active rheumatic disturbanbe in some other form and occurs chiefly in the marginate or urticarious form. It is not unfrequently associated with endocarditis and pericarditis in the more serious cases.

Erythema nodosum.—Although it has an arthritis of its own yet it is associated sometimes with true articular rheumatism. The eruption is attended with pain of joints and sometimes swelling, possibly from pressure. The tendency of the erythema to occur in young girls—who are also most liable to rheumatic arthritis, to endocarditis and to chorea—is in agreement with the view of its rheumatic nature; yet although often rheumatic it is often set up by other causes. It should be regarded as evidence of some irritant matter in the circulation (*e. g.* its presence in cholera, septicæmia and in poisoning by certain drugs), the rheumatic poison being regarded in that light.

Purpura rheumatica.—This may arise as a separate disease or in the course of a general acute tuberculer rheumatism, but usually it occurs independently. Purpura rheumatica is probably a minor expression of the rheumatic state, altogether far less common than exudative erythema.

Chorea.—When associated with articular rheumatism it usually follows the arthritis, sometimes is concurrent with it and sometimes precedes it. All are agreed that there is a certain connexion between chorea and rheumatism. The point in dispute is the nature of the relation, its closeness and con-stancy. "I do not think the evidence warrants the assumption that chorea is invariably of rheumatic origin. I must say of chorea, as of tonsillitis, erythema, endocarditis, pericarditis and arthritis, in fact of the whole of the rheumatic series except subcutaneous nodules, that it is produced by other causes as well as rheumatism. But I am convinced that rheumatism is the most common and potent factor." Children never acquire chorea by imitation. It is a "time-honored fallacy in the etiology of chorea." "I have not seen a single instance spread by imitation."

In true chorea there is, even in rheumatic cases, often something more than the constitutional basis of mobility of the nervous system, influenced and played upon by the rheumatic poison. There is frequently another factor—nervous shock. Witness the case of J. T—, eminently rheumatic, yet having two attacks of chorea ascribed to fright long before the first arthritis; and this shock or excitement is a common exciting cause in rheumatic cases. Fright chorea and rheumatic chorea should not be spoken of as distinct. The rheumatic state is the most common predisposing cause, a nervous shock stirs it suddenly into action; fright acts equally on rheumatic and non-rheumatic.

As to the degree of closeness and constancy of the connection between chorea and rheumatism, in addition to the evidence afforded by the occurrence of acute articular rheumatism either preceding or accompanying the chorea, there is still more of recent development bearing upon the question. Firstly, the records of the Collective Investigation Committee, as previously stated, show that between the ages of ten and fifteen girls have a remarkable proclivity to acute articular rheumatism as compared to boys, which is that of the maximum incidence of chorea. This corresponds with a similar greater proclivity during that same period of girls as compared with boys to organic heart disease associated with chorea, and to articular rheumatism associated with chorea. This similar harmony of relative incidence is possible of more than one interpretation, but it is *primâ facie* very suggestive of close pathological connection.

Secondly, there is the evidence afforded by the association of chorea with other conditions which are themselves found in close relation to articular rheumatism—the other members of the rheumatic series, *e.g.*, endocarditis or pericarditis in association with chorea. "There is no other general morbid state so closely associated with chorea as rheumatism. There are only two diseases largely and closely associated with endocarditis, viz.: chorea and rheumatism. Explanations more or less plausible have been suggested as to the cause of the endocarditis of chorea apart from rheumatism, but no dynamic theory will explain the *pericarditis* of chorea when it occurs without articular affection. The significance of this fact has, I think, been overlooked.

The association of erythema nodosum or tonsillitis with the endocarditis or pericarditis would greatly strengthen the presumption of the rheumatic nature of an accompanying chorea; while the presence of nodules so absolutely associated with rheumatic activity, would be in itself conclusive. Dr. Cheadle cited several cases in illustration and as a general result of his investigations and experiences arrives at the conclusion that in the majority of cases at least chorea is a phase of rheumatism.

Subcutaneous tendinous nodules.—"I have long been familiar with them as occurring occasionally in the course of articular rheumatism; but the credit of pointing out their frequency and great importance as clinical signs in the various manifestations of rheumatism belongs to Dr. Barlow and Dr. Warner. Fibrous nodules are common in children but much more rare in adults. They are often overlooked because of this rarity in adults, because they are not looked for and because often they are of small size. They are sometimes to be felt rather than seen. The collective investigation records give but a small percentage of cases in which they were found, yet at the moment there are seven cases at Great Ormond Street Hospital. All these are, except one, of articular rheumatism, cases of chorea. The nodules vary in size from that of a hempseed to that of an almond or larger; in extreme cases they may attain that of half a walnut. The nodules lie under the skin and are connected with fascia or tendons—in relation with fibrous tissues. They are not tender except slightly in rare instances. There is no redness of the skin over them except occasionally from friction or pressure. They are found most commonly upon the back of the elbow, over the malleoli, and at the margin of the patella, not infrequently upon the head, especially along the superior curved line of the occiput, the temporal ridge and now and again upon the extensor and flexor muscles of the hands, on the extensors of the feet, the vertebral spines, the spine of the scapula and the crista ilii. In extreme cases nodules may be found in nearly all these positions. Once Dr. Cheadle saw them the size of almonds studded over the flexor tendons, on the palms of the hands, and once in great numbers over the tendinous structures of the intercostals on the front and sides of the thorax. There may be only one of these nodules but more, usually three or four, are to be found. Sometimes the number is large, as many as thirty or forty. Sometimes there is only a single crop; sometimes several crops appear in succession. They develop to perceptible size in the course of a few days. Large nodules have an existence of months, Their evolution is unaccompanied by pain or fever. They consist of nuclear growth in process of development into fibrous tissue in all stages of transformation.

The connection of these nodules with rheumatism is extremely close, and I believe absolute. They owe no other origin or connection. "In all cases in which I have seen them there has been either rheumatic joint affection at the time or at some period of the child's history or such a con-currence of rheumatic events one or more—such as endo-carditis, pericarditis, chorea and erythema—that there could be no doubt as to the nature of his condition." Not only are the nodules connected with rheumatism but they are specially connected with the graver forms of it; and they are signs, serious apparently, in proportion to their size and number. "I regard the eruption of large nodules (such as are shown in the sketch) as almost equivalent to a sentence of death." They mean persistent cardiac disease, generally uncon-trollable, and marching almost infallibly to a fatal ending. General experience agrees as to the grave significance of these fibrous growths, at first looked upon as unimportant curiosities. In twenty-seven cases (Barlow and Warner) there was organic heart disease in all; in eight there was pericarditis; in twelve there was progressive valvular disease, and eight were fatal in spite of all treatment. Money has found nodules in half the cases of rheumatism in which well-marked heart disease occurred. Dr. Cheadle's experience is quite in accord with these observations: "I could give examples of the association of these nodules with every other phase of the rheumatic series as well as with endocarditis and pericarditis and chorea and pleurisy, already mentioned ; and in all these cases the evidence they afford as to the rheumatic nature of the affection is of the highest value, and I believe decisive. But their greatest interest lies in the fact of their frequent association with endocarditis and pericarditis of the most deadly, although subacute, form, and in their connection with chorea.

Pleurisy occurs in association with rheumatism in two different ways. It arises frequently towards the end of rheumatic heart disease—partly as a result of the mechanical congestion of the pleura caused by the valvular defect, or pericarditis or by extension of the latter. But pleurisy likewise occurs in rheumatism as an initial phenomenon, coming immediately before, together with, or immediately after arthritis as a direct result of the rheumatic influence. Probably many idiopathic pleurisies and pleuropneumonias are of rheumatic origin.

Pericarditis.—Pericarditis may appear at any point in the rheumatic procession of events—first or last, alone or in combination with other phases. Most often it comes late after endocarditis, especially when the heart is hypertrophied and dilated. Sometimes it is associated with valvular inflammation, it is often accompanied by the evolution of nodules and not unfrequently arises in connection with chorea. The development of pericarditis in association with chorea, apart from articular rheumatism, is a link of association between them which is of considerable significance. But the acute general pericarditis of rheumatic fever is not representative of the disease in children. The classical signs are sometimes wanting. Pericarditis in children occurs insidiously ; a slight rub is noticed which may cease or continue without much change ; the child is restless and uncomfortable ; pain in præcordial region ; the pulse quickens to 120 or 130 ; anæmia increases ; the chorea, if present, increases a little, or curious emotional attacks come on, the child being moved to tears or laughter by a word ; the temperature is slightly raised, perhaps to 100° or 101°, but often remains normal if there be no arthritis, pleurisy or pneumonia; and with this a mitral murmur develops or an existing one grows rougher, and subcutaneous nodules begin to appear on the elbows and knees, or ankles and occiput. The pericardial rub may disappear for a time or it may continue, but in spite of treatment the rapid action of the heart continues; fresh nodules come out; the cardiac dulness is increased; the sounds are muffled in the mid-cardiac region, but there is no sign of effusion; the heart is growing more bulky and the pericardium thicker, emaciation and anæmia proceed apace; pulse becomes more feeble; and so without extreme dyspnœa or dropsy, the patient sinks from exhaustion and heart failure.

Rheumatic pericarditis, then, in early life, is apt to be subacute, persistent, recurrent and progressive; going on not for days only, but for weeks or months, the inflamed membrane slowly or intermittingly exuding not serum but adhesive lymph, causing adhesions more or less complete, and development of fibrous tissue, so that the pericardium becomes thickened, sometimes enormously. This subacute, progressive form might almost be called "nodular," so frequent is the evolution of these significant bodies associated with it.

What is the pathological relation of the fibrous nodule to the fibrosis of the pericardium? The same virus seems to stir up inflammation alike of fibrous sheaths and of the fibrous tissue of the pericardium. The pericardial thickening has even been found nodular (Barlow and Angel Money). "I believe that the fatal issue is largely dependent upon the tightening grip of the adherent contracting pericardium." Possibly, also, there is fibrous interstitial invasion of the heart muscle and concurrent myocarditis; hence the rapid pulse and the progressive feebleness or cardiac action.

Endocarditis.—Endocarditis occurs acutely in the course of articular rheumatism in children just as it does in adults; yet in childhood it often occurs quite apart from any concurrent affection of the joints, and it may develop at any period in the rheumatic procession of events, early or late, in combination with arthritis or pericarditis or chorea or nodules, with any or all of those combined. Usually it comes early in the series and recurs later, towards the end. "The rule is endocarditis early, pericarditis late." But as with pericarditis, so with endocarditis; the acute form in connection with severe articular rheumatism is far less common than one slight and trivial apparently at the time, accompanying an equally slight articular affection and chorea, all sign of it perhaps disappearing for a season, yet recurring and persisting until the injury to the valve becomes serious and finally fatel. It is not, as it is so commonly with adults, a sharp attack of endocarditis accompanying the articular affection, ceasing with it, and followed slowly by chronic after-changes in the valve or muscle; but subacute, insiduous, progressive.

Valvulitis may often be overlooked owing to the mildness of the articular affection. Children are nearly twice as liable to this complication as are adults. Excluding cases arising from congenital causes, as well as those arising from the other fevers there remain three classes, (1) the valvular affection arises in association with distinct attacks of rheumatism, (2) those associated with chorea in which no articular affection is observed, (3) those in which no connection with any other morbid condition of any kind can be traced—what may be called the "unexplained cases."

Now, with regard to the first class, the organic change is due to rheumatic endocarditis, and statistics show that these form the largest proportion. The only question with regard to the second class, those associated with chorea, is whether they are the result of rheumatic endocarditis. "In my judgment most of these are to be regarded as examples of rheumatic endocarditis. The cardiac affection of chorea is, as a rule, organic, not merely functional. Functional murmurs do, no doubt, arise occasionally in chorea, e.g., the ordinary hæmic murmur of the pulmonary orifice. But that the mitral murmur of chorea is not usually of functional origin seems to be established by the following considerations : 1. If the mitral murmur were hæmic it is strange that it should be mitral, such function disturbances being in other conditions associated with pulmonary and aortic orifices; and further, if a mitral hæmic murmur did exist a fortiori, a pulmonary one should exist also, but it does not. Morcover, the mitral murmur of chorea comes early as a rule, before anæmia and debility arise. 2. The hypothesis that the mitral murmur of chorea is commonly spasmodic or paretic is unsupported by positive evidence. It is improbable because the murmur does not arise in connection with irregular action of the heart. The general immunity of all involuntary muscle is against the theory of spasm (Osler); while as to paresis, the murmur has no special association with paretic chorea. 3. In chorea endocarditis is almost invariably found *post mortem*. There is no other disease in which it is so constant. 4. In fatal cases of valvular disease arising in association with chorea the changes found in the valves *post mortem* are identical with those from endocarditis from other causes, while the valve chiefly affected is the mitral, the one most liable to endocarditis.

Careful clinical observations bear out these observations (Osler, Stephen Mackenzie). The valvular affection in chorea is, in a vast number of cases, due to endocarditis. Is the endocarditis due to rheumatism? The evidence is strong. (1), the frequent association of articular rheumatism with chorea and endocarditis together; (2), the frequent association of articular rheumatism with the two independently with chorea on the one hand, and with endocarditis on the other; (3), the especial association of endocarditis with those cases of chorea which are also associated with articular rheumatism. The great proportion of cases of endocarditis which arise in connection with chorea arise in choreas connected with articular rheumatism. Endocarditis picks out the rheumatic cases.

It has been suggested that strain or shock or violent action of the valves is the source of choreic endocarditis. For many reasons this is untenable: (1.) The heart does *not* act violently in chorea, but feebly; tension is lessened, not increased. (2.) In diseases such as Graves' disease, where the valves flap to with great force, valvulitis is not set up, although a functional murmur is sometimes set up. (3.) Heart disease does not arise especially in connection with chorea associated with fright, when a sudden strain might be postulated, but in connection with chorea associated with rheumatism equally whether fright is or is not present as a co-factor. But the most cogent argument is that drawn from

pericarditis. Pericarditis arises in chorea quite apart from
any articular affection as often in proportion to its general
frequency as endocarditis. This cannot be accounted for
either by the strain hypothesis, the paretic hypothesis or the
spasm hypothesis. The active morbid change in the valves in
subacute endocarditis appears to be analogous to that in the
subcutaneous fibrous tissues giving rise to nodules. Such
nodules are frequently developed without concurrent articular
rheumatism, but with endocarditis in the course of chorea.

The eruption of subcutaneous nodules is associated with
grave progressive endocarditis as closely as with progressive
pericarditis. The inflammatory process in the valves appears
to be identical with that met with in nodules, viz. : nuclear
proliferation, cell infiltration, spindle cells in process of transformation into fibrous tissue, wavy bands of fibres and vessels.
(Microscopical specimens of valves were shown). The chief
change—the greatest and most important—that which causes
the thickening and rigidity—is the proliferation of fibrous
tissue, which is the leading feature of the morbid process seen
in the subcutaneous nodule. " This correlation of nodules and
valvulitis gives the appearance of the former great clinical
significance, as probably indicative of a similar change going
on in endocardium or pericardium or both."

Ulcerative endocarditis is most rare in the rheumatism of
children, since it is met with chiefly in patients broken down
by drink and disease.

It was formerly taught that mitral stenosis is less often
rheumatic than any other valvular affection. As a matter of
fact, this form of heart disease—in children at any rate—is
especially rheumatic. It is the special product of the slight,
subacute, slow, recurrent, rheumatic endocarditis which is
characteristic of childhood. The stenosis does not usually
reach the degree when it is proclaimed by the loud, vibrating
presystolic murmur, until a few years have passed.

Hypertrophy and dilatation.—These secondary changes occur
more rapidly in children than in adults. Compensation is
usually for a time exceptionally complete ; and as a further
result of this effective compensation, great enlargement of the
liver and spleen, pulmonary apoplexy and extreme dropsy are
rare in the younger children, becoming more common as age

advances. It is an unusual thing to see a little child, blue, turgid and waterlogged, as in adults. Instead of engorged liver and lungs, with blueness, extreme dyspnœa and general dropsy, there is rapid wasting, progressive anæmia, feebleness, and death from asthenia rather than from the direct injury to the mechanism of circulation, unless it be the strangling grip of pericardial exudation and adhesion.

Scarlatinal rheumatism.—Articular inflammation appears now and again in the course of scarlet fever which can in no way be distinguished from that of acute rheumatism. It is often accompanied by endocarditis or pericarditis and sometimes by chorea. This scarlatinal rheumatism, although it may come late, in most cases arises early and does not appear to be due either to uræmia or to septicæmia. The special liability of girls to acute articular rheumatism extends to this scarlatinal form.

Treatment.—Minimize the danger of cardiac complication by being constantly on guard against an insidious attack of endocarditis or pericarditis. " It is essential then to examine the heart carefully in every case of the slightest articular effection, even a stiff neck or a stiff knee; and in chorea, in tonsillitis, in erythema, in an evolution of nodules, and indeed, in every pyrexial condition of every form. Enforce absolute rest in bed whenever there is suspicion of rheumatic inflammation. Heroic treatment by salicylate of soda is rarely called for in childhood, for the salicylates appear to exert no favorable influence upon any rheumatic phase, except only arthritis and tonsillitis. Salicin is less depressing and may be given with alkalis."

NASAL OBSTRUCTION IN ITS RELATION TO THE ADMINISTRATION OF ANÆSTHETICS.

By J. Fredk. W. Silk, M.D. (Lond.), &c.,

Anæsthetist to the Great Northern Central Hospital; to Guy's Hospital (Dental School); and to the National Epileptic (Queen's Square).

There are but few morbid conditions which have received of late years more careful attention than that of nasal obstruc-tion, and it has frequently been shown that the condition is by no means one which concerns the specialist alone, but, on the contrary, that the patency or the mere or less complete closure

of the naso-pharyngeal airway may greatly influence the
general health. The production of artificial anæsthesia by inhalation is so frequently resorted to that I hardly need to offer
any excuse for attempting to point out how important are the
bearings of such obstruction upon the process of administration.
Unless the indications to the contrary are very obvious, the
administrator naturally concludes that the anæsthetic vapor
reaches the lungs by the usual channels, i.e., the nose and mouth,
and mainly the former. If, however, nasal obstruction exists,
this double-barrelled or oro-nasal airway is converted into a
single or oral one in direct proportion to the degree of obstruction.   In this connection I would point out—

1. That such anæsthetics as ether, and, in a lesser degree,
nitrous oxide, by increasing the turgescence of the mucous
membranes, tend to accentuate any slight obstruction that may
already exist, or may convert what was originally a partial,
and maybe unnoticed, obstruction into a complete one.

2. That with all anæsthetics, extreme degrees of relaxatien
likewise accentuate pre-existing nasal obstruction by permitting of the falling of the velum palati towards the posterior
wall of the pharynx. The proper explanation to give of the
apparent superiority of chloroform for children appears to me
to be that partial nasal obstruction is then of very frequent
occurrence, and that such obstruction, on account of the depressing action of the chloroform, is somewhat less likely to
be rendered absolute than with ether; but I think that when
the condition in question is fully recognized by those administering anæsthetics, and precautions taken to obviate any possible difficulty which may arise from this cause, one, at any
rate, of the most serious objections to the use of ether in the
young will be removed.

The conversion of an oro-nasal into an oral airway should
not, of course, under ordinary circumstances, give rise to the
slightest anxiety or trouble; difficulties may, however, then
arise under the following circumstances, viz.:—

1. During the stage of induction, on account of the swelling
of the tongue, which then tends to fill up the only remaining,
or oral, airway. This condition is often aggravated by the
abundant secretion of mucus and saliva, and by the spasmodic
closure of the jaws and mouth, as a result of the action of the

anæsthetic employed; not only is the inhalation prevented under these circumstances, but a certain degree of asphyxia is also developed;

2. During the maintenance of the narcosis. Short of absolute occlusion of the glottis by the base, mere contact of the tongue (even if not swollen) with the roof of the mouth, by obstructing the *oral* airway, is sufficient to add materially to our difficulties. Spasmodic closure of the mouth and jaws likewise ensues in these cases, but rather as a result of the partial asphyxia than as a cause of that condition.

If the true nature of these difficulties is recognized at the outset, it is comparatively easy to prevent their occurrence or to overcome them when developed. In the first place, then, if nasal obstruction is known, or is suspected to exist, it is always wisest to place a prop between the teeth before commencing the inhalation. Not only is it then easier, subsequently, to insert a gag or mouth-opener, if necessary, but the mouth will be held sufficiently open to enable us to seize the tongue should it be desirable to do so.

In the second place, the frequency of more or less complete nasal obstruction, and its tendency to be accentuated under an anæsthetic, should be borne in mind, especially in administering to children. If no prop has been inserted, and if asphyxial troubles arise which do not yield readily to simple measures, *e.g.*, pushing forward the lower jaw, we should endeavor to secure a proper oral airway by the use of the mouth-opener or gags. I am inclined to place the importance of opening the mouth second only to compression of the chest or artificial respiration. With the mouth open, we are rendered independent of the nasal passages; we can clear away mucus, etc., and pull forward the base of the tongue; we can command the glottis, and, if need be, proceed to intubate the larynx.

I have been led to devote a good deal of attention to the subject, because of the occasional occurrence, in my own practice, of cases of which the following is almost a typical example, viz.:—

The patient was a lad aged 10; chloroform was administered by means of a Skinner's frame, and he passed fully and quietly under the influence of the anæsthetic in four minutes, half a drachm being used. The narcosis was maintained subsequently for about ten minutes, towards the end of which time the breathing became slow and shallow, but with nothing approaching stertor; lividity of the lips then appeared, deepened, and extended to the nose and cheeks, but the pulse remained good, became almost bounding in character, and the pupils did not dilate; obviously the danger was due to asphyxia and not to syncope. Dr. Howard's paper upon apnœa had just then appeared, and this case seemed one in which good might be expected to result from the procedure therein advocated. The child's head was accordingly brought over the edge of the bed, the shoulders raised, and the neck extended to the very utmost limit, but without appreciable result. I then endeavored to open the mouth, but the spasm was by that time extreme, and I could only succeed in introducing my forceps just sufficiently to seize hold of the tip of the tongue and draw it forward. Momentary relief was thus afforded, but, unfortunately, the jaws were not sufficiently wide apart, the tongue became jammed between the teeth, and the last condition of that boy was decidedly worse than the first. It was not until the jaws were widely opened and the full extent of the oral airway was established that the patient could be considered out of danger.

As I say, this case is but typical of others that have occurred to me and, I doubt not, to other anæsthetists. The usual explanations given of the phenomena (e.g., arytæno-epiglottidean relaxation) did not appear to me to be quite satisfactory, and it was not until some little time after, that the possibility of nasal obstruction being at the bottom of the mischief impressed itself upon my mind. If my views upon the subject are correct, it might be useful in similar cases—i.e., when oral supervenes upon nasal obstruction—to pass into the pharynx via the nostrils a good-sized gum-elastic catheter, in order to furnish means for the passage of air beyond the oral obstruction; at any rate, the manœuvre is worth trying. Such a catheter might well be added to the armamentarium of the anæsthetist, for it is quite possible to intubate the larynx with such an instrument should that proceeding be necessary.

If the naso-pharynx itself is the region involved in the operation, additional elements of difficulty in administering are introduced, such as:—

(1) The manipulations of the surgeon. When the post-nasal

...and the finger, or an instrument, is thrust
...channel by which the anæsthetic can be adminis-
...hardly surprising that the patient tends to
...that, at best, the narcosis is fitful and uncertain;
...profuse hemorrhage attendant upon most operations
... Apart from the possibilities of syncope (*e.g.*,
..."bleeders") and complete asphyxia, an accumulation
...mucus, etc., in the pharynx and upper parts of the
...set in other ways, not the less dangerous because
...Thus the glottis being partly occluded, the actual
...air passing into the lungs is sensibly diminished,
...vapor of the anæsthetic employed is, as a rule,
...air, the diminution takes place (especially in the
...tion) mainly at the expense of the latter; the vapor,
...sheer force of gravity, gradually tends to displace
...to accumulate in the upper part of the larynx.
...lation explains, I believe, in great measure, how
...cases we are considering are particularly prone
...development of what I have termed elsewhere
...apnœa."
...with a diminution of inhalatory power is of neces-
...diminished expiratory function and pulmonary
...and consequent accumulation of anæsthetic vapor
...and blood. Hence it is not uncommon for attacks
...syncope to occur some little time *after* the ad-
...has been discontinued.
...although I have happily had no experience myself
...matter, it is usually taught, and seems quite possible,
...may be inhaled in such quantities as to give rise
...tly to atelectasis, pneumonia, and other troubles.—
...*Laryngology and Rhinology.*

...th from Hydrophobia.—The following
...of a case of death from hydrophobia in Birmingham
...forwarded to us by Dr. Richard Drury. The sufferer,
...15, who had lately resided in Ceylon, arrived three
...in Birmingham. In November, 1888, he and his
...) were bitten by a stray dog. As a precau-
...e, the wounds were sucked and cauterized. It
...nat the dog was rabid, as before that fact could

be ascertained it was drowned. On July 13th the elder lad complained of not feeling well. The following day he kept the house and had a slight shivering fit. On July 17th Dr. Drury was summoned. He was told there was difficulty in swallowing, and that the patient seemed in danger of being choked. He found a very well-developed young fellow in bed, who had a sullen and apprehensive aspect, and was very reticent. To test his vocalisation he was asked his name, which was not clearly heard until he had repeated it several times. No redness or swelling of the fauces was perceptible, and nothing abnormal was revealed to the touch. On the right side there was a slightly swollen submaxillary gland. A cup of water was then handed him to drink to try his powers of deglutition, and here the first suspicion was aroused, for the moment he saw the water he was seized with spasm of the pharynx, and it was only on pressing him to drink after much protestation on his part that he managed to take two or three gulps. There was no headache, no heat of skin, and the pulse was calm. As the pharyngeal spasms kept constantly recurring chloroform inhalations were ordered. During the day he had short intervals of sleep, and took some solid food His condition at night did not seem worse. He passed a bad night, but took nourishment freely; and in the morning he stated he had drunk easily two cups of tea, and said if he could only get "this lump" out of his throat he would "feel as happy as a bird." He made frequent attempts to vomit and to eject the viscid mucus from his fauces. His mind was perfectly clear. Receiving a hurried message saying that the lad was worse, Dr. Drury, on his arrival, found the patient struggling for breath. The spasms of the throat had greatly increased. He was vainly attempting to get rid of the glairy mucus that kept constantly filling his throat, which could not be removed by any effort on his part, and had to be wiped away from time to time with a handkerchief. Later on Mr. Bennett May saw the case in conjunction with Dr. Drury, when the lad was found to be in great anguish and distress, excessively restless, at times struggling with maniacal frenzy, but lucid at intervals, recognizing those surrounding him, and able to articulate clearly. His features were of a dusky leaden hue and the pupils widely dilated. The spasms commencing in the pharyngeal muscles affected also those of respiration. The muscles of the trunk and limbs were flaccid. There was no trismus. The tenacious mucus became excessively copious and deeply stained with a coffeeground-looking material. Gradually the pulse began to fail, the extremities became cold, and in a few hours death ended a most painful scene.—*Brit. Med. Journal.*

Hæmatoma Oris, a Sign of Spinal Injury.

—Dr. B. Lee, in the *University Medical Magazine* for February, gives an interesting record bearing on this point in the case of a child eight months old who fell four feet, striking on the head and thigh. Examination later revealed what seemed to be hip-joint trouble on the right side, which was treated by various mechanical devices for three weeks. At that time the mother noticed a slight swelling of the gum above the right central incisor in the upper jaw. This gradually increased, and as it did so, became of a livid purple color. It had no tendency to ulceration, nor did it seem painful, except at times when it would cause the child to refuse her bottle for a few hours. After a time it showed itself on the inner side of the jaw as well, and extended laterally in both directions; and bulging down over the teeth, completely hid them. Occasionally there would be a slight hemorrhage from it, which was followed by a reduction in size. By the 1st of December both hips had improved most encouragingly, and permission was given for the child to sit up. This was followed in a few days by most serious results. The attacks of screaming were renewed, sleep was much disturbed, appetite lost, and a certain amount of febrile action set up. It was evident that the upright posture caused her great pain, and it was also observed that the movement of the right arm was painful to her. A day or two later the power of motion in this arm became impaired. It was then remembered that occasionally, all along through her illness, movement of this arm had been painful. On the 18th of December, a careful examination demonstrated that there was disease very high up in the cervical spine, possibly between the atlas and the skull. The shoulder soon became slightly elevated and the left arm also began to lose power. Every attempt to place her in the erect position for the purpose of adjusting mechanical support in-

duced paroxysms, threatening convulsions, in which the face
became livid and the respiration difficult. She was kept flat
on the back, with the head slightly lower than the shoulders,
extension being made upon the occiput horizontally, sometimes
including the chin. This was maintained continuously, and
manfestly added much to her comfort. Emaciation now progressed rapidly, and her face became excessively pallid and
lips colorless. The tumor of the gums steadily increased and
hemorrhage became more frequent. Toward the middle of
January a slight purple discoloration manifested itself below
the left eye; later under the right eye. A few days later the
eye began to protrude, and it was evident that there was a
hæmatoma of the orbit. Loss of power in the lower extremities was now very apparent. In order to employ more efficient
extension a padded steel collar was now applied, acting upon
the occiput and chin. This was not well borne, however, and
it was soon removed. Symptoms of meningeal inflammation,
slight convulsive movements, alternating with stupor, and constant vomiting now supervened. As a last resort, another
effort was made to apply the spinal splint with an attachment
for head extension. In order to do this the child was placed
face downward upon the knees and kept in that position for
possibly five minutes. At the end of that time it seemed as if
all the blood in the brain had rushed into the face. It was
streaming from the mouth. The turgescence of the gums was
excessive. Both eyes were prominent, the left frightfully so.
It seemed as though all inhibitory power over the circulation
had ceased, and the blood flowed simply in obedience to gravity.
After this time the excessive restlessness abated, and there was
little suffering, but the patient steadily sank and death ensued
within twenty-four hours.—*Alienist and Neurologist.*

Enormous Hydatid Cyst of Right Kidney ; Autopsy.

(By Dr. A. L. Stavely.)—A Russian
Pole, aged 43, was admitted to the Reading Hospital, Penn.,
March 3, 1889, with a temperature of 101.5°F., pulse 88, respirations 24, and suffering intense lancinating pain anteriorly,
just below the thorax and extending round to the back. About
two months before admission he first became conscious of something wrong from severe pain that he experienced whenever

he would attempt to work. The patient was quite well preserved, though his eyes were sunken and the face indicative of
suffering. Inspection revealed a very marked prominence of
the lower part of the thorax and the upper part of the abdomon,
with labored inspirations and pulsation below the ensiform
cartilage. On palpation, a large, firm mass could be felt, extending about four inches below the margin of the ribs. Percussion gave the following results: Over the sternal region
the line of dulness was seven inches, the lower limit being
from two to three inches above the ensiform cartilage. The
length in the right nipple line was ten inches, dulness beginning at the nipple. In the right mid-axillary region dulness
extended seven inches, beginning at the eighth intercostal
space. Posteriorly, on the right side, decided dulness began
at tenth rib, the lower boundary being obscure. Dulness extended over to the left mid-axillary line, where it began at the
seventh intercostal space and extended to the edge of the
thorax. Auscultation demonstrated encroachment of the mass
upon the right lung. The pain continued after admission, and
had to be relieved by hypodermics of morphine and atropine.
The stools, with one or two exceptions, were loose, varied from
light to dark green in color, and were about normal as to frequency. His urine was slightly darker than normal, and contained no albumin nor anything else that could be of assistance
in making a diagnosis. There was no jaundice nor anything
but the stools which would indicate any hepatic disturbance.
The pulse varied from 72 to 100, the respirations from 19 to
30, the temperature averaging about 99°F. On April 11th he
complained of excruciating pain, and frequent resort was made
to the hypodermic syringe. On the morning of the 12th he
went to the bath-room for a wash, and was there only a minute
when he came rushing out, and, dropping on the floor by his
bed, expired.

On opening the abdomen a large, tense, fibrous sac was seen,
and, by manipulation, was found to have liquid contents. All
the organs were found to be displaced by it. On feeling for
the right kidney, it was discovered that its position was occupied by this enormous body, and the kidney was not to be
found. In trying to remove the cyst the manipulator's finger
forced its way through a weak spot and over nine pints of a

clear, odorless, serous-like fluid escaped, and floating in the fluid was found a solitary daughter-cyst about half an inch in diameter. After great difficulty the cyst was removed, and was found to contain a thick, white, membranous mass floating in some liquid. The membrane, or more properly the cyst-wall, was distinctly laminated, and looked something like boiled albumin. One surface was slightly roughened, and had on it here and there aggregated nodular masses, which proved to be ecchinococci buds. The other surface of the cyst-wall was smoother, and had on it thin layers of a jelly-like consistence, which were easily detached, and which seemed to be of more recent formation. Examination of the sac that contained the hydatid cyst demonstrated the fact that it was nothing but a dilated kidney, the ureter of which had become entirely occluded, and the lateral halves of which were imbedded in the walls of the sac at about two inches distance from each other, and feeling like masses of muscular tissue. The walls were composed of bands of fibrous tissue running regularly in every direction, being thinner in one place than another. The inside of the sac, or what presumably corresponds to the pelvis of the kidney, was smooth. Microscopic examination of the cystic fluid revealed a number of echinococci hooklets, and crystals of chloride of sodium were discovered on evaporation. The fluid was somewhat acid and gave a slight albuminous reaction. The left kidney was much enlarged, weighing over 12 ounces. There was no degeneration as yet, and the hypertrophy was due entirely to vicarious action. The spleen weighed $12\frac{1}{2}$ ozs., was very brittle in consistence, and deeply congested. The heart was somewhat dilated, and there was some fibrinous deposit about the mitral and aortic semilunar valves. No apparent lesion of any other organ was recognizable.—*The Epitome.*

Chronic Poisoning by Arsenic.—In a recent communication to the Académie de Médecine of Paris, Professor Brouardel gave the results of a very careful inquiry into the symptoms of chronic poisoning by arsenic, basing his investigations mainly on an outbreak of arsenical poisoning which recently occurred at Hyères, owing to the accidental poisoning of some wine with arsenic. Professor Brouardel

onic poi-
rm, only
e remark-
entry of
man is alive
of chronic
equally cogni-
criterion as
rious green colour
ene, other sources
witness the cases at
where violet powder
cal symptoms, various
for wrapping them in,
may have in numerous
of poisoning. In the
people engaged in making
how the wearers fare
presumably go com-

depend somewhat on the
less gradual than in those
be found to bear a definite
inquiry be made, either to the
or medicine, or to the times
person. A simple *malaise*, with
disturbance, perhaps trivial, per-
ptoms suggestive of typhoid fever,
indication. The vomiting is more or
any rate, it is independent of, and unac-
in the stomach; it is generally copious,
by diarrhœa, and especially if the
with blood, we have a condition which
at once suggest the possibility of arsenical
existence of vomiting and diarrhœa, with
ptoms, is in an adult indicative of poi-
e; in a child such a combination of
import. Constipation is, how-
mmon than diarrhœa. In the
iratory tract generally makes

its appearance; there is a certain amount of mucus expectoration, and the patient has symptoms of laryngitis. Coryza, more or less lachrymation and injunction of the conjunctiva will probably also be present, with swelling of the eyelids. Patches of erythema, a vesicular eruption, urticaria, and a branny desquamation are amongst the manifestations that may be expected at this stage, as also the tendency to pigmentation to which attention has frequently been drawn in this country in the case of choreic children treated by arsenic. A persistent headache, numbness in the legs and feet, and sometimes cramps in the legs will also be generally found; the special senses are unaffected. Up to this period it is more than probable that the case will have been misinterpreted, but when, in addition to the above phenomena, paralytic symptoms are developed, the true nature of the case should at once suggest itself to the careful observer.

At this stage the patient is easily tired, has a difficulty in going upstairs, and gradually loses all power in his legs, so as to be unable to stand without assistance. The group of muscles on the front and outer side of the leg are the ones principally affected, and after a time they waste, their faradic excitability in advanced stages is lost, and the response to galvanism is diminished. The muscles of the arms are also affected, but to a less extent; the muscles of the face and the sphincters always escape. The tendon reflexes are absent, and the plantar reflexion diminished. Even when the condition is recognised it does not always follow that recovery will take place, death sometimes occurring suddenly from heart failure when the patient appeared to be doing well. Cases in which paralysis has supervened are always tedious. The paralytic symptoms have been shown to be due to peripheral neuritis.

In a doubtful case, examination of the vomited matters or the motions might, of course, reveal the presence of poison, but in a criminal case it might not be possible to obtain these, or we might not wish our suspicions to be known. The examination of the urine is quite as efficacious as the examination of the vomit, as arsenic is sure to be present in it if the case is one of arsenical poisoning. Arsenic has been found in the urine a few minutes after its ingestion, and Professor Brouardel states that in one case he found arsenic in the urine forty days after its administration had been stopped. He also recommends that the hair should be cut and examined; in one case in 100 grammes of hair he found 1 milligramme of arsenic. As regards the discovery of arsenic in the tissues after death, authorities have been by no means agreed. Scolosoboff and others have asserted that arsenic accumulates to the greatest extent in the brain and spinal cord. Ludwig found that it was most persistent in the liver; the bones, according to him, might retain the poison for some time, but not so long as the liver. Professor Brouardel, however, finds that when the poison has been taken into the body slowly in small repeated doses it is apt to be deposited in the spongy tissue of the flat bones, for example, of the cranium, vertebræ, and scapula, and that it is eliminated from these very slowly indeed; in the more rapid cases it is found in the bones rich in compact tissue, that is, the femur, and this fact no doubt explains the apparent discrepancy between his results and those of Ludwig.—*British Medical Journal.*

Spontaneous Rupture of the Heart.—

Dr. Mallet of Paris described before the Société Anatomique of that city a case of this accident which occurred last May in the Hôpital Tenon. The patient was a man aged 79, with pulmonary disease. He died suddenly after rising to micturate. A rent, almost vertical and over two inches long, was discovered in the anterior aspect of the wall of the left ventricle. The pericardium was full of blood, the aorta atheromatous, and the left coronary artery nearly obliterated. All the valves were normal. Dr. Mallet quotes Odriozola's statistics of spontaneous rupture of the heart. That observer could only collect 176 authentic cases. In many instances the patient was old, being between 60 and 70 in thirty-six, and between 70 and 80 in forty-five. The accident appears most frequent in women. As a rule, the escape of blood into the pericardium is considerable. The rent in the wall was unusually large in Dr. Mallet's case. In nearly every instance in Odriozola's statistics, the rupture was in the anterior part of the left ventricle. The original report of the case deserves study. The rupture apparently took place fifty-three hours before death, when the patient was seized with dyspnœa and epileptiform convulsions marked in the upper extremities ; his face turned pale.   The exertion of rising to micturate caused immediate death, probably by sudden escape of blood into the pericardium.   A similar history has been recorded in other cases of spontaneous rupture of the heart.—*Brit. Med. Journal.*

New Skin Remedies.—Schwimmer has lately, in the *Wiener Medizinische Wochenschrift*, published the results he has obtained in certain skin diseases by the use of salol, oxynaphthoic acid, salicylate of mercury, and anthrarobin. Salol mixed with starch in the proportion of two to one he finds a very effective remedy in all forms of venereal sores and in the buboes resulting from them.   Iodoform seems to have a more rapid action, but salol has the superiority of possessing no smell.   The drug also appears useful in conditions of the mucous membrane of the bladder, when given internally in doses of forty-five to ninety grains distributed through the day. Oxynaphthoic acid did not give good results in venereal cases, acting as an irritant.   In scabies, however, it did not irritate, and was an effective remedy.   It may be mixed with chalk and soft soap, each 10 per cent., with lard.   It acted well also in the secondary eczema of scabies, and allayed itching in prurigo.   Salicylate of mercury possesses no superiority over the ordinary remedies used in gonorrhœa and venereal sores. Given internally in doses of one and a half to two grains, it was an effective anti-syphilitic drug, although apt to cause irritation of the intestine and stomatitis.   Anthrarobin was found to have no beneficial effect in psoriasis, but in herpes tonsurans, eczema marginatum, and pityriasis versicolor it acted well, being mixed with collodion in the strength of one in ten.—*Brit. Med. Jour.*

TREATMENT OF CORNS.—The following is an extract from a standard English surgical text-book, which is much in use in England and America, but especially well-known in the neighborhood of Guy's Hospital : "Soft corns are best treated by taking away pressure by means of the introduction of *cotton* wool—that directly off the *sheep* being the best—between the toes, and the use of some dry powder, etc., etc."

THE

Montreal Medical Journal.

| VOL. XVIII. | AUGUST, 1889. | No. 2. |

THE MORTALITY OF ACUTE LOBAR PNEUMONIA.

Within the last twelve months or so attention has been drawn to the mortality rate of pneumonia, and several essays have been published mainly with the aim of demonstrating that the mortality for the last fifty years was steadily on the increase, and one of the writers attempted to prove that the present plan of treatment was mainly to blame. Hartshorne's figures were so arranged as to show an increase in the mortality from 6.25 per cent. in 1845–1847 to 31 per cent. in 1884–1886. The statistics of Osler collected from the Montreal General Hospital, as well as from others, show a different result, viz , in 1848–1850 a mortality of 37.9, and in 1878–1880 a mortality of 32 per cent. More recently Drs. Townsend and Coolidge of Boston have examined the records of the Massachusetts General Hospital from 1822 to the present date, making out a mortality for the whole number of cases taken of 25 per cent., but showing that the mortality has gradually risen from 10 per cent. in the first decade to 28 per cent. in the present. They argue that this increase is deceptive, and for the following reasons, all of which were shown to be a cause of a large mortality : (a) The average age of the patients has been increasing from the first to the last decade. (b) The relative number of complicated and delicate cases has increased. (c) The relative number of intemperate cases has increased. (d) The relative number of foreigners has increased

We may add to the above considerations some others which suggest themselves to us. Improved methods of diagnosis have enabled us to exclude other diseases producing symptoms resembling those of pneumonia, such as bronchitis and pleurisy, of which many cases in pre-stethoscopic days were probably counted in as cases of pneumonia, and so have reduced the mortality. The clinical thermometer has drawn the line between typhoid fevers of rapid onset and pneumonia. Some cases of typhoid fever with high temperature and cough bear a strong resemblance to pneumonia, and without a thermometer or a stethoscope a mistake might easily be made. Added to these, there are a number of cases of pneumonia met with in hospital practice, secondary to other morbid conditions, usually fatal ones, which now-a-days are recognized, while they may formerly have been classed as " shock," " blood-poisoning," " purulent infection," and the like. The only true method of comparing the results of treatment in different decades would be to select a number of cases of the same age, same sex, cases where there was no history of alcohol and no complication, and to exclude from this list all cases where the diagnosis had not been verified by post-mortem examination.

THE CREOSOTE TREATMENT OF PULMONARY TUBERCULOSIS.

At the present time the creosote treatment of pulmonary tuberculosis is attracting considerable attention. It is no new treatment, for it has been alternately used and discarded for more than a century as a remedy in pulmonary consumption. Some of the recent statements made as to its action by most authorities are of such a character that we consider it to be our duty to place them before our readers. Prof. Sommerbrodt of Breslau, in the current number of the *Therapeutische Monatshefte*, gives the result of his experience of the treatment of upwards of five thousand cases of pulmonary tuberculosis with creosote. Sommerbrodt advances very extraordinary claims for this drug. He says it not only is of marked value as a symptomatic agent, but that it actually is truly and directly curative. He claims that it so influences the diseased epithelial structures that they no longer are adapted for the proper nourishment of the tubercle bacilli ; that, in other words, creosote is an indirect as well as direct poison to the cause of the tuberculosis. The appetite improves, the expectoration lessens, and the cough becomes less troublesome are the results by the use of creosote. Guttmann maintains, from the result of experiments, that in order to bring about a directly poisonous action on the tubercle bacilli it is necessary to introduce into the blood a quantity of creosote that will bear the following proportion : creosote, 1 part ; blood, 4,000 parts. In an ordinary-sized adult this would require at least one gramme to be in the blood. Sommerbrodt claims that he is able to introduce into the blood that quantity of creosote. Details of a case are given where 5,400 creosote capsules, each containing 0.05, were taken between the 1st of September, 1888, and the 1st of June, 1889. In a period of eight months 270 grammes of creosote were used. The result was very marked. The author insists on the administration of large doses, for, in his experience, he finds little good from small ones.

CANADIAN MEDICAL ASSOCIATION.

The following papers are promised for the meeting of this Association at Banff, N.W.T., August 12th to 14th :—

(1) The Endemic Fever of the North-West Territories (Mountain Fever)—Dr. A. Jukes, Regina.

(2) The Climate of South Alberta, with special reference to its advantages for Patients with Pulmonary Complaints—Dr. G. A. Kennedy, McLeod, N.W.T.

(3) Traumatic Inflammations of the Eye and their Proper Treatment —Dr. John F. Fulton, St. Paul, Min.

(4) Hæmatonia of the Vagina and Vulva—Dr. A. H. Wright, Toronto

(5.) A Case of Empyema Successfully Treated by Free Incisions—Dr. James Ross, Toronto,

(6) The Early Recognition and Treatment of Epitholioma—Dr. L. Duncan Bulkley, New York City.

(7) The Relief of Pain in Eye and Ear Affections—Dr. R. A. Keen, Toronto.

(8) Sulphonal—Dr. James Stewart, Montreal.

(9) Nephro-Lithotomy—Dr. F. J. Shepherd, Montreal.

(10) Vertigo, an Eye and Ear Symptom—Dr. J. W. Stirling, Montreal.

(11) A Resumé of a few Surgical Cases—Dr. E. A. Proeger, Nanaimo, B.C.

(12) Varicella—Dr. Whitaker, Cincinnati.

(13) Renal and Vesical Colculi in the Museum of McGill University— Dr. Fenwick, Monreal.

THE CHAIR OF ANATOMY AT ABERDEEN.

The following names have already been mentioned as probable candidates for this chair, now rendered vacant by the resignation of Dr. Struthers : Dr. R. W. Reid, of St. Thomas's Hospital ; Mr. Arthur Thomson, M.B., of Oxford ; Dr. Symington and Mr. J. Macdonald Brown, of Edinburgh. We feel certain that were the profession in Canada allowed to vote, Dr. Reid would be the successful candidate. Successive generations of Canadian students who have attended the classes at St. Thomas's Hospital Medical School have found in Dr. Reid a sound anatomist, a good teacher, and a kind friend. The governors of the University of Aberdeen in appointing Dr. Reid will not only select an anatomist and teacher of the very first rank, but they will have the satisfaction of being able to fill this important chair from amongst their own alumni.

A GOOD MOVE.—The medical department of the University of Buffalo now demands a matriculation examination. True, it is not a very searching ordeal, but it represents, such as it is, the beginning of a movement to advance the general education of the profession in the United States. Students who join in the coming session will be required to pass an examination in arithmetic, geography, the elements of natural philosophy, and in English composition, including orthography, penmanship and grammatical construction.

Medical Items.

REPORT OF THE AUSTRALIAN COMMISSION ON M. PASTEUR'S PROPOSALS.

The Melbourne correspondent of the *British Medical Journal* writes that the Commission on Pasteur's method for exterminating rabbits has forwarded its report. While rabbits are killed by the addition of the microbes of chicken cholera to their food, the disease does not spread freely from infected to healthy rabbits. The disease in rabbits differs widely in this respect from chicken cholera as seen amongst fowls, where it is virulently infective. Fowls thus infected suffer not only from blood poisoning, but also from severe diarrhœa, and the droppings have power to spread the disease. On the contrary the infected rabbits with few exceptions, remain free from diarrhœa, and die of pure blood poisoning. The microbes are chiefly in the blood. If these microbes are to infect other rabbits in any number, the bodies of the rabbits dead from the disease must be broken up by decomposition or by the agency of carrion birds, etc., and the microbes so set free must contaminate the food of other rabbits. If the dead bodies lie in burrows, it will be remembered the rabbits do not feed there. If they lie open and the microbes are set free at a temperature of 125° or by the mere process of drying at a much lower temperature, it will suffice to destroy their virulence. Moreover, the experience of Dr. Katz indicated that while microbes retain their virulence for a time when mixed with putrifying matter, there is a limit to their power of survival. Generally, therefore, it appears that the destruction of rabbits on a large scale by the chicken cholera can be obtained only by feeding the rabbits with microbes of disease. Other poisons such as arsenic and phosphorus will kill the rabbits to which they are administered. The Commission cannot recommend that permission be given to disseminate broadcast through Australia a disease which has not yet been shown to exist in these colonies, and which in other countries prevails in disastrous epidemics among fowls, but which has never been known to prevail naturally among rabbits. The Commission has found no evidence to warrant the belief that any known disease can be so employed as to exterminate rabbits. Amongst other things the Commission found that chicken cholera will not affect domestic animals other than birds, and that wild birds are not so subject to it as fowls and rabbits. They are therefore not prepared to recommend the Government to forbid M. Pasteur to experiment with chicken cholera in an infested country, subject to certain restrictions. From this, however, Professor Allen dissents, as he objects to any such experiment.

TAR WATER.—The ghost of Bishop Berkeley would be delighted to find that tar-water is once more receiving attention and being used as a remedial agent in many diseases.

Tar-water contains thirty grains of tar to a quart of water. Locally it is unirritating, and slightly astringent and stimulating. Recently it has been used as an anti-septic injection in the puerperal state, as well as in leucorrhœa, vaginitis, pruritus vulvæ, and in chronic cystitis. Dr. Murrell has been using tar in the treatment of chronic bronchitis, and speaks of it in the highest terms. At first he used two-grain pills, but has latterly prescribed the syrupus picis liquidæ, U. S. P., of which the dose is about a tablespoonful given frequently. "A mixture of two parts of syrup of tar and one part of syrup of Virginia prune is an ideal cough mixture. It has a sweet, agreeable taste, and patients as a rule like it. When the cough is very irritable and there is very little secretion, the addition of three minims of liquor morphiæ acetatis will be found most useful. I have used with some success aromatic oil of tar, which is apparently a solution of tar in old Jamaica rum. The results have been good, and the preparation is popular with patients. When a more decided expectorant action is required, I add a small dose of hydrochlorate of apomorphine about one-tenth of a grain."

DEATH UNDER CHLOROFORM.—A man aged 36, described as an actor, died last week at the Middlesex Hospital when under the influence of chloroform. The evidence given at the inquest by the house-surgeon was that the deceased was first admitted in March last, when he remained in the hospital a month. Meanwhile chloroform was administered to him twice. On July 15th he again sought assistance. He was put to bed, and subsequently witness had administered about a drachm and a half of chloroform, when the deceased expired quite suddenly. Before he died he struggled violently. A post-mortem examination showed he had congenital malformation of the heart. Death was due to syncope while the deceased was under the influence of chloroform and suffering from a malformation of the heart and extensive kidney disease. The jury returned a verdict of "death from misadventure."—*Brit. Medical Journal, July* 27, 1889.

THE

MONTREAL MEDICAL JOURNAL.

| VOL. XVIII. | SEPTEMBER, 1889. | No. 3. |

Original Communications.

THE PRESIDENT'S ADDRESS

AT THE TWENTY-SECOND ANNUAL MEETING OF THE CANADIAN
MEDICAL ASSOCIATION, HELD AT BANFF, N.W.T.,
AUG. 12TH, 13TH AND 14TH, 1889.

BY H. P. WRIGHT, M.D.,
President of the Association.

Gentlemen of the Canadian Medical Association :

Contrary to the usual custom on such occasions as these, I
will ask you to share with me a few moments to consider the
loss the country, the profession, and the Canadian Medical Association have this year sustained in the death of Dr. Robt. Palmer
Howard. My reasons for alluding to this sad circumstance in
the very earliest stage of my remarks are, because of the long
standing and deep-seated affection I feel towards my teacher,
my friend, and my ideal physician, and because of the prominent
position he held in this Association and the feeling of admiration
entertained towards him by its every member. I wish, indeed,
I felt equal to the task of doing justice to such a theme as the
one I have now before me, but any attempt of mine must fall so
far short of even mediocrity, that I shall only try to outline some
of the principal events of his active and exemplary career. He
spent a portion of his youth in the city which has been my home
for the past twenty-three years, and those who recollect him
describe him tersely as having been upright, energetic, and
studious. These are the traits which characterized his youth
and which dwelt in the memories of those who knew him nearly

11

fifty years ago, and these are the traits which characterized his
life and made him what he was—a good Christian, a good citizen,
and a great physician.   In 1848 he graduated at McGill University, and then devoted about a year to hospital work abroad.
Soon after his return he was appointed demonstrator of anatomy
in his own college.   His teaching powers were soon recognized,
and in 1856 he was appointed to the chair of Clinical Medicine,
together with a position on the staff of the Montreal General
Hospital.   Later, on the death of Dr. Holmes, he was elected
to the chair of Practice of Medicine.   With this he became
identified.   For nearly thirty years not only did he lecture on,
but *taught* the practice of medicine.   As he eloquently discoursed
on some given disease, he artistically painted perfect pictures
and brought his subject so vividly before the student's imagination, that after contact with pathological conditions in the hospital wards he soon made himself, if he chose, master of the situation.   In 1882 he became Dean of the Medical Faculty on the
death of Dr. Geo. W. Campbell.   In this position, as in all others,
his far sight and good judgment, and his knowledge of the rapid
strides being made in every department of science, enabled him
to recognize the necessities of the times, and, with a steady and
unswerving hand, to develop the college into a great scientific
workshop, to be filled with busy teachers and demonstrators
rather than didactic lecturers.   When, in 1884, the present able
incumbent of the chair wholly relinquished the practice of his
profession for the teaching and culture of the department of
animal physiology, the Dean gave him and his subject the moral
support he so fully appreciated.   In alluding to the circumstance
in a brief obituary, Dr. Mills tells us he supported him with a
gigantic moral strength, which he felt like the " shadow of a
great rock in a weary land."   The University showed their high
estimate of the Dean's valuable work and conferred on him the
honorary degree of LL.D., but the greatest of all a teacher's
rewards is his, for he dwells for ever in the memories of the
hundreds of grateful students who received their early and most
valued instruction from his lips.   The Canadian Medical Association has certainly lost in Dr. Howard one of its bright and

shining lights. From its very birth until it attained its majority did he take a deep and active interest in its welfare, which, if shared in by even a tithe of the profession in Canada, would have made the Association a tower of strength in the country for the country's good and one of the world's recognized scientific institutions. With untiring zeal he tried to hold together the different elements of which every truly national society in this country must consist. He always maintained that science knew no creeds and had but one language, and that our French-Canadian *confrères* should have withdrawn themselves and have ceased to unite with us in advancing the interests of our common profession was to him a source of the deepest regret. In 1880 he was elected president of this body, and previous to that time held many offices of responsibility. To each and all he devoted the greatest attention, for he had no mentor equal to that of duty. He steadily fought for needed reforms through the medium of the national association, and faithfully, though unsuccessfully, endeavored to bring about the organization of a Central Examining Board for the Dominion, believing that such a scheme would be alike in the interests of the profession and the public. His regular contributions to the scientific part of our annual feast were listened to with pleasure, and I have no hesitation in saying, with profit, by every one who had the privilege of hearing them. His close reasoning, his familiarity with the latest researches, and his careful analysis of new theories, often filled the minds of his hearers with wonder. He possessed the great power of taking in the whole and separating the wheat from the chaff. In his private capacity as a physician I know of no words to describe him, and as a friend, my personal feelings demand absolute silence. How well he endeared himself to his patients by his untiring care and skilful management of their ailments, his naturally kind and sympathetic manner, and his ever faithful adherence to the truth, can in some measure be understood by all who know him. He died on the 28th day of March, after a fortnight's struggle with an attack of acute pneumonia—strange to say, the disease, perhaps of all others, with which he was most familiar, and of which he had been for many years a keen ob-

server and faithful recorder.   He was cut down in the midst of
his usefulness.   He fell at the post of duty : and it was better
so, for, to a temperament like his, a long sickness or a life of
inactivity would have been worse than death.

> " But when we muse on all thy great heart hunger
>   For knowledge and for light,
> How thy keen intellect was always searching
>   For deep things hid from sight,
> We smile to think how clear is now thy vision,
> · Thy face——how bright."

At the annual meeting of this Association in 1887, Dr. Graham
of Toronto, in his presidential address, earnestly advocated periodical rest and change for the steadily working medical practitioner.   His successor, and my immediate predecessor, feeling
that advice from such a source deserved attention, took a trip
in the summer of '88 to the Pacific coast, and was so impressed
with the panoramic magnificence of the country through which
he passed, and so strengthened and invigorated by the pure dry
air of these vast plains, that when it became his duty to address
the Association, he suggested, with a great deal of feeling, having the welfare of his *confrères* at heart, that Banff should be
our next place of meeting : so that to these two presidents are
we indebted for the trip we are now enjoying.   Who can say
he is disappointed ?   May we not justly expect to return to our
homes refreshed and strengthened in mind and body, readier
than ever for the varied and onerous duties our chosen and loved
profession demands of us.   Yet we must not forget that these
same healthful and invigorating surroundings justify us in expecting a great deal of this meeting.   Such a pure, bracing
atmosphere must quicken the wit, and such a rare combination
of the grand and beautiful in our surroundings must stir up
within us all that is eloquent and poetical.   This meeting will,
I hope, be characterized by good work and by brisk and fearless
discussion, for, no matter where situated, the voice of the Canadian Medical Association should be heard and its influence felt
throughout the whole length and breadth of our country.   I
hope that resolutions passed here to-day may affect legislation
in the near future.   It is high time our Parliaments recognized

Medical Associations, and if they do not, we ourselves only are to blame. And we are blameworthy, to our reproach be it said; for, are we not, as the belligerents of disease, the natural guardians of the public health? And should we not be a unit, not of apathy, but of earnest activity, in all matters of sanitary legislation? Can anyone for a moment imagine that if each medical practitioner would exert himself in favor of some one movement, which has for its sole objects the prevention of disease, the protection of the people and the prolongation of life, that that object would not soon be attained! Gentlemen, it is our duty to exert ourselves. It is our duty not only to support measures affecting the public health, but, as medical associations, to bring them before the notice of the different governments, and, as individuals, to gain the personal attention of our representatives in parliament, for surely we should be familiar with the necessities of sanitary reforms long before a body of legislators composed chiefly of lawyers, men of commerce and agriculturists. Let us then be up and doing, and while others go before the electors preaching national wealth, let our watchword always and for ever be—*national health.*

This brings me, rather sooner than I expected, to a subject which has often occupied my thoughts, and which has already, on several occasions, been alluded to from this chair—more particularly by the gentleman who occupied it in 1880. The great desirability, indeed the necessity, of establishing a Central or National Board of Health has long been felt by the profession, but until within the past year the question was never raised on the floor of the House of Commons. It has now been freely talked over by the medical members of Parliament, and a notice of the following resolution was given by Dr. Roome on the 11th of last March: "That, in the opinion of this House, the time has come when the Federal Government should establish a Central Board of Health, with a responsible head, for the purpose of educating the people in health matters, preventing the spread of disease, and perfecting, as far as possible, the return of vital statistics." The importance of such a movement as this can hardly be over-estimated. In the early history of this

Association many and lengthy were the discussions on this question, with, however, so little satisfaction, and at the cost of so much ill-feeling, that in its fourth year a resolution was brought in stating that as all matters of public health belonged to the Provincial Parliaments, the question should not, for the present, be discussed by the Canadian Medical Association. In 1880, nothing daunted, Dr. Howard again brought this matter before this Association, and so earnest was his appeal, and so clear and concise his plan, that when a national board of health becomes an actual fact his name should be for ever associated with its foundation. He suggested that each Province should have its own Board of Health, and that there should be a Central or National Board at Ottawa, all to work together for the public welfare. That amongst other duties should be assigned to the National Board " the preparing of a comprehensive plan for a national public health organization to be submitted to the Federal and Provincial Legislatures for their approval ; the obtaining information upon all matters affecting the public health ; the advising the several departments of the Government and the Executives of the several Provinces on all questions submitted to them, or whenever, in the opinion of the Board, such advice may tend to the preservation and improvement of the public health ; the securing the establishment of a board of health in each Province, whose functions shall be performed in accordance with the plan prepared by the central board ; the guiding, advising and assisting provincial boards, and securing their co-operation in the obtaining of regular periodical reports upon all matters of State medicine ; the combining and summarizing in annual reports all the information and facts contributed by the several provincial boards of health, and by any municipal organization or other source." Further on he says the board should consist of a physician, a surgeon, a physician with practical experience as a health officer, a chemist, a veterinarian, a statistician, and a sanitary engineer and architect, all first-rate men, and to receive compensation during the time when actually engaged in the performance of their duties. Here is a scheme which every one must admit is as practical as it is comprehensive. In Ontario to-day we have a board of health in good working order, faithfully performing its duties in guarding the health interests of its own Province. If each Province was equally well equipped, and all united to assist such a central board as I have indicated, the number of lives annually saved to the country would be very great, though difficult to estimate. Dr. Roome's scheme is much like that proposed by Dr. Howard. He tells me he purposes laying before the Federal Parliament a plan for the establishment of a Department of Health, presided over by a responsible head as a minister of health, or, if associated with the department of agriculture, or with the department of the Secretary of State, by a deputy minister, with an advisory board of, say, five or more of the members of the House, the majority being medical men. The department would have for its objects the education of the people in all matters of health, the prevention of the spread of disease, attention to sanitary regulations and the adulteration of food and drink, the perfecting of the system of collecting vital statistics, and the establishment of a hygienic laboratory for investigating the causes of disease. All these, with the exception of, perhaps, attention to sanitary regulations, come under the jurisdiction of the Federal Government. To a body of scientific men such as I have the honor to address, argument is almost unnecessary. That such a department, properly administered, must soon become a great life-saving, health-giving organization cannot be doubted. Bacteriology, though yet but a new and imperfect science, has already taught us that many of the most important diseases we meet with are communicable. Could the progress of tuberculosis, to which I shall have occasion to refer later on, alone be arrested, when we consider that over 15,000 of our people succumb to its lethal influence every year, the reward would be sufficient. The well-known epidemic and endemic diseases, some of which are constantly in our midst, and how far they could be controlled by prompt and effective legislation, I need not allude to. The great prophylactic properties of vaccination are admitted on all sides, and as long as the world lives will Jenner be regarded as one of the greatest benefactors of the human race ;

yet, as most of us hold that, with a better knowledge of the nature
of contagion and the laws governing contagion, smallpox ought
to be controllable, the necessity for inoculating each individual
with virus from a possibly tubercularized cow may be, in the
near future, open to question. Under such a department, whose
cause I am now maintaining, such important questions would
have to be considered. Such a bureau should be in communication with all others of a like kind throughout the world, for all
scientific institutions have a common cause ; so that, in addition
to the good gained by original investigation, such a body should
be an epitome of universal knowledge on all matters affecting
public health. Some will say that a department of this kind,
with such an extensive programme, could not be conducted with
the limited allowance likely to be granted to a new undertaking ;
but, if we regard the question in its proper light, the difficulties
are not insurmountable, for we, as a profession, ought to consider
ourselves one great department of health, ready, as individuals,
to devote some of our time and energies to the development of
its aims, and, through the medium of our Medical Associations,
to convey to our official chiefs in the central bureau information
from all parts of the Dominion. Now is the time to act. Let
us have petitions signed in every district throughout the country.
Legislators are willing to listen, and, among the medical members
of parliament, never was there " such a strong feeling aroused
as to the necessity of some central responsible body to look after
the health interests of the Dominion." The great merit of this
subject is my excuse for dwelling on it at such length. I hope
it may not prove to be a " vain repetition," and that my successor may be able to announce from this chair next year that
something has been accomplished.

With your leave I will touch again upon an old topic, and say
a few words on the Canadian Medical Association *as an organization*. It was framed twenty two years ago after the model of
the British Medical Association. It had to be built after some
model, and certainly none better could have been chosen than
that of the greatest of the world's medical societies. But the
circumstances of the two countries are so different—the mother

compact and thickly populated, so that every member is within easy touch, whereas we are scattered over an area equal in extent to the whole of Europe, with a population about the same as that of the city of London. In Great Britain nearly all the smaller societies are branches of the greater, and are governed by the same rules and regulations. Here, in the nature of things, each medical society is a complete entity, and no one is in any way related to the other. Though this may look like a commendable independence, it is a source of weakness, and cuts us off from a great deal of useful information. The Canadian Medical Association should be a more or less synthetical body, built up by representatives of every medical association in the country—not that I would exclude any registered practitioner. Let every medical man who can, feel it to be his duty to attend, but let us have delegates. I would suggest that the secretary of every medical association in the country bring, or send, a condensed report of the year's proceedings to be read at the annual meeting of the parent society ; that good papers be re-read and fully discussed—the papers would be new to many and the discussions more general and more valuable. I would suggest that the travelling expenses to the general meeting of the secretary be paid out of the funds of his own local association (excepting, probably, when we meet in the neighborhood of the Rocky Mountains). The amount of information thus to be gained would make these meetings extremely attractive and successful, for, believe me, though the social feature of these meetings is in nowise to be despised, few men will annually leave their homes and their work for such an inducement alone. Their health can be recruited at some more convenient place or in some more economical way. The only one lasting incentive is the amount of good gained, the number of new facts brought home, and the practical lessons learned. This only will command good attendance and ensure success.

Education, professional and general, has so often been dealt with, that I approach the subject with considerable hesitation ; and yet its importance compels me to bring it to your notice. I should like to remind you that we are all shareholders in this bank, whose capital is knowledge, and not till each one appreciates his responsibility can we expect to perfect a system of education already good, but not faultless. In Ontario the system of medical government is thoroughly representative, and as the council, elected every three years by the registered practitioners, has the appointment of the examiners for the license, and full control over the choice of subjects for examination, we should be careful to vote for the best men, and aid them in every way to raise the standard of education, as the growth of the country and the advancement of science render it necessary. This system has now been in working order for about twenty years, and is so successful that I cannot express a better wish for the sister provinces than that they may follow Ontario's example. Dr. Holmes, in his address in 1886, dwelt at some length on the importance of a more thorough and liberal early education. To use his own words : " The future of the medical profession in this as in every other country will largely depend upon the natural ability, and the mental and moral training in childhood and youth, of those entering its ranks ; so that in considering any scheme for the creation of a high standard of medical qualification, domestic training and the plan of education pursued in the public schools must be recognized as bearing an important part." And he goes on to tell us that, instead of children being taught to reason and think, their memories are overburdened with facts and figures. I am strongly of the opinion that elementary physiology and chemistry should be carefully and practically taught in our public schools, and that these subjects should form a part of the curriculum for the entrance examination to the study of medicine. Without some knowledge of these sciences, the student enters upon the study of his profession seriously handicapped, and the teacher labors under equally serious disadvantages. A greater part of the first year is wasted in becoming familiar with new terms ; such a loss as this cannot be sustained by a four years' course. The entrance or matriculation examination throughout all the Provinces is about the same, and represents a fair general education. This was well enough twenty years ago, but it is not enough now.

Such progress has been made in every department of science, that a higher and broader culture is necessary to those entering these fields of labor. Many consider a B.A. degree a necessary qualification, and with the increased facilities offered by our Universities, this is not, at least in the older Provinces, an impractical suggestion. No doubt some of our best men in medicine, particularly on this continent, had to battle against the opposition offered by the want of means in their early struggles. All honor *to them!* But these men are made of such stuff that success is part of themselves, and the mere increase of the standard of the entrance examination, even to such an extent as I have just mentioned, is only putting on another bar to the fence they have to climb; but for all that, the climbing will be successfully accomplished.

Of our medical schools in Canada we have good reason to feel proud. They are under the care and management of thoughtful, hard-working and self-sacrificing physicians and surgeons. In most instances the teachers are necessarily active practitioners, for few in our ranks have private means, and the instructors' pecuniary rewards are but pittances. As a country, we do feel proud of our schools, and, as a people, grateful to our teachers; but, we know, as institutions they are not yet perfect. These imperfections are not faults controllable by the teachers; they are the silent appeals to the wealthy and philanthropic. To quote from Dr. Alfred L Loomis in his magnificent address to the New York Academy last year : " Why is it that men of wealth do not realize their great opportunities for wise liberality in this direction, liberalities which will not only shed lustre upon themselves, but will mitigate the sum of human misery as certainly, and in many ways far more effectually, than our hospitals and charities for the sick and suffering poor.' He blames the profession for not having tried to direct the stream of accumulated wealth in this direction, for, " next to religion, education is the corner-stone of our civilization." Then, after alluding to the noble gifts recently made to some of the medical colleges, he is inspired by the hope that the stream of emotional benevolence for the sick and suffering is being turned into intellectual channels for higher educational needs. *We* have not yet to complain of emotional benevolence, as they have in the city of New York, where they have so many hospitals and dispensaries that patients are at a premium ; but we know that public attention has not been sufficiently directed towards the endowment of chairs in our educational institutions, for the provision for scholarships to help on the needy and industrious student, or for the establishment of a general fund for the purpose of erecting and maintaining laboratories at different points to further original investigation and research. All these are necessary if we are to have a perfect system of medical education " in order that those who teach may, by personal and familiar contact, gain such intimate knowledge of each student and firm control of his mental processes " as will enable them to become teachers in the good old Anglo-Saxon sense—to be educators, and not simply instructors " pouring out their daily dole of wisdom into unreceptive ears."

Within the past year several strong appeals have been made, through our medical press, in favor of more practical instruction, and that every student may have books in his possession giving a careful digest of the subject he is studying. The teacher's duty, in so far as the method of imparting knowledge is concerned, is changed. When books were scarce and biology was a nursling, twenty or twenty-five years ago, didactic teaching was a necessity and note-books were valued possessions. Now, our teachers should be expert demonstrators, appealing largely to the senses in the hospital wards and laboratories.

The question of reciprocity between the Provinces and between each and the mother country has frequently been before us, and last year a committee was appointed to make all possible enquiries and to report at this meeting. I am afraid such a report is not forthcoming, because of the scattered positions of the members of the committee. The matter is altogether in the hands of the Provinces, and whether it would be well or not to discuss the subject at this meeting in order to let the proper authorities know how we think about it is for you to decide. In this connection, I might mention that since our

last meeting the College of Physicians and Surgeons of the
Province of Quebec, under the presidency of Dr. Hingston of
Montreal, has succeeded in bringing about satisfactory recipro-
cal arrangements with Great Britain.

When it was decided that the Association should meet at
Banff, it occurred to me that, to be in tune with the place and
its surroundings, I might discuss at some length Canadian climatology and, in connection with it, the Canadian mineral springs.
These subjects had for me the attractiveness of novelty, as well
as being of some considerable importance; but the deeper I
dipped into the well from which I sought information on these
branches, the more difficult I found it would be to do them justice and not to tax the patience of even the most indulgent
audience. Those who are interested in the subject will find a
graphic and almost poetical description of the country and its
climate in Dr. Hingston's brochure entitled "The Climate of
Canada," and, I understand, a work will shortly appear on the
mineral springs of Canada by my painstaking fellow-townsman,
Dr. Beaumont Small, the author of the article on Medicinal
Springs in the *Reference Handbook of the Medical Sciences.*
That the first meeting of the Canadian Medical Association outside the limits of what is now known as the older provinces
should commend itself to our thoughts is most natural; and were
I not to devote some time and attention to the development of
the North-West and British Columbia from a medical point of
view, I should feel myself unworthy the position I occupy to-day,
and derelict in my duty, at least towards the nominating committee of last year. When we consider that the whole of this
vast country, as far west as the Rocky Mountains, but twenty
short years ago, was looked upon by the world, not excluding
Canada, as a barren waste, a great lone land unfit for civilized
human habitation, we must, indeed, be the prototypes of its
original inhabitants if we are not moved with wonder and surprise at the present extraordinary evidences of advanced modern
civilization as we passed through flourishing cities, active towns
and villages, great tracts of country under the highest cultivation, comfortable homesteads occupied by a healthy, happy and

thrifty people hailing from " all the four corners of the earth," and then, when we remember that we have been conveyed hither by a railroad spanning the continent, superlatively well equipped, and the most extensive in the world, and that its first sod was not turned fifteen years ago, we ought to feel proud of our citizenship. We must also acknowledge that this is a favored corner of the earth, designed by nature to be peopled by a great people. Practical observation has demonstrated to us the superiority of a high altitude, with a dry, cold and well sunlit atmosphere, over and above all others, to prevent the development of tuberculosis in those who are predisposed ; and the *curative* properties of medium altitudes with somewhat similar atmospheric conditions. How these atmospheres prevent and cure consumption is an interesting question for consideration. Till recently it was accounted for by Jaccoud's explanation, by bringing the idle portions of the lung into activity owing to the lessened supply of oxygen. Now it is more generally held to be owing to the absolute purity of the air—the absence of microbic life. Here we have the perfection of aseptic atmospheres—a condition recognized by the aborigines, who cure their meat by drying it in the sun without fear of putrefaction. It was also observed by our volunteer surgeons during the troubles of '85, who found wounds to heal, without special dressings, by first intention. This particular spot is most favorably situated, and seems to me to offer greater protection to the weak-lunged than to any other class of the ailing community—situated, as it is, at an elevation of 5,450 feet above the sea level, with a temperature never oppressively high and not subject to rapid diurnal changes, a freedom from moisture, an almost cloudless sky, and surroundings whose beauty and grandeur beggar description. Before, however, this section of the country can be regarded in the light of a first-rate sanitarium, a well-managed signal station will have to be established. This, I am satisfied, will not long be delayed by the Government. The mineral springs of this district, and from this to the Pacific coast, are said to be very numerous and mostly thermal. The best known are at Banff and Harrison's Lake. They enjoy a wide reputation, particularly for the treatment of syphilitic and rheumatic affections. Their waters are chiefly saline and alkaline.

Great as has been the material development of this new country, scientific and professional advancement have not lagged behind. Medicine is abreast with the others, and now in every settled part of these territories are to be found active and energetic doctors willing to work and anxious to grow with the country's growth. In the city of Winnipeg there are two hospitals, an insane asylum, and a medical college affiliated with the University of Manitoba. Belonging to the Province is the College of Surgeons and Physicians, which is composed of every registered practitioner, and is the sole licensing body. The medical college is well equipped and conducted by a staff of teachers of known ability and exceptional energy. By an Act passed in 1886, all the examining powers formerly belonging to the College of Physicians and Surgeons were vested in the Manitoba University, and in lieu thereof seven members of the College of Physicians and Surgeons became members of the Council. The requirements for the degree of M.D. are much the same as in the several universities of Ontario, including the matriculation examination. Having passsd the necessary ordeals elsewhere to the satisfaction of the Council, the candidate may register, when, on the payment of $25, he becomes a member of the College of Physicians and Surgeons of Manitoba. The presence of seven members of the College in the Council is a wise arrangement, as it guards the interests of the outside profession and makes a second examination unnecessary.

A perusal of the last report of the Winnipeg General Hospital leaves no room for doubt as to the good work being done by that institution. It is built according to the most approved methods, and, besides having a lying-in hospital and wards for contagious diseases in separate and distinct buildings, it has a well-appointed Nurses Home and Training School, built at a cost of $10,000, and accommodates twenty-two nurses. This is an excellent plan, and might with advantage be adopted by many of our eastern hospitals. I know of only one, the Toronto General Hospital, having such an annex.

The medical history of the North-West Territories is, though brief, not uninteresting. But a short time ago the only " medicine man" was the Indian, who used roots and herbs to heal the sick, and, in the words of a narrator, in all serious cases clothed himself in fantastic garments and invoked the bad spirits to leave their victims. In 1874 the first properly qualified medical men came into the North-West Territories with the mounted police, under the command of Colonel McLeod. Eleven years after, in the month of December, the Medical Act of 1885 became law. This Act was passed by the North-West Council, and shows a great deal of care and judgment. Under it a license was granted to all qualified men from other licensing bodies within Her Majesty's domains, and to those from the United States who could show that a full two years course had been taken. Even to those who had been practising without a license the Council gave an opportunity of passing an examination before two of its appointed examiners. In 1888 the Act of 1885 was repealed, and now the medical law is much the same as in Manitoba. Every registered practitioner is a member of the College of Physicians and Surgeons of the North-West Territories. There is a council of five elected every five years; an examination held annually, and fixed fines imposed on all the unqualified. So you see the people of these Territories have lost but little time in protecting themselves against the certain invasion of quacks and charlatans.

The Province of British Columbia was well known long before Confederation. The magnificence of its scenery, its grand mountains and rivers, its fine harbors, great mineral wealth, and delightful climate, have made the country familiar to every schoolboy. I hope some of the profession hailing from that envied province will give us facts relating to its climate, which, I have always understood, admits of as much variety as it does in that wonderful island whose northern extremity is John-'o-Groats and whose southern is the Land's-End. In it our profession is well represented, and working under a good Medical Act. The Council numbers seven, and is elected by the registered men of the province. It meets once a year, and during its sitting examines candidates.

That satisfactory progress has been made in the science of medicine during the past year is beyond dispute, and is of such an extent that even a short commentary on each new fact brought to light, or on the several new theories claiming our consideration, would lead me into regions beyond the limits of an address of this kind. There are one or two points, however, I feel called upon to allude to, and without any intention of interfering with the gentlemen who have been asked to address the Association on the different branches of medicine. Considering that we are, with very few exceptions, general practitioners, each one of us bound to give a great portion of his time to the practice of midwifery, it is to be regretted that so few papers are brought before the different medical associations by those whose opinions may be looked upon as more or less authoritative, because of special study or extended experience. I venture to say graduates, as a whole, go out into the world knowing less of this subject than of any other, and yet an obstetrical case is among the first they have to deal with. I do not propose to discuss the methods of teaching midwifery; it, like other branches of our profession, has of late years been more practically and properly taught. I claim that we should, at our different gatherings, talk more freely of and about what is new and good in this particular field of observation. The life-saving claims of antiseptics in midwifery are generally, I think I may say universally, recognized, and in some cases probably over-estimated, for, as Dr. Galabin aptly puts it, not even the most fashionable antiseptics of the day would be a sufficient compensation for allowing unnecessary lacerations of cervix or perineum, for omitting to secure good contractions of the uterus, for leaving a ruptured perineum unsewn, or for bruising tissues needlessly in operations. What accounts for the large mortality among children in footling presentations? I unhesitatingly say *ignorance* of the more recent methods of treatment. How often is the chin depressed without any regard to the position of the head in the pelvis, and how many know how to diagnose the position of the head? The recent opinions about extra-uterine fœtation, its early recognition and treatment, and the possibilities of faradization in such cases,

12

tain that blocked the way was reduced to a hill that might be climbed. Feeling that I must be brief, and in order to condense what I have to say, I shall make the following statements :

1. Koch's bacillus is the ever-present and irrefutable witness of tuberculosis.
2. So far, no difference has been discovered between the human bacillus and that of the lower animals.
3. It is capable of direct transmission, in the human being and in lower animals, from parent to offspring.
. It is communicable from man to man.
. It is also communicable among the lower animals.
. It is communicable from man to the lower animals.
7. It is found in all the domestic animals, more particularly among the bovine race.
8. It is communicable from animals to man.

That the bacillus is always present has been demonstrated by so many experts since Koch's announcement, that further proof is unnecessary. On the question of heredity, Dr. Johne of Dresdren gives the most conclusive evidence. He found an eight-months fœtus, taken from a tuberculous cow, to be affected with the disease. The placenta and uterus showed no visible signs of the disease, but in the lower lobe of the right lung a tubercle as big as a pea was detected, containing the characteristics of the disease. The bronchial glands and also the liver were affected, and microscopical examination revealed the tuberculous bacilli. In the child the tuberculous germ first appears under the name of scrofula. This is nothing but a particular form of tuberculosis, all of whose manifestations contain Koch's bacilli. Sometimes, indeed oftener than in the lungs, the tubercular disease shows itself in children in the brain or the intestines, producing meningitis or enteritis. We know, also, since the curious researches of Landwizy and Martin, that the placentary blood contains the germs of tuberculosis. The inoculation of that blood produced tuberculosis as if tuberculous matter itself had been injected. That the disease is transmitted from man to man cannot be doubted, though circumstances make direct experiment impossible. Yet the many instances in which a tuberculous husband

has affected a non-tuberculous wife, and the not infrequent instances in which the children of non-tuberculous parents successively become the victims of the disease, render further proof
on this point almost unnecessary.   There is a great deal of convincing evidence in favor of the next assertion as to its communicability among animals.   The histories of several well observed
outbreaks among herds are highly suggestive.   At the State
College Farm, at Orono, in Maine, in the autumn of 1885, a
cow was attacked with a husky cough, which increased in severity, and becoming much emaciated, she was killed about the last
of January, when her lungs were found to be badly diseased.
About the same time three others were affected with a slight
husky cough, and by the end of February most of the animals
in the herd commenced coughing almost simultaneously.   The
whole herd was ordered to be slaughtered, and an examination
made by Drs. Michener and Bailey revealed the fact that they
were nearly all affected with consumption.   There are several
familiar examples showing its communicability from man to the
lower animals.   Hens, by eating the sputa of a tubercularized
patient, have become tubercular.   Koch fed guinea-pigs on dried
tubercularized sputa which had been kept for two, four and eight
weeks, and in each instance tuberculosis was induced.   Brush
fed hens on tubercularized lung, and soon they became diseased.
It has lately been noticed that the disease prevails chiefly among
cows, and this to the human family, if it be communicable, is of
vital importance.   Considering that beef, milk, butter and cheese
enter so largely into our dietary, we may well be dismayed at
such a contemplation.   Dr. Brush of Mount Vernon, N.Y., in a
paper read before the New York Medical Academy in February,
1889, says that after several years of close study of the affection,
and consulting all accessible statistics and the habits of the people
where the disease prevails, the only constantly associated factor
is found, in his opinion, in the inbred bovine species, without any
regard to the social position of a community, its geographical
habitation, terrestrial or atmospheric condition.   He says if a
community *is closely associated with inbred cattle tuberculosis
prevails.*   Though Dr. Brush produces an enormous quantity of

evidence in support of his theory, some of which is very striking, it is not quite convincing. We might ask him, for instance, why the disease prevails among our North-West Indians? They have no cows! Yet that it does prevail among cows is undoubtedly the case; the circumstances of their surroundings favor the development of any such predisposition. Often kept in close stalls under the impression that the greater the amount of heat the greater the quantity of milk, fed on all sorts of swill, and sometimes allowed to remain in these places for years till their hoofs grow too big to allow of locomotion. The bacillus has been found over and over again in the milk of tubercular cows, though only where the udder is affected with tubercular disease. It is an undoubted fact that the close inbreeding of cattle favors the development of tuberculosis. The steer that took the prize at a recent exhibition in Paris was found tuberculous.

Is the disease communicable from the lower animals to man? This is *the* important question in connection with this subject, and though it has not been proved with certainty, yet, as the bacillus of man has been demonstrated microscopically to be the same as that of the lower animals, and as the disease it produces in each presents the same clinical features, even obeying the same laws of heredity, we must believe they obey the same laws of contagion. We know the disease is capable of being communicated to the lower animals through the ingesta and by the inhalation of divided particles of dried sputa; and we know it is readily transmitted by inoculation. Considering that the chemical and physiological conditions of domestic animals and man are sufficiently alike to afford to the bacillus the same means of cultivation, we should certainly adopt every possible method of protecting the human family against such a source of evil. Physicians and veterinarians must unite to battle the common enemy. Professor Ferland, of the Massachusetts Agricultural College, in an exhaustive paper, warns the community that the disease is intercommunicable between man and animals, *contagious* as well as *hereditary*, and is conveyed by using, for food, the milk or meat of diseased animals. In cases mentioned, he found, in public markets, that more than half the carcases showed signs of has affected a non-tuberculous wife, and the not infrequent instances in which the children of non-tuberculous parents successively become the victims of the disease, render further proof on this point almost unnecessary. There is a great deal of convincing evidence in favor of the next assertion as to its communicability among animals. The histories of several well observed outbreaks among herds are highly suggestive. At the State College Farm, at Orono, in Maine, in the autumn of 1885, a cow was attacked with a husky cough, which increased in severity, and becoming much emaciated, she was killed about the last of January, when her lungs were found to be badly diseased. About the same time three others were affected with a slight husky cough, and by the end of February most of the animals in the herd commenced coughing almost simultaneously. The whole herd was ordered to be slaughtered, and an examination made by Drs. Michener and Bailey revealed the fact that they were nearly all affected with consumption. There are several familiar examples showing its communicability from man to the lower animals. Hens, by eating the sputa of a tubercularized patient. have become tubercular. Koch fed guinea-pigs on dried tubercularized sputa which had been kept for two, four and eight weeks, and in each instance tuberculosis was induced. Brush fed hens on tubercularized lung, and soon they became diseased. It has lately been noticed that the disease prevails chiefly among cows, and this to the human family, if it be communicable, is of vital importance. Considering that beef, milk, butter and cheese enter so largely into our dietary, we may well be dismayed at such a contemplation. Dr. Brush of Mount Vernon, N.Y., in a paper read before the New York Medical Academy in February, 1889, says that after several years of close study of the affection, and consulting all accessible statistics and the habits of the people where the disease prevails, the only constantly associated factor is found, in his opinion, in the inbred bovine species, without any regard to the social position of a community, its geographical habitation, terrestrial or atmospheric condition. He says if a community *is closely associated with inbred cattle tuberculosis prevails*. Though Dr. Brush produces an enormous quantity of flesh does not contain any bacilli. Dr. Arlving contended that in his experience virulent bacilli existed in the muscles of tubercularized animals in one-fifth of the cases. He desired to see tuberculosis inscribed among the infectious diseases, and thought the flesh of tuberculous animals should be prohibited as food till means were found to render it harmless. He suggested the creation of a permanent committee to carry out, in cities and towns, the realization of a complete sanitary organization. It was learned that in Paris, Brussels, Constantinople and other large cities the meat is condemned if the disease is generalized and the cattle emaciated. After a lengthened discussion, which brought out a great many interesting facts in relation to the etiology of tuberculosis and its communicability, the following resolution was voted upon and carried almost unanimously : " It is necessary to carry out, by all possible means, including indemnification of those interested, the general application of the principle of seizure and total destruction of all meat coming from tuberculous animals, whatever may be the gravity of specific lesions found in those animals." Chauveau, president of the congress, suggested that simple instructions should be printed and widely distributed throughout the cities and towns and in the country, explaining the danger of drinking tuberculous milk and eating tuberculous meat, and the ways of rendering the meat inert. Though much has yet to be learned on this vital question, enough proof has already been adduced to warrant the adoption of active measures towards the extermination of tuberculous cattle. Is not the Government called upon to deal with tuberculosis as it does with pleuro-pneumonia ?

Gentlemen, I fear I have already shown too little consideration for my audience. Before concluding, however, I must say a word of welcome to our visitors. In the name of the Canadian Medical Association 1 beg to offer them the right hand of good fellowship. Though most of us have travelled from two to three thousand miles to attend this meeting, we do not for a moment forget that we are still in our own country. It is our earnest desire that they shall be one with us in everything, not only in this room, where we hope to hear from them on matters of professional interest and in discussion with full member's privileges, but on our further journeyings and in our social life. We cannot offer them the hospitality of our homes, but we can give them a warm welcome and earnest expression of the hope to see them again. We feel honored by the presence of so many eminent men from the United States, and can assure them that the dotted line, of which we heard so much the other night, does not separate them from us. We hope, in all seriousness, this visit may be one of thorough enjoyment, and that their personal experience and the information they may gain of this section of Canada may enable them to regard it as a health resort deserving of the highest consideration.

In thanking you for the great honor you have conferred on me by electing me your presiding officer for the ensuing year, I need not tell you how highly I appreciate this mark of your esteem and confidence. I am painfully conscious I have done nothing to merit the one or the other, and were I not consoled by my desire to perform the duties of the office to the best of my ability, by my loyalty to the Canadian Medical Association, and by the knowledge I possess of your forbearance and generosity, I should be inclined to insist on immediate retirement or retreat.

Retrospect Department.

QUARTERLY RETROSPECT OF SURGERY.

BY FRANCIS J. SHEPHERD, M.D., C.M., M.R.C.S., ENG.

Surgeon to the Montreal General Hospital; Professor of Anatomy and Lecturer on
Operative Surgery. McGill University.

Trephining for Cerebral Hemorrhage.—At a meeting of the
Clinical Society of London, held April 12th, 1889, Mr. Herbert
Allingham read a paper on a case of cerebral hemorrhage in
which trephining was done. The patient was shown. He was
a man, aged 40, who was admitted into the Great Northern
Hospital in the following condition: He had fallen off a tram-
car while semi-intoxicated and was taken into hospital. When
examined he complained of pain in the left shoulder, but there
were no external signs of injury to the head. Next morning,
Dec. 8th, he was rather drowsy, and complained of headache on
the right side of his head. The pupils were equal and reacted
to light. There were no signs of paralysis, and no vomiting.
On the evening of Dec. 13th his breathing was noticed to be
rather labored and stertorous, and he became more drowsy and
apathetic, not noticing things about him. At 6 A.M. he had a
convulsion. It began in the muscles of the left side of the face,
the mouth being drawn upwards, and the eyelids moved in clonic
spasm. The muscles of the neck were next affected, the chin
being drawn towards the right shoulder. Subsequently the left
arm and leg passed into a state of clonic spasm. The eyes were
not noticed to deviate to either side. Urine acid, no albumen
or sugar, and was passed unconsciously. There was no optic
neuritis. The fits recurred at frequent intervals. On Dec.
14th Mr. Allingham decided to operate. A curved incision was
made, ascending from the external angular process to the malar
process, and a large semi-lunar flap turned down so as to expose
the temporal muscle ; the muscle was divided from its origin
and also turned down ; a crown of bone was then removed over
the right fissure of Rolando—about 2½ inches behind and one
inch and a half above the external angular process. The posterior branch of the middle meningeal artery was exposed. The

artery and dura mater were found intact, but the dura mater bulged and did not pulsate. It was divided, together with the artery; a large blood-clot was exposed, and about three ounces of black clot removed by the finger and irrigator. On inserting the finger, the brain was felt to be compressed and the cavity extended forwards and backwards as far as the finger could reach. The pia mater was intact, except at the right frontal lobe, where the cerebral hemisphere was felt to be lacerated and soft. The cavity was well irrigated with carbolic solution (1–40), which came out clear. One catgut suture was introduced into the dura mater and two drainage-tubes inserted into the skull, one going upwards and the other downwards to its base; the ends were brought out through a hole mode in the lower part of the skin flap. The wound was dressed with carbolized gauze. Next day the patient had a slight fit, confined to the face. On Dec. 16th he was quite rational and began to move the left leg. On Dec 17th paralysis had gone; he moved both arm and leg well and was quite sensible. From that date he made an almost uninterrupted recovery. On Feb. 18th he left hospital quite well. Mr. Allingham was of opinion that the case was unique, as it was one of cerebral hemorrhage and not due to hemorrhage between the skull and dura mater.

Trephining for Spinal Injury.—At a meeting of the Medical Society of London, held April 8th, 1889, Mr. Herbert Allingham (*Lancet*, April 20th, 1889) read a paper on fracture of the spine treated by trephining. Two cases were reported. The first was injured by a fall of forty feet, and was completely paralyzed, having lost all sensation from a point on a level with the ensiform cartilages. As he did not improve a month after the accident, Mr. Allingham trephined the spine, making an incision about ten inches in length over the 5th, 6th and 7th vertebræ. The muscles were then turned aside and it was seen that the laminæ of the 6th vertebra was very badly fractured and depressed. The spinous processes and laminæ of the 5th, 6th and 9th were removed with cutting bone forceps, and the cord was exposed for about four inches; it was rather bruised. The theca was not opened, and the operation took one hour and a half. Sutures were put in the skin only ; no deep sutures were used. A large drainage-tube was inserted and antiseptic dressings applied. The wound healed in ten days, and for a while improvement took place, the line of sensation recovering to within an inch of the umbilicus, but since then it had remained stationary. In the second case the patient had fallen from a house and was paralyzed from a line seven inches above the umbilicus six days after the accident. No improvement occurring, the spine was trephined, and the spinous processes and laminæ of the 3rd, 4th, 5th and 6th vertebræ were removed. The cord was found crushed, so the dura was opened. In two weeks the wound had healed. The patient died seven months after the accident of bedsores and cystitis ; and at the autopsy the cord was found to be almost divided into two parts, both ends tapering down to a fine point. Mr. Allingham drew the following conclusions from these cases :

(1) That by trephining, it was evident from these cases that inflammatory ascending changes were prevented.

(2) That no bad symptoms followed from the opening of the spinal dura mater and allowing the cerebro-spinal fluid to escape.

(3) The operation, though tedious, is not a difficult one to perform, and does not in any way diminish the chance of recovery.

He suggested that in all cases of spinal injury followed by paralysis and loss of sensation, trephining should be done at the end of a week if the patient showed no sign of improvement, so that if symptoms were produced by pressure of blood on displaced bone they might be removed before ascending and descending changes came on.

In the discussion which followed the reading of the paper, Dr. Beevor alluded to the difficulties that arose in consequence of the fact that the anæsthesia began much lower down than the seat of injury would lead one to suppose. He said that the question as to the points in the cord at which the sensory fibres were given off required elucidation.

Mr. Shattock has lately been working at this point, and has arrived at fairly definite conclusions as to the origin of the sensory nerves.

Mr. Wm. Thorburn of Manchester publishes a short note on *Spinal Localizations as indicated by spinal injuries in the lumbo-sacral region.* (*Brit. Med. Jour.*, May 4, '89.) From an analysis of a number of cases of spinal injury, certain definite conclusions as to the functions of the various nerve roots have been published in the form of a table.

Subdural Division of Posterior Roots of Spinal Nerves.— Mr. W. H. Bennet, at a meeting of the Royal Medical and Chirurgical Society of London, held April 23rd, 1889, read a paper on a case in which acute spasmodic pain in the left lower extremity was completely relieved by subdural division of the posterior roots of certain spinal nerves, all other treatment having proved useless, and in which death resulted from sudden collapse and cerebral hemorrhage on the twelfth day after operation, at the commencement of apparent convalescence. A laborer, aged 45, was admitted into St. George's Hospital, under Mr. Bennet's care, August 29th, 1888, suffering from acute pain, sometimes spasmodic, in the left leg, apparently due to syphilitic thickening of the tibia of nine years duration. The patient was submitted to the following treatment without relief, viz , (1) the administration of drugs, *e.g.*, iodide of potassium, mercury, anodynes and narcotics ; (2) trephining and linear osteotomy of the thickened tibia; (3) amputation through the knee-joint; (4) stretching of the sciatic nerve ; (5) resection of two inches and a half of the same nerve. By December 8th the patient's condition was much worse ; he had lost strength and was much emaciated, the pain was much worse, the spasms being violent and frequent. By Dec. 23rd it was clear that death must soon ensue if the suffering could not be relieved by some surgical proceeding. Mr. Bennett therefore proposed to lay open the spinal canal, examine the membranes and, if necessary, the cord itself over the region of the lumbar enlargement in order to see whether any lesion existed. In the event of this exploration proving negative in result, it was proposed to divide the posterior roots of these spinal nerves, the distribution of which seemed to correspond to the areas over which the pain was felt. The operation was performed Dec. 24th, and the pos-

terior roots of the 1st, 3rd, 4th and 5th lumbar, and 1st
and 2nd sacral nerves being divided. The patient was entirely
relieved of his pain. For two days the patient's condition was
critical, and later there was troublesome diarrhœa. By January
3rd the wound had healed, except a small sinus which discharged
cerebro-spinal fluid. On the 4th, patient felt discomfort in his
head, vomited, became collapsed, and died in a few hours. At
the autopsy a large clot was found over the left occipital lobe of
the brain. The cord was healthy, but opposite the 7th and 8th
dorsal vertebræ was a well-defined thickening of the arachnoid.

Prof. Korteweg (*Archiv für Klin. Chir.*, Hft 4, '89), in an
interesting article on *Statistical Results of Amputation of the
Breast for Cancer*, shows from the tables of Winiwarter, Olde-
kop, Sprengel, Hildebrand and Küster that recurrence is more
frequent in cases operated on early, and that the whole length
of life after operation is shorter. He explains this by stating
that the more malignant the cancer the earlier it is operated on
the earlier it returns. In these cases the glands are usually
affected early. He states that the great majority of the cases
of return occur in the cicatrix and seldom in the glands of the
axilla. In the more malignant and rapid cases the glands are
early affected. In the more benign cases, where the glands
have not become involved, extirpation of the breast alone has
been followed by a comparatively large number of cures.

Some years ago, according to statistics, a much larger number
of cases existed of simple cancer of the breast without involvement of the axillary glands. In 1870, in 60 cases of breast
cancer, there were 24 where the axillary glands were not
affected ; in two only of the 24 cases was there a permanent
cure. At present, in 60 cases, only 10 are without involvement of the glands, and out of these, two are permanently cured.
He explains this by the fact that now the glands are removed
when they are not actually involved but merely inflamed, when
formerly they would not have been removed. Hence the result
is the same. The 14 additional cases which were regarded as
simple mammary cancers would now, because the glands are felt
to be slightly enlarged when the axilla is opened, not be re-

garded as simple, hence there apparently existed a larger number of cases where the glands were not involved than at present. Again, formerly very severe and advanced cases were not operated on as at present. He urges strongly the thorough removal of the growth locally as well as the axillary glands, and favors early operation in all cases.

On the Causes of the Local Recurrence of Cancer after Extirpation of the Mammary Gland.—Dr. Heidenhain of Berlin, at the recent congress of the German Society of Surgery in Berlin, read a paper on the above subject. (*La Semaine Médical*, May 1, 1889, and *Medical News*, June 1, 1889.) He had made a histological examination of eighteen cases of cancer of the mammary gland for primary cancer. In all cases in which there had been a recurrence he was able to make out by microscopical examination that fragments of cancer had remained in the wound after operation. If it is easy to see infiltrated lymphatic glands, it is not easy to see by the naked eye if the tumor has been completely removed. In the eighteen cases which he examined, he had tried to ascertain whether in the section of the tumor which was in contact with healthy tissues he would find healthy or diseased tissues; on the presence of healthy or diseased tissue would depend the recurrence of the disease. He had in this manner examined several fragments of each tumor; in twelve cases he had found the tissues infiltrated with epithelial rays, and out of these twelve cases there had been eight recurrences, one death, one patient had disappeared, and two others remain well. In six cases he had found only healthy tissues, and in those six cases up to date the cancer has not reappeared. In cancer of the breast, the epithelial extensions follow the lymphatic vessels and extend often to the pectoral aponeurosis; it is therefore most important to take away the aponeurotic covering of the pectoral muscle, and even to cut into the muscle so as to be sure that the lymphatic vessels, which cross the aponeurosis perpendicularly, are not infected. Dr. Küster has been in the habit of taking away this aponeurosis, because of the bad prognosis presented by cancerous tumors which are adherent to the pectoral aponeurosis. In Von

Volkmann's practice, out of sixty-five cases in which the tumor was adherent to the pectoral aponeurosis two were cured, and in all the others the disease has returned.   Out of twenty-one cases of the same kind operated on by Küster but a single one is still alive, and she had a return of the trouble ; hence when the tumor is adherent, it is well to take away a good part of the muscle and to clean it thoroughly so as to be sure that the whole growth has been removed.

Statistics of Cancer of the Breast.—Dr. Fink of Prague has collected the histories of 194 cases of cancer of the breast treated in Prof. Gussenbauer's wards from 1878 to 1886, tracing after histories to the end of September 1888.   He found that at the 41st year the frequency of cancer suddenly increased, slowly rising towards the age of 60 ; 128 of the cases occurred between 40 and 60, 38 between 60 and 80, and 28 between 20 and 40. Activity of the sexual functions had a marked etiological influence, especially in regard to long periods of activity of the functions of the mammary glands ; 72.1 per cent. of all cases had borne children, 62.8 per cent. had suckled them.   In 22 per cent., mild or severe inflammatory disease had attacked the affected breast.   In only 12.7 per cent. could a clear history of injury or prolonged mechanical irritation be obtained.   Direct hereditary predisposition was only substantiated in 8 out of 194 cases.   Both mammæ were affected with equal frequency.   The disease was found to begin in the superior external segment of the breast in a very large majority of the cases—in 104 out of 171 which were carefully and early inspected.   In 53 cases, metastases were detected on an average of twenty-five months after the beginning of the disease.   These were situated in the pleura, lungs and liver.   One hundred and fifty-three of the cases underwent amputation of the breast with clearing out of the axillary glands ; the mortality was 3.3 per cent.   Ninety of the cases died of recurrence of the cancer, but Dr. Fink states that most of the women did not apply for relief until the disease was far advanced ; 21.6 per cent. remained free from the disease for two years, and 16 per cent. for three years.   The patients who had undergone operation lived seven months longer than those whose breasts were not removed.—(*British Medical Journal*, June 1, 1889.)

Dr. J. Collins Warren, in an article on the *Diagnosis and Treatment of Cancer of the Breast* (*Boston Med. and Surg. Journal*, April 11, '89), says that the most important part of the operation for removal of cancer of the breast is the careful dissection of the fascia from the pectoral muscle, for it is in this tissue that capillary lymphatics are concealed, which form hiding places for the outposts of the disease. Careful attention should also be paid to the margin of the pectoral muscle; not only should the fascia which covers the axilla be dissected off from it, but its lower border should be well freed from fat and connective tissue. The axilla is best opened by a cut through the skin along the edge of the pectoralis, until we come to the edge of the coraco-brachialis; continuing down on this muscle a short distance with the knife, the skin and superficial fat drop away sufficiently to disclose the great vessels lying beneath a thin fascia; opening this fascia backward along the line we have come exposes the contents of the axilla, and especially the branches of the vessels, which can now be secured. A pyramidal mass of fat is now dissected out, the apex reaching sometimes to the clavicle, the base frequently extending deeply into the subscapular group of muscles. The glands which lie near the clavicle will have to be removed separately, and can best be enucleated from the neighborhood of the vessels by the finger. If they are numerous, the pectoralis can be separated on the line selected for the ligature of the axillary artery below the clavicle, and the glands and some of the loose tissue can then be readily removed.

Excision of the Scaphoid for Flat-foot.—Mr. Richard Davy (*Lancet*, April 9th, 1889) says that this static deformity is so commonly met with in debilitated subjects as to suggest many points of consultative interest. He referred to Prof. Ogston's paper read before the Medical Society of London in January, 1884, on *Flat-foot and its Cure by Operation*, which recommended the excision of the astragalo-scaphoid articulation in a wedge-shaped manner and pegging the scaphoid and astragalus together, and stated that Prof. Ogston's paper led him to again investigate the subject. The result was that he found that excision of the scaphoid fulfilled all the requirements necessary and resulted in giving the patient a useful foot. Should any difficulty be experienced in removing the scaphoid, the easiest plan is to chisel the bone in a wedge-shaped form and then carefully clean the bone out, leaving the cartilage on the head of the untouched as well as the cartilage on the cuneiform bones. The foot is then wrenched inwards so as to press back the astragalus into place, and make the cartilage of the astragalus touch the cartilages of the cuneiform bones. No little spicula of bone must be left behind between these two opposing sets of cartilages. The utmost cleanliness, of course, should be observed, and after the first stage of inflammation is passed a plaster of Paris splint is advocated. The operation is reserved for advanced and rare forms of club-foot only, where bony deformity and dislocation have occurred, and the distortion cannot be reduced by the manual efforts of the surgeon.

Mr. Golding Bird (*Lancet*, April 9th, 1889), in a paper on *Operations on the Tarsus in Confirmed Flat-foot*, says there is a class of cases where the arch is so fallen that a convexity rather than a flatness takes its place, due to two tubercles projecting downwards the scaphoid and head of the astragalus ; along with these objective symptoms there is a most wearying and constant aching under the external malleolus. The pain is always present on standing, and after a few hours it becomes a physical impossibility to stand any longer. The continued deep-seated pain the author declares to be due to the fact that, since the arch of the foot is sunken and its piers are now wider apart on the inner side of the foot, a corresponding crowding or mutual pressure of the bony structures forming the outer or supporting edge of the sole takes place, which mere reposition of the foot will not improve. It is in these cases tarsotomy in some form is called for. Mr. Bird operated on four such cases in 1878-80. All were between 12 and 17 years of age. In two the scaphoid bone was removed, and in the other two the scaphoid and head of astragalus. In all the results were good ; all were relieved of pain, but in only one was the arch restored.

Inflammation of the Seminal Vesicles.—Every surgeon has met with cases of supposed prostatis and cystitis which resist all treatment. Frequent and painful micturition characterizes these cases, and they go from one surgeon to another seeking relief but not obtaining it. Such cases are always obscure and most commonly follow an attack of gonorrhœa. An explanation of this condition is offered by Mr. Jordan Lloyd. In an article published in the *British Medical Journal* of April 20th, 1889, he calls attention to the part played by inflammatory disease of the seminal vesicles in these obscure cases of vesical prostatis one so often meets with. He considers " seminal vesiculitis" analogous to Fallopian salpingitis, and states that this is dependent on similar causes. The disease is usually secondary to simple or gonorrhœal urethritis, the latter constituting the most frequent cause. It may also follow simple urethritis due to the passage of a sound, urethral stricture, or coitus with a woman suffering from leucorrhœa. It is also common as a complication of gonorrhœal epididymitis. The severe type sometimes, but not frequently, ends in suppuration. The tendency is to resolution, but if suppuration occur, pus may burrow laterally into the ischio rectal fossa or into the deep circumrectal tissues, or it may escape by the ejaculatory duct, or the abscess may rupture into the bladder or rectum. The disease sometimes runs a chronic course, and results in cystic enlargement of the vesicle due to obstruction of the duct. In one of Mr. Jordan's cases the cyst contained ten pints of fluid. The symptoms of " seminal vesiculitis " are essentially those characteristic of vesical irritability, inflammation of the neck of the bladder, and of acute prostatitis, with the additional symptoms of almost constant painful erection of the penis. Nocturnal emissions are common, as is also blood in the seminal fluid. Physical examination per rectum reveals the presence of an elongated tumor, situated above the prostate, at the base of the bladder, running obliquely upwards and outwards. The presence and size of this tumor are made more manifest to the exploring finger if a large metallic sound is passed into the bladder and moved from side to side over the tumor. In the acute form, heat, tenderness and swelling are felt over the prostate, and if accompanied by the symptoms of vesical irritability, with no urinary evidence of cystitis, this sign should make the diagnosis certain. Mr. Lloyd recommends incision through the perineum rather than through the rectal wall for evacuation of pus when suppuration occurs. He urges digital examination of the rectum in all cases of gonorrhœa or epididymitis which present vesical symptoms, and believes that in most of such cases this disease will be found.

The subject is one of great interest to surgeons, and it is hoped that more light will be thrown on the subject by investigations which are sure to follow the publication of Mr. Lloyd's paper.

Surgical Treatment of Pulmonary Cavities.—Mr. J. D. Harris (*Brit. Med. Jour.*, May 4, 1889) reports the case of a gentleman, aged 33, who, in 1887, suffered from abscesses of kidney, which broke in four or five places in the loin, and from which he was convalescent, when in March, 1888, he was seized with a rigor, and a pneumonia of the left lung rapidly developed. The pneumonia ran a very unfavorable course, and instead of undergoing resolution, broke down into abscesses. In May he was rapidly emaciating, and had an incessant hacking cough with considerable expectoration, which, towards the end of the month, became fœtid.   There were now all the physical signs of a cavity of the lung posteriorly, just below the angle of the scapula, on the inner side. By the end of June he was in a highly critical condition and was much run down. Operation was advised and consented to. On July 2nd, without any anæsthetic, an incision was made through the skin at the lower border of the intercostal space, which ran through the centre of the area of loudest pectoriloquy. An aspirating needle was introduced, and pus flowed through the tube ; the tissues were now cut through down to the pleura ; this was then cut through, and following the aspirating needle the lung was incised. A silver tube was introduced and afterwards a large gum-elastic catheter. Considerable discharge came away. On account of the fœtor the cavity was daily syringed out with a weak solution of carbolic acid. The tube was kept in a month, and then a rubber tracheotomy tube was substituted. The patient went on well. His cough ceased and he increased in weight. By Christmas, 1888, only one small renal fistula existed, and the pulmonary fistula had completely healed.

Renal Surgery.—The progress of abdominal surgery has been especially marked of late by the increasing number of records of operations on the kidney. Since Mr. Thomas Smith, twenty years ago, advocated the removal of a renal calculus by operation, and Professor Simon proved, after making a series of experiments on dogs, that the removal of one kidney did not necessarily produce acute or chronic disease of its fellow, a whole series of operations on the kidney have come into vogue. There are nephrorrhaphy, or sewing up a floating kidney by its capsule to the parietes ; nephrotomy, or incision of the kidney ; and, lastly, nephrectomy, or removal of the kidney entire. Notwithstanding the truth of Simon's theories, and the encouraging results claimed by several surgeons, nephrectomy must still be considered a very serious undertaking.

There is a great difference of opinion amongst the few really experienced operators as to the right manner of performing nephrectomy. Some, like Mr. Lucas, advocate the lumbar, and some, like Mr. Thornton, the abdominal incision. An instructive discussion took place at a meeting of the Royal Medical and Chirurgical Society on April 9th, 1889. Mr. Lucas considered it necessary to estimate for some time the amount of urea excreted daily. If this were found to be less than half the normal quantity, then nephrectomy, he maintained, would be a very serious operation. Mr. Knowsley Thornton said that if a large suppurating kidney be treated medically, not surgically, the labor thrown upon its fellow would be possibly greater than that entailed by the operation ; he also quoted one of his cases where both kidneys were diseased, yet when one containing twenty pints of pus was removed, the operation was borne well. To form anything like a correct estimate of the excreting power of the healthy organ in cases where the diseased kidney is not absolutely obstructed is very difficult in actual practice. Dr. Tuchmann's ureter forceps, for temporarily blocking the orifice

of one ureter for a time, may prove of service, but many find
them difficult to apply. Catheterization of the ureter, practised
by Newman of Glasgow, and others, requires much special training. Lastly, physicians, physiologists and chemists have possibly
more to discover as to the import of each constituent of the
urine. As yet, much in respect to calculating the powers of a
healthy kidney when its fellow is diseased is theoretical or
empirical.

Separation of the Lower Epiphysis of the Femur.—In an
interesting article on this somewhat rare accident by Mr. Mayo
Robson (*Annals of Surgery*, Feb. 1889) the meagre description
given by surgical authors is alluded to. He does not think the
accident is as rare as the standard works on surgery would lead
us to believe. In the museum attached to the Yorkshire Medical
College two interesting specimens exist. In both, amputation
was performed for gangrene. The epiphysis lies with its articular
surface forwards, and the lower end of the shaft of the femur
(the diaphysis) is directed backwards and presses on the popliteal
vessels ; the gastrocremius is attached to the diaphysis. The
second specimen was from a primary amputation of the thigh
performed by the late Mr. Samuel Hey on account of a compound diastasis of the lower epiphysis of the femur. In this
case the lower end of the diaphysis projected through the wound
in the popliteal space, whilst the epiphysis was directed forwards.
Mr. Robson relates a case which came under his own observation.
A boy, aged 16, was kicked by a horse on the outer side of the
left knee-joint. When admitted to hospital there was considerable swelling with fluctuation around the knee. The leg and
foot were enormously swollen. The foot everted and the leg
rolled outwards. No pulsation could be felt in the tibial arteries,
the circulation being interrupted by the sharp edge of the lower
end of the diaphysis of the femur, which was pressing on the
popliteal vessels and making the skin bulge in the popliteal space.
The joint was in a state of semi-flexion, and extension was most
painful. A marked depression was felt immediately above the
patella, beneath which could be felt a movable mass with rounded
edges. There was one and a half inches of shortening. Under

ether the leg was fully flexed and the parts forced into proper position, then the leg was extended and placed on a McIntyre splint. Pulsation at once returned in the tibial vessels and the engorged vessels emptied themselves in a few hours. Two months after the leg could be fully flexed and there was no deformity. Mr. Robson mentions two other cases in the practice of his colleagues, in one of which excision was performed, and in the other a good result followed reduction. In most cases the diagnosis is not difficult. The shortening of from one to two inches, the projection of the lower end of the diaphysis into the popliteal space, the displacement of the epiphysis in the front of the femur, and the interference with the circulation of the leg, form a group of symptoms which are not easily mistaken. The prognosis is serious unless the injury be diagnosed and treated at once ; the dangers arise from the pressure of the lower end of the diaphysis on the popliteal vessels, interfering seriously with the circulation of the leg and producing great œdema or gangrene. In one case reported secondary hemorrhage ensued.

Mr. Robson draws attention to the fact that this injury differs from transverse fracture of the lower end of the femur ; in transverse fracture the upper end of the lower fragment projects into the popliteal space, whereas in diastasis the lower end of the upper fragment projects into the space. The treatment is reduction under ether, and if reduction is impossible, excision. I have seen two cases of this accident. In both the accident had occurred several years before, and the patient had good use of the limb. One case under the care of one of my colleagues, the diaphysis had been displaced outwards and caused a remarkable obliquity and deformity of the lower end of the femur which interfered with the lad's progression. The limb was straightened by Macewen's osteotomy. The other case was kindly shown to me by Dr. Elder of Huntingdon. A boy, aged 7, fell and injured his leg. When the doctors arrived they found the lower end of the femur projecting through the flesh on the outer side of the popliteal space. They advised amputation, but this being refused, and failing to reduce the protruded bone, they sawed off two inches. The boy ultimately did well, and was able to go about in three months. Now (ten years after the accident) he has perfect use of his leg, and the knee has as wide a range of motion as the other. He walks with only a slight limp, and measurement gives some two inches of shortening.

Extirpation of Goitre.—Dr. Eugene Hahn (*Archiv f. Klin. Chir.*, bd. 36), in a paper on a *Method of Partial Removal of Goitre without Tamponade or great loss of Blood*, says this method has been carried out on several patients affected with struma. A median incision is made from the incisura jugularis to the cricoid cartilage; to this is added a lateral incision dividing the sterno-hyoid and sterno-thyroid muscles, and then the superficial veins are ligated. In this way the whole gland is exposed. The left upper lobe is then released and lifted forward, the left superior thyroid artery tied; the inferior thyroid is clamped, and the middle artery tied by first exposing it in lifting forwards the gland and then passing a ligature about it. The same is done on the opposite side. After securing these vessels the capsule is divided in its whole extent, avoiding visible veins, and the glandular tissue is drawn forward with a hook. It is thus possible to remove sections of the gland with scissors so as to leave very little behind. There is very little hemorrhage. The inferior thyroid arteries are only secured by a clamp having a weak spring; this is done to avoid securing the recurrent nerve in a ligature. If disturbance of speech follows the operation, the clamps can be immediately removed. A weak clamp will control the circulation, but not injure the nerve. The wound should be stuffed with iodoform gauze, the clamps removed at the end of twenty-four hours, and secondary sutures applied.

Resection of Intestines.—At the meeting of the Edinburgh Medico-Chirurgical Society, held Dec. 5th, 1888, Mr. Cotterill reported a successful case of *Resection of a Gangrenous Transverse Colon*. The patient, a very stout woman, aged 38, had been subject to umbilical hernia for seven years. When seen by Mr. Cotterill she was seven months pregnant. The rupture was a bright red and angry-looking prominence about 14 inches in diameter. The patient vomited coffee-colored fluid mixed with blood. The sac was opened and found to contain a large coil of gangrenous transverse colon, much sloughy omentum and free from fæculent matter. The gangrene appeared to be due, not to strangulation, but to pressure of structures in the sac between the pregnant uterus below and a firm binder which had been worn above. Fifteen inches of colon were cut away and the ends of the gut stitched to the edge of the skin-wound. Three days after the operation the woman gave birth to a child. A few months later an operation was performed for uniting the cut ends of the intestine. The upper end was first ligatured to avoid the escape of fæces. Traction was then made on the two ends until normal gut, covered with peritoneum, protruded sufficiently for resection. Instead of using a clamp, the operator passed a piece of thin India-rubber tubing through a small hole in the mesentery and round the gut, fixing it there with a pair of catch-forceps. Four inches of the upper segment of the colon and three of the lower were then cut away with portions of the mesentery. As the lower portion had been unused for five months it was very narrow and hard to join to the upper piece. By careful introduction of over 100 stitches, the ends were brought satisfactorily together. Fine curved needles were used, round, not flattened, and threaded with fine Chinese twisted silk, and the Czerny-Lembert suture was employed. The cut edges of the mesentery were sutured together, and the gut returned to the abdomen. The operation took three hours. On the third day fæces passed. In the two operations 22 inches of intestines were removed.

I have space only to refer to the following :—

A Successful Case of Immediate Resection of the Intestine for Gangrene, by Robert H. M. Dawbarn, M.D. (New York *Medical Record*, April 20th, 1889.)

Resection of Gangrenous Intestine occurring in Strangulated Herniæ, and the Report of a Successful Case : by A. J. McCosh, M.D. (New York *Medical Journal*, March 16, 1889.)

Free Division of the Capsule of the Kidneys for the Relief of Nephralgia.—At the recent meeting of the American Surgical Association, held in Washington, May 1889, Dr. McLane

Tiffany read a paper on the above subject. The author had suggested this mode of treatment four years ago. The patient was a married woman, aged 49. Had gonorrhœa and syphilis. Three years ago had a severe and sudden pain in right loin. These attacks occurred at regular intervals, the periods becoming shorter and pain more severe. Blood was seen at rare intervals ; pain was characteristic from loin to groin increased by exertion. Pressure over right kidney caused severe pain. No tumor could be made out. Kidney calculus was diagnosed and operation was performed January 12th, 1889. The kidney was reached and incised, and a sound passed into its pelvis and a systematic exploration made, but no stone detected. The capsule was freely slit open for three inches and the wound closed. It soon healed. Since the operation no attacks of pain had been felt. In the discussion which followed the reading of the paper, several similar cases were related, several speakers stated that the relief of pain was often only temporary.

I very much doubt the existence of these cases of nephralgia. In nearly all these cases a stone would be found if thoroughly searched for. It has been my misfortune to cut down several times on the kidneys and fail to find a stone. The kidney was always explored in the usual way by sound, needles, and touch. In some of the cases pain was relieved, in others not. In a case where I cut down on the kidney in November, 1888, I failed to find a stone, the pelvis of the kidney was thoroughly explored with a short-beaked sound and the kidney punctured with needles, also handled freely, yet no stone was detected. The patient made a good recovery and was relieved of his pain for a couple of months, but then it returned with renewed violence, utterly incapacitating him from work. I determined to cut down, and if I failed to find a stone, to remove the kidney. The operation was performed in June, 1889, and the kidney carefully examined as before with sound, needles and by palpation; no stone was felt. It was then freely incised, the finger introduced, and at the upper end was felt a hard body encapsuled or rather floating freely in a separate compartment, the intervening tissue was scratched through with

diminishing. *20th*—Patient left the hospital to-day feeling quite well.

[In this case, which was one of the glandular variety of endometritis with almost constant bleeding, I adopted Vulliet's method of packing the uterine cavity with iodoform gauze after thorough curetting with the sharp instrument. If this method is carried out properly and the packing allowed to remain *in situ* for four or five days, I think better results can be obtained in such cases than from the method of injecting the cavity of the uterus with iodised phenol. It is also, I think, a safer method of dealing with them, the gauze ensuring more perfect drainage. In this case it proved most satisfactory.—T. J. A.]

CASE IV.—*Recto-Vaginal Fistula.*

Aged 32 ; admitted June 2nd, 1889, complaining of pain in interscapular and lumbar region ; bearing-down pain in pelvis ; burning pain in vagina ; leucorrhœa. These symptoms have lasted more or less since the birth of her first child, about four years ago.

History:—Menses began at 18 ; always regular, never painful until after marriage. Married six years ; two pregnancies at full term ; labors natural : last labor one year ago.

Examination.—Found large recto-vaginal fistula ; cervix lacerated ; uterus enlarged and hard.

June 10th—Emmet's operation on the cervix and Tait's flap-flap-splitting perineorrhaphy were performed by Dr. Alloway, and the vagina packed with iodoform gauze. *14th*—Patient doing well. *19th*—Allowed up to-day. *21st*—Patient has been up and walking about the ward ever since ; fistula completely closed. Discharged to-day. *27th*—Sutures removed from the cervix to day ; union good.

[This was a very interesting case regarding the rarity of recto-vaginal fistulæ of this nature. A full description of the case can be read in the July number of this JOURNAL embodied in a clinical lecture delivered at the hospital.—T. J. A.]

CASE V.—*Trachelorrhaphy.*

Aged 26 ; admitted June 7th, '89, complaining of continuous

and profuse bloody discharge from vagina with very fœtid odor ;
pain in right inguinal and hypogastric regions ; sensation as of
a lump falling down in rectum, which seems to partially occlude
the vagina. The discharge has lasted about six months, the
pain about three months. Pain began during a menstrual period
and has remained constant ever since. She continued at her
work till the pain became so severe that she had to come to
hospital.

History.—Married nine years ; two pregnancies to full term ;
labors were easy, last one six years ago.

Examination.—Extensive bilateral laceration of cervix, with
considerable hypertrophy and ectropion.

Emmet's operation on the cervix was performed on the 10th
of June by Dr. Alloway.

June 17th.—Sutures removed.

July 6th.—Discharged to-day quite well.

CASE VI.—*Curetting for Menorrhagia*.

Aged 46 ; admitted June 17th, 1889, complaining of profuse
flooding. About a week after her last regular period she noticed
a slight bloody discharge coming from vagina. This discharge
continued, but was slight until about eight days ago, when it
became very profuse. Before this attack came on she had severe
bearing-down pain, but since the flow has had little or no pain.
At present blood comes in gushes and large masses of clot along
with it.

History.—Menses began at 14 ; always regular but painful
before marriage. Married eleven years ; ten pregnancies, eight
to full term and two at third month ; labors easy. First miscarriage about twelve years ago ; had severe flooding following
it. Has had an attack of flooding every year for the last nine
years, but at present it is more profuse than ever.

Examination.—Slight bilateral laceration with ectropion.

June 19th.—Dr. Alloway curetted uterus and filled cavity
with iodoform gauze. *22nd*—Iodoform gauze removed, free
from odor. *24th*—No discharge to-day ; patient feels well.

July 1st.—Discharged, quite well.

Patient came back about a week later saying discharge was

as profuse as ever, and had commenced the day after she left the hospital. The uterus was injected with iodized phenol. Patient reported several days later that discharge was gradually lessening.

[This case left the hospital much too soon, which accounted for the return of the discharge. The injection of iodized phenol undoubtedly arrested it for the time, which it always will do, but if she had had sufficient rest after the curetting the bleeding would not have returned abnormally.—T J. A.]

CASE VII.—Aged 53 ; admitted June 14th, 1889, complaining of profuse and over-frequent menstruation, and frequent and painful micturition.

Examination.—Chronic metritis and endometritis ; right unilateral laceration with extensive hypertrophy and cystic degeneration of cervical glands ; retroversion of uterus, and lacerated perineum.

June 17th.—Schrœder's operation on the cervix, Tait's flap-splitting operation on the perineum, and Alexander's operation to shorten the round ligaments were performed by Dr. Alloway at one sitting.

July 1st.—Perineal sutures removed ; union good. *3rd*—Sutures removed from abdominal wound to-day ; union perfect. *9th*—Patient has continued to improve ; sat up in bed to-day for the first time. *12th*—Walked round the ward a little to-day. *21st*—Discharged to day feeling well and free from feelings of discomfort. Vaginal examination with patient in erect posture, found uterus anteverted and high up in the pelvis.

[The bladder irritability must have been due to traction upon it by the retroverted uterus, in sustaining the weight of the intra-abdominal pressure. When the uterus was brought forward and elevated on the pelvis, the pressure passed behind the uterus and the bladder was no longer influenced. It will be noticed in this case that the three operations were done at the one sitting in about an hour and a quarter. This is not by any means a difficult procedure, and should always be done when necessary in preference to subjecting the patient to a second etherisation and invalidism.—T. J. A.)

Society Proceedings.

CANADIAN MEDICAL ASSOCIATION.

BANFF, August 12th, 1889.

The twenty-second annual meeting of the Canadian Medical Association was called to order by Dr. Ross, at 11 a.m.

Dr. Hingston, a past president, was invited to a seat upon the platform.

The following members, by invitation, were introduced by Dr. Ross: Drs. Whittaker and P. S. Connor, of Cincinnati; Drs. Bulkley and Gibney, of New York; Dr. Marcey, of Boston; Dr. Gordon, of Quincey, Mass.; Prof. Barker, of Philadelphia; Dr. Hannon, of Hoosac Falls: Dr. Lathrop, of Dover, N. H.

Dr. BRETT, of Banff, on behalf of the citizens of Banff, presented the following address of welcome :—

" *To the President and Members of the Canadian Medical Association:*

"Gentlemen, we the members of the Citizens' Committee, representing the community of Banff, on this the occasion of your assembling here for the purpose of holding the twenty second annual meeting of your important association, desire to express our appreciation of the honor which the gathering of so learned a body implies, and, in the absence of a demonstration worthy of the occasion, beg to tender you through this unpretentious address, a sincere and cordial welcome to our midst.

"We venture to assert that the selection of this spot for your place of meeting is singularly felicitous, inasmuch as you, as members of an association distinctively national, could find no more appropriate place in which to conduct the important and useful affairs of your association than this little town of Banff, the heart of the Canadian National Park.

"We hope that your brief stay here may not be altogether without interest to you, that in the grandeur of the scenery, the extent and diversity of mountain, forest and river, or in the healthful qualities of the springs which abound in these parts, and whose sanative properties are now so well known, you may find something worthy of more than a passing notice, worthy in fact of being treasured, when this short visit is over, among the memories which it shall be a pleasure to recall.

"Assuring you of our desire to make your sojourn among us as agreeable as possible,

"We have the honor to be

Yours, &c.,

(Signed)   R. S. BRETT,

F. J. BOSWELL,

R. B. C. O'DONOGHUE.

On behalf of the Citizens' Committee.

Banff, August 12, 1889."

The following gentlemen were next elected permanent members, the President having declared an adjournment of ten minutes to allow the candidates to send in their names and pay the annual fee to the Treasurer.

Proposed by Dr. Cameron and seconded by Dr. Roddick, that the following gentlemen be elected members of the Association:—

Dr. Spencer, Brandon, Man.; Dr. J. W. Smith, Galt, Ont.; Dr. G. A. Kennedy, McLeod, N. W. T.; Dr. W. A. Ross, Barrie, Ont.; Dr. H. B. McPherson, North Sydney, N. S.; Dr. Geo. Riddell, Crystal City, Man.; Dr. A. J. Rutledge, Moosomin, Man.; Dr. H. L. McInnis, Edmonton, N. W. T.; Dr. D. Young, Selkirk, Man.; Dr. G. Fleming, Chatham, Ont.; Dr. W. J. Mitchell, London, Ont.; Dr. Lewis Johnston, Sydney Mines, C. B.; Dr. Samuel Webster, Norval, Ont.; Dr. W. P. Chamberlain, Morrisburg, Ont.; Dr. Alex. Thompson, Strathroy, Ont.; Dr. John J. Farley, Belleville, Ont.; Dr. P. Robertson, St. Andrew, Que.; Dr. G. Loughead, Petrolia, Ont.; Dr. C. Selby Haultaine, Maple Creek, N. W. T.; Dr. W. J. Lindsay, Calgary, N. W. T.; Dr. P. Aylin, Calgary, N. W. T.; Dr. James Hayes, Simcoe, Ont.; Dr. D. Eberts, Nanaimo, B. C.; Dr. G. A. Praeger, Nanaimo, B. C.; Dr. S. J. Tunstall, Kamloops, B. C.; Dr. Fagan, New Westminster, B. C.; Dr. R. J. Bentley, New Westminster, B. C.; Dr. F. H. Mewburn, Lethbridge. N. W. T.; Dr. A. Olver, Medicine Hat, N. W. T.; Dr. Reginald Henwood, Brantford, Ont.; Dr. A. J. Henwood, Brantford, Ont.; Dr. A. Jukes, Regina, N. W. T.: Dr. I. Harkness, Iroquois, Ont.; Dr. Webster, Kentville, N. S.

The Committee on Reciprocity of Registration was not prepared to report.

The following gentlemen were appointed as a Nomination Committee:

Dr. Stewart, Pictou, N. S.; Dr. Armstrong, Montreal, Que.; Dr. Roddick, Montreal, Que.; Dr. Lachapelle, Montreal, Que.;

Dr. Henderson, Kingston, Ont.; Dr. A. H. Wright, Toronto, Ont.; Dr. Grasett, Toronto, Ont ; Dr. Chown, Winnipeg, Man.; Dr. O. C. Edwards, Qu'Appelle, N. W. T.; Dr. LeFevre, Vancouver, B. C., and also the President and Secretary, *ex officio.*

The Secretary then announced the programme to the meeting, explaining why there were no printed programmes prepared for this meeting.

Dr. WRIGHT then read his Inaugural Address. (*See page* 161.)

The meeting then adjourned until 8 p. m. for discussion of the amendments to the by-laws.

BANFF, August 12th, 1889, 8 p. m.

After a prolonged discussion the By-laws of 1874 were amended It was then decided that the by-laws, as amended, should be brought up for adoption at the next annual meeting.

DR. TRENHOLME, of Montreal, gave the following notice of motion :—

"That the Nominating Committee shall be appointed by and for each Province by the members present thereof at the annual meeting."

The meeting then adjourned.

———

BANFF, August 13th, 1889.

The meeting was called to order at 9.30 a.m, Dr. Wright presiding.

The minutes of the previous meeting were read and confirmed.

Mr. Niblock, Assistant Superintendent of the Western Division of the Canadian Pacific Railway, was introduced by the President, and addressed the meettng on behalf of the new hospital now being built at Medicine Hat.

DRS. F. W. CAMPBELL and T. A. RODGER, of Montreal, gave information on behalf of the Committee on Reciprocity of Registration.

DR. CAMPBELL expressed the opinion that it would be impossible to secure reciprocity between England and Canada under existing circumstances.

The Committee was continued.

Without dividing into sections, the reading and discussion of papers was then proceeded with.

The first paper was read by Dr. A. H. Wright on "Hæmatoma of the Vagina and Vulva."

Discussed by Drs. James Ross, Muir, Marcey, Roddick, Trenholme and Sloan.

Dr. Wright spoke in reply.

Dr. G. A. Kennedy, of McLeod, N.W.T., next read a paper on "The Climate of South Alberta," with special reference to its advantages to those suffering from pulmonary complaints.

Discussed by Drs. Oldright, McInnis, Praeger, Bentley, Henderson, McLellan and Spencer.

Dr. Whittaker, of Cincinnati, spoke on this subject, dealing chiefly with the origin of tuberculosis.

Dr. Ross (Toronto) reported a case in which he had discovered gross evidences of tubercular disease in an eight-months fœtus, which died soon after delivery.

Dr. Kennedy replied.

Dr. V. P. Gibney apologized for not having his paper with him, but opened a discussion upon the subject upon which he had intended to write: "The Management of Hip Joint Disease." He proposed to call the disease "Tubercular Ostitis of the Hip Joint," and recommended absolute immobilization. The American idea of traction with motion had become obsolete. Axillary crutches with spica plaster bandage, including pelvis and calf, or, if a splint is desirable, a crutch splint from the perineum.

Discussed by Dr. P. S. Connor, who stated that 95 per cent. of all cases of hip joint disease were tubercular. For treatment he recommended in early disease immobilization; in later stages of the disease he recommended arthrectomy, excision, or amputation, the essential principle being complete removal of tubercular matter.

Dr. Strange did not favor excision. He considered traumatism a common cause.

Dr. Roddick agreed with the previous speakers and suggested traumatism as a special cause in addition to the ordinary cause, tuberculosis. He believed in extension.

Dr. Oldright related two cases.

Dr. Praeger related a case caused by a blow upon the left hip.

Dr. I. H. Cameron recommended the American plan of

treatment. Recommended Buck's extension until rigidity of the muscles is overcome, then splints and movement.

Dr. Shepherd drew a distinction between the treatment of hospital cases and those who have the means of resorting to climatic and other hygenic conditions.

The meeting then adjourned till 2.30 p.m. for lunch.

The first paper after lunch was by Dr. Buller upon "Preventible Deafness."

Dr. Reeve spoke upon the desirability of keeping the post-nasal and pharyngeal cavities clean and healthy.

Dr. Grasett read a paper upon "Colles' Fracture," dividing the subject into three sections. (1) Those in which the fracture is complete. (2) Where there is great displacement which is hard to reduce. (3) The form occurring in old people.

This was discussed by Drs. Roddick, Sloan, McLellan, Geikie, I. H. Cameron and Stockwell.

Dr. Ross read a paper upon "Empyema Successfully Treated by Free Incisions." No discussion.

Dr. James Stewart read a paper upon "Sulphonal."

Dr. Whittaker corroborated the remarks of Dr. Stewart in his paper. He considered sulphonal and paraldehyde the best hypnotics we have, and they are harmless.

Dr. Whittaker then read a paper upon "Varicella."

Discussed by Drs. Geo. Ross and Bulkley.

Dr. Reeve, of Toronto, read a paper on "The Relief of Pain in Eye and Ear Affections."

Dr. Shepherd read a paper on "Nephro-Lithotomy."

Discussed by Drs. Connor, Dupuis, Bell and Roddick.

Dr. Bulkley read a paper on "The Early Recognition and Treatment of Epithelioma," dealing with the subject from a clinical standpoint. He deprecated the use of mild caustics, such as nitrate of silver, and recommended soothing and mildly stimulated applications in early cases, and in the more advanced cases, excision, curretting or cautery, claiming good results from Marsden's Paste, which consists of arsenious acid and gum acacia in equal parts by measurement.

Discussed by Drs. Muir, Dupuis, Chamberlain, Wright of Ottawa, Shepherd, Roddick and Connor.

Dr. Bulkley replied.

The meeting then adjourned until 8.30 p.m.

Dr. Stewart, of Pictou, convener, reported on behalf of the nominating committee as follows : —

OFFICERS.

President, Dr. James Ross, Toronto, Ont.
Secretary, Dr. James Bell, Montreal, Que.
Treasurer, Dr. W. H. B. Aikins, Toronto, Ont.

Vice-Presidents—

For British Columbia, Dr. D. Eberts, Nanaimo, B.C.
For the North-West Territories, Dr. Brett, Banff, N.W.T.
For Manitoba, Dr. R. Spencer, Brandon, Man.
For Ontario, Dr. Bruce Smith, Seaforth, Ont.
For Quebec, Dr. E. P. Lachapelle, Montreal, Que.
For New Brunswick, Dr. Holden, St. John, N.B.
For Nova Scotia, Dr. L. Johnston, Sydney Mines.
For Prince Edward Island, Dr. McLeod,Charlottetown, P.E.I.

Local Secretaries—

British Columbia, Dr. Fagan, New Westminster, B.C.
North-West Territory, Dr. Rutledge, Moosomin, N.W.T.
Manitoba, Dr. H. Higginson, Winnipeg, Man.
Ontario, Dr. J. J. Farley, Belleville, Ont.
Quebec, Dr. John Elder, Huntingdon, Que.
New Brunswick, Dr. Raymond, Sussex, N.B.
Nova Scotia, Dr. W. S. Muir: Truro, N.S.
Prince Edward Island, Dr. Wraburton, Charlottetown.

The following standing committees were appointed :—

Necrology—Drs. Hingston, A. H. Wright and Geo. Ross.

Medical Education and Literature—Dr. Dupuis, Kingston; Dr. Cameron, Toronto, and Dr. Mullin, Hamilton.

Prize Essays—Moved by Dr. Bell, seconded by Dr. Stewart (Pictou), that no committee be suggested this year, as there are no prizes offered.—*Carried.*

Climatology and Epidemic Diseases — Drs. Oldright and Bryce, Toronto; Campbell and Lachapelle, Montreal; Parker, Halifax; Jukes, Regina; Robillard, Ottawa; Patterson, Winnipeg; Milne, Victoria; Kennedy, McLeod, N.W.T.

Ethics—The president and president-elect and the eight vice-presidents.

Committee of Arrangements—Drs. James Ross, W. B. Geikie, Oldright, Graham, Strange, Grassett, A. H. Wright, O'Reilly and W. H. B. Aikins, Toronto.

Publication Committee—Dr. A. Morrow, Halifax ; Dr. James Stewart, Montreal ; Dr. Sheard, Toronto.

The report was adopted and the above named officers and committees declared elected for the ensuing year.

The meeting was re-opened at 8 30 p.m. by the reading of a paper by Dr. I. H. Cameron, on "Hernia," in which he gave the views of Mr. Lockwood.

Discussed by Drs. Marcey, Gardner, and H. P. Wright,

Dr. Cameron replied.

Dr. Praeger narrated several surgical cases.

The President announced that Dr. Jukes had withdrawn his paper on "The Endemic Fever of the North-West Territories."

Dr. Dupuis was called upon to read his paper, "Some improvements in Medical and Surgical Instruments." As the hour was late, he contented himself with showing and explaining the instruments without reading his paper.

The following papers were then declared read by title, the authors not being present.

1. "Mineral Springs," by Dr. H. P. Small, of Ottawa.

2. "Vertigo: an Eye and Ear Symptom," by Dr. J. W. Stirling, of Montreal.

3. "A Common and Easily Preventible Cause of Retro-Displacements," by Dr. A. L. Smith, of Montreal.

4. "A Case of Necrosis following a Compound Fracture," by Dr. John Campbell, Seaforth, Ont.

Dr. Stewart of Pictou, moved, seconded by Dr. Roddick, that the president nominate a committee to confer with the provincial and local societies and approach the federal and local governments with a view of reducing the tariff on surgical instruments.—*Carried.*

Dr. P. S. Connor, on behalf of the American visitors, in a happy manner, thanked the Association for having invited the American delegates.

Cheers were then given for the American delegates.

The treasurer's report, audited by Drs. Buller and Lachapelle, was received and adopted by motion.

The treasurer's report is as follows:—

Fees received by acting-treasurer from members (82).	$164.00

Liabilities.

Balance due Dr. Sheard, former treasurer.............$ 2.07	
Times Printing Co., Hamilton....................... 13.00	
Somerville, Benallack & Co., Montreal.............. 52.50	
Secretary for post stamps, stationery, &c.......... 30.75	
Moulton's Theatre Co............................... 20.00	
Burland Lithographic Co............................ 2.75	
	$121.07
Balance...	$42.83
Reduction in charge for use of theatre.............	5.00
	$47.83

Examined and found correct.

The following resolutions were then proposed, seconded and carried.

Moved by Dr. Buller, seconded by Dr. Chas. O'Reilly :

"That this Association has great pleasure in conveying to the Canadian Pacific Railway Company its most cordial acknowledgements, for the facilities that they have been accorded in coming to Banff, and the kind attention they have received from all the employees of the company with whom they have had to deal, as well as for the superb accommodation and the great enjoyment they have derived from their sojourn in the world renowned Banff Springs Hotel. Taking into consideration the length of the journey, the season of the year, and the unavoidably imperfect information as to the location and numbers of those who formed the main body of the excursion, the arrangements, as carried out by the company, have been such as to excite the admiration and grateful recognition of the Association. The thanks of the Association are especially due to Mr. William Whyte, general superintendent of the road, for his exceeding kindness in accompanying them from Winnipeg to Banff and giving his personal supervision in all matters concerning their safety and welfare."

Moved by Dr. Geikie, seconded by Dr. Bruce Smith:

"That the cordial thanks of the Association be and are hereby given to the citizens of Banff, for the kindness and courtesy exhibited towards the Association during the annual meeting just held, and especially for the address of welcome presented by the citizens to the Association at its first session, which contained so many expressions of interest in the Association and of good will towards it."

Moved by Dr. Ross, seconded by Dr. McLellan :

"That this Association hereby tender to His Honor, Dr. Schultz, Lieutenant-Governor of Manitoba, its grateful thanks for his cordial reception of them at the Government House during their passage through his province. That they rejoice to observe that the press of political duties has not interfered with the continuance of a keen interest on the part of his Honor in everything calculated to advance the interests of that profession in which he is so proud to number himself amongst its loyal members. That this association assures Dr. and Mrs. Schultz that their generous hospitality in Winnipeg has been highly appreciated, and will in retrospect make one of the brightest memories of an ever memorable meeting."

Moved by Dr. Farley, seconded by Dr. Edwards :

"That this Association appreciates and will gratefully remember the Grand Trunk Railway Company for kindly co-operating with the Canadian Pacific Railway in making our trip to Banff a pleasant one."

Moved by Dr. Oldright, seconded by Dr. Lachapelle :

" That the Canadian Medical Association do respectfully submit to the Government of the Dominion that it is highly desirable in the public behalf, as well as in the interest of medical science, that members of the profession should be in possession of reliable statistics of the climatic conditions of Banff and other resorts in the North-West territories, as well as of the chemical composition of the soil and waters of the district, in order that they may act with greater confidence in sending patients to these resorts, and that the Association do further memoralize the Government to establish a signal station at Banff with branches at such other points as may be found jnccessary, a competent person being appointed to superintend the observation at such station or stations."

Moved by Dr. W. S. Muir, Truro, N. S., seconded by Dr. Shepherd, Montreal:

"That the Local Provincial Secretaries be requested to ascertain the feeling of the medical societies of their respective Provinces on the subject of affiliation with the Canadian Medical Association."

A vote of thanks to the medical men of Winnipeg was moved by Dr. W. S. Muir, of Truro, N. S., seconded by Dr. Geikie.

Moved by Dr. Lachapelle, seconded by Dr. Oldright:

" That this Association hereby declares its opinion that it is the duty of all practitioners to loyally comply with the regulations in force in the different Provinces, and to report cases of contageous disease to their respective local authorities, so as to enable these authorities to give suitable advice and take such measures as might be required in order to prevent the spreading of contagious diseases and prevent epidemics."

Moved by Dr. Strange, seconded by Dr. Henderson:

'·That the cordial thanks of the Canadian Medical Association be tendered to the Manitoba and other Clubs of the City of Winnipeg for the privileges conferred on its members."

Proposed by Dr. Shepherd, seconded by Dr. Lachapelle:

"That the thanks of the Association be conveyed to Mr. Lalonde for his great care and attention and unfailing kindness to the members during the trip from Banff to Montreal."

Moved by Dr. Campbell, seconded by Dr. Preston :

" That the thanks of the meeting are hereby tendered to Dr. Wright, the President, for the impartial and business-like way in which he has conducted the Canadian Medical Association.

Moved by Dr. Campbell, seconded by Dr. Sloan :

" That the thanks of the Association are tendered to Dr.

Bell, General Secretary, for the able and courteous manner in which he has performed the large amount of work which has of necessity fallen to him in organizing what has been the most remarkable meeting in our history.

The following letter was received from his Honor the Lieutenant-Govertor, Dr. Schultz, of Manitoba:

GOVERNMENT HOUSE. Winnipeg, Man., Aug. 12, 1889.

MY DEAR SIR,—In answer to the wish expressed by the officers and many of the members of the Association that I would be present at your Banff meeting, I regret to say that I find other duties will, for a time at least, call me in another direction, though I will make an effort to meet you all in British Columbia before your return. Kindly allow me to say to the Association through you, how gratified I am personally, and how pleased I know the profession here to be, at the choosing of a place in the North-West for the meeting of the Association this year. To my mind Banff is particularly appropriate, for it is one of our National Sanitariums. There are questions of medical and other scientific importance which may be better observed and discussed there than almost anywhere else in Canada. You are on a range of mountains memorable with recollections of several great men. Doctor, and afterwards Sir John, Richardson followed their course down our mighty northern river till their grand heights slowly descended to the flat plain which forms the shore of the Arctic Sea. This worthy companion of the great Arctic voyageur, whose dust is sepulchered in the snows and ice of the Arctic archipelago, first gave to the world the knowledge of the animal life of the great northern wilds. Dr. Hector gave most valuable information in tha same direction, and of the diseases of the Northern tribes, when with Captain Palliser he explored the Rocky Mountain passes to the south of the one in which your meeting is now being held. Dr. Cheadle, surgeon to Lord Milton's party, wrote that most interesting aed valuable book, "The North West Passage by Land," describing one of the passes to the north of where you are; and I feel sure that so many men learned in the profession to which I am proud to belong, when discussing in council can not fail to throw light upon many of the questions which will naturally present themselves for solution, such as, for instance, whether the high temperature of these springs is due to the disintegration of the sulphites and sulphates, or is the result of volcanic action; and whether, if from other of these causes, the temperature varies and the proportion of chemical constituents changes from the published analysis. The effect of high altitudes upon the bacilli of phthisis and upon other disease germs, and the effect of large areas of non-absorbable granite rocks upon the life of such bactoria as may be found at these elevations; and I would ask my learned confreres, when in discussion of more scientific questions shall have been completed, to pause and reflect for a moment that for economic purposes Canada is widest and no longer a mere arable strip on the banks of the St. Lawrence, where on the east (and northward from the boundary line) Canada measures thirteen hundred miles of arable and pastoral land, and to the west nearly an equal north and south width of one of the richest mineral districts in the world.

I am, Dear Sir,

very faithfully yours,

JOHN SCHULTZ.

The Secretary Canadian Medical Association,
    Banff, N. W. T.

As the meeting had been concluded, it was decided by the President and Secretary to acknowledge the receipt of the letter, and to request the various medical journals to publish it in full in their next issues.

MEDICO-CHIRURGICAL SOCIETY OF MONTREAL.

Stated Meeting, May 31st, 1889.

WM. GARDNER, M.D., PRESIDENT, IN THE CHAIR.

On motion by Dr. Roddick, seconded by Dr. Shepherd, Dr. Joseph Workman of Toronto was elected an honorary member of the Society.

Drs Low, Campbell, Booth, England and Brown, resident medical officers of the Montreal General Hospital, were also elected members.

Removal of Appendix Vermiformis.—DR. BELL exhibited the patient on whom he had operated and gave the following history :—

G. D., aged 28, a young Englishman, with a markedly tubercular family history and a small area of tubercular deposit in one lung, had suffered for four and a half years with repeated attacks of pain, tenderness and swelling in the right iliac region, with fever and digestive disturbance. These attacks had been coming on more and more frequently, and were each time more imperfectly recovered from. There had been eight or nine such attacks in all, and the patient had been confined to his room for nine months, when the last attack seized him about the middle of April, 1889. This attack came on with severe pain, radiating from the right cæcal region, griping and diarrhœa. When seen, thirty-six hours after the onset of the attack, the patient lay with his knees drawn up, suffering great pain all over the abdomen, but most severe over the cæcal region, with paroxysmal exacerbations. The abdomen was swollen, tympanitic and very tender, and a resisting mass could be felt just internal to and above the antero-superior spine of the right iliac crest. Pulse 100 ; temperature 100°F. Patient was sent to hospital, but would not consent to operation which was immediately proposed to him. He was treated with hot applications and opium in large quantities.* (The diarrhœa had only lasted a few hours and occasional vomiting occurred.) The opium failed to relieve his pain and all the symptoms increased in severity, so that he consented to the operation, which was performed twenty-four hours after admission. An incision about five inches long was made from just above the middle of Poupart's ligament almost vertically upwards—inclining slightly outwards—exposing the cæcum and lower two inches of the ascending colon. A small abscess cavity containing from two to four drachms of thick, creamy pus was formed by the cæcum, appendix vermiformis, and a mass of swollen omentum in front. The appendix was bent upon itself, swollen to the size of an ordinary index finger, with a gangrenous spot about midway from its base. The small intestines (as far as seen during the operation) were greatly congested and distended, but no lymph nor adhesions were observed in the abdominal cavity. The appendix was ligatured and removed with the mass of swollen omentum. A sharp attack of pneumonia supervened and endangered the patient's life for a few days, but the abdominal symptoms immediately subsided, and the patient recovered perfectly. Three months after operation he remained quite free from abdominal symptoms of any kind.

Rupture of the Ileum.—DR. BELL exhibited a portion of the ileum and said that the patient, a coachman, aged 47, strong and healthy, became intoxicated on the evening of the 3rd of May. He was last seen by his friends about 8.30 p.m. of that

15

day. During the night he was arrested and next morning tried and sentenced to ten days in jail (failing to pay the fine imposed). That same afternoon he was removed to the jail, which he entered complaining of pain in the abdomen. He was put to bed in the jail hospital, and at four o'clock in the morning was found dead in bed. An autopsy revealed the following conditions: (1) a couple of quarts of blackish, turbid fluid with a fæcal odor in the abdominal cavity ; (2) intense congestion of the intestines ; (3) matting together of the small intestines in the right pelvic and iliac regions, and adhesion of this mass to the abdominal wall and the base of the bladder with recent lymph in large quantities ; (4) a tear obliquely across the free surface of the ileum about twelve inches from the ileo-cæcal valve. This wound was about an inch long, with the mucous membrane everted on both sides. There was no loss of mucous membrane anywhere nor evidence of recent or old ulceration of the intestines, which were carefully examined. There were no marks of violence externally. Dr. Bell expressed the opinion that the rupture of the bowel was undoubtedly the result of traumatism, almost certainly a violent blow upon the abdominal wall, giving the following reasons for this opinion : (1) the man was perfectly healthy until within thirty-six hours of the discovery of his death ; (2) the absence of any ulcerative or other disease of the intestines ; (3) the position, the length, and the direction of the lesion of the bowel and the eversion of the mucous membrane.

Tubal Pregnancy with Rupture.—DR. ANGUS MACDONELL gave the following history of the case :—

Between five and six o'clock in the evening of the 28th April he was called to see a young woman suffering from violent cramps in the bowels. He found her in bed in a state of collapse, with a pallor and expression of face suggesting hemorrhage as the cause. She complained of intense pain in the hypogastric region, which came on suddenly while in the act of ironing some clothes. She had been feeling quite well all day up to that moment. She had been losing no blood ; there was no tenderness on pressure in any part of the abdomen ; nothing in her history would lead one to infer peritoneal rupture or perforation. He therefore concluded that the pain from which she was suffering was merely neuralgic, that the apparent collapse was due to the intensity of the pain, and that she would soon rally. He accordingly prescribed an anodyne ; pill of opium gr. i, to be followed by antispasmodic doses of chloric ether and spirits of camphor. In the meantime he gave her a glass of spirits, which speedily revived her, and finding her sufficiently improved, he left her. At half-past eleven the same night he was called again to see the patient. On arriving at the house he found that the patient was all but actually dead ; she gasped but two or three times at short intervals, when life entirely ceased.

DR. FINLEY, who performed the post-mortem, exhibited the uterus and appendages. On opening the abdominal cavity he found an effusion of blood in the peritoneal cavity. The quantity he estimated at about two gallons. The right tube presented a sacular swelling near the uterus about half an inch long, with a rent on its posterior surface. The interior of the sac was lined with a granular membrane which proved to be villi on subsequent microscopic examination. The corpus luteum was situated on the opposite ovary. The uterus admitted a probe for 3½ inches, the cervix was lacerated, and the parts about the lacerations indurated. No fœtus was found.

DR. MACDONELL stated that as the patient had menstruated twenty-seven days previously, and was daily expecting her monthly period, the fœtation could not have been, at the outside, more than a month old.

Pale, contracted Kidneys in a young girl. Death from Peritonitis.—DR. FINLEY exhibited the kidneys of a young girl aged 19, who had died of acute peritonitis. The organs were much diminished in size, being less than half the normal weight. Although the surface presented numerous small puckered areas, the capsules were neither adherent nor thickened. On section, they appear to be of about normal consistence ; the cortex slightly increased in depth, and of a pale yellow color, mottled with reddish patches. The pyramids are also pale, with reddish streaks, giving them a somewhat darker color than the cortex. Microscopic examination showed moderate fibroid thickening of the Malpighian capsules, and hyaline necrosis of many of the tufts. The renal epithelium was for the most part normal, but presented areas of degeneration. The arteries were much thickened, and there was a moderate increase of fibro-nuclear tissue between the tubules. The spleen, which was increased in size, was bound to the surrounding parts by old adhesions. The peritoneal cavity contained about a pint of pus, and the intestines, liver and other viscera were covered with recent lymph. The appendix vermiformis, abdominal and pelvic organs were normal, and no cause for the peritonitis could be found except the condition of the kidneys. The heart was not hypertrophied, and there was no endocarditis. The other organs were normal, with the exception of a few old caseous nodules in lungs.

DR. WILKINS stated that the girl had come under his care in hospital four weeks before her death for an attack of subacute rheumatism in the ankles and shoulder, rapidly yielding to treatment. The patient was expected to leave hospital in a day or two. About five days before death the temperature rose, varying from 102° to 104½°, and forty-eight hours before death the ordinary symptoms of acute general peritonitis developed. The urine was examined on admission, but no albumen found. Dr. Wilkins commented on the absence of hypertrophy of the heart and on the latent character of the renal affection.

Papillomatous Fibroma.—DR. McCONNELL exhibited microscopic preparations from a tumor removed by Dr. Roddick showing an excess of fibrous tissue in papillomatous tumor. The tumor was removed from the breast of a middle-aged woman some weeks before, and presented many unusual features on section. The prepared sections showed it to be a papillomatous fibroma, a very rare form of growth.

Case of Spastic Paralysis in a Pigeon.—DR. MILLS exhibited a pigeon, taken from the nest, affected with *spastic paralysis* of the right leg. It was congenital. He had in his loft another nestling of the same variety of pigeon (owl) similarly affected, and last year another case, though in a different breed. In none of these instances did the general health seem affected. The point of greatest interest to himself was the causation. In every case these young ones were the offspring of parents that had been much buffeted about in the loft and unable to find a resting place amid the struggle for choice for a considerable time. The disease was the result, probably, of the disordered condition of the nervous system of the parents in consequence of this excitement, and if so, illustrates how the strains of our own civilization may account for the increase of nervous instability.

Dr. Mills also exhibited a specimen of a flying tumbler pigeon which had died a couple of days previously, manifesting psychic derangement. It had just hatched out a pair of young, and was possibly then the more readily affected, for pigeons, owing to the secretion of a kind of milky fluid from the crop at such times, seem occasionally to suffer from what corresponds to milk fever. An autopsy showed inflammation of the duodenum, apparently from round worms. It was likely that the irritation of these worms had given rise to the inflammation, and also contributed to the mental derangement at this critical period. In another case he had taken twenty of these worms (1½ inches long) from the upper intestine of a barb pigeon. They had apparently been the sole cause of death.

Dr. Stewart remarked that the case of spastic paralysis presented many features commonly seen in the human species, but differed inasmuch as in the case shown the affection was unilateral and confined to the posterior extremity.

(*To be continued.*)

Selections.

The Maybrick Case.—The trial of Florence Elizabeth Maybrick for the wilful murder of her husband, James Maybrick, by poisoning him with arsenic last May, commenced on Wednesday, the 31st July, and ended on Wednesday, the 7th August, in a verdict of guilty and sentence of death. It was tried at the Crown Court, Liverpool, before Mr. Justice Stephen. Mr. Addison, Q.C., M.P., Recorder of Preston, led for the prosecution, with Mr. W. R. McConnell and Mr. Swift; Sir Charles Russell, Q.C., M.P., with Mr. Pickford, appearing for the defence. The greatest interest was taken in the proceedings, the court being crowded each day. The case for the prosecution occupied three days and a half; that for the defence nearly a day and a half. The learned judge's summing up took up the whole of Tuesday, the 6th, and more than one half of the next day, and a more exhaustive recapitulation of the whole case could not have been made. The following is a condensed history of the more important medical features of the case as given in evidence.

The deceased was a Liverpool cotton-merchant, having an office in the city, and a residence at Aigburth, a suburb situated a few miles south of Liverpool. His age at the time of his death was fifty; he had been married eight years, the issue of the marriage being a boy aged seven and a girl aged three. The deceased and his wife lived apparently on happy terms until the day of the last Grand National Steeplechase, when they had a very serious quarrel, which was, however, on the intervention of Mr. Hopper, the family medical attendant, apparently made up. The deceased's health was described by Mr. Hopper and his relatives as being fairly good. His brother denied positively that he was in the habit of taking arsenic, and it appeared that the deceased had indignantly denied it. The deceased's family history was good, and his life was insured. On Sunday, April 14th, Mr. Fuller, of Albany street, London, saw the deceased at the residence of his brother, Mr. Michael Maybrick, Wellington Mansions, Regent's Park. He complained of a little pain in his head and numbness in his legs; he was apprehensive of paralysis. Mr. Fuller spent an hour with him, examined him fully, and expressed his opinion that there was nothing the matter with him beyond indigestion, for which he prescribed acid. nit. mur. dil. with nux vomica and syrup. He also ordered a compound camomile pill, and in a second prescription extract of carcara, some glycerine, and cream of tartar. The deceased called at Mr. Fuller's residence the following Saturday, April 20th, and expressed himself as much better; the prescriptions were varied a little. Mr. Fuller never prescribed arsenic, and nothing was said to him about it. On Sunday, April 28th, Dr. Humphreys, who resides not far from the deceased's residence, was sent for, and found him in bed. Except for a trifling injury, he had not previously attended him. He complained of some peculiar condition of his chest and heart, was afraid he would be paralysed, and referred his symptoms to a strong cup of tea, adding that upon several previous occasions tea had produced similar inconveniences. He complained of the dirty state of his tongue, which he said had been furred and dirty for a long time, and that he could not get it clean. He had been at the Wirral races the day before, had dined with a friend, and while at dinner his hands were so very unsteady and twitching that he spilt some wine, which distressed him very much, as he feared his friends might think him drunk. Dr. Humphreys prescribed dilute prussic acid, and advised him to have nothing that day except milk and soda. He was called again to him that evening, and found him suffering from stiffness of the legs, for which he prescribed bromide of potassium and tincture of henbane. He called the next day; the deceased was better, but remained in bed, and concluding that it was a case of chronic dyspepsia, Dr. Humphreys ordered him a dietary in writing and Seymour's preparation of papain and iridin, one teaspoonful a day. On May 1st the deceased was much better, his tongue was clean, and the headache had disappeared. On Friday he complained of being worse, and that the medicine did not agree with him. Dr. Humphreys assured him he was better, and at the deceased's request allowed him to go to town and to have a Turkish bath. He met him in town that afternoon, but had no conversation. At midnight Dr. Humphreys was again sent for; the patient was in bed in great pain, which he referred to his thighs, hips, and knees. He had been sick, which he attributed to inferior sherry put into his Revalenta Arabica food. The sickness continued, and on the following Sunday, May 5th, Dr. Humphreys proposed a consultation, to which Mrs. Maybrick objected on the ground that he had had so many doctors and that they had done him little good. But Dr. Humphreys being puzzled with the case, and the deceased's brother insisting upon a second opinion, Dr. Carter was called in and saw him on Tuesday, the 7th. He examined him thoroughly, and found nothing wrong with the heart, lungs, liver or brain; diarrhœa was just commencing; the throat was much inflamed, red, dry, and glazed. The deceased complained of a sensation as of a hair in his throat, and some vomited matters and fæces were shown. Drs. Carter and Humphreys agreed that it was a case of acute dyspepsia resulting from improper food or drink, or both. On the 9th tenesmus was present, and there was looseness of the bowels, examination of the rectum causing such pain that it had to be abandoned. The symptoms strongly suggested some irritant, and about this time, circumstances exciting strong suspicions against Mrs. Maybrick having arisen, nurses were in attendance, with strict orders that the deceased

was to have no food except what they themselves prepared in
the rooms.   Dr. Humphreys tested some urine and fæces, with
a negative result ; Dr. Carter tested some Neave's food, with
the same result; but in a bottle of Valentine's meat juice he
got distinct evidence of arsenic, both by Reinsch's and Marsh's
tests.   It was too late, however, to save the life of the unfortunate man, who sank and died on Saturday afternoon.   On
Monday a post-mortem examination was made, Dr. Barron,
pathologist of the Royal Infirmary, representing Mrs. Maybrick.   There were no indications of any natural cause of
death, and the appearances of the stomach, intestines, and
rectum were those which would be produced by an irritant
poison, such as arsenic.   That the cause of death was an irritant poison was the opinion of all the three gentlemen who
made the post-mortem examination ; but Drs. Carter and Humphreys also expressed a decided opinion that it was a case of
death from arsenical poisoning after hearing the result of the
chemical examination by Mr. Edward Davies, analyst.   That
gentleman found arsenic in the liver, in the intestines, and in
the kidneys, the total quantity in the abdominal viscera being
estimated at one-eighth of a grain.   Mr. Davies also found
arsenic in the bottle of meat juice handed to him by Dr. Carter,
the quantity being about half a grain.   He found arsenic in
many other articles sent him from the house, including a bottle
of mixture made up from Mr. Fuller's prescription by Messrs.
Clay and Abraham, a firm of Liverpool chemists, and proved
the absence of any arsenic in another bottle of the same mixture found at the deceased's office, as also in all the bottles of
ingredients from which the prescription had been made up.
In the jug, basin and pan from which the deceased warmed
and took his lunch at the office, Mr. Davies found distinct evidence of arsenic, from which he inferred that there must have
been a very decided quantity of arsenic in the whole of the
food, as he had obtained crystals of arsenic from the small
fragment which remained adhering to the jug even after it had
been washed.   On comparing the specific gravity of the fluid
in the Valentine's meat juice bottle with that of a fresh sample,
Mr. Davies concluded that the arsenic had been introduced in
a fluid form.   A basin containing fly-papers soaking in water
was found by the housemaid in Mr. and Mrs. Maybrick's bedroom covered over with a towel.   It was shown that Mrs.

Maybrick had purchased fly-papers from several chemists, alleging that the flies were beginning to be troublesome, which was not correct. Arsenic was also detected on the front and in the pocket of a dressing-gown, on a handkerchief, and a bottle contained liquid with from twelve to fifteen grains of solid arsenic, also water and powdered charcoal. It was identical with some powder found in a packet and labelled "Poison for cats." A tumbler containing milk and a handkerchief was found to have between twenty and thirty grains of arsenic in it. A bottle of Price's glycerine also contained arsenic. Mrs. Maybrick was seen by one of the nurses to remove the bottle of Valentine's meat-juice into another room—afterwards found to contain arsenic,—to return with it in a very suspicious manner half hidden in her hand, and to replace it on the table. The nurse gave it to Mr. Michael Maybrick, who delivered it to Dr. Carter. The lunch taken on May 1st was wrapped up in brown paper and given by the prisoner to Mr. Edwin Maybrick, who gave it to his brother. The latter ate it in his presence, and complained of it as having made him ill. It was in the remains of this that Mr. Davies found the arsenic.

Dr. Stevenson, Professor of Forensic Medicine in Guy's Hospital Medical College, and Analyst to the Home Office, received some of the viscera to examine, and was the last witness called for the prosecution. His analysis confirmed that of Mr. Davies, with the exception that he estimated the proportion found in the liver as larger. He expressed his opinion that death resulted from poisoning by arsenic.

For the defence, Dr. Tidy, the Lecturer on Medical Jurisprudence at the London Hospital Medical College, who was called on the same day as Dr. Stevenson, contended that it was not a case of arsenical poisoning. He argued that the four symptoms—vomiting, purging, pain in the stomach, and soreness of the eyes—were absent, and that the small quantity of arsenic found in the body of the deceased was accountable for by the alleged habits of the deceased. Evidence from America was brought by two witnesses, who testified to the deceased having taken arsenic some years ago, and by a retired Liverpool chemist, who identified the deceased by means of a photograph, who deposed to the fact of the deceased having gone to his shop to have "pick-me-up's" containing doses of Fowler's solution. Dr. Rawdon Macnamara, of Dublin, also gave evidence for the defence, contending that the deceased's symptoms did not correspond with those of patients suffering from poisoning by arsenic. Mr. Paul's evidence went to show that there was arsenic in the glazing of the pan in which the lunch was warmed, which might be set free by muriatic acid. He also contended that if arsenic had been present in the urine it must have shown itself by Reinsch's test which Dr. Humphreys employed.

Mr. Justice Stephen, in summing up, alluded to the partisan character of expert evidence, quoting also the old saying that "a physician was a man who put medicine, of which he knew little, into a body of which he knew less." He deprived the sarcasm of its sting, however, by the compliments which he paid to the various medical witnesses, the whole of whose evidence, as well as that of others, he went carefully through. At her own own request the prisoner was allowed to make a statement. She stated that the solution of fly-papers was for a cosmetic, as her mother and some friends in Germany could have testified. She added that she put some white powder in the meat juice at her husband's request, and, as some of it was spilt, filled it up with water.

The jury were only absent from court about forty minutes, and returned with a verdict of "Guilty." Sentence of death was pronounced upon the unhappy woman, who throughout the whole of the long trial, and in a close court, in sultry weather, bore herself with remarkable firmness.

The case resembles in some points that of Wooler, in others that of Madeline Smith; but it has its own peculiar features. As in Wooler's case, the poison was arsenic, and it was suspected during the deceased's lifetime. But there was not the same delay in coming to a conclusion as to the real nature of the case, or the same performance of Reinsch's test with acid contaminated with arsenic. The cosmetic theory set up in Madeline Smith's case was again set up here.—*London Lancet*, Aug. 17, 1889.

THE

Montreal Medical Journal.

VOL. XVIII.   SEPTEMBER, 1889.   No. 3.

QUARANTINE.

From the report of the Minister of Agriculture of the Federal Governmnnt for 1888 we learn that a more efficient medical inspection of incoming vessels is now maintained at the different Canadian ports. At Grosse Isle no less than seventeen vessels were reported as having infectious disease on board, and of these nine belonged to leading passenger lines. The diseases so reported or discovered were smallpox, yellow fever, enteric fever, scarlet fever, diphtheria, measles and variola. The quarantine superintendent reports that the necessary precaution for the vaccinal protection of steerage passengers had not been thoroughly carried out by the ship surgeons for various reasons mentioned, such as absence of instructions from owners or agents, neglect of the ship surgeon, and inadequate supply of vaccine. In such cases the steerage passengers were examined at quarantine, and where necessary, vaccinated in accordance with the regulations which direct that no steerage passenger shall be allowed to pass the inspecting stations without furnishing evidence to the satisfaction of the quarantine medical officer of having been vaccinated within the seven previous years or having had the smallpox within that period. Five persons objected to being vaccinated. They were accordingly put ashore and kept at Grosse Isle under medical supervision until the period of incubation from the date of their last possible exposure to the infection of smallpox had expired. All told, there were 4,000 persons vaccinated at Grosse Isle last season, and smallpox was reported on one steamer. Vessels with smallpox on board were also detained at Halifax, St. John, N.B., and Victoria, B.C.

Whatever views may be held as to the efficiency of quarantine, there can be no doubt of the advantage, in a country like ours, of insisting upon rigid medical inspection, vaccination of immigrants, isolation of suspicious cases, and the disinfection of ships and clothing. By carrying out measures such as these we may hope to prevent the ingress of diseases not now known in the country, and prevent the spread by immigrants of the more common infectious diseases.

LEAD POISONING.

When Sir George Baker discovered that the cause of the Devonshire colic was the presence of lead in the cider for which that county was so justly famous, it was thought that lead-poisoning would become one of the things of the past. Unfortunately, however, the study of the various manifestations of saturnism lead us to the opinion that although there may now-a-days be less colic in Poictou and Devon, yet lead poisoning is still prevalent in both town and country to an extent truly alarming. Within the last few years we have published several well reported cases occurring in rural districts. Country practitioners are not too fond of putting their experiences into print, and the few reported cases represent a large number which have never seen the light. Again, it is reasonable enough to suppose that both in town and country very many cases fail to come under the notice of the medical man at all, while other cases may be treated without being recognized as being of saturnine origin. In Montreal the various forms of lead poisoning are very prevalent. The wards of the General Hospital are seldom without three or even four severe cases, and a still larger number are to be found in attendance at the out-patient department.

Moreover, we are of opinion that lead-poisoning is largely on the increase, and that preventive measures should demand the immediate attention of the local Board of Health. The origin of the poisoning, as related by the patients themselves, is in some instances to be found in the defective arrangements for the ventilation of those workshops where lead is used. Not long ago a paint factory in the city sent a case to the General Hospital which ended fatally, and at this moment there is a workman dying in hospital from lead poisoning.

The local Board of Health should take this matter in hand, ask for reports of cases, investigate the alleged causes of the poisoning, and, where it is possible, do away with them.

THE ROYAL VICTORIA HOSPITAL.—The work of blasting the rock for the foundation of the new hospital is in active progress. The outline of the base of the building can now be made out. The approach to the hospital will be the head of Upper University street.

IMPROVEMENTS AT THE MONTREAL GENERAL HOSPITAL.—At a recent meeting of the governors of this institution it was decided to construct nurses' quarters by the addition of a Mansard roof to the building. By this means comfortable bedrooms will be provided for the hard-worked nursing staff as well as for the servants of the hospital. An efficient staff of trained nurses is an essential requirement of a modern hospital, and to secure recruits for such a staff, as well as to enable the committee to retain the services of reliable nurses, it is an absolute necessity that they should be well housed and, more particularly, well fed. A nurse's hours of duty are long, and are spent in an atmosphere not of the purest, it should therefore be an object with committees to provide every means of enabling these deserving women to pass their hours of rest in a wholesome as well as a pleasant atmosphere. The scaffoldings are already erected, and it is expected that the whole work will be completed by the 1st of November. It is probable that the old nurses' rooms in the annex of the Morland wing will be made to serve as isolation wards for cases of erysipelas.

APPOINTMENT.—Dr. H. S. Birkett has been appointed one of the Demonstrators of Anatomy in the Medical Faculty of McGill University. The college career of Dr. Birkett was one of great distinction. His accurate knowledge of anatomy, and the care and attention he bestowed upon his dissections, won for him the Demonstrator's Prize in Practical Anatomy. In the session of 1884–85 he did good work in the dissecting-room as prosector and as student assistant demonstrator. In 1886 the Holmes Gold Medal was awarded him. After graduation, Dr. Birkett served one year on the house staff of the Montreal General Hospital, and subsequently spent two years in study in England and Germany. The appointment will go far to strenghthen the teaching staff of this important branch of the medical department of the University.

Medical Items.

SPECTACLES AND EYE-GLASSES.—Dr. G. J. Bull, M.D., of the Faculty of McGill University, Montreal, has lately taken his degree in Paris, and chose for the subject of his inaugural thesis, "Spectacles and Eye-glasses." After having practised about twenty years in America, the greater part of which time Dr. Bull practised ophthalmology in New York, he came over to Paris, and perfected himself in this branch under the guidance of Dr. Javal, the celebrated ophthalmologist, with whom he worked at the laboratory of the Sorbonne. Those who wish to learn how to wear spectacles and eye-glasses should read Dr. Bull's newly published work, which is the reproduction of his thesis, containing, in addition, an introduction by Dr. Javal. The work is most interesting, and of great theoretical and practical value, particularly to those affected with astigmatism. According to the author, for some years a more precise knowledge of astigmatism has produced a complete revolution in the science of ophthalmology. He says it is important to draw the attention of the public to the existence of this optical defect, which is more frequent than myopia and than presbyopia, and which is corrected by means of special glasses, cut to measure, after the indications of the oculist. As regards myopia, Dr. Bull states that infants are not myopic; with very rare exception they become so with age, and more frequently because they acquire the habit of reading and writing at too short a distance. The eye, therefore, becomes developed in a defective manner. It is often said that myopia and presbyopia are two affections opposed and incompatible; but the author affirms that this is not the case, the real state opposed to myopia being hypermetropia. Dr. Bull is the inventor of a new optometer, a full description of which will be found in his work, where other useful hints are given for the preservation of the eyesight.—*Paris Correspondent of the London Lancet.*

A DICTIONARY OF MEDICAL SPECIALISTS.—There was recently published in London a classified list of London practitioners who chiefly attend to particular departments of medicine and surgery. The editor is a member of the legal profession, and the principal result of the work is to demonstrate how dangerous it is to meddle with affairs of which one knows nothing. Practically it is a trades list, or what is called a classified business directory. We have not seen this work, but from what is said about it in the *Lancet*. the reading of it must be entertaining. The venerable President of the College of Physicians, Sir Andrew Clark, to take an example, is exactly defined in this dictionary. He is no longer the broad, general physician refusing to be shut out of any corner or cavity of the body where he can find any disease to battle against ; he is a specialist, or rather he is three specialists in one. He is a specialist for children, he is great on the eye, and he is to be consulted specially on midwifery and the diseases of women. The profession must not expect to be able hereafter to consult him on general matters, but may take their cataract cases to him, or fly to him at night for assistance in cross-births. How convenient this book will be to the medical profession, and how helpful to the British public ! Strange to say, we are not told the hours at which Sir Andrew Clark may be seen.

DOGMATIC RECTITUDE.—To many practitioners whose student days were passed at the medical school of McGill University, it will be a mournful piece of news that a trusty servant of the college has been stricken with a malady which, regarded even in the most favorable light, is one of gloomy prognosis. It was, we believe, in 1883 that the present incumbent of the post of janitor, Mr. James Cook of Brighton, Sussex, England, succeeded the late Mr. Thomas Cook, formerly of Her Majesty's army. Students who were in college at the period of his assumption of office will remember that Mr. James Cook came provided with an efficient and painstaking quadrupedal assistant whose honesty of purpose and power of governing men equalled that for which his master is so justly famous. All who have ever attended classes at McGill will grieve to hear that Cook's dog is suffering from symptoms of a very serious nature. The patient was at first submitted to the consideration of the members of the Faculty of the Veterinary School, and a diagnosis of *carcinoma recti* of the infracaudal variety was given. The constitutional symptoms, however, not being grave, it was decided by Mr. Cook that an expectant attitude suited the exigencies of the case. As time wore on, the general condition improved somewhat, and Mr. Cook became dissatisfied with the opinions of the veterinarians. The University Professor of Surgery was called in, and we understand that certain features in the case have arisen of such a nature as to enable this distinguished practitioner to give a more favorable prognosis, and to hold out the sufferer some hopes, if not of actual recovery, at least of mitigations of his suffering. This interesting patient has an intimate connection with the Medical Faculty. He is the son of the dog of the father of the Professor of Anatomy, by whom he was given to the Professor of Ophthalmology, who presented him to the janitor of the college, and he is the uncle of the dog of the Professor of Clinical Medicine.

BABY *was* HUNGRY.—A physician was called out of a sound slumber the other night to answer the telephone. "Hallo! what is it?" he asked, little pleased at the idea of leaving his comfortable bed. "Baby is crying, doctor; what shall I do?" came across the wire. "Oh, perhaps it's a pin," suggested the doctor, recognizing the voice of a young mother, one of his patients. "No," was the reply; "I'm sure it can't be that." "Perhaps he has the colic," returned the doctor, with well-simulated solicitude. "No, I don't think so," replied the anxious mother; "he doesn't act that way." "Then perhaps he is hungry," said the doctor, as a last resource. "Oh, I'll see," came across the wire, and then all was still. The doctor went back to bed and was soon asleep again. About half an hour afterwards he was again awakened by the violent ringing of the telephone bell. Jumping out of bed and placing the receiver to his ear, he was cheered by the following message—"You are right, doctor; baby was hungry."

THE

MONTREAL MEDICAL JOURNAL.

| VOL. XVIII. | OCTOBER, 1889. | No. 4. |

Original Communications.

ON THE MANAGEMENT OF HIP DISEASE.

BY V. P. GIBNEY, M.D., OF NEW YORK.

(*Remarks before the Canadian Medical Association, at Banff, N.W.T., Aug. 13, 1889.*)

MR. PRESIDENT AND GENTLEMEN :—It was my intention to present at this meeting a paper on the above subject, but, for many reasons, I have decided to detain you only a short while with some remarks, which, I think, will at least open a discussion that may prove profitable. On my way across the continent I learned that Dr. Cameron of Toronto would read a paper on Bone Tuberculosis. I thought, therefore, that mine would be superfluous, and I contented myself simply with a desire to participate in the discussion which Dr. Cameron, I knew, was so competent to open. Furthermore, from the impressions I have gathered, it seems that long papers would be out of place on the present occasion.

So much, then, for an apology. Into the spirit of the views expressed this morning I naturally fall. At once, therefore, I array myself on the side of the tubercular origin of what is commonly known as hip-joint disease. I have long since abandoned the traumatic theory. I believe that all cases occurring in children, with very few exceptions, are tuberculous. The researches of pathology during the last decade have, to my mind, abundantly established this theory. Clinical experience furnishes irresistible proof that the lesion here encountered is almost identical with the lesion encountered in pulmonary tuberculosis. Mr.

16

Savory of London, a few years ago, drew a very happy analogy between pulmonary and epiphysial tuberculosis. The cancellous structure of bone, apart from its hardness, is in structure almost identical with the parenchyma of lung. When the bacillus is lodged in lung tissue there radiates from this focus an inflammatory areola. If the focus is near the pleura the areola extends to this tissue, and may light up an ephemeral pleuritis. This pathological process is usually known by the symptoms produced. When the bacillus lodges on one or the other side of the epiphysial line, there radiates from this focus an areola just as we find in the lung. The signs produced are lameness, stiffness of the hip, possibly a rise of temperature, pain at the knee, reflex spasm, etc., in proportion to the degree of the inflammatory process. After a little while this process—exacerbation, we call it—undergoes resolution, for it is often ephemeral, and only a small spot of bone around the bacillus remains involved. This tissue, through which the inflammatory excursion, so to speak, has traversed, becomes more vulnerable. Recurring exacerbations destroy a larger area of tissue, and ultimately this central abscess cavity breaks through into the environment. In the disease under consideration it breaks, usually, into the capsule of the joint near the digital fossa, and we have suppurative synovitis, just as we have an empyema or a pyopneumothorax. A large clinical experience gives one a pretty intimate knowledge of the course, and the explanation of the various pathological processes becomes very easy. I can fully sympathize with fellow-practitioners who have members of their family thus afflicted, and can readily see how they cling to the traumatic theory. Few of us like to admit that any tuberculous process has invaded a member of our family. If the treatment of the traumatic hip disease differed from that of the constitutional disease, a differential diagnosis might be desirable. I am familiar with a great number of so-called traumatic cases. The families insist on this, the family physician likewise, and yet the course of the disease is identical with that occurring in a notoriously tuberculous subject.

There is another good reason, too, for belief in the tuberculous theory ; it forewarns us, and, of necessity, forearms us. The ravages of tuberculosis throughout the world have impressed all physicians alike. Even the laity looks with dread upon this decimating disease. If we, therefore, at once recognize the tuberculous lesion in the bones that enter into the formation of the joint, and if we recognize the disease sufficiently early, the responsibility will become very great. We will feel that we have a dread disease to combat ; we will adopt prompt measures of relief ; we will insist on these measures being protracted ; we will know that the disease does not run a short course ; we will not be eluded by remissions ; false hopes will not tempt us to omit protection of the joint ; our duty to ourselves and to the patient, above all, will be emphasized. This much, then, on the etiology and the pathology.

I recall the title announced, and shall proceed to tell you how I would manage a given case. Let me first, however, dwell just a little on early diagnosis. When a case comes to you for examination, take advantage of all the means that nature has given you. Remember that you have a hip with which you can compare the hip suspected. Have the clothing removed. Test the functions of the sound joint fully and carefully. By so doing you will gain the confidence of the child, and remember that the confidence is the *sine qua non* in a physical examination. Spend the time that you have in making observations. Don't waste valuable time with irrelevant talk. Observe whether there be any difference in the size of the limbs. If so, record this difference. Note any inequality in the functions of the two limbs—that is, try flexion, extension, hyper-extension, rotation inward and outward, abduction, adduction. There is no occasion for any violence. Striking the foot or the knee with the palm of the hand to test the tenderness of the joint is not only valueless, but actually harmful. In the first place, it destroys the child's confidence ; in the second place, the muscular rigidity, which is at once excited, shuts out all information. Again, if it were possible to bring the joint surfaces suddenly into contact, an abscess in the bone might be ruptured, and a destructive joint lesion follow, So that such a procedure is, as I have just

remarked, not only valueless, but hazardous. Many physicians
take a limb carelessly and move it up and down and from side
to side, and if they find a pretty fair range on motion, they say
the child has no hip disease. Many a case, both in large cities
and in provincial towns, is thus hastily passed over, and an
opinion given that there is no disease. The doctor waits for the
mother to make the diagnosis. It is she who observes the persistent lameness, expression of pain, the tenderness on moving
the limb, especially in putting on the stockings or the shoes. It
is she who hears the shriek at night. All these facts can be
brought out by a careful examination, and every patient threatened with hip disease is certainly entitled to this careful examination. Let men get into a routine method of examining. Pass
nothing over hastily. The issues are too great. The public
expects this of us. We claim to belong to an enlightened profession. In making the examination, therefore, look for atrophy
and reflex spasm—that is, an involuntary spasm which occurs
in certain groups of muscles when they are passively put on the
stretch. Look for a persistent lameness,—once lame, always
lame. Regard suspiciously any statement of the mother that
the child has been perfectly free of lameness for a certain period.
Cross-examine, and find whether it is a fact or not. We attach
very little importance now-a-days to the ilio-femoral crease or to
the shape of the nates. So much, then, for diagnosis.

While I employ the long splint known as the Davis-Taylor
splint, and while I find this very satisfactory, I am convinced
that it is not so satisfactory outside of large cities, or, at least,
away from the instrument-maker. The difficulty in securing a
fit, a knowledge of the details, putting on adhesive plaster, for
instance, adjusting the peroneal straps, getting the pelvic band
at the proper angle with the stem, getting the stem sufficiently
long,—all these points require a little practice, and he who
seldom sees cases does not get this practice. I am in the habit,
therefore, of advising, for country practice, a plaster-of-Paris
bandage, applied from the calf up over the hip in the shape of a
spika, extending up to the free ribs. Then put the patient on
a high shoe for the sound foot, and a pair of axillary crutches.

This secures protection to the joint, maintains the limb in good position, and approximates, as nearly as we can approximate, that great desideratum—absolute and unqualified rest to the joint.   The old opinion prevails, I find, throughout the country, that immobilization produces ankylosis.   This is a fallacy. Ankylosis is produced not by immobilization, but by imperfect immobilization.   The slight amount of motion that is allowed in all splints is just enough to induce adhesions about a joint, and these adhesions are what produce the ankylosis.   I have long since demonstrated that the best protection against ankylosis is immobilization while the disease is present.   If the case be taken early, before deformity has arisen, there is no occasion for any deformity occurring.   Plaster and felt, or anything that maintains the limb in a normal position and maintains it for a long time, will be a powerful factor in resolution.   If deformity is present, then secure the limb in the plaster at the angle found. After a week or two the plaster can be removed, and the deformity, with a little manual force and without pain, be reduced to a certain extent.   Secure this by plaster, and later on gain more motion and a better position.   I am aware that there are plaster bandages, and plaster bandages.   I am aware that very few men know how to put on a plaster-of-Paris bandage, but still this does not prevent me from urging them to learn how to apply a bandage.   A skin-fitting bandage can be applied just as well as one with a lot of cotton intervening.   The main thing is to have good plaster, that sets well, and is fine in quality. The best plaster is known as the dental plaster.   The Dental Manufacturing Company supplies this in six or twelve quart cans, hermetically sealed.   It needs to be kept dry, and then salt and alum are unnecessary.   Next in importance is a good crinoline bandage.   The salient points may be protected by cotton batting, but this should not be thick. The bandage should be rubbed plentifully and be rubbed glossy, and then all inequalities will have been rubbed out.   I have treated a number of cases of double hip disease by this method, and the results have been gratifying in the extreme.   Time and again I have reduced a deformity by immobilizing the joint in plaster for a

few weeks. I do not expect to cure a case in a short time.
The case must be managed. If abscesses form and become
alarming, then get rid of the abscesses by incision and evacuation. If the abscesses give rise to no constitutional disturbance,
or pain, or inconvenience, especially, do not take fright and make
a grave prognosis, but let the abscess take care of itself. Many
cases open spontaneously and good results are obtained. Bad
results take place because the joint is not protected ; not because
the abscesses are present, but because the bone and joint are
not attended to. The question of excision of the joint or gouging I shall not discuss, because I see many surgeons about me
who are more competent to discuss this matter, and shall close
my remarks by urging upon you the importance of early diagnosis—the diagnosis made before any deformity has arisen,—
the importance of regarding the lesion as tuberculous, and the
importance of protecting the joint first, last and all the time.

In conclusion, I trust none of my hearers will accuse me of
belittling the so-called American mode of traction with motion.
I simply say that traction with motion is not only bad practice,
but it is difficult to obtain. My observation is that those who
employ this method do it only in name, not in practice. The
joints of the splint are usually rusty, and the patients are not
taught to keep them in order. Good results are obtained by the
traction. The traction produces fixation. With fixation and
traction to the joint, therefore, we have the best attainable treatment. I employ traction in all of my well-to-do cases.   In my
charity cases I frequently omit this element because of the
expense, and I must confess that these do about as well as my
well-to-do cases, sometimes better. I seldom find it necessary
to confine the patient to bed. I do not use a splint by day and
a weight and pulley by night. The splint is used night and day.
I aim to keep the protection continuous. The peroneal straps
that pass from the pelvic band of the splint serve as peroneal
crutches. The constitutional treatment employed is cod liver
oil, hypophosphites, and iron in its various preparations, according to the needs of the patient. The digestive functions must
be good ; when these fail, remedies to correct. In other words,

I aim to keep my patient's health above par, and great import-ance is attached to climatic influence. It is just as important to have a patient with hip disease in a climate where bacilli are in high dilution as it is to have a phthisical patient in this alti-tude. With such advantages, then, the prognosis ought to be good. We can control a tuberculous epiphysis better than we can a tuberculous lung. By means of axillary and peroneal crutches the patients can live in the open air.

I thank the gentlemen of the Association for the attention they have given me, and I trust that I have made myself well understood.

THE CLIMATE OF SOUTHERN ALBERTA AND ITS RELATION TO HEALTH AND DISEASE.

By G. A. KENNEDY, M.D., FORT McLEOD, ALBERTA.

(*Paper read before the Canadian Medical Association, at Banff, N.W.T., August, 1889.*)

It appears to me that no apology is necessary in introducing the subject of this paper. It is only a few years since the opening of our great national highway brought the North-West Territories into touch with the rest of the world. And only a few years further back since these vast plains and mountains which are now so quickly becoming the home of civilized man were regarded as an inhospitable desert, fit only for the buffalo which roamed their solitudes and the Indians subsisting on the chase. The past five years have been epoch-making, so far as our great west is concerned. Coincident with and following on the building of the Canadian Pacific, a flood of light began to illumine the eastern intelligence, and, as a consequence, settle-ment has steadily and in a gradually increasing stream poured into the territories, and cities, towns and villages, surrounded by cultivated farms, now occupy the places once sacred to the Indian tepee or the half-breed camp.

As a matter of course, this progress has been marked by a corresponding increase of knowledge with regard to our climate. We are no longer supposed merely to exist Esquimault-like for the greater part of the year. It is conceded that our winters are bearable, even, in some enlightened minds, that they may

possess a charm of their own, but beyond this, serene and un-
bounded ignorance is the rule.   Furthermore, so far as I have
been able to ascertain, no observations have yet been published
as to the effects of the climate of the North-West on the human
system.   It is in my mind a subject of almost national importance, and I have an earnest hope that my temerity in venturing
to introduce it in this discussion will inspire others better fitted
than I to follow it up.

It will be readily understood that a country almost equal in
area to Russia must have many diversities of climate.   As I
cannot undertake to speak for the whole of the North-West, I
have limited my remarks to that part with which I am best
acquainted—viz., that strip of country lying along the eastern
base of the mountains, and more particularly the southern part
of this, bounded, say, on the north, by the Caanadian Pacific
Railway.   I make the eastern limit a line drawn north and south
through Lethbridge, although, for all practical purposes, this line
can be extended as far east as Medicine Hat; on the south is
the international boundary line, and to the west the summit line
of the Rockies and British Columbia.   This Southern Alberta
comprises an area of 150 miles square of mountain, foothill and
prairie.   It is intersected every few miles by mountain streams,
where clear and sparkling waters rippling over their gravelly
beds are as yet unpolluted by the filth and garbage of more
thickly settled communities.   Its general character is treeless,
save along the valleys of these streams, which are fringed by
the willow and cottonwood, and on the sides and bases of the
mountains, whose rocky framework is clothed by the grateful
germ of the spruce and fir.

To the outside world, this is known as Canada's grazing
country, whence England will draw a large part of its future
beef supply.   As a sort of corollary to this, it has also been
known, in a general way, that it was reputed to have a milder
climate than the rest of the North-West Territories.   To most
of you, the following description will be not only interesting but
necessary to a proper understanding of what follows.   It is
taken from an admirable paper by Mr. C. C. McCaul of Leth-

bridge, published in the August number of the *American Meteorological Review*. After noticing that winter really sets in about the middle of December, he goes on to say—

" It is characterized by a maximum of bright, still, cloudless days, a scanty snow-fall, and frequent and prolonged breaks of warm weather, heralded by the chinook wind, of which more hereafter. Occasionally a bad snow-storm will cover the prairie to a depth of eighteen or twenty inches ; this, however, is very exceptional. The winter generally breaks up in February by a grand blow from the west, followed by a period of from one to three weeks of warm, bright weather, which may fairly be called the beginning of spring.

" Spring, here as elsewhere, is the most variable and capricious season of the year. On the whole, it may, perhaps, be described as cold and damp, with frequent rain-falls, varied by bursts of the most gloriously bright, warm weather, lasting sometimes a fortnight or three weeks.

" May is generally fine, warm and bright ; June and the earlier part of July, rainy ; the remainder of July, August, September, October and November, warm and very dry.

" The summer, July to September, is characterized by hot days and cool nights, with very little rain, but the warm, hazy days of autumn often lasting well into December, are the glory of the year.

" The grand characteristic of the climate as a whole, that on which all weather hinges, is the chinook wind. It blows from west to south-west, in varying degrees of strength, from the gentle breeze, that just lowers the heads of the daisies, to the howling gale, that carries off contributions of chimneys, barrels, shingles, hats and miscellaneous rubbish to our neighbors in Assiniboia. In winter the wind is distinctly warm ; in summer, not so distinctly cool. Its approach is heralded by the massing of dark, cumulus clouds above the mountain tops, and a distant wailing and rumbling from the passes and gorges. Its effect in winter is little short of miraculous. When the real chinook blows, the thermometer often rises in a few hours from 20° below to 40° above zero ; the snow, which in the morning may have been a foot deep, disappears, and before night everything is dripping. But before another night falls, all the water is lapped up by the thirsty wind, and the prairie is so dry that a horse's hoof hardly makes an impression, as you take your first welcome canter, after a prolonged and tedious spell of 'settin' round the stove.' "

It may be added to this that the elevation above sea level of the plains here varies from 2,700 feet at Lethbridge to 4,500 feet at the entrance to the Crow's Nest Pass, which may be taken as the base of the mountains proper.

Now, as to practical details, I might say that winter and early spring are characterized by the coughs and colds incident to their seasons in almost any country. Summer is very healthy, and in autumn there are occasional cases of malarial fever of a remittent type, of which more hereafter. Rheumatism is remarkably rare, when we consider the sudden changes of temperature that often occur and the fact that most of the male population have led lives of the greatest exposure. When it does occur it is almost always in the subacute and chronic forms. Affections of the lungs are also very infrequent. During eleven years' practice I never had a case of pneumonia until last winter, when four cropped up, two each of croupous and catarrhal. Summer disorders are almost unknown—a fact which must be attributed partly to the sparseness of population, but which is largely due, in my opinion, to the cool nights, which allow exhausted nature to recuperate even after the hottest days. About nervous affections I am hardly in a position to speak, but I judge that the rarified air and the sometimes high winds would not be beneficial. During the past four years I have had three cases of paralysis—hemiplegia—occurring in patients otherwise perfectly healthy, cowboys in the prime and vigor of manhood, who have had no specific disease, who were quite temperate, and whose family history the most careful inquiry found irreproachable. These cases were and are a puzzle to me, and I can imagine no cause but excessive riding. A cowboy's life, as you know, means often ten, twelve and fourteen hours in the saddle, day after day, week after week, and month after month, and it has seemed to me possible that this might in time produce the above effects.

I have alluded to the existence of an endemic malarial fever occurring principally in the fall.   This is general throughout the Territories, and has given rise to much comment and some difference of opinion among medical men. Its character is variously modified by the season, climate, soil and immediate surroundings of the locality in which it is present.   It has been called remittent, intermittent, malarial, typho-malarial and typhoid, according as a certain set of symptoms predominated, and is known throughout all the West by laymen as "mountain fever." During the past ten years, and while acting as surgeon in the Mounted Police, I have been stationed in different parts of the Territories, and have had occasion to observe this fever in all its different forms.   I have seen it at its lightest, characterized only by a chill and the symptoms of a heavy cold, and broken up at once by free diaphoresis and a dose of quinine.   On the other hand, I have attended cases in which all treatment was of no avail, cases badly affected by environment, that would go on from bad to worse until finally they would sink into the typhoid state— too often only the beginning of the end. Between these extremes all grades of severity are met with, their most general characteristic being, however, their atypical character. Routine treatment is therefore impossible, except, perhaps, at the beginning, when I made it a rule to relieve the bowels by a calomel purge, promote free diaphoresis by pulv. ipecac. co. or antipyrin, sometimes a combination of the two, and give two or three large doses of quinine,—subsequent treatment on general principles.

I have alluded to the different names by which this fever has been called and the consequent confusion.   The cause of this is, I believe, the tendency to regard it as a distinct typical disease, which it is *not*.   The cause may be the same (no one, I believe, has ever questioned its malarial nature), but the variations in the course, symptoms and severity are important enough to entitle them to be called almost distinct types.   These variations are due to locality, to the season, to differing conditions of soil, climate, atmospheric moisture, etc., and to the individual.   Another cause of the confusion has been the occasional occurrence of typhoid fever and the incautious use of the unfortunate term " typho-malarial." I say unfortunate, because I believe that from the time of its coinage in 1861-2 it has never ceased to be a cloak for uncertainty, an unknown quantity in statistics, and an added difficulty to the struggling and inexperienced practitioner. It would be a good thing, in my opinion, if it were expunged from the nomenclature of diseases ; for, notwithstanding the care that was exercised in its definition by the U. S. Commission, wherein it was distinctly pointed out that it was " *not* a specific or distinct type of disease, but a term conveniently applied to the compound forms of fever which result from the combined influences of the causes of the malarious fevers and of typhoid fever," there *has been* a tendency to elevate it into a distinct type of disease. In the North-West, while I have often seen severe cases of malarial-remittent falling into the typhoid state, and cases of typhoid marked at first by malaria, while, I confess, I have been sometimes at a loss at first to classify my case, I can hardly recall an instance in which waiting a few days did not clear up the diagnosis. A case in point is the following :

A man came into Macleod from a ranche twenty miles distant, last fall, suffering from all the symptoms of quotidian intermittent. He had, some years before, lived in a malarious district of Michigan, and been subject to ague. He had been sick for three or four days, the chills, fever and sweating well marked and definite, but there was more depression than is the case in an ordinary intermittent. I treated him for three or four days, and broke up the periodicity. The fever became remittent then, and four days after there appeared the rose-colored spots and other symptoms of typhoid, which ran its course to recovery. I may say in passing, that a case like this illustrates the difficulty in understanding how typhoid fever never occurs *de novo*, but always from the presence of a pre-existent specific germ. The ranche from which this man came is isolated, and had only been established some two or three years. The water supply was from a spring. There had never been a case there before, and the place has been free from it since.

In 1886 I made an attempt to have collected detailed reports of all cases of fevers occurring throughout the North-West, so that the special features of each district might become better known. This attempt was frustrated through ignorance or misapprehension of my motive. It is a matter of regret to me that my suggestions were not adopted, for I am not one of those who believe that we have reached the sum possible of attainable knowlege with regard to malaria. We owe much to the researches of Thommasi, Crudeli and Klebs, Laveran, Osler and Carter, in tracing out the life history in the blood of the malarial plasmodium. But I believe the future has still something to unfold to us of its nature, mode of action outside of, and entrance into the human system. And I believe we have yet much to learn of the relations between the paludal and typhoid poisons. I find it difficult to believe the story of the statistics which tells us that typhoid fever, pure and simple, is three, four and five times more fatal than the same fever complicated with malaria. And I believe that more care in the diagnosis, which is now rendered somewhat easier by the application of Ehrlich's test, more thoroughness in the recording of cases, and more attention to etiology, will help us to clear up these doubtful points which few will question are stumbling-blocks in our path.

I trust that I have not been misunderstood—that while remarking on the fever at greater length, perhaps, than its importance warrants, I have not led you to the belief that it is a constant menace to life and health in South Alberta. I should be sorry to have made this impression, which would be an entirely false one. Some years the country is entirely free from fever, and generally it is mild and readily amenable to treatment. And severe cases will no doubt become rarer when greater care is exercised in personal and domestic sanitation. I believe that I have now said the worst that *can* be said of the climate of Southern Alberta, and I consider that in doing so I have earned the right to dwell briefly on what appears to me its distinguishing characteristic. I allude to its freedom from diseases of the lungs and its value as a resort or place of living for phthisical patients. I have already spoken of the

rarity of pneumonia and other lung affections. I know of two
cases of phthisis commencing in the country—one of acute
tuberculosis, strongly hereditary, and which proved fatal, and
another of fibroid, the cause of which I believe to be the fine
dust of the corral acting in the same manner as stone-mason's
and knife-grinder's phthisis. This latter steadily improved on
ceasing work, and is now nearly well. On the other hand, I
have known of a great many cases of incipient consumption that
have come to Alberta, and in some the disease has been arrested,
and in others the sufferer restored to perfect health. These facts
will not appear strange when the conditions are considered, for,
according to the latest consensus of opinion among climatologists,
the climate treatment of phthisis requires—

1. A dry aseptic atmosphere.

2. A dry soil.

3. The greatest possible number of clear, sunshiny days during which the invalid can exercise in the open air.

4. A certain amount or degree of elevation above sea level.
Equability of temperature within certain limits is not considered
necessary.

I believe I may assert, without danger of contradiction, that
Southern Alberta possesses all these requisites in a most eminent
degree.   The dryness of the atmosphere is insured by the character of the country. A great, grassy, undulating, treeless
plain, elevated from two to five thousand feet above sea level,
and distant some hundreds of miles from any considerable body
of water.   Accurate meteorological data are wanting, but it is
sufficient to say that Alberta is not different from the whole
strip of country lying along the eastern base of the continental
watershed, and which the absence of a sufficient rainfall has
caused to be devoted principally to the raising of stock. This
dryness of the air, combined with its elevation, almost necessarily renders it aseptic in a wonderful degree.

Elevation is not now considered by some an essential feature
in the climatic treatment of phthisis. The altitude theory, which
Miguel did so much to bring into favor, and which was so great
an advance in the indiscriminate employment of places like

Madeira and Havana—places where warmth and equality of temperature and a certain degree of moisture were prevailing features—is now slowly going out of fashion. But it is doubtful if even the immense power of fashion—which, it is to be deplored, is almost as great in medicine as in millinery—will ever be able to seriously affect, in the medical mind, the value of elevation. The reason it is not so much considered new is that it was found that the curative properties were the dryness and purity of the air, not necessarily elevation. But it is difficult, almost impossible, to find a dry aseptic atmosphere* without the elevation, or near sea level, and for this reason, if for no other, patients in search of a climate will still throng to the elevated regions. Besides the other physiological effects of elevation, the increased respiratory activity and expansion of the lungs and chest walls, the consequent increased nutrition, the cool nights, almost compelling sound and refreshing sleep, are all factors of no little value in the altitude treatment.

As before mentioned, the elevation in Southern Alberta varies from two to five thousand feet, and the patient can therefore choose the locality which seems to suit best his particular case. Laennec, Bowditch, Buchanan and others having made it very clear that soil moisture is one of the chief causes of phthisis, a dry soil must be considered a necessity for any place putting forward claims to be regarded as a resort or place of living for consumptives.

While I am not able to give the geological formation of South Alberta, I *can* assert, without fear of contradiction, that its soil must be regarded as pre-eminently a dry one. While water is easily obtainable in and near the mountains, and in certain places elsewhere throughout the greater part of the district, and particularly from where the foothills merge into the plains, it is difficult to get it near the surface, and it is not unusual to hear of wells having to be bored to the depth of one, two and three hundred feet.

Perhaps a more important point than any of the foregoing—certainly a most necessary one—is the number of days during which patients can take exercise in the open air.

* Excepting Aiken, Ga.

Here the want of meteorological observations is again surely felt, but from a private record kept during the five years, ending December, 1888, I am able to state the following.

The number of days which are recorded as overcast, raining and storming, is respectively, 51, 49, 56, 53, and 44, being an average of a fraction over fifty, all the rest being noted as fine. Over fifty per cent. of these (fifty) are simply overcast, so it is fairly presumable that in the large majority, confinement to the house would be unnecessary.

These observations were taken, moreover, very close to the mountains, where local storms are more prevalent than on the plains.

As to the class of cases for which Southern Alberta is suitable, I am content to take Dr. Knight's selection, which is, I believe, approved by the great balance of authority on the subject. It comprises :

I. Those presenting the earliest physical signs of tuberculosis of the apex, who have as yet shown little if any general disturbance from the disease, and who complain only of morning cough and expectoration.

As Dr. Knight very truly remarks, the prognosis in this class has been changed from very bad to very good by the improved ideas of treatment.

II. Hemorrhage cases without marked febrile reaction or much physical evidence of disease.

III. Certain cases of fibroid or interstitial pneumonia.

IV. Patients recovering from acute pleurisy or pneumonia in whom the erruption of the tubercle is dreaded.

For these classes of cases Southern Alberta offers inducements hardly excelled by any place on the continent. I trust I have already satisfied you that the necessary climatic conditions are present, the dry aseptic atmosphere, the dry soil, the clear sunshiny days, and the necessary elevation. I have not dwelt on other points, but I should exceed the limits of an article of this kind, but there are one or two which I feel compelled to mention. One is that seekers after health are not obliged to remain for a few months, at the approach of winter or summer, only, and then go away again. They can live here with equal benefit all the year round. Another is that, being a stock-raising country, it is easily possible to spend almost all one's time in the saddle. It was Sydenham who said that "unlimited horseback exercise is almost as good a cure for phthisis as quinine for ague." Another is that Alberta is in Canada, so why should Canadian physicians send their patients to Colorado, when they have a climate equally as good within the confines of their own Dominion ?

The general conditions of life are those of any new and growing country. Many of the pleasures of the east have to be dispensed with. Our embryo cities do not yet possess the theatres, opera houses and pleasure resorts of their more pre-tentious eastern sisters. But to most people the bright sunny skies, the pure, bracing, intoxicating air, the exhilarating freedom of outdoor life, and the unrivalled scenery of Alberta will amply compensate for the artificial pleasures they are obliged to forego.

17

Retrospect Department.

QUARTERLY RETROSPECT OF OBSTETRICS.

PREPARED BY J. CHALMERS CAMERON, M.D.,

rofessor of Obstetrics, McGill University ; Physician-Accoucheur to the Montreal Maternity, &c.

A Variety of Post-Partum Shock.—The notes of the following three cases were read before the Edinburgh Obstetrical Society by Dr. Ferguson in May last (*Edin. Med. Journal*).

1.—Patient æt. 28, IV-para, had a neurotic family history and was herself of a highly nervous temperament. Previous labors were normal ; present labor was rapid and easy, terminating four hours after the onset of pains. In the absence of the medical attendant, the nurse conducted the case, grasping the uterus firmly after the delivery of the child, and keeping it compressed till a physician arrived. The patient complained that the kneading of the uterus caused her much pain, and soon after the expulsion of the placenta she suddenly lost consciousness. For three hours she lay in that state, with face pinched and pulse imperceptible, then gradually the pulse began to flutter, and shortly afterward she swallowed some stimulant and regained consciousness. Thenceforth convalescence was normal.

2.—Patient æt. 27, I-para, healthy, had a normal labor, except that rigidity of the outlet necessitated the low forceps operation. The placenta not coming away, an anæsthetic was sparingly administered, and Credé's method tried. After repeated fruitless attempts, the placenta had finally to be removed manually. The patient complained of great pain while pressure was being made upon the uterus. Immediately after the placenta was delivered, she suddenly became pulseless, cold, pale and gasping. Ether was injected hypodermically, and she rallied for a time but soon again collapsed. Throughout the whole night rectal injections and hypodermics of ether had to be administered, and she did not rally permanently till the following morning. Convalescence was uninterrupted.

3.—Patient æt. 27, healthy and well developed, but of nervous temperament, had a tedious labor, requiring chloroform and forceps.   After anæsthesia had passed off, she complained loudly of pain when the uterus was grasped, and felt sick and faint.   Just as the placenta emerged from the vulva, she became unconscious, pulse and respiration scarcely perceptible and she seemed moribund.   She remained in that state for three hours and then slowly recovered consciousness.   The uterus was well contracted and there was no hemorrhage.

These three patients were all young, healthy, and of nervous temperament, their labors were not specially difficult, there was no hemorrhage, cardiac disease and eclampsia could be excluded, and yet they all suddenly developed symptoms of syncope and shock.   They became unconscious, with rapid, feeble and irregular pulse, dilated pupils, shallow, irregular breathing and cold clammy perspiration.   The face was at first anxious, then vacant and torpid, and sensibility to pain became entirely obliterated.   This alarming condition lasted about three hours, and it was with great difficulty that the patients were restored to consciousness in eight to twelve hours by means of hypodermics, rectal injections, stimulants, frictions and hot applications.   No ill effects were felt afterwards, nor did the women have any recollection of what they had passed through.   They felt exhausted and complained of tenderness in the lower abdomen.   In two cases the convalescence was quite normal, in the third there was persistent sleeplessness, with occasional incoherence developing into mild melancholia, from which recovery eventually took place.   The shock occurred either during or immediately after the expulsion of the placenta while the uterus was being grasped and manipulated through the abdominal wall.   In all probability squeezing or bruising of one ovary (or perhaps both) took place during the manipulations.   Analogous symptoms have been described during operations for removal of the appendages when it was found difficult to bring the ovaries near the abdominal wound, and when they were pretty roughly handled.   Credé's method should always be used gently ; rough handling of the uterus and too vigorous friction can do no good and may cause serious harm.   The post-partum uterus should be grasped as nearly as possible *antero-posteriorly*, always remembering the usual rotation of the uterus upon its own axis to the right. A *lateral* grasp is apt to include the ovaries and subject them to injurious pressure. Lateral grasp is only required during intra-uterine injections post-partum, in order to compress the fallopian tubes and prevent the entrance of fluid into the abdominal cavity.

Can the Typhoid Fever Germ be transmitted from the Mother to the foetus in utero ?—The whole question as to the passage of infective germs from mother to child is still under discussion. While the possibility of such an occurrence must be admitted, it by no means follows that germs have the power of penetrating and traversing the *healthy* placenta. It is more than probable that some lesion must exist in the placental structure before such an interchange can become possible.

Eberth has recently published an important case bearing upon this point. (*Die Fortschritte der Medicin*, 1889, No. 5.) A woman, æt. 30, five months pregnant, contracted Typhoid fever and aborted three weeks afterwards. Eleven hours after birth the fœtus and placenta were sent to Eberth for examination. Samples of blood from the heart, lungs and spleen were examined microscopically and gelatine cultures prepared from them. A large number of typhoid bacilli (Gaffky) were found in the villosities of the placenta, as well as in the gelatine cultures. Did they pass from the mother to the fœtus, and, if so, how ?

Causes of Placental Retention after Full-time Delivery.— In the Strassburg Policlinic, Freund has observed retention of the placenta 7 times in 780 cases (*Zeits. f. Geb. und Gyn.*, Bd. XVI. Hft. 1), and in all the seven cases he found great contraction of the internal os. In three there was congenital anteflexion of the uterus, and in one an acquired anteflexion. He considers marked narrowing of the os to be one of the characteristic symptoms of anteflexion. In such cases he considers that flexion, narrowing of the os and an unyielding condition of the walls may be early recognized. He considers that this theory has a practical bearing, and insists that in all cases where anteflexion has been made out before or shortly after the beginning of gestation, the attendant should be very careful in the management of labor; in the third stage especially he should avoid everything which would tend to promote constriction of the contraction-ring, to which a predisposition already exists. The bladder and rectum should be emptied before and during labor; ergot and all irritating drinks or medicines should be avoided; the treatment of the third stage should be strictly expectant. All manipulation, friction and compression of the uterus, pulling upon the cord, and untimely or violent efforts to express the placenta should be avoided.

Ahlfeld says (*Zeits. f. Geb. und Gyn.*, Bd. XVI., Hft. 2) that when the placenta is allowed to separate and come away naturally without making any attempt to excite uterine contraction by friction or other manipulation, retention will not occur more frequently than 5—8 times in 1000 cases. He states that in 1500 births in the Marburg Clinic, from 1883 to 1889, the whole placenta had to be removed 11 times (7 per cent.), and small pieces of placenta twice, making 13 cases in all (8 per cent.) When any artificial method is employed (such as Credé's), and the placenta is subsequently retained, it becomes a question whether we have to do with a primary retention or with an incarceration due to the manipulation. Retention may be due to (1) spasmodic constriction of the uterus below the already separated placenta, (2) adhesion to the uterine wall, (3) both causes combined. The site of the constriction may be anywhere between the contraction-ring and the external os. In order that a constriction may keep back a wholly-separated placenta, it must occur soon after the passage of the breech from the uterus, and there must have been some irritation of the contracting part either before or after delivery. Such irritation may be caused by the use of the forceps, especially in case of eclampsia, or by forcibly dragging the fœtus through a partially dilated os, or by the use of very hot or very cold vaginal douches before the placenta has left the lower uterine segment. Touching, rubbing or irritating the puerperal cervix will sometimes cause such a degree of constriction that even fluids are retained in the uterine cavity for a time. He says that in the

Marburg Clinic the most frequent cause of retention has been manipulation of the cervix and lower uterine segment (instead of the fundus and upper portion of the body), while Credé's method was being practised by unskilled persons. He agrees with Credé that, in the majority of cases of so-called *adherent placenta*, there is simply incarceration without adhesion ; but he thinks that cases of true adhesion are not as infrequent as Credé and others affirm. Morbid adhesion of the placenta is most apt to occur when the attachment is low, especially in placenta praevia. The morbid adhesion between the maternal decidua and the fœtal portion of the placenta is the result of inflammatory action, either in the placenta itself or decidua. He believes inflammatory action to be set up by cell-elements migrating from the cervix into the uterine cavity and making their way beneath the placenta. The prognosis of adherent placenta is worse than that of simple incarceration. When the hand has to be passed into the uterus and the placenta peeled off, more or less elevation of temperature usually follows, no matter what antiseptic precautions are adopted. Out of 13 such cases, only four made a normal convalescence, free from fever—*i. e.* 30.8 per cent., against 70 per cent., the average in uncomplicated cases. With regard to treatment, he says that if incarceration only is suspected, he tries to draw down the placenta by means of its presenting part and avoids passing his hand into the uterine cavity if possible. He agrees with Freund in recommending the expectant treatment in the third stage, but does not agree with him as to the ætiology of incarceration. He considers Freund's anteflexion of the puerperal uterus to be a normal condition, and attributes the retention to other causes.

The Treatment of Retained Membranes.—Eberhardt, of Halle (*Zeits. f. Geb. und Gyn.*, Bd. XVI., Hft. 2), finds a wide divergence of opinion among authorities as to the ætiology, significance and treatment of retained membranes. *Ahlfeld* thinks that self-infection may follow the retention of even a very small portion of decidua, and attributes retention to the use of Credé's method. *Lazarewitsch* considers the retention of chorion and decidua more dangerous than of ammion, because they offer less resistance to decay. *Olshausen* believes the retention of even the whole chorion to be free from danger, and advises passing the hand into the uterus only when there is reason to believe that a placenta succenturiata exists. *Credé* says that retention of membranes is not dangerous. *Kaltenbach* reconciles these differences of opinion by maintaining that the danger does not consist in the retention of membranes or blood-clots *per se*, but in bacteria gaining access to them within the uterine cavity. Clinically he has not been able to find bacteria inside the healthy uterine cavity *post partum*, and his clinical observations have been subsequently confirmed by the bacteriological investigations of Döderlein and Winter. From his examinations of uteri removed by the total extirpation operation or the supravaginal amputation, Winter concludes, " the genital canal of the healthy woman contains micro-organisms in the vagina and cervix, while the uterus and tubes are free ; the boundary line between the bacteria-holding and the bacteria-free portions is about the margin of the internal os uteri." Döderlein's observations prove that, under normal conditions, bacteria do not exist in the lochial flux as it comes from the uterus, but that bacteria enter it in the vagina. Applying these observations to the question of retained membranes, Kaltenbach concludes that as long as the membranes are enclosed in the uterine cavity, and not brought in contact with infectious germs without, they will remain free from putrefactive changes ; but they will begin to putrefy as soon as bacteria enter the uterine cavity and reach them. If the membranes protrude partially into the cervix or vagina, the entrance of bacteria is facilitated and the danger of infection increased ; he therefore removes manually only those portions which protrude through the cervix into the vagina. He lays great stress upon the prophylactic disinfection of the vagina before and during labor. While carrying out this strict prophylaxis for four years in Giessen, and one year and a half in Halle, he has had no parametritis, no severe endometritis, no endocolpitis, no peritonitis, although the sanitary condition of the Giessen hospital was bad. In Halle the treatment of the third stage is expectant; if the placenta does not come away in 1½–2 hours, Credé's method is employed. Retention of membranes is very rare; but when it does occur, two or three fingers are passed into the vagina (never into the uterus) and those portions which protrude from the cervix are removed. The prophylactic treatment consists in washing the external genitals thoroughly with soap and water and irrigating the vagina before the first vaginal examination is made, and at intervals till the conclusion of labor. If the membranes are retained, the vagina is irrigated twice daily with a sublimate solution (1×3000) and ergotine administered till they come away. Intra-uterine injections are avoided for fear of introducing bacteria into the uterine cavity. The essential points in Kaltenbach's treatment are (1) removal of only those portions of the membranes which protrude into the vagina, (2) keeping the vagina aseptic during the puerperium by repeated irrigations, (3) the administration of ergotine to hasten the separation of the adherent membranes.

The Micro-organisms of the Umbilical Cord and Stump.—Cholmorgoroff, of Moscow, has recently published the results of his elaborate investigations upon this subject (*Zeits. f. Geb. und Gyn.*, Bd. XVI., Hft. 1). In ordinary practice the cord is washed, dried and wrapped up in a fold or two of singed or dry linen, and changed once or twice daily till the cord falls off. Under this method the cord separates slowly, and if it happens to be very thick there may be considerable odor for three or four days; it may not come away for 8 to 10 or even 12 to 14 days; a large open surface is then frequently left which is often difficult to heal, and through which there is liability to septic infection. Pus from the child's eyes, foul compresses, sponges or bath water, septic matters from the mother, may be the medium of infection. Von Holst has proved that the puerperal virus may enter the child's body through the unhealed navel-stump, as well as through wounds of the skin or mucous membranes. It is, therefore, better for the nurse to make a daily practice of washing and dressing the child before she attends to the mother. It must be borne in mind, however, that the matter from a foul suppurating cord may prove injurious to the mother, so that the nurse should always wash and disinfect her hands after dressing such a cord before she attends to the mother.   The cord separates either by dry mummification or by moist gangrene ; mummification is favored by high temperature, and dryness of the air and dressings which come in contact with the cord ; gangrene is favored by moisture and exclusion of air.   The infection of the child through the umbilical stump is best prevented by aiding the dry mummification of the cord ; dry dressings seem most suitable for this purpose. Some use absorbent cotton or gauze, plain or medicated ; others use powdered starch, or powdered salicylic acid and starch (1×5), or fine plaster of Paris.   Cholmogoroff made a series of observations upon the cord at the time of birth to ascertain whether micro-organisms are normally present ; and as mummification does not proceed with equal rapidity in all cases or under all dressings, he investigated the development of bacteria under different methods of treating the cord.   His conclusions may be summarized as follows :—

1.—The navel-cord of the new-born child is absolutely free from bacteria ; if subsequently present, they must have been introduced from without.

2.—In the stump the organisms which are found are—
   Non-pathological : Sarcina lutea and bacillus subtilis.
   Pathological : Staphylococous albus, aureus and citreus
      and streptococcus pyogenes.

3.—The stump undergoes mummification or mortification according to its surroundings.

4.—An increased development of both the pathological and non-pathological bacteria is favored by fœtid mortification.

5.—During dry mummification, the greater portion of the cord (the hard dry external portion) develops only non-pathological organisms, while a very small segment (next the navel) develops a few pathological as well as the non-pathological organisms.

6.—Under the plaster dressing, mummification takes place

more completely than under other dressings, and fewer pathological bacteria are observed.

7.—The pathological bacteria of the navel-cord are identical with those of puerperal fever.

8.—The appearance of pathological bacteria in the navel-cord is independent of puerperal fever in the mother and ophthalmia in the child.

Precocious Marriages and Their Consequences (Annales de Gyn. et d' Obstet).—Prof. Rouvier, of Beyrouth (Syria), during a prolonged residence in the East, has had abundant opportunities of studying the effect of precocious marriage upon the general health of the mother and child. Out of 1400 married women who applied for treatment at his clinic, he found 79 under the age of 15 years. He divides these into four groups:—

1.—*Nulliparæ*, comprising 11 women, 5 of whom had married before having menstruated (two at 11 years, one at 12 and one at 15). In these five women the menses first appeared on the average 24 months after the consummation of marriage.

2.—Women who had accouchements at full term only—29 women, 8 of whom had married before the establishment of menstruation.

3.—Women who had both accouchements at full term and abortions—32 women, of whom 9 had not menstruated before marriage.

4.—Women who had had abortions only—7 women, of whom one had married six months before menstruating.

These 79 women, all married before their sixteenth year, during seventeen years of married life had 316 pregnancies, of which 76 were abortions (24 per cent). Inflammatory affections (metritis and endometritis) occurred 40 times; displacements and flexions, 33 times, retroversion being the most frequent; dysmenorrhœa, amenorrhœa, metrorrhagia, fibromata, cancer, polypi, &c., 20 times.

His conclusions respecting the effects of early marriage are—

1.—The absolute fecundity is diminished.

2.—The proportion of abortions is increased.

3.—Sexual intercourse and labor at too early an age favor

the development of inflammations and displacements of the uterus, and alterations in its shape.

Prof. Rouvier says that it is erroneous to suppose, as is commonly done, that the very early marriages in the east are the logical result of precocious puberty. Marriage is contracted regardless of puberty.

Shoulder Presentation Thirteen Times in the Same Woman. —Dr. G. Eustache, of Lille, reports a remarkable case (*Nouv. Arch. d' Obst. et de Gyn*). Shoulder presentations are relatively rare, but it is rarer still to find this abnormality recurring a number of times successively in the same patient. Only a few such cases are on record.

Gery reports one case where the shoulder presented in *nine* successive pregnancies.

Walter reports one of shoulder presentation in *five* successive pregnancies, the fourth being a case of twins, each foetus presenting by the shoulder.

Léchryse reports one of *three* successive shoulder presentations.

Danyan reports several cases, one of *five* and another of *nine* consecutive shoulder presentations.

Joulin confined a woman *four* times with shoulder presentation; in two subsequent pregnancies the vertex presented and labor terminated spontaneously.

Nægelé had one case of *five* shoulder presentations in *six* pregnancies.

Meissner, the elder, relates a case where the first pregnancy was a vertex and the *eleven* subsequent ones were shoulder.

Eustache's case is even still more remarkable. The patient was married at the age of nineteen, and two years subsequently bore her first child (1870). The vertex presented, labor was tedious and difficult, but terminated spontaneously. The perineum was completely torn through and the cervix lacerated on the left side up to the vaginal junction ; both healed badly. In 1871 she became again pregnant, shoulder presenting, version. The same again in 1873, 1875 and 1876. In 1877, a seven months' child, still-born, shoulder presenting. In 1878, abortion at the third month. In 1879, a seven-months' child, still-born, shoulder presenting. In 1880, 1882 and 1883, living children at full term, shoulder presentations, version. In her next three pregnancies she miscarried, twice at seven months and once at eight months and a half, the children all presenting by the shoulder, and delivered by version still-born. Her fifteenth pregnancy, also a shoulder presentation at full term, was terminated by version (April, 1889). A careful examination was made of the uterus by external and internal manipulations without finding any evidence of malformation, such as the *uterus septus*. Here was a woman who in her first pregnancy had a normal vertex presentation and was delivered spontaneously ; then thirteen times consecutively the shoulder presented and version had to be performed. In such a case one can hardly suppose that the abnormality was always accidental or by chance ; it is more rational to infer that the shoulder presentation was the regular and normal one, "*franche,*" as Pinard would call it. The explanation, however, is not easy. In accidental cases the abnormality is usually explained by the absence or derangement of some of the factors of accommodation, such as small size of the fœtus, dropsy of the amnion, twins, deformity of pelvis, abnormal insertion of placenta, abnormal laxness of the uterine or abdominal wall, frequent child-bearing, &c. It is hard to admit the action of such purely contingent causes when the malpresentation recurs so repeatedly. It has been suggested by Wigand, Hergott and others that a special primitive malformation of the uterus may exist, by virtue of which the long diameter of the uterine ovoid is transverse instead of vertical. This might be the case in a cordiform or partially bilobed uterus. Eustache attributes the recurrence of the malpresentation in his case to the relaxation of the uterine walls and fibromuscular structures at the pelvic brim, caused by the enormous cervical laceration of the first confinement. He intends performing trachelorrhaphy, and, if the operation succeeds, it will be interesting to note whether the malpresentation recurs in future pregnancies. If the author's theory is correct, we will have still another argument in favor of Emmet's operation.

The Diagnosis of Placenta Prævia by Abdominal Palpation.—Dr. Herbert Spencer, of University College Hospital, read a paper before the London Obstetrical Society recently (*Brit. Med. Journal*) which provoked considerable discussion. After shewing the possibility of making out the placental site by abdominal palpation when situated in the upper segment of the uterus, he described seven cases of placenta prævia in which he had diagnosed the presence or absence of the placenta from the anterior wall of the lower segment, the diagnosis being subsequently verified by vaginal and intra-uterine examination. The seven patients were all multiparæ, the vertex presented, and the examination was made without anæsthesia before the rupture of membranes and onset of pains. In four cases it was made out that the placenta was not attached in front ; in the remaining three its exact site was determined, in two cases before it could be felt per vaginam. As the result of this experience Dr. Spencer concludes that the following information can be derived from abdominal palpation, the patient being in the dorsal position with rectum and bladder empty :—

1.—In ordinary vertex presentations, the placenta being in the upper segment under favorable circumstances, the occiput, forehead (at a higher level) and the side of the head can be distinctly felt in the lower segment.

2.—In *placenta-prævia*, with vertex presenting, the head cannot be felt where the placenta is situated, but may be distinctly felt where the placenta is absent. If the placenta is in front, the examining fingers are kept from the head by an elastic mass of the consistence of a wetted bath-sponge. If its edge can be felt, it has the shape of the segment of a circle ; within the circle everything is obscure to touch, but outside the head may be plainly felt. Impulses to the head are not clearly felt through the placenta ; impulses to the head through the placenta are distinctly felt wherever the placenta is absent.

In the discussion which followed, opinions varied greatly. Braxton Hicks and Barnes agreed with the speaker. Barnes said that when the placenta is situated in the upper zone in front, the uterine wall is thickened and raised at the area of placental attachment, forming a sort of hillock, rising above the smooth uterine surface. Matthews Duncan believes the diagnosis of the healthy placenta during pregnancy, by palpation, to be impossible. In order to know what to expect to feel, the mind must be divested of the appearance and feel of the born placenta ; one must learn the feel of an attached living healthy placenta in utero. The born placenta is a thrombosed cake, while the living placenta is ill-defined, soft, with fretted vesicular surface not easy to recognize by touch. Champneys and others pointed out that the placental site can not be diagnosed by auscultation. In reply, Dr. Spencer admitted that the placenta (in p. prævia) is more easily made out when the head presents ; but, judging from actual measurements of specimens, he did not think that the prævial placenta is usually thin and spread out. In one of his cases at the eighth month the part felt through the abdominal wall was one inch and a half thick near the edge.

QUARTERLY RETROSPECT OF GYNÆCOLOGY.

PREPARED BY T. JOHNSON-ALLOWAY, M.D.,

Instructor in Gynæcology, McGill University ; Assistant Surgeon to the Montreal General Hospital ; Gynæcologist to the Montreal Dispensary.

Discussion on Treatment of Pedicle in Myoma.—A most interesting discussion took place recently at one of the meetings of the British Gynæcological Society relating to the best method of securing the pedicle of a myoma uteri:

Dr. BANTOCK said there could be no doubt that the question of the treatment of the pedicle was all-important in fibroids of the uterus. He agreed that certain cases of pedunculated fibroid might be treated by ligature of the pedicle, but if Dr. Fenton thought that the matter could be settled in the easy way suggested by him, he was very much mistaken. Some pedicles would be insecure and dangerous, no matter however carefully they were tied. An allegation of careless-ness was not a sufficient explanation. He had tried both plans, and it was his want of success with the ligature that had led him to have recourse almost invariably to the extra-peritoneal treatment. He had used the most powerful forceps. He had compressed the pedicle to an eighth of its original volume. He had applied the double ligature, transfixing it in addition to a circular ligature, and even stitched the peritoneal edges together; yet before the operation had been completed oozing had often begun. He insisted on the fact that patients did not usually die from the hemorrhage as such, but from septicæmia, due to the decomposition of the ooze. That was why the use of a drainage tube was advised. It must be that they feared the oozing from the stump of the pedicle, for there was nowhere else it could come from. He would be very glad if a method could be devised to overcome the difficulties and drawbacks, as the recovery took much less time. Hitherto, however, he had heard of no such method which would give them such assurance against hemorrhage as they could obtain from the extra-abdominal method.

Mr. TAIT said he heartily endorsed the remarks made by Dr. Bantock, but he thought it was necessary to refute somewhat more categorically the allegation that patients died in consequence of carelessness in trying the ligature. He said that if Dr. Fenton visited his armamentarium and saw the numberless contrivances and devices for the purpose of tying the cord more tightly than it could be tied by the human hand, he would relieve them from such a charge. He said that even the most tempting-looking pedicles could not be relied on, because uterine tissue was so laden with serum that even if tied ever so tightly it would begin to bleed in twenty-four hours. He had tied some five or six thousand pedicles, and while he had never had hemorrhage from ovarian pedicles, except in one or two cases, it was quite another thing with the pedicles of fibroids. He regretted nothing so much as having been induced to try the intra-peritoneal treatment of the pedicle. Even hydraulic pressure would not render them secure, and he had employed pressure up to two or three tons. At present, all that his nurses had to do was to give a turn to the next nut whenever oozing set in. They were not secure until the lapse of eighty or ninety hours. It was true that certain cases might be safely treated by ligature, but as it was impossible to distinguish them prior to operation, that knowledge was not of much service. To illustrate the peculiarity of uterine tissue, he mentioned that it was his habit in applying the *serre nœud* to tighten the wire all he could; indeed, all that the wire would bear without cutting through the tissues. Then, in the course of trimming the stump he tightened once more, and again when he had got the tumor completely away. When he closed the stitches he tightened again, and so on several times. Yet they were not secure against oozing. They showed how the tissues shrank, and how utterly impossible it was to control these extraordinary tissues.

Case of Delayed Operation in Extra-Uterine Gestation: Death. —Dr. EDIS related the following circumstance in connection with a fatal case of extra-uterine gestation:

Mrs. W., aged thirty-two, married five and-a-half years; sterile. Last normal menstruation December 2nd, 1888. Generally very regular every twenty-eight days, but she missed the period due at the end of December and saw nothing for forty-five days, *i.e.*, January 15th, 1889. During this time she felt perfectly well. On January 14th she experienced a sudden attack of excruciating pain in the right iliac fossa; she was almost collapsed, but after lying down on the bed for two hours, although she felt weak, she was able to get up, but could not fasten her dress without discomfort. On the following day, 15th, a sanguineous discharge from the vagina occurred, and continued uninterruptedly until February 5th, the day before she was first seen by Dr. Edis. She remained in bed on the 16th, and on the 17th passed two clots *per vaginam*. These were examined, but consisted merely of coagulated blood. On the 20th she hurried to church, and when there became so ill that she could not move, even to come out, but remained until the service was over. On the 21st she experienced another severe attack of pain at 5 p.m., accompanied by a rigor. At this time there was pain on micturition and defæcation. On examination, *per vaginam*, the uterus was found to be bulky—anteflected— pushed over to the left side by a tense cystic mass in the right. On careful conjoined manipulation some slight tenderness was experienced in the right iliac fossa. The cervix was somewhat softer and more fleshy than normal. The uterus was mobile, as also the cyst, which was about as large as a hen's egg. The mamæ were only slightly developed, but more so lately than usual, according to both the patient's and her husband's account. As the patient was in no present discomfort, and according to my calculation was at the furthest ten weeks advanced in pregnancy, it was decided to keep her quietly in bed for a few days and watch her symptoms; the operation being fixed for Monday, the 11th. On the 9th there was some local pain in the right lower abdomen, which was relieved by a poultice, the sanguineous discharge continuing. At 11.45 a.m. she had an acute attack of pain together with vomiting, the pain not being so distinctly localized as hitherto, but extending up to the navel. At 5.45 p.m. another attack of pain occurred, which was sharp and severe, the patient becoming blanched and cold; pulse 90, temp. 97.3°F.

Operation.—On opening the abdomen there was a rush of thin, dark, venous blood, which evidently had nearly filled up the abdominal cavity. Some sixty ounces of this were collected, but there was probably much more all told. The right broad ligament was at once transfixed and tied securely in two portions. The peritoneal cavity was then washed out thoroughly with hot water at 110°F., and the cyst and tube removed. All superfluous fluid was sponged out, a drainage tube inserted, and the abdominal wound closed with silver sutures. The patient never thoroughly rallied, the heart's action being very feeble, and she ultimately sank at 6.45 a.m., ten hours subsequent to the operation. On examining the specimen it was seen to consist of an ovarian cyst, the size of a hen's egg. Above this the right Fallopian tube was enlarged to the size of a walnut by an extra-uterine gestation cyst, which had ruptured at the other end. The orifice of the Fallopian tube itself was patulous and blood exuded from it.

Mr. TAIT said the case was very instructive. Dr. Edis had emphasized everything he had said in reference to extra-uterine pregnancy except in one respect, as to which he had misrepresented him. He had never said that extra-uterine gestation had never been recognized prior to the period of rupture. What he did say was that he himself had never recognized them. There was a very good reason for that, for with one exception he had not seen them until rupture had taken place, and in that one case he had mistaken it for something else.

18

Dr. RUTHERFORD said the case was another which brought into relief the uselessness of electricity. If electro-puncture had been employed the needle would have gone through the ovarian cyst and left the extra-uterine gestation untouched. Another point worthy of remark was the practical value of Mr. Tait's direction to go straight for the broad ligament and so put a stop to the hemorrhage. Although the tube looked healthy, on making a microscopical section, he found that the columnar ciliated epithelium was gone and the mucous membrane swollen and full of inflammatory leucocytes.

Extra-uterine Gestation of five months duration: Rupture between layers of Broad Ligament: Complication of an Intra-uterine Fœtation: Operation: Death.—Dr. EDIS related the following case of much interest and rarity.

He said he was called upon to operate upon a case of four or five months extra-uterine pregnancy, which illustrated the differences between rupture into the peritoneal cavity, when there was a considerable amount of hæmorrhage, and rupture between the layers of the broad ligament, that is, extra-peritoneal. Mr. Lawson Tait, who was an authority upon the subject, had laid it down as a law, that in cases of rupture into the peritoneal cavity one was called upon to operate *instanter;* but in cases of extra-peritoneal rupture he discountenanced the primary operation, except the life of the mother was menaced. He preferred to leave the case to go on to full term. It was one of those peculiar cases in which an extra u erine gestation starting in September was followed by an intra-uterine gestation early in October. It was situated upon the left side; and the child's head was low down in the pelvis and pressed upon the rectum; causing almost total obstruction together with extreme intolerance of urine. The patient was exceedingly emaciated, suffered from persistent vomiting, and her life seemed to be in danger. He made an incision in the median line from the umbilicus nearly to the symphisis, and there he found the uterus distended to about the fourth month of pregnancy, and running off from this on the left side was the extra-uterine fœtation, the fœtus from which he produced. Carefully avoiding the intra-uterine tumour, he made an incision through the cyst and extracted the fœtus, which seemed to be about five months old. He left the placenta intact and stitched the walls of the cyst to the abdominal wound, so as to be able to irrigate and drain. The operation was performed February 12th, the pressure on the rectum was immediately relieved. The only complication so far was the formation of a fæcal fistula. There were symptoms of threatened abortion during the first few hours following the operation, but they had passed off and the case promised to do well.

Treatment of Fibroid Tumours and Twisted Pedicles.—In a discussion on fibroids and their treatment, the question had been raised as to the class of cases most suited for removal of the appendages, and those best dealt with by hysterectomy. Dr. BANTOCK said the case in hand belonged to the class of soft fibroids which sometimes attained such enormous dimensions and demanded removal. They were very rapid in growth. In the case in question, the existence of the tumour had only been noticed a few months before. It was situated in the right broad ligament and was adherent to the right side of the uterus. It was shelled out of the broad ligament with the greatest readiness, until he got down to the pedicle, when he had to apply a ligature. The patient recovered without a bad symptom. She was a single woman forty years of age. The tumour weighed three pounds three ounces. The second specimen illustrated another subject of recent discussion. It was a case of twisted pedicle of a dermoid cyst. The patient had been brought to him about three weeks ago in a very distressed condition. She had been seized a week before with sickness, accompanied with severe abdominal pain and some shock. He discovered a tumor in the lower part of the abdomen, and at once ventured on the diagnosis that the symptoms were due to the twisting of the pedicle of an ovarian tumour. It was only on that day that he had been enabled to operate on her. He recalled that, when the matter was under discussion, he had expressed the opinion that it was not advisable to operate upon the patient while she was suffering from the immediate symptems of twisting of the pedicle, and particularly to the accident that usually accompanied twisting of the pedicle, viz: hæmorrhage into the sac, which appeared to have more to do with the production of the shock than the twisting itself. In this patient the pedicle was twisted about one and a-half turns. It was not absolutely strangulated; but it was pretty nearly so, and there had been hæmorrhage into the cavity at the time of the accident. He thought that it was unwise to operate during the continuance of the shock and acute symptoms. He thought that it was best to allow such patients to remain quiet for some time, in order that the acute symptoms might subside. A tumor, if completely strangulated, would contract adhesions to surrounding structures, and its death would thus be prevented. This conclusion had been the result of his invariable experience. He had never seen a patient die from a twisted pedicle, or from hæmorrhage into the interior of the sac, nor had he ever heard of such a case.

Mr. LAWSON TAIT said he could give a melancholy example of the results of leaving uterine fibroids alone. A lady, sixty years of age, was sent to him from Nottingham with an enormous soft œdematous myoma. The tumor and symptoms dated twelve years back. The patient went on bleeding continuously, her menstruation being practically continuous. The tumour increased in size, and when she came to him on the 10th of December last, it was of an enormous size. He advised immediate operation, warning, however, the patient that in her exhausted condition recovery was materially interfered with. She nevertheless eagerly requested the operation, as did her husband; he therefore operated, shelling it out as easily as possible, but the shock was so great that the patient never rallied from the operation, she died about thirty-six hours after. He asserted that if the patient had been operated upon ten years earlier, when she was fifty, instead of sixty, and with ten years less of suffering and hæmorrhage, her chances of recovery would have been materially increased. As to the other points, he and Dr. Bantock were not so much agreed; he had seen thirty or forty cases of twisted pedicles of par-ovarian tumours, and he was strongly of opinion that it was the twisting that caused the shock. He had seen the severest shock without a drop of hæmorrhage. In a case he had to operate upon a few days ago after rupture, he had seen serious hæmorrhage with shock, but the balance of evidence was in favour of twisting as the cause of the shock. His rule was to operate as soon as he could get to the patient.

Cysto-Fibro-Myoma of the Uterus, (Dr. HENRY T. BYFORD: Chicago).—A fibro-cystic tumour of the uterus weighing thirty pounds. It was surrounded by forty-five pints of ascitic fluid, so that the patient was relieved of seventy-five pounds of weight at the operation. What was left of her weighed about ninety pounds. On the right side is a plain fibroid growth; on the left side it has undergone myxomatous degeneration. A peculiarily is that the uterine cavity is completely obliterated half an in inch below the normal sized fundus by the tumour, and begins again lower down. The patieut was about forty-four years old and menstruated scantily. The tumour, which is known to have been growing over fifteen years, started below the fundus in the posterior uterine wall. The broad ligaments were ligated separately, and the uterine stump treated extra-peritoncally. Formerly, when I was an adherent of the intra-peritoneal method of treating the stump, I stood in great awe of abdominal hyster-ectomy for fibroads, but since adopting the extra-peritoneal method I find that the mortality is but little greater than after ovariotomy.

A case of Epileptoid Seizure in which Erotic Symptoms were manifested to a marked degree.—In the August uumber (1889) of the *British Gynæological Journal,* Dr. Routh gives the history of a very remarkable case of an epileptic, exhibiting unpleasantly amorous manifestations towards him after the application of a galvanic current within the uterus. The interest in such cases bear towards us in a medico-legal light, and it is well known that many an innocent physician has been made the victim of hallucinations of an epileptic woman, under similar circumstances as those described by Dr. Routh. She is now forty-five : the catamenia having been unusually copious, and very irregular. The uterus is very large, fibroid tumor reaching above the pubes and heavy, pro-gression is difficult, always accompanied with backache. There were head symptoms, confusion, headache, &c., and violence of temper with something more doubtful displayed in her actions. I therefore determined to pass a negative

electrical continuous current through the womb, the positive
pad being placed on the belly. She bore it well up to about 90
milliampères, when, to my annoyance, I noticed that sexual orgasm occurred. I, of course, pretended not to perceive it, but as
soon as completed she began to wander, imagining some terrible accident had occurred to her husband. I removed
the electrical apparatus and stopped the current as soon as I
could, but before I could place her on a chair she went off
into a regular epileptoid attack, foaming at the mouth and
convulsed. The attack was soon over, and she became
somewhat comatose, but not to any very marked degree. I
removed her to an adjoining room, and left her in
charge of a young lady and relative, while I attended to
my other patients. She became excessively amorous
towards this young lady, frequently asking to be kissed,
throwing her arms round her neck, probably not altogether
conscious of how she was acting. In about an hour she came
completely to herself, and was ready to return home in cab.

Remarks.—The case I was anxious to record as one in
which epilepsy was preceded and succeeded by marked sexual
excitement. We are all acquainted with those cases in which
epilepsy precedes a catamenal period, and many women will
tell you that the sexual orgasm is also strongest before or
after a period. As a period did follow in this case, it might
be ascribed to this cause, but the fact that an ordinary
conjugal relation had frequently before induced a fit without
a period following, points rather to the sexual orgasm as the
cause of the epilepsy, *plus* some peculiar condition not otherwise discovered, especially although epilepsy often followed
conjugal relations, it was by no means a universal occurrence.
Did the electrical current induce it? In one other I think
I saw it imperfectly developed. But I have seen far more
marked symptoms under the delirium of chloroform, or even
ordinary examinations. The one important feature, however,
is the erotic symptoms which not only proceeded, but continued
after the epileptiform seizures. Two cases of a similar kind
in which charges were brought against medical men not very
long ago followed the same course. Perhaps, had I not been
an old friend, and judged by herself incapable of abusing her
confidence, my patient might have supposed or believed that

I had taken undue liberties with her person. She seemed even with the lady friend subsequently to have no control over her amorous inclinations, and retained but a shadowy remembrance of the occurrence. So far, this case is one of a class of which I think it would be well if our judges knew more than they do, where patients firmly believe and detail with "much minuteness events which deviate so little from what is possible that on several occasions trials have been instituted upon such accusations, and in a few instances convictions have followed" (Ziemsen vol. 14, 584)—one of the most cruel that can occur to a medical man.

Mr. TAIT referred to the well-known case of Dr. Bradley, who was accused by an epileptic woman of having assaulted her. He pointed out that the woman was a confirmed epileptic, and was not of irreproachable morality, and there was every reason to believe that there was some peculiar sexual excitement in connection with her attacks. The assault was alleged to have taken place in a branch surgery, the floor and ceiling of which were so thin that it was impossible that the persons above and below would not have heard the noise of anything like a struggle. The woman had an attack in the presence of the accused, and doubtless firmly believed, in virtue of the sexual excitement which accompanied her attacks, that she had been assaulted. Dr. Bradley, strong in his innocence, had neglected to bring forward any medical witnesses to deal with this feature of the case, and he was found guilty by the jury and sentenced to two years' imprisonment. Ultimately, however, some new facts in the case were brought under notice of the Lord Chief Justice and he was released. Mr. Tait said that it was important to notice the association of a certain form of epilepsy with an erotic condition, an association which was as certain as possible. He mentioned also that some patients, in passing through the stages of anæsthesia, were subject to the same excitement. He had seen that happen over and over again, and in one case the patient had mentioned the matter to him afterwards, probably because she had some misty recollection of having done something which called for an explanation. These things ought to be widely known. They ought to be in the text books, and men should not be sent to prison on charges made by women who were very likely subject to sexual disturbances of this kind. He added that another curious point was the charges brought by children under the new law. He had been engaged by the Birmingham police to investigate these cases, and in only one out of twenty or thirty was there reason to believe that such an offence had been committed.

Dr. BARNES said it was important that this case should be put on record. He mentioned that some years ago he had gone down into the country to give evidence at the assize on behalf of a highly-respectable practitioner, who was accused of having committed an assalt on a female patient in a room in his own house, which was so surrounded by doors on every side that if anything of the kind had taken place it would certainly have been overheard by those in the adjoining rooms. The complainant was apparently a respectahle woman, and in support of that statement it was given in evidence that she had formerly been in the employ of a lady of position. He gave evidence strongly in his favour, and the accused was acquitted.

Chlorosis and Menstruatioa: An analysis of 232 *eases.*—Dr. W. STEPHENSON, University of Aberdeen, the author of this paper, observed that, in the rapid progress of uterine specialism, chlorosis, in its relation to menstruation, has been too much neglected. This constitutional disease has been investigated by the physician and the pathologist, but not by the gynæcologist. The paper is based on an analysis of 232 cases carefully noted by the author. The cases were divided into two groups: the first, where tho illness was primary and occurred before tho twenty-third year, comprising 183 cases; and the second, where the attacks were of the nature of relapses after a period of good health: these number forty-nino cases. Chlorosis is regarded as due to a constitutional state; bnt it is shown that the diathesis is not necessarily associated with an impairment of the development of the body, and is not. to any marked degree, eonnected with defective health previous to the onset of the disease. First is considered tho influence of the chlorotic constitution on menstruation before chlorosis sets in. Tables are given which show that the tendency of the chlorotic diathesis is to accelerate the age at which menstruation first appears, and that chlorosis by itself is not the cause of retarded appearauce of the catamenia. At the same time, in one-half of the cases the functional activity is defective, and is chiefly character-ized by lengthening and irregularity of the intervals and scantiness in the amount of the flow. The author's statistics are against the opinion that there is a menorrhagic form of chlorosis. In 96.6 per cent. the effect was to diminish the activity of the function ; the remaining fraction were com-plicated with ovarian irritation. In 58.7 per cent. menstrua-tion became scanty and irregular, and in many cases painful, while in 38.8 per cent there was amenorrhea for various periods.

Chlorosis and Age.—A table is given which shows that there are two marked chlorotic periods: the one of primary attacks, from 14 to 21; the other, of secondary attacks, from 24 to 31. The number of cases of the disease presents a regular curve, beginning at 14 and rising steadily to a maximum between 18 and 28, then rapidly falling, to disappear altogether at 22. The tendency to secondary attacks manifests itself first at 24, rises to a maximum between 26 and 28, to again disappear at 32. That there may be a third period is probable, as two cases are recorded at 39 and 41. This law applies to attacks of the disease with distinct intervals of good health between, as distinguished from the simple relapses, after periods of imperfect convalescence, frequently met with after a primary attack. The curve of menstrual age, compared with the curve of the onset of chlorosis, does not bear out the opinion that " foremost in etiological importance is the period of the first appearance of the catamenia." The fact of a periodicity in the attacks is also against it. The cause of this periodicity is considered ; and the general conclusion arrived at is that imperfect evolution of menstruation, as evidenced by scanti-ness of the flow and irregularity of the periods, is as regular a feature of chlorosis as the imperfect evolution of the red corpuscles of the blood ; that these contestants are not related to each other as cause and effect, but are independent one of the other, at the same time there is a close relationship between them whereby the reproduction and development of the red corpuscles of the blood are governed by, or form part of, the menstrual cycle.

Syphillitic Disease of the Cervix Uteri.—Dr. E. RODE, in *Brit. Med. Jour.*, has observed three cases of ulcerating gummata of the vaginal portion of the cervix. They appeared from ten to twelve years after infection. In all these cases there was extensive œdema of the pelvic connective tissue. Diagnosis was based upon the distinct history of syphilis, which was readily obtained from the patient. There were, moreover, no symptoms of cancer, tuberculosis, or simple erosion. The patients all recoved rapidly after the administration of iodide of potassinm. No local treatment beyond simple cleanliness was thought desirable. Dr. Rode's experience are of considerable interest. A good monograph on the ulcers of the uterus, written by a recognized authority, would prove of great utility to practitioners and specialists. The "ulcer" is hardly even an erosion; it is rather the replacement of the natural squamous epithelium of the outer part of the cervix by a layer of the columnar epithelium proper to the cervical canal. The severe symptoms once attributed to "ulcerated womb" are due totally different causes. Nevertheless, there are such things as ulcers of the cervix, due to cancer frequently, to syphilis occasionally, to tubercle rarely.

Sterility: (Dr. OUTERBRIDGE, in *Medical Era*).—For the cure of sterility I have devised a cervical dilator made of steel wire, and silver or gold plated. This is introduced five or six days before the menstrual period, and removed at a like interval after it. The instrument is self-retaining, dilates the cervical canal, and gives the spermatozoa ready access to the uterine cavity.

The reviewer, after a trial of this instrument, would say that it is worthless, unsatisfactory and cannot be recommended.

Cholocystorrhaphy.—Dr. HOWARD A. KELLY reports a case of cholocystorrhaphy followed by cholocystotomy and evacuation of one hundred and eighty-eight gall-stones, and recovery. Frau B., a wizened, brown-skinned, little German woman, fifty years old, is the mother of a nun ber of children, and aside from a single attack of jaundice when thirty years of age, enjoyed good health up to twelve years ago, when she lay many weeks abed with a severe febrile attack diagnosed as typhoid fever. She noticed at the same time the appearance of a well-defined tumor in the right hypochondrium. Since this time she has always been a sufferer with abdominal pains, indigestion, and constipation. The pains, although not located in any particular spot, were very definitely referred as arising from the right side. She suffered from menorrhagia two years ago, for which I was called in consultation by Dr. A. K. Minich, a year ago. After dilatation and curetting and a conrse of arsenic prescriptions by Dr. Minich, this disappeared, and she improved very markedly in every way. Last January (1889) I was again called in consultation by Dr. Wintter to consider the nature of her abdominal complaint. The lobes of a distinctly enlarged liver, also displaced downwards, 10 cm. below normal, with a gall-bladder greatly distended, elastic and projecting far beyond its fissure, were easily detected, and the diagnosis of obstructed gall-bladder made. I operated on the 28th January, in the presence of Dr. Wintter, assisted by Dr. Hunter Robb. As the liver was freely movable, and the gall-bladder lay 3 cm. to the right and 4 cm. above the navel, an incision 4 cm. long was made in the linea alba. It was found to be a large, tense cyst about 13 cm. in length. Upon palpating the rest of the abdominal viscera through the opening, I found extensive mesenteric, small intestinal, and colonic adhesions, made up partly of the union of broad surfaces and partly of sharp bands from 4 or 5 to 10 cm. in length. These were all carefully separated and broken up by the fingers used as a wedge between the broad adhesions, and bringing the sharp bands into view when they were cut. The oozing which followed this separation was but slight. The next step was to suture the gall-bladder to the abdominal wall, so as to expose a part of its surface for subsequent incision. This was done by means of a series of fine interrupted silk sutures about an eighth of an inch apart, introduced so as to catch up the serous and subserous coats of the bladder and the visceral peritoneum.

The completion of the operation left a small wound, at the floor of which lay exposed a part of the gall-bladder, 3 by 1½ cm. The whole operation lasted to completion ten minutes. Iodoform gauze was placed in the wound, and absorbent cotton and bandage over the whole. On the third day the dressing was removed and the exposed bladder opened in its length by

Paquelin's cautery knife. About 300 gr. of clear, sticky fluid like synovia escaped. On the fifth day I removed one hundred and six gall-stones of varying size by means of a pair of small stone forceps. Three days after forty more were removed, and on the eleventh day forty-two stones more appeared. A stillicidium of fluid commenced with the opening of the bladder, and lasted eighteen days, when the wound closed. The length of the gall-bladder measured by a sound was 11½ cm. On the twelfth day she sat up, and on the twenty-sixth day she went home. The relief following the operation was perfect. She had no more pain, recovered her appetite, and became bright and cheerful in disposition.

Rapid Curative Treatment of Cystitis. (THOMAS MORE MADDEN, M.D.)—Within the past year twenty-eight cases of cystitis have come under observation in the gynæcological wards of my hospital; and in nearly every one of these cases the patient was discharged free from the disease, which in some of them had resisted years of other treatment. In women cystitis is, not only from the special causes incidental to the sex, more frequent than in men, but is also more urgent in its symptoms and more liable to lead to grave pathological consequences.

General Treatment of Cystitis.—I may say a few words with regard to the general principles which should guide our management of these cases, as well as on the ordinary plans of treatment and palliative measures generally recommended in cases of cystitis in women. It is obvious that in this, as in every other disease, our primary business is to ascertain and to remove, if it be removable, whatever may be the exciting cause of the morbid condition of the bladder. Thus, if the disease be dependent on extension of vulvar or vaginal inflammation, either gonorrhœal or non-specific, this must be at once allayed by appropriate treatment. If due to the mechanical pressure of a displaced uterus, this should be rectified by a suitable pessary. In the same way, the weight of a uterine fibroid pressing on the bladder, if it cannot be otherwise got rid of, must be at least lifted well above the pelvic brim, and there maintained. If vesical calculus be present, or if, as ascertained by careful examination of the urine, renal disease exists, and has extended from the kidneys along the uterus, it will be useless to attempt the topical treatment of the consequent cystitis until in either instance its cause has been removed. Presuming the case to be one of uncomplicated cystitis, we have then an abundant choice of suggested remedial measures which (save that advocated by Dr. Emmet, to which I shall subsequently refer) are all equally useless, as far as probability in concerned, of thus curing any extreme case of cystitis. Nevertheless, some of these measures are unquestionably of value as palliative expediments, and may possibly even prove curative in exceptionally mild cases of the disease. The most generally useful in this way are long continued warm baths, washing out the bladder through a double catheter with plain warm water, thin flax-seed tea, or a solution of boroglyceride; conjointly in all instances with absolute rest in bed, the free use of diluents, together with the administration of the old-fashioned Dover's powder in small, frequently repeated doses, as the best opiate in these cases; and lastly, above all, by the use of boracic acid in 10 or 15-grain doses three or four times a day, by which the generally fœtid ammoniacal urine is deprived of its fœtor and rendered less irritating to the endovesical mucous membrane.

Curative Treatment of Cystitis.—These measures may relieve, but will not cure well-established cystitis, nor am I aware of any method by which this result can be obtained except by primarily giving the diseased lining membrane of the bladder and its sub-mucous muscular walls absolute physiological rest. This may be secured in either of two ways,—namely, first, by that advocated by Dr. Emmet, which consists in the formation of an artificial vesico-vaginal fistula through which the urine may drain away as fast as secreted, and by the consequent removal of the immediate source of irritation to the unhealthy and hyperæsthetic endovesical mucous membrane thus affords the patient a fair chance of escape from ultimate extension of the disease to the kidneys. The objections to this plan of treatment are, however, so grave as to render any rational alternative that may be suggested for attaining the same object by less heroic means deserving of fair consideration and full trial. These objections are, first, the general difficulty of keeping the fistulous opening patulous for a sufficient time to allow the diseased bladder to regain its normal condition; secondly, the irritation often occasioned by the button commonly employed for this purpose ; and thirdly, the more serious trouble, which we meet with in some exceptional instances, of closing the fistulous opening when the desired object has been attained, and the consequent misery resulting from this mischance, by which the patient's last condition may thus possibly be rendered worse than her former state. I have abandoned this operation, and believe that we may obtain all its advantages more easily and more safely, simply by so thoroughly dilating the urethral canal as to enable us to pass the index into the bladder, and thereby paralyze the contractility of the sphincter or of the canal for a time, which may be indefinitely extended by repeating expansion in the same way as often as may be necessary. It may, moreover, be advisable in some instances to remove the proliferating vesicle mucous membrane by the cautious employment of a dull wire curette, which I have used with advantage in cases of this kind. And, lastly, whether the curette be required or not, the method of dilation should, in all cases, be conjoined with the topical application of carbolic acid to the mucous surface. The latter is best employed in the form of glycerine of carbolic acid of the Pharmacopœia, which is quite strong enough for the purpose, and introduced by the ordinary stilette, armed with a piece of absorbent cotton saturated in the application, and passed through my dilator so as to avoid any of the acid being brushed off in the canal until it reaches the fundus vesicæ, where it should be retained for a couple of minutes until every part of the vesical wall contracts firmly upon it. The urethral canal is then to be similarly brushed out by another application of the carbolized glycerine. The pain caused by this procedure may be prevented by previously introducing in the same way a 10 per cent. solution of cocaine, The plan of treatment recommended seldom requires to be repeated more than two or three times, at intervals of a week, to effect a cure of even the most aggravated cases.

Cysts and Abscesses of Bartholini's Glands. (Dr. BONNET, of Paris, in *Gaz. des Hôpitaux.*)—The diseases of the vulvo-vaginal or the glands of Bartholini are abscesses and cysts. Cysts arise from an occlusion, obstruction or adhesion of the duct of the gland, produced by catarrh, cicatrices, cancerous neoplasms, etc. The affection generally attacks only one, and that the left side. The contents of the cyst is a viscid fluid, sometimes clear, other times of a blackish green or a bloody color. The pathological anatomy is yet but little known. The phenomena which the cysts give rise to during their growth are usually but slight. They are painless, and trouble the patient but little when walking. The seat of the tumor is, if its duct be affected, a superficial one ; but if the gland itself be implicated, the swelling is deeper. It may undergo a change into an abscess, if, for example, a gonorrhœic vulvitis be complicated with it, or various manipulations to induce its healing, may also induce this change. All methods of treatment, as catheterization, puncture, incision, or excision of a portion of its wall, as well as drainage, are not sufficient, and it reoccurs as a rule. Bonnet proposes, as the only remedy for its cure, which will be followed by lasting success—extirpation of the gland. This is to be done under chloroform, or by the use of cocaine locally. The abscesses may, as already mentioned, originate in the cysts or in traumatism, but in the most cases they are dependent upon an acute or chronic vulvitis. Its symptomatology is well known, as well as the bad results obtained by simple excision, with or without cauterization. Here also the writer is in favor of a radical treatment, i.e., an antiseptic extirpation of the gland.

Uterine Cough. (DR. MULLER of Paris, in *Gaz. Méd.*)—The uterine cough is physiological at the time of menstruation, pregnancy, and the menopause. It becomes pathological in diseases of the uterus of every kind. It is not to be mistaken for the hysteric cough, as it appears in women who show no trace of hysteria. The prognosis of uterine cough is very favorable, if one finds and cures the affection of the uterus upon which it depends.

Strangulation of the Clitoris. (DR. BOKAI, in *Central-Blatt fur Gynækol*)—A girl ten years of age, who for quite a long time had practiced masturbation, had for the same purpose ligated the clitoris so tightly with a thin thread that that organ swelled up to the size of an Italian hazelnut. The thread was removed by Bokai fourteen days later, whereupon the sensitiveness and œdema gradually disappeared. The ulcerated line of strangulation healed after proper treatment. Yet the clitoris remained even after the removal of the thread still

the size of a hazelnut, so that this hypertrophy, which was
regarded as a result of the masturbation, had to be removed by
means of thermocautony.

Abdominal Pregnancy. (*Lancet.*)—It has always been a cardinal rule of operation in abdominal pregnancy that the
placenta should not be disturbed but should be allowed to dis-
integrate and come away piecemeal, the cyst cavity being
carefully and thoroughly drained until suppuration ceased.
The reason for this rule was the obvious danger of hemorrhage
from the placental site if forcible removal should be made,
there being nothing corresponding to the contractions of the
uterus after the third stage of labor, to check the hemorrhage.
But Lawson Tait has successfully hazarded the immediate
removal of the placenta after operating upon a case of abdominal pregnancy, checking the hemorrhage from the placental
site by the application of the perchloride of iron. Tait does
not advise this method in both cases, but has simply shown
that it is not as dangerous as was feared. It has obvious advantages, and if its safety be established will be a great improvement on the old method.

Operative Methods for Retroversion of the Uterus. (H. T. B.)
—After having exhausted our medical knowledge and mechanical skill in unsuccessful attempts at the cure of retroversion,
it occasionally becomes necessary to resort to surgical operations. These may be divided into three kinds: (1) Those
intended to restore the uterus to a normal condition; (2) to
restore the uterine supports to normal function; (3) to fix, by
unnatural means, the fundus in front, or the cervix back, of
the axis of the superior strait—operations of expedience. The
second class interests us because there is a question of choice
of methods for the patient before us. The normal action of the
uterine ligaments is to draw the fundus in front, and the cervix back, of the axis of the superior strait. The round ligaments are the main ones that accomplish the former, and the
sacro-uterine ligaments the latter. Hence operations directed
to the restoration of the natural action of these ligaments may
be considered rational and justifiable.

Alexander's operation for shortening the round ligaments
has now been performed several hundred times, and is established as a safe and effective procedure. The position of the

uterus obtained is one of moderate or normal anteversion. Relief of symptoms is not always immediate, since the traction • of the shortened round ligaments upon the tender or contracted tissues about the broad ligaments, or, contrariwise, the dragging of the rigid resisting tissues and uterus upon the newly healed round ligaments, may give rise to discomforts for some weeks or months. Adjustment of the parts takes place after a time, however, and all symptoms due to uterine displacement, together with many others, eventually subside. Much unmeaning argument has been trumpeted throughout the scientific world about the inadequacy of the round ligaments to support the uterus against abdominal pressure, and about the part other structures beside the round ligaments play in causing retroversion. It is not pretended that the round ligaments support the womb in its natural position—they merely draw the fundus in position so that its weight and abdominal pressure will act to antevert the uterus. The effect of their action upon the uterus may be likened to the effect of the action of the rudder upon the boat—directing merely, not antagonizing the displacing or propelling powers. This brings us to the methods by which the fundus has been fixed in front of the axis of the superior strait. Koeberle was the first to stitch the uterus to the abdominal wall by suturing the stump, after abdominal oöphorectomy, in the wound. Olshausen recommended suturing the broad ligaments to the abdominal walls by a laparotomy performed expressly for this purpose. Since then Kelly and Saenger have prominently associated their names with this operation. By it the uterus is dislocated toward the front of the pelvis and swings on a somewhat rigid fundal attachment near the reflection of the peritoneum over the bladder. The position of the uterus is not at all comparable to that after Alexander's operation, since there is a dislocation forward and a fixation of the fundus. The Germans call it ventro-fixatio-uteri, or ventral fixation of the uterus, while Kelly has named it hysterorrhaphy. Laparo-hysterorrhaphy, or anterior fixation of the uterus, as it might more properly be called, must be reserved for those cases in which Alexander's operation may not be available or practicable, or for those in which it may become necessary to perform laparotomy for breaking up of adhesions or other purposes.

19

The Early Diagnosis of Cancer of the Cervix. (Dr. H. C. Coe, in *Med. News.*)—The majority of the cases of cancer of the cervix uteri do not come under the observation of the surgeon before the disease has progressed so far that it is impossible to perform a successful radical operation. The attending physician is too often responsible for this delay, although he is not entirely inexcusable for misinterpreting the initial symptoms. The symptoms of incipient malignant disease of the cervix are seldom characteristic, but they are such as to awaken suspicion and to justify an examination. Slight, irregular hemorrhages, especially after coitus, are always significant, above all in women who have passed the menopause. Pain is seldom characteristic. There is no offensive discharge in the early stage. Hypertrophy and general induration of the cervix, accompanying an erosion which bleeds easily to the touch, should lead the physician to confirm the diagnosis by excising a fragment of the suspected tissue and submitting it to microscopical examination. A positive opinion regarding the presence of malignant disease is justified only by the finding of processes of atypical epithelium which invade the subjacent muscular tissue. Excision of the cervix should be performed in every case of extensive erosion with general induration, whether cancer has actually developed or not. This is often sufficient to ensure a cure, and thus to render a radical operation unnecessary. If the disease recurs, the uterus may be extirpated subsequently.

Hospital Reports.

MONTREAL GENERAL HOSPITAL.

CONDENSED REPORTS OF CASES IN DR. MACDONNELL'S WARDS.

CHRONIC LEAD POISONING.

Lead Poisoning a very common condition. A case in which the poison inhaled in a factory was followed by Colic, Wrist-drop, Gradual Impairment of Mental Functions, Chronic Interstitial Nephritis, with Hypertrophy of the Heart, High Tension Pulse, Transient Hemiplegia and Uræmic Manifestations.

Cases of chronic lead poisoning are very commonly met with in the practice of the Montreal General Hospital, indeed we are scarcely ever without two or more cases in the medical wards. Six cases have been admitted into ward 11 since May 1st, and not very long ago five cases were reported in the *Canada Medical and Surgical Journal* by Dr. Molson, in all of which the nervous system was attacked. I feel convinced that if lead poisoning were made the subject of investigation that it would be found to be of very common occurrence amongst those engaged in the various manufactures in which lead is used. So far lead poisoning has never in this country received at the hands of the health authorities the attention it deserves. For every case severe enough for admission to the hospital wards, there must be a large number of cases in which the poison has been less active, and in which the patient is still able to earn some kind of a living without being obliged to seek help at a hospital. Indeed, when a case of lead poisoning comes to my wards I always make a point of enquiring whether there are other people in the same employment suffering in the same way. In several instances the answer has been that many of the employees have had to leave, owing to attacks of colic, wrist drop, or other saturnine manifestations. At the moment there are three cases of lead poisoning in ward 11.

W. S , aged 58, a steel plate printer, had been employed in a lithographic establishment in this city for many years. He

had enjoyed good health until 1876, when he suffered from a
mild attack of colic with constipation, followed in three days by
a very severe attack. At the same time there was great
oppression about the chest. During the last twelve years he
has had four distinct attacks of colic. In 1882 the arms first
became involved. At that time there was distinct wrist drop,
and he was five weeks in hospital and had to abandon
his occupation altogether and go to live in the country.
Having regained the use of his arms he returned to Montreal,
and worked more or less steadily at his trade, without any
return of the symptoms, until six weeks ago, when he again
suffered from colic and weakness of the arms. On 19th March,
1888, he was admitted to the Montreal General Hospital. The
symptoms present were constipation, colicky pains in the abdomen, great emaciation, feebleness in both arms, but no marked
wrist-drop. At that time the urine was in a healthy condition.
He remained 49 days in hospital, and was discharged considerably improved. On the 11th May of the present year he was
again admitted, but now the symptoms were mainly mental, and
there was evidence of advanced renal disease. The patient
is thin, anæmic and of sallow complexion. No distinct lead line
is visible, but the gums are soft and have receded from the
teeth. He is very dull and listless, and has an air of dense
stupidity and lack of expression. There is great difficulty in
walking, unaided he feels dizzy and staggers. The memory is
greatly impaired, he cannot remember faces. The speech is
thick ; voice husky and weak, there is stammering ; somewhat
deaf ; cannot write, partly from actual weakness, partly from
inability to control the pen. There is general impairement of
muscular power, which is especially evident in the extensors of
the forearm ; the superficial reflexes are slow ; deep reflexes over
active ; no ankle clonus ; co-ordination of muscular movements is
impaired ; cannot walk unassisted across the ward ; in the finer
movements co-ordination is also very defective. He has a great
deal of difficulty in feeding himself. Pain and soreness in the
head and neck is complained of and there is a feeling of pins
and needles in the hands. Sight is greatly impaired and the

pupils are dilated. He cannot distinguish more than the outline of a person's form. The ophthalmoscope shows the presence of the characteristic changes of albuminuric retinitis. Hearing is very dull. Taste and smell appear to be normal. There is a considerable degree of paralysis of the seventh nerve ; he cannot whistle, cannot wrinkle the forehead, and the facial muscles of the left side appear to be somewhat weaker than those on the right. There is stiffness and pain on moving the muscles ; all the joints are said to move stiffly, but there is no distinct swelling or pain. The action of the sphincters has not been interfered with.

The apex beat is displaced downwards and outwards. Pulse, 64 : regular, forcible, visible at the wrist, showing a condition of high tension in the arteries, which is confirmed by the tracing of the sphygmograph ; the curve is suggestive of general arterio sclerosis plus a moderate degree of hypertrophy of the heart. The physical signs of the lungs are negative.

The urine is of a pale amber color ; specific gravity, 1017 ; small trace of albumen ; no sugar. The proportion of urea nearly normal. The total quantity passed per day varies, but it is usually not much above or below the normal quantity. Hyaline casts are present.

So far the case presents evidence of the poison having permeated every part of the nervous system, and exerted its influence over brain, cord and cranial nerve alike. The general condition seems hopeless. There is no doubt that the kidneys and the arterial system are beginning to suffer. There were no morbid changes in the urine when he was last in hospital, and no note was made to the effect that the heart was enlarged or the pulse of high tension.

August 20*th.*—Up to date several interesting changes have taken place. On the 18th May there was transient right hemiplegia, with very marked aphasia ; great mental distress and a sense of impending death. This sensation occurred several times during the day and then passed off gradually. There has been great variation in the rate of the pulse, which at times has been counted at 60 and 70, and at other times at 100 and 120.

August 31st.—Condition slightly improved; left the hospital yesterday.

CHEYNE-STOKES RESPIRATION.

N. C., an old French-Canadian, aged 70, was admitted June 22nd, 1889, under Dr. Stewart, and came under my care on the 27th July. On admission the patient complained of very great dyspnœa, of choking sensations, and a sense of weight in the chest. His health was excellent up to about three weeks ago, when, while engaged in cutting grass, he suddenly felt a sharp pain in the chest, and began at once to experience a choking sensation, symptoms from which he has suffered more or less ever since. He is a shrivelled up, little, old man. Expression very anxious and indicative of great suffering. The eyes are watery, and there is unusual redness of the conjunctiva. The pupils are contracted and react to light and accommodation. The skin is universally dry and scaly. The nails are curved, the finger-ends clubbed and rather blue.

The remarkable feature of the case is the rhythm of the respiratory acts, which is distinctly of the Cheyne-Stokes character. For thirty seconds all movements cease, then they become gradually deeper and more frequent, the head is thrown back, and the respiratory muscles are brought into play. Then by degrees the respirations become less deep, until they finally cease, to begin again. The interval from one pause to another is about one and a half minutes. The area of the heart's dulness is normal in extent, the impulse feeble, and apex beat not perceptible. No murmurs. The sounds are feeble. Pulse 78; irregular in volume and rhythm, every fourth or fifth beat being omitted. The arteries are tortuous and hard. Urine is of a pale color, acid reaction; specific gravity 1022; albumen present in small quantity, no sugar; passes 7½ grains of urea to the ounce; granular and hyaline casts are present; total quantity of urine daily, 28 ounces.

Shortly after admission the albumen and casts disappeared and the specific gravity became reduced to 1012. Five days after admission it was noticed that the Cheyne-Stokes breathing was no longer present. It was again noticed on one or two occasions, but in a less marked degree; it lasted but a few minutes at a time. Over both lungs sibilant and sonorous râles are heard, but much more readily in front. Improvement in the symptoms and general condition took place, so that at the end of a month he was discharged comparatively free from dyspnœa and any of the unpleasant sensations in his chest for which he had entered the hospital. The pulse became regular and the tracings assumed, to a certain degree, the characters of irregularity of the heart's action.

He was readmitted August 25th, 1889, complaining of pain, dyspnœa, weakness, cough, swelling of the legs and feet. A week ago began to suffer from constipation and dyspnœa, and in a few days relapsed into his former condition. The skin seems to be more shrivelled. The legs are slightly œdematous, skin dry and scaly, extremities blue and cold. Pulse weak and irregular in volume and rhthym. The respirations are 32 to 22 to the half minute, and the rhthym is of the Cheyne-Stokes character. In the period of dyspnœa the breathing is very rapid and the distress very great. At the climax there is generally a violent fit of coughing followed by scanty expectoration. The period of dyspnœa lasts ½ minute, that of apnœa ½ minute also. The chest sounds are similar to those previously observed. The cardiac impulse is weak; orthopnœa, sleeplessness. Urine is pale and clear, specific gravity 1015, acid; trace of albumen, but none of sugar; 6 grains urea to the ounce; hyaline casts were found in four specimens.

The chief interest of the case centres itself in the Cheyne-Stokes phenomenon. To what condition is it due? To the heart or to the kidneys? Probably the latter. The sphygmographic tracings are likely to be delusive, owing to the atheromatous condition of the arteries. The general characters of the tracings show (1) a short line of ascent; (2) the presence in a marked degree of the dicrotic wave; (3) the obliteration of the predicrotic wave. A comparison of the tracings, taken during the stages of apnœa and dyspnœa, show that during the interval of apnœa the tracings are comparatively regular and of the character above-mentioned. As the period of dyspnœa begins the tracing becomes disordered, the line of ascent becomes length-ened in some beats, shortened in others, and two beats at times run into one. The dicrotic wave is well marked in each tracing. As the dyspnœa reaches its height, the irregularity becomes greater, and, at the beginning of the period of rest or apnœa, the tracing suddenly becomes regular. As to whether there was any difference in tension between the periods of dyspnœa and apnœa it is not easy to say, but, judging from the various tracings obtained, it seems that during the interval the tension was less than during the dyspnœa. We failed to make out any difference in the frequency of heart's beat.

Cheyne-Stokes breathing is not a commonly observed pheno-menon. It is curious that we should have two cases in a small ward of 15 beds.

The second case is that of a stout French-Canadian farmer, 60 years of age, and is well marked. A dilated heart is the probable cause. Sphygmographic observations were not easily made, owing to the fatness of the forearm and the restless-ness of the patient. Changes in the pupil during apnœa and dyspnœa were observed. When the breathing was full and laboured the pupils dilated to a slight extent. In the first case this was not observed. In neither case was any contraction of the limbs noticed during dyspnœa,* as was recently described by Robertson, of Glasgow.

GYNÆCOLOGICAL CASES UNDER CARE OF DR. ALLOWAY.

(*Continued from page 213*—Reported by *Dr. Low*).

CASE VIII.—*Emmet's Trachelorrhaphy and Alexander's Round Ligament Operation.*

Admitted into hospital April 2, 1889 ; age 33 ; married ten years ; four pregnancies, two went to full term, one to 7th month, and one to 2nd month. Last full term labor took place five years ago. Menstruation for some years past has been irregular and scanty, accompanied with severe pain, violent headache and vomiting. She at present complains of severe pelvic pain ; painful and frequent micturition ; recurring

---

* On Rhthymic Contraction of the Pupils and Muscles of the Limbs with Cheyne-Stokes Respiration, by Alex. Robertson. *Lancet*, Nov. 27th, 1886.

paroxysms of violent headache, followed by distressing vomiting. On examination there was found a bilateral laceration of the cervix; extensive glandular hypertrophy, ectropion, endometritis and retroversion of the uterus. The uterus could easily be replaced, but would return again when supporting pessary was removed.

Dr. Alloway performed Emmet's trachelorrhaphy upon the cervix, and Alexander's operation of shortening the round ligaments, at the one sitting. This patient did very well, with the exception of a few localised points of suppuration in each inguinal wound, which appeared on the fifth day after the operation This circumstance necessitated the removal of sutures, but notwithstanding, the ligaments had united firmly in the wound, the uterus was well anteverted, and symptoms relieved when the patient left the hospital one month afterwards. In connection with the suppuration accident in this case, it may be mentioned that all other cases operated upon on that day had also exhibited evidence of wound infection, and, on enquiry, it was found that a foul-smelling empyaema had been opened in the theatre the previous afternoon. As an incident, however, in Dr. Alloway's case, it proved of value in showing that fairly firm union of the ligaments can take place in so short a time without the further aid of the sutures.

CASE IX.—*Trachelorrhaphy vnd Perineorrhpphy.*

Age 21 ; unmarried ; admitted into hospital June 21st, 1889. Had one full-term child six years ago, and has not been well since ; complains of profuse and over-frequent menstruation, accompanied with severe pain. Leucorrhoeal discharge also profuse.

Examination.—Perineum and lower part of vaginal wall extensively cicatricial and adherent, although the outer integument of perineum was intact ; cervix elongated and extensively eroded ; inflammatory remnant in left broad ligament, exhibiting much tenderness on pressure. This patient was kept in bed on preparatory treatment for four weeks. At the end of this time the uterus was thoroughly curetted with the sharp instrument, the cervix amputated and the cicatricial perineum and posterior vaginal wall were operated upon after Tait's method. Patient left hospital eighteen days afterwards in excellent health.

CASE X.—*Trachelorrhaphy and Perineorrhaphy.*

Age 25; married 6 years; 2 pregnancies; admitted into hospital June 25th. Ever since marriage has complained of severe pain over hypogastrium and left side; painful defecation; dysmenorrhœa; leucorrhœa very profuse; general debility and ill-health.

Examination.—Uterus low down and retroverted; bilateral laceration of cervix with eversion; pelvic floor somewhat fixed and very tender. This patient was kept in bed for several weeks on preparatory treatment. The pelvic floor became movable, free from tenderness, and the uterus regained its normal position.

July 28th.—Dr. Alloway performed Schrœder's trachelorrhaphy and Tait's permeorrhaphy.

August 20th.—Patient discharged well.

CASE XI.—*Curetting and Trachelorrhaphy.*

Aged 28; married 6 years; 2 miscarriages, no full term children; admitted July 9th, complaining of severe headache, pain in side and hypogastric region; menstruation every two weeks, accompanied with severe pain; leucorrhœa very profuse, and external parts irritated by discharge. This patient had been under the usual medical treatment for the past two years, consisting of hot medicated vaginal injections, rest in bed, etc., without benefit.

Examination.—Cervix lacerated bilaterally to the vault of vagina, everted and enormously hypertrophied. There was chronic metritis and endometritis; pelvic floor fixed and very tender; uterus anteverted.

After a few days rest in bed and the usual preparatory treatment, Dr. Alloway dilated the cervical canal with steel dilators, sharp curetted the diseased endometrium, and performed Schrœder's trachelorrhaphy. Three weeks afterwards left hospital perfectly well.

[This case clinically demonstrates the eteology of many such

cases of pelvic inflammation. The condition is kept smoulder-
ing by irritation and septic infection afforded by a diseased
endomentrium, associated with a virulent muco-purulent leucorrhœa. The only treatment at all satisfactory consists in
thoroughly removing every vestige of diseased endometrium
with Martin's sharp curette, and exsecing the cervix by
Schrœder's method. The cervix in such a case only serves as
a channel for infection, and can never be of any other use.—
T. J. A.]

CASE XII.—*Emmet's Trachelorrhaphy and Alexander's
Round Ligament Operation.*

Age 21 ; married four years ; 2 pregnancies, last child born
2 years ago ; menstruation regular, but profuse and very painful. Admitted July 1st, complaining of severe pain in back,
constant bearing-down pain, painful and frequent micturition,
painful defecation, and general debilitated condition of health.

Examination.—Bilateral laceration of cervix, eversion of
cervical segments, and retroversion of uterus. The displacement was easily corrected, showing no adhesions present.

July 18th.—Dr. Alloway performed Emmet's trachelorrhaphy
and Alexander's operation of shortening the round ligaments,
at the same sitting.

This patient had an uninterrupted convalescence, and left
hospital three weeks after operation had been performed. The
inguinal wounds healed by primary union, the uterus was found
anteverted when examined in the standing position, and the
patient was in excellent health when discharged.

CASE XIII.—*Emmet's Trachelorrhaphy and Alexander's
Shortening of the Round Ligaments.*

Age 21 ; married four years ; 2 pregnancies, one miscarriage
two years ago. She complains of severe pains in lumbar region,
of bearing-down character ; leucorrhœa profuse ; dysmenorrhæa
and dyspareunia ; micturition painful and frequent.

Examination.—Bilateral laceration of cervix, with extensive
glandular hypertrophy and ectropion, uterus enlarged, hard,
tender and retroverted to third degree. The uterus could easily

be replaced, but through relaxation of uterosacral and round ligaments, would not remain so.

July 18*th.*—Dr. Alloway performed Emmet's trachelorrhaphy and Alexander's operation of shortening the round ligament at same sitting.

July 30*th.*—Sutures removed from inguinal wound and cervix to-day ; union perfect, and uterus anteverted and firmly held in that position.

August 6*th.*—Discharged in excellent health.

Reviews and Notices of Books.

A Text Book of Animal Physiology. With Introductory Chapters on General Biology and a full Treatment of Reproduction. For Students of Human and Comparative (Veterinary) Medicine and of General Biology. By WESLEY MILLS, M.A., M.D., L.R.C.P.L., Professor of Physiology in McGill University and the Veterinary College, Montreal. With over 500 Illustrations. New York : D. Appleton & Co. 1889. Montreal, E. M. Renouf.

It was with no ordinary degree of interest that we opened the pages of this work. From the author's distinguished position and well-known reputation, much is expected of him, and we have the fullest confidence that the verdict of the profession in his own country and elsewhere will be that he has produced a work of great merit. In many ways the work differs from the ordinary text books on this subject. The first and most important point of difference that we will notice is that, although mainly intended for students during their college course, it is peculiarly adapted for the needs of the practitioner. Of how few text books on physiology can this be said.

The older and rustier a practitioner becomes, the deeper he sinks into grooves. For such, and very few are otherwise, we would recommend a perusal of this treatise. Few could arise from the perusal of the chapters on metabolism, physiological research, the laws of habit and periodicity, &c., &c., without being awakened to the thought that physiology is the very ground work of true practice, and without catching some of that spirit of enthusiasm and abiding love of work, which so markedly characterize the author.

Prof. Mills' work differs from other works on physiology in being essentially founded on the comparative method and in the introduction of the principles of evolution and the teachings of embryology for the full elucidation of the subject. It is an "attempt to do, in some degree at least, for physiology what has been so well done for morphology." The field of biological science is made to contribute to this end. We find frequent references throughout the text to the differences in function for different groups of animals. Through this means the student will be better able to appreciate and understand the ever varying pictures of disease that come up before him in the wards of the hospital. He will be compelled to pause and think.

In turning to the chapter on the circulation we find a very full and thorough representation of the most recent knowledge on this subject. Dr. Mills, through his experimental investigations on the hearts of tortoises and turtles, has done much to bring this knowledge about. It is, however, very apparent that a great deal yet remains to be cleared up, especially on the relation between the nervous system and the heart. There is abundant evidence to prove that there is a marked difference between the hearts of different groups of animals, and that we know less about the intricate relations of the nervous system to the heart of man than any other. It is so difficult to interpret the nature of functional cardiac affections in man, that we are deprived in a great measure of the value accruing from clinical investigation. The physiology of the circulation is greatly in advance of our clinical and pharmacological knowledge. Physicians may appear to be slow in making practical application of much of what is known. The time, however, will no doubt soon arrive when the recent advances in the physiology of the circulation will bear fruit even in every day practice.

The nervous system is considered with that thoroughness which its great importance demands. The following quotation expresses the author's view on the important subject of cerebral localization :—"There is in the cerebral cortex a

localization of function, variable for each group of animals, and
to some extent for each individual; that it is not of a character to be mapped out by mathematical lines; that in case of
disease or injury one part may, to a certain extent, take up
the functions of another; that the functions of any part, however limited, are only to be understood when taken in connection with all other parts of the cortex of the brain, and in fact
of the entire body. These views we believe to be borne out by
the facts of physiological experiment, clinical medicine, operative surgery, pathology, sleep, dreaming, hypnotism, the
nature of the cerebral circulation, and the general truths of
biology." To the firm believer in strict localization, the above
statement may appear to be short of our acquired knowledge
on this subject. It is certainly cautious.

There appears to be no doubt whatever that the earlier
experimenters in the field of cerebral localization took too narrow a view of the subject, in mapping out very distinct territories as the seat of certain functions. In the light of the
recent investigations, it is plainly evident that there are no
sharp lines of functional distinction in the motor cortex. The
variability of motor and other functions in different groups of
animals is shown, at least in the dog, from Goltz's very
recent communication to the Society of German Physicians
and Naturalists, at their late meeting in Heidelberg. He succeeded in keeping a dog alive for many months after the
entire removal of the cerebrum. After recovery from the
effects of the operation, and up to its death, this animal did
not present any trace of motor defect.

How are these results to be explained? Can they be
brought into conformity with the dominant ideas of cerebral
localization? There appears to us to be great force and truth
in the remarks made by the author that the comparative
method has been as yet too little studied, and that conclusions
from experiments on one class of animals should not be applied
to another class. There is abundant evidence to show that
the cortex of the monkey's brain cannot be destroyed or removed without the production of paralysis.

As a text book for students this work will undoubtedly take a
high place, not altogether because it is a succinct and clear record of the latest knowledge in animal physiology, but also on

account of its being founded on the true principles of teaching. Especial care is taken to point out what is really known; to separate the known from the unknown; to show what directions our investigations must take in order that our knowledge may increase. The work is well printed and profusely illustrated, and reflects great credit on the publishers.

Natural Inheritance. By Francis Galton, F.R S. London: MacMillan & Co., and New York, 1889.

Mr. Galton has produced so many works bearing on the subject of heredity, which have been well received by the reading public that this last one cannot fail to receive a warm welcome.

This investigator has brought a method of his own to bear upon this important subject, which may be denominated perhaps as the physico-mathematical.

Many readers will be interested in the results who are unable to criticize the methods.

We think ourselves that mathematics must be applied with a good deal of caution to the problems of biology in the present stage of the development of that science. In this age the tendency to seek for accurate, precise and systematic results, and grouping is so great that we are in not a little danger of sometimes cramping the truth in order to adorn a page. However, Mr. Galton deserves all praise for his attempts to bring results within precise statements, even within the bonds of formulæ. Time will test the method and the results. Perhaps no worker has done so much for evolution in relation to man as the author of "Natural Inheritance." And not a little that he has brought to light is great interest to the physician.

His method is one that the physician applies himself in chemical and pathological investigation, though we are afraid not always with the thoroughness and precision of Mr. Galton. The chapter on "Family Faculties," "Eye-colour" "Stature,' &c., are all worthy of study both for the facts and the method, as well as the chapters on "Marriage Selection," "Heredity in Disease" and others.

The present work is not bulky but its reading requires close attention. There are a good many tables and appendixes.

Altogether it is perfectly plain that an enormous amount of work must have been done before the material was available for publication in the present neat form.

Those who are willing to look carefully into the subject will find Mr. Galton's latest work an interesting study. To the thoughtful it cannot but prove highly suggestive.   W. M.

The Physician Himself. By D. W. CATHELL. Philadelphia: F. A. Davis. 1889.

That Dr. Cathell's book has made a happy hit, is proved by the fact that it has now reached its ninth edition. It gives much valuable information in a pleasant chatty way, and the hints respecting business and ethical relations will be found particularly useful by the young practitioner. In the present edition the entire work has been revised and some new matter introduced. The publisher's part is well done ; the paper is good and the print large ; altogether it is a very readable and enjoyable book.

Lectures on Obstetric Nursing. By THEOPHILUS PARVIN, M.D. Philadelphia : P. Blakiston, Son & Co., 1889.

The two lectures delivered recently by Professor Parvin at the Philadelphia Hospital Training School for nurses were so highly appreciated that an urgent demand was made for their publication. The author has added an appendix, in which he treats several important matters not included in the original lectures. Much valuable information is given in small compass ; the teaching is sound and quite in accord with modern antiseptic practice.

Exploration of the Chest in Health and Disease. By STEPHEN SMITH BURT, M.D. New York : D. Appleton & Co. 1889.

It seems to be a necessity that every teacher of physical diagnosis should produce a little text-book, just as it is indispensable that every gynæcologist should be godfather to a pessary and every obstetrician should be the inventor of a special modification of the forceps. All these manuals have a strong family likeness the one to the other, and the family is a large one. The work before us, like many of its brethren, is the result of a request for publication coming from the writer's own pupils; so was the last one we noticed, and so was the one before that.

Dr. Burt has succeeded in condensing into small space nearly all that is really essential to a practical knowledge of the examination of the chest. The introductory chapter, which undertakes to give an account of the landmarks of the thoracic viscera, is meagre, the information given is scanty and insufficient, and a student who has to depend solely upon this chapter for his knowledge of the relations of the viscera to the chest wall will, indeed, be badly off for information, but the body of the book shows that much care has been bestowed upon its preparation. There is accuracy and commendable conciseness. The original illustrations are useful and instructive, but would be improved by enlargement.

Naturally, in a work of this character there will not be found much original matter to criticise. The section on adventitious sounds in the lungs is well written and the subject clearly put in a simplified form which will help the student greatly. Dr. Burt does not deal with dry or moist râles, but places all of them under one or other of the following headings: sibilant, sonorous, crepitant, subcrepitant, bubbling, tracheal, gurgling, and clicks (air and fluid in excavation). It is not unworthy of note that Dr. Burt is influenced by the teaching of Leeming, Loomis and Hudson in his acceptance of the theory of the intra-pleural origin of the crepitant râle. " The sound (crepitant râle) probably originates in the pleura, for crepitation is not heard until the two surfaces of this membrane move one upon the other; it ceases when movement becomes impossible, and commonly returns with returning pulmonary mobility."

We have no doubt that Dr. Burt's work will be found very useful to senior students. We recommend it to them and wish it every success. When a second edition is called for, it is to be hoped that the author will dispense with the use of that new and ugly word "calormetation" which pervades the book. The coining of new words must not be encouraged.

A Student's Text-Book of the Practice of Medicine.
By ANGEL MONEY, M.D., Lond.　London : H. K. Lewis.

The author states in his preface that he has attempted to produce a very concise book of modern medicine which may, he hopes, prove useful to those who are beginning the practice of medicine, to those who are preparing for examination, and to practitioners who have no time or inclination to peruse treatises. We specially recommend the work to the first class of readers. A student in his third year, who is just beginning his study of the final subjects, will find Dr. Money's book of great value. It is concise, fairly comprehensive, very readable, and, if it be well studied during the first year of hospital attendance, the knowledge thus gained will prove a great assistance to the reading of more extensive treatises. Let the student thoroughly master such a book as this before attempting the larger text-books such as those of Bristowe or Flint. To the candidate for final examinations such a book as this is not sufficient, and we say this because we doubt if examiners would accept as answers some of the statements to be found here. For example, suppose that a candidate were asked the treatment of Graves' disease, he would, armed with the knowledge gained in Dr. Angel Money's book, make answer : " The best treatment is perfect rest and plenty of belladonna." And all other treatment is disposed of in six lines. " Plenty" of belladonna is a somewhat vague quantity. And so, again, in the treatment of gallstones. " A mixture of sulphuric ether (twenty minims) and spirits of turpentine (five minims) in the compound almond mixture, three times a day, is very nasty and not at all efficacious." Students preparing for examinations can surely dispense with the knowledge of formulæ both nasty and ineffective. Why mention it at all ? In fact throughout the whole work the sections on treatment are very carelessly written. The few pages on prescription writing will, however, be found very useful.

We cannot help noticing one or two points which show a

certain degree of hurry and want of care in the preparation of the work. Measles, for instance, is omitted from its usual place amongst the eruptive fevers and placed at the very end of the whole book, amongst the skin diseases and the medicinal rashes. And this is the more strange, since the author begins his description by saying that "measles is best compared and contrasted with smallpox." Again, at page 407, in the chapter on Saturnism, the writer seems to think that *painters' colic* and *colica pictonum* mean the same thing. " Plumbers, painters (colica pictonum), type-founders and color-grinders are the usual sufferers from Saturnism." Colica pictonum is the colic from which the Pictones or inhabitants of Poictou suffered, and the term has nothing to do with painters, as the passage above quoted certainly implies. But certain parts of the book are very well written, and those are mainly upon subjects to which he author has given special attention, and in connection with which he is regarded as an authority. The chapter on rheumatism contains, in compressed form, some new and valuable information specially interesting in connection with recently published articles on that subject by Cheadle and others.

In conclusion, we trust that, with a few corrections, the work will pass through many editions and prove very useful to the junior final student.

Diseases of Women : A Manual of Non-Surgical Gynæcology. For use of students and general practitioners. By F. H. DAVENPORT, A.M., M.D., (Boston). Philadelphia : Lea Brothers & Co. 1889.

This little book will certainly fill a place in usefulness, although it would have been better if the author, in his determination to write a book early in his professional career, had written upon " diagnosis of pelvic disease in women," and set his title to that key. Medical gynæcology is a branch of the " Healing Art" not exactly understood by scientists, and is, therefore, not entitled to a place in literature.

Dr. Davenport's work will prove very useful in enabling the student to familiarise himself with the methods of examination of patients, and aid him in the diagnosis of pelvic disease.

Society Proceedings.

MEDICO–CHIRURGICAL SOCIETY OF MONTREAL.

Stated Meeting, May 31st, 1889.—Continued.

WM. GARDNER, M.D., PRESIDENT, IN THE CHAIR.

Microscopic Changes after Section of the Extra-Cardiac Nerves.—DR. MILLS then read for himself and Dr. Workman a paper on the above subject, which appeared in the June number of this JOURNAL, page 881.

Discussion.—DR. WILKINS said that a paper involving such important changes in accepted theories required careful consideration. The results regarding the action of the trophic fibres of the cardiac nerves seem quite opposed to the conclusions arrived at by Goltz in his experiments on the sciatic nerve. Section of this nerve caused paralysis of the leg, dilatation of the blood-vessels, loss of strength, and wasting of the extremity, but no microscopic changes in the muscles could be found, even the muscular coats of the vessels remaining unchanged.

DR. STEWART asked if Dr. Mills considered the histological changes to be degenerative, or at first inflammatory, followed by degeneration. He could cite several cases of atrophic paralysis where the cause was inflammatory.

DR. GIRDWOOD related a case in which a bullet under the gluteus maximus produced pressure on the sciatic, resulting in coldness with lividity of the limb, followed by wasting and weakness. The bullet, which gravitated to the lower edge of the muscle, was removed, with complete recovery from all the symptoms.

DR. MILLS, in reply, explained that the experiment of Goltz referred to was instituted to settle the question of the nature of the vaso-motor fibres in the sciatic nerve and not the trophic nature of nerves. Sympathetic fibres entered into the composition of the vagus in all animals thus far examined. Besides, the accelerators of the heart were, in all animals, derived from the sympathetic. These fibres emerged from the spinal cord in the upper dorsal region, proceeded upwards, and might be given off to the heart either from the stellate ganglion or the inferior or the middle cervical ganglion. In man, the most important in all probability come from the middle cervical ganglion. The accelerator (sympathetic) fibres were the motor nerves of the heart. In reply to Dr. Stewart's question, Dr. Mills stated that he thought degenerations following section of nerves were usually not inflammatory, and do not seem to have been such in this case, though on *à priori* grounds he did not see why they might not be of that character, seeing the important part the nervous system plays in inflammations generally.

***

Stated Meeting, June 14th, 1889.

WM. GARDNER, M.D., PRESIDENT, IN THE CHAIR.

Two Cases of Lead Poisoning.—DR JAS. STEWART presented to the Society two patients from the Montreal General Hospital suffering from lead poisoning. He said they were both typical cases of chronic lead poisoning, and exhibited the usual symptoms—marked anæmia, emaciation and nervous symptoms, paralysis of the extensor muscles of the forearm being marked in each case. The particular interest attached to the cases was due to the modes by which the lead had been introduced into the system. In one case the patient was a workman in a shot tower and had inhaled the oxide of lead from the melted metal. His face, hands and other portions of his body were constantly blackened by the lead while at work. It would appear that in this case the lead was absorbed through the skin and lungs. The patient in the second case is a bar-tender, and habitually drank a number of bottles of cream soda every day. These bottles were stoppered by a metallic button, which, together with the soda-water, was analysed by Dr. Ruttan and found to contain lead.

DR. RUTTAN stated that his attention had been called to this case by Dr. Stewart, and that he obtained a number of bottles of soda-water stoppered by this particular contrivance, and had found the stoppers to be made of a solder, an alloy of tin and lead, and in every bottle of soda-water with these stoppers lead was found in solution. The bottles and stoppers were exhibited. The stopper consists of a metal button attached to a wire loop, which projects beyond the mouth, and so contrived that it does not drop into the bottle further than about half an inch when open. The button is fitted gas tight to the shoulder of the bottle by means of a rubber ring. These bottles, when filled with soda-water, are immediately inverted, so the liquid remains in constant contact with the lead and becomes impregnated. The carbonate of lead at first formed is probably taken up by the excess of carbonic acid and held in solution ; but, besides this mode of solution, many samples of soda-water contain alkali as carbonate of soda, which aids the solution. He further said that he considered these stoppers to be very dangerous, and had written to the manufacturer informing him of the fact.

DR. GEO. ROSS related a case of lead poisoning where the patient was a druggist and took a glass of soda-water from a soda fountain early every morning. The fountain was fed from a reservoir by a lead pipe, and the liquid remaining in contact with the lead over night took up sufficient of the metal to cause serious symptoms. He had had a number of cases of plumbism from the shot works of the city. He asked Dr. Ruttan if he could account for the common occurrence of lead poisoning among the men working in the British America Bank-Note Company.

DR. McGANNON said he had a number of cases of painters suffering from plumbism; one case traceable to drinking beer from bottles in which the shot used in cleaning had been left.

DR. REED had seen large doses of strychnia recommended for the treatment of the chronic forms.

DR. TRENHOLME had seen marked symptoms of lead poisoning follow the use of acetate of lead in vaginal douches.

DR. WM. GARDNER related a case similar to that given by Dr. Ross. Intense lead colic was caused by drinking from a soda fountain in the morning.

DR. MILLS said that the number and variety of the cases referred to were very instructive, and brought up some interesting questions. He referred to a case of poisoning from shot boiled in milk, where the symptoms were those of lead poisoning. The patient also suffered for some time from crops of boils one after another. He further remarked that the chemistry of the body could not be measured by that of the laboratory. The conditions under which the chemical reactions occur within the system cannot be even approximately imitated outside the body, because they are quite unknown. He further suggested that perhaps the lead salt, rendered insoluble by the action of therapeutic agents, is picked out by the tissues from the circulation like grains of indigo are. He also raised the question as to whether the colic, anæmia, etc., of plumbism were due to the direct action of the lead or entirely to secondary changes. He favored the latter view.

DR. HINGSTON said that some years ago he followed a practice then highly recommended of treating phthisis by large doses of acetate of lead, a half to one drachm three times a day. He found, when accompanied with acetic acid to insure its solution, no toxic effects followed these large doses. He was inclined to the opinion that it was not lead that was toxic, but the particular salt. Observation had shown that the carbonate and chromate were both highly toxic, while the acetate was not so.

DR. GEO. ROSS said he had been induced to try acetate of lead for abdominal aneurism, but he found that small doses (five to ten grains) brought on colic and other toxic symptoms.

DR. RUTTAN, in reply to Dr. Ross, stated that the yellow and green dyes used in printing postage stamps contained chromate of lead, and he had been able to trace several cases to this source. He believed that there was much still to learn regarding the pharmacology of lead salts. A favorite hæmostatic among obstetricians was two-drachm doses of acetate of lead, repeated, if necessary. Excess of acetic acid could not be a preventative, as he knew of several cases of lead poisoning from using vinegar that contained lead dissolved from the glazing of the jar that was used to hold it. In one case there was less than two grains to the fluid ounce of vinegar, yet the colic and other toxic symptoms were well defined. The lead in these cases must have been in the form of acetate in solution.

DR. STEWART said that where acetate of lead is given in medicinal doses some escape and some are affected; all patients are not equally susceptible to the action of lead. And, again, the toxic effect of the drug occasionally manifests itself by its action on the blood, or may attack the nervous system or the intestinal ganglia. The treatment is generally an alterative one. He thought that iodide of potassium acted as an alterative and not as a chemical antidote to the lead. He regarded the œdema so frequently a marked symptom in these cases to be due to vaso-motor paralysis.

ASSOCIATION OF AMERICAN PHYSICIANS.

The fourth annual meeting was held in the Army Medical Museum and Library, Washington, D. C., September 18, 19 and 20, 1889. The Association was called to order at 10 a.m. by the President, Dr. Francis Minot, of Boston.

The first business was the reading of the President's address, which dealt with the progress of medicine during the last fifty years. He reported the deaths of the following members: Drs. H. D. Schmidt, New Orleans; John C. Dalton, New York (honorary member); Robert Palmer Howard, Montreal; and Edward T. Bruen, Philadelphia.

Dr. C. F. FOLSOM, of Boston, read a paper on *The Early Stage of General Paralysis*. The author first reported a number of cases illustrating the early stage of the disease, in which the motor disturbances were very slight, and might readily be overlooked and escape detection. The striking loss of muscular control or power, generally considered a part of the disease, was not found until a late period of the disease. The mental symptoms consist in impairment of a peculiar quality, often so slight as to be made out with difficulty. The disease arises most commonly under prolonged strain, particularly when associated with unaccustomed excesses. At least two-thirds of the general paralytics have had syphilis. The relation of the disease with syphilis is too frequent to be accidental. The disease is, however, not a stage of syphilis, and is not benefitted by specific treatment. The prognosis is probably not so hopeless as it is generally considered to be. The common early treatment is hurtful. Foreign travel is injurious. The only hope of at least partial cure or marked amelioration is in entire mental and physical rest.

Discussion.

Dr. ROBERT T. EDES, of Washington, reported the case of a man suffering now from pronounced general paralysis, in whom the first symptoms of the disease made their appearance some twenty years ago. If the anatomical view of general paralysis is accepted, he did not consider it strange that mental symptoms might precede the motor, depending upon the seat of the lesions.

Dr. S. WEIR MITCHELL, of Philadelphia, was sure that certain cases of general paralysis began most markedly with motor trouble, while others began most decisively with mental conditions. In regard to syphilis he agreed with the author, except that he had seen cases due to syphilitic disease in which cure followed specific treatment. He had also seen cure follow in a small number of cases where the treatment was begun in the early stages, but where the motor disturbance and the mental incapacity were sufficiently marked to render the diagnosis reasonably certain. In all of these cases there had been a total abandonment of all previous pursuits with absolute mental and physical rest. He agreed with the author that foreign travel was often injurious.

Dr. JAMES J. PUTNAM, of Boston, remarked that the fact that syphilis acts in this disease, not by producing a direct lesion, but in an indirect manner, justified us in looking for other causes of degeneration which might act in a similar manner. He asked if the reader had seen any cases in which chronic lead-poisoning was the apparent cause of the general paralysis, and related a case in which the imperfect and slow speech, the imperfect handwriting, and the expression of apathy and indifference, suggested a diagnosis of general paralysis. In this case there was, however, a history of drinking-water contaminated with lead, and there were certain local symptoms indicating lead-poisoning.

Dr. WM. PEPPER, of Philadelphia, believed that he saw these cases from a different standpoint than that of Dr. Folsom. They come to him as cases of dyspepsia, lithæmic disturbance, and the like, and are under his care for some time before symptoms leading to recognition are developed,— sometimes for years before the paretic symptoms appear. He could not regard syphilis as in any way essential in the causation of general paralysis. In regard to the early stage of the disease, there was not one symptom mentioned by Dr. Folsom or described by others as indicating the early stage, which he did not often find in cases of nervous lithæmia. There may be a grouping of these symptoms, or a delicacy on the part of the diagnostician which will enable a finer and finer shade of these differences to be recognized, which does constitute a basis of diagnosis. He thought that general paralysis could be initiated by many disturbing, depressing or irritating causes, and that, in its early stages and slight degrees, it was capable not rarely of being entirely cured. If these cases are permitted to go on, with neglect of hygeine, and with excesses (sexual, alcoholic or business), a notable proportion will end with symptoms of general paralysis.

Dr. C. F. FOLSOM, of Boston, said, in regard to lead, that while he had seen cases in which this agent had produced symptoms of general paralysis, he had not seen a case in which the terminal symptoms of general paralysis had been produced. As illustrating apparent cure after specific treatment, he referred to a case in which the use of large doses of iodide of potassium apparently produced complete recovery, and the patient returned to his previous business. The symptoms, after several months, reappeared, and have continued to steadily progress. Whether this is the result in all such cases, he was unable to say.

Dr. JAMES STEWART, of Montreal, read a paper on *Tetany*. The details of the following case were referred to: The patient, a male, aged forty, has been troubled during the past eight years with regularly recurring attacks of tetany. He served as a soldier during the American civil war. Suffered at that time and subsequently from chronic dysentery and malarial attacks. For upwards of ten years he has been troubled with diarrhœa. Patient is tall, emaciated and anæmic. The first subjective symptom of his tetany is usually double vision, which is quickly followed by the characteristic contractions of the flexor muscles of the hands. Occasionally the flexor muscles of the fore-arms and the abductors of the arms become spastic, muscles of the face almost constantly suffer, muscles of the lower extremities rarely. The affected muscles are the seats during the attacks lactation and removal of the thyroid, can induce similar symptoms. It appears probable that impoverishment of the nerve centres is one of the main factors in its production.

Dr. JOHN T. CARPENTER, of Pottsville, Pa., read a paper on *Tetany and a New Principle of its Pathology* The author defined tetany as a nervous disorder accompanied by tetanic spasms of an intermittent character, which may extend from the extremities to the muscles of the jaw, and is reproduced during the periods of intermission at will by pressure on the track of the affected nerve trunk or over the blood vessels obstructing the circulation. An historical view of the disease was given. Tetany was regarded, not as a special disease, but as a sequel of precedent phenomena only. The affection was regarded as the result of septic absorption. The diminution of cases of tetany coincident with the successful treatment and the prevention of septic poisoning was regarded as an argument in favor of the connection between septicæmia and tetany. Cases illustrating this view were cited. The views previously held in regard to the pathology of tetany were discussed and considered.

Discussion.

Dr. FRANCIS P. KINNICUTT, of New York: I have seen but two cases of intermittent tetany, both occurring in patients with dilatation of the stomach. In one the dilatation was due to pyloric stricture resulting from cancer. In the other there was non-malignant stricture. In both of these cases the conditions were favorable to absorption of poisonous matter.

Dr. F. T. MILES, of Baltimore, reported the case of a young woman aged twenty-two years. She had suffered from six to eight years from dilatation of the stomach. She had vomited acid matters but never offensive. She had several times had numbness of fingers and toes. She suffered her first attack of tetany twenty-four hours before her death. In this case the stomach had never been washed out.

Dr. A. JACOBI, of New York, had been struck with the stress laid by the readers upon sepsis as the cause of tetany. In one of the cases reported by Dr. Stewart, which he thought was due to the absorption of putrid material, the stomach was twisted; and Dr. Jacobi suggested that the intermittent contracture was due to nervous influence resulting from the twisting rather than to absorption. He did not doubt that there were cases in which septic absorption produced such symptoms; but when we recall the fact that the contracture is temporary, we must conclude that the influences given rise to that attack were also temporary. Many of these cases are, I think, the result of nervous irritation. In some of these cases reported I should attribute the condition to anæmia.

(To be continued.)

THE

Montreal Medical Journal.

| VOL. XVIII. | OCTOBER, 1889. | No. 4. |

ANTIPYRINE IN WHOOPING COUGH.

During the past few months a great deal has been written about the alleged efficacy of antipyrine in the treatment of whooping cough. From a careful perusal of a number of these articles, we think an unbiased observer must be led to the conclusion that this treatment is not only practically inoperative, but is attended by greater or less dangers.

In Monti's Klinik, in Vienna, twenty-eight cases were carefully treated with antipyrine, in doses ranging between five and thirty grains in the 24 hours, with an entirely negative result; the average duration of the twenty-eight cases being 50½ days. Neither the intensity or the number of paroxysms were in any way influenced. Baginsky records a very similar experience. Tuczek treated his own child, a boy aged four, who was suffering from whooping cough, with 6 grains of antipyrine 3 times daily. Towards the end of the third week the little patient became soporose, had violent convulsive attacks resembling cortical epilepsy. The heart's action was weak and frequent. The pupils were dilated and the temperature subnormal. A maculous exanthem made its appearance. During the whole period of treatment the urine contained acetone. Tuczek attributes all the untoward symptoms to the antipyrine. The case certainly teaches the valuable lesson that antipyrine should always be given with caution, especially to children, when a continuous action is desired. From its direct influence on the albuminous constitutents of the blood, its prolonged use is certainly attended with considerable danger.

BANFF AS A HEALTH RESORT.

It is unfortunate that no paper was read at the recent meeting on the virtues of the Banff springs and air, in the treatment of disease. That this place is destined within a short period to become an important health resort appeared to be the almost universal verdict of the numerous practitioners present at the meeting. Banff air and Banff sulphur water are, however, powerful for evil as well as good, and until the Government appoints a physician who is thoroughly conversant with modern balneotherapy, the evils are as likely as not to predominate. A motion was introduced at the late meeting with the object of attaining this end, but it was withdrawn, owing to the opposition of a few men who certainly should have known better. We have heard of numerous instances where great and irreparable mischief was caused by the too free use of the hot sulphur bath. No one who understands the profound functional changes induced by the frequent use of such water, but will at once see the advisability and urgent necessity there is for scientific direction, and until this is done, practitioners from a distance should exercise the greatest possible care in advising anyone to this resort. It is impossible for the family physician, even were he competent, to so instruct his patient in all the numerous details of hygienic and dietetic treatment which should be carried out at such places, in order that the fullest benefit and the least evil should result.

THE CLIMATE OF SOUTHERN ALBERTA.

The important paper on the Climate of Southern Alberta, by Dr. Kennedy of Fort McLeod, which we have great pleasure in publishing, deserves the serious attention of all Canadian practitioners. As yet, unfortunately, no exact observations of a general character have been made on the climatic conditions of the North-West. Dr. Kennedy, from his own observations, is able to show however the adaptability of this region as a climatic resort for many diseases, especially for the earlier stages of pulmonary tuberculosis. Dr. Kennedy well lays stress on the importance of a dry, bracing, clear atmosphere in the treatment of these cases. Alberta fulfils these necessary conditions apparently as well as any climate on the continent. The unsuitability of the climate for neurasthenic patients is noted. Several instances came under our own observation where the truth of this assertion was brought out.

The comparative rarity of typhoid fever is what we should naturally expect, and if ranchmen understood better the value of cleanliness it would be still rarer. If the microscope was used more frequently in the diagnosis of fever, we would hear less about typo-malarial fever all over the American continent. It has been well said by Osler that "the characteristic changes in malaria are as distinctly determined in the blood as are those of tuberculosis of the lungs in the sputa." Laveran's researches on the blood in malarial fever have now been confirmed from so many sources, that we may say that by means of a microscope we can usually determine in a very few minutes whether we have to do with malarial poisoning or not.

THE INDEX CATALOGUE.

The tenth volume of the Index Catalogue, recently published, contains references from the letters O to Pfutsch. It is hardly necessary to add that the same care and thoroughness characterize this volume as the previous issues. It is impossible to overestimate the usefulness of the great work so ably conducted by Dr. Billings. The present volume includes 7,658 author titles, representing 2,905 volumes and 7,282 pamphlets. It also includes 14,265 subject-titles of separate books and pamphlets, and 29,421 titles of articles in periodicals.

Medical Items.

MEDICAL DEGREES ACQUIRED IN THE UNITED STATES WITH ALARMING FACILITY.

The *North American Review* for October contains a very instructive, if somewhat alarming, article by Drs. Eggleston, Flint and Doormus, in which, under the title "The Doors Open to Quackery," the writers discuss the present methods by which professors of the art of healing are manufactured in America, and turned loose upon a luckless community. Dr. Eggleston says that there are "not a dozen American medical colleges out of 117 that would be tolerated for a moment in any country that pretends to be civilized;" and this despite the efforts of the best men in the medical profession, which are openly combatted or secretly thwarted by quacks, charlatans and low-class colleges. It clearly is not for want of degree-granting colleges that the American doctor is less informed than his brethren in other countries, for it seems that taking the average of all other countries as a fair average, there are schools enough in America to educate medical men for 300,000,000 people, but in most of them the standards for matriculation and graduation are put down so low as to make an American diploma almost a reproach in other countries. It will be remembered that Dr. Rauch, of the Illinois Board of Health, visited Montreal during the small-pox epidemic that raged in this city some years ago. Dr. Rauch was able to speak in terms of high commendation of the general sanitary regulations of Montreal, and the means it has at command for coping with zymotic disease. Dr. Rauch, it seems, put up a young journalist of Springfield, Ill., to try for a medical diploma from the Bellevue Medical College, Boston, Mass., the president of which was a rabid anti-vaccinationist. The diploma was granted, and the reader will be interested by the perusal of the thesis on the strength of which this license to kill was issued.

VACINATION.

The Grate increase of Disease in thease Late years Calls for Explanation Undoubtedly the Doctors of this day is to blame for very much of it. But more than anything Else in my opinion is the Inseartion into the Pure Blood and Vitle fluid of our Inosent offspring of that vile Diseas of the Animals cowpox So grate has the Curse Became that Privelidges of School Edication is Denide in this and Many other States to those who wisely Refuse to Submit to this Curse that is just a Peace of the Nonsensikal Medical teachings of the Day when Theory and Imagination Rool instead of Practical Expearance and which keaps its Studends in close Confinement a Big part of three or four years to hear the Nonsens which is thear peddeld out to them consumtion Siffles and Skin Disease Runn Wild among the People This calls for a Strong kick on the Part of our noble Proffession which should seak to Build upp the Health and Streangth of the People instedd of Planting the Seeds of Diseas in them To Prove that Vacination Don't do no good we nead ondly to say that Thear has Been More Small Pox in this Place in the last

year than thear was in the last Nineteen or Twenty
year and more deaths from it I neadnt say no more
About a Thing that is so Plane to Eny thinking Man
or Woman Eather we should all Band ourselves togather in all
Parts of the Country to Shut off this Cursed Practise the people
Should be tought Better But the Days is Cuming when Enlightenment will take the Place of Ignoranse and Prejudice and
when that Time Comes these fannatics who live by Scaring
People will have to step aside and Vacination will not be Heard
of any more. (*Montreal Star.*)

—George C. Stephen, M.D. (McGill '87), after a course of
study in Vienna, has received the L.R.C.P. Lond., and L.S.A.
Eng. He has begun practice at 88 Sutherland Avenue, London, Eng.

—Through the great liberality of the late Thomas Workman
of Montreal, McGill University is to receive the sum of $120,-
000, to be devoted to extending and perfecting the facilities
for teaching Applied Science.

—The seventeenth annual meeting of the American Public
Health Association will be held in the hall of the Brooklyn
Institute, Washington and Concord streets, Brooklyn, N.Y., Oct.
22, 23, 24 and 25. Addresses of welcome will be delivered
by Hon. Alfred C. Chapin, Mayor, on behalf of the city, and
by Alexander Hutchins, M.D., on behalf of the medical profession. The following topics have been selected for consideration
at the meeting :—

1. The Causes and Prevention of Infant Mortality.

2. Railway Sanitation.—(a) Heating and ventilation of railway
passenger coaches; (b) water-supply, water-closets, etc.; (c) carrying
passengers infected with communicable diseases.

3. Steamship Sanitation. 4. Methods of Scientific Cooking.

5. Yellow Fever—(a) The unprotected avenues through which
yellow fever is liable to be brought into the United States; (b) the
sanitary requirements necessary to render a town or city proof against
an epidemic of yellow fever; (c) the course to be taken by local health
authorities upon the outbreak of yellow fever.

6. The Prevention and Restriction of Tuberculosis in Man.

7. Methods of Prevention of Diphtheria, with Results of such
Methods.

8. How far should Health Authorities be permitted to apply known
Preventative Measures for the Control of Diphtheria.

9. Compulsory Vaccination.

10. Sanitation of Asylums, Prisons, Jails, and other Eleemosynary
Institutions.

'ion of the members of
governments, with
practice and pre-
their dangerous
-piter's stork,
-umed the
-ist teach
-ed the
ered
-is-

)A.

ABER, 1889.

Communications.

INTRODUCTORY ADDRESS

AE OPENING OF THE FIFTY-SEVENTH SESSION
MEDICAL FACULTY OF McGILL UNIVERSITY,
OCTOBER 1ST, 1889.

BY R. L. MacDONNELL, B.A., M.D.,
Professor of Clinical Medicine.

At the beginning of a new session it has always been the custom in this college for the members of the Faculty to select one of their number to address words of welcome to the new-comers and to those who have already embarked upon their medical career. This year my turn has come. On such occasions it is customary for the lecturer to introduce himself with an apology for his general and special unworthiness, but it is not my intention to do anything of the kind. On the contrary, I think myself peculiarly well fitted to welcome and give advice to new students. Firstly because, not being yet stricken in years, though scarcely juvenile, I fancy I can still think and act as a young man and look upon the world from the stand-point of a medical student; and, secondly, because it has been my good fortune to have spent ten years of my professional life in daily companionship with students. And indeed it would be a strange thing if I did not, during that time, learn to know how students thought, how they lived and moved and had their being. It is for these reasons that I think my advice may be of some service to those who are about to begin the work of the 57th session.

21

year than thear was in the last Nineteen or Twenty
year and more deaths from it I neadnt say no more
About a Thing that is so Plane to Eny thinking Man
or Woman Eather we should all Band ourselves togather in all
Parts of the Country to Shut off this Cursed Practiss the people
Should be tought Better But the Days is Cuming when Enlightenment will take the Place of Ignoranse and Prejudice and
when that Time Comes these fannatics who live by Scaring
People will have to step aside and Vacination will not be Heard
of any more. (*Montreal Star.*)

—George C. Stephen, M.D. (McGill '87), after a course of
study in Vienna, has received the L R.C.P. Lond., and L S.A.
Eng. He has begun practice at 88 Sutherland Avenue, London, Eng.

—Through the great liberality of the late Thomas Workman
of Montreal, McGill University is to receive the sum of $120,-
000, to be devoted to extending and perfecting the facilities
for teaching Applied Science.

—The seventeenth annual meeting of the American Public
Health Association will be held in the hall of the Brooklyn
Institute, Washington and Concord streets, Brooklyn, N.Y., Oct.
22, 23, 24 and 25. Addresses of welcome will be delivered
by Hon. Alfred C. Chapin, Mayor, on behalf of the city, and
by Alexander Hutchins, M.D., on behalf of the medical profession. The following topics have been selected for consideration
at the meeting :—

1. The Causes and Prevention of Infant Mortality.

2. Railway Sanitation.—(*a*) Heating and ventilation of railway
passenger coaches ; (*b*) water-supply, water-closets, etc.; (*c*) carrying
passengers infected with communicable diseases.

3. Steamship Sanitation. 4. Methods of Scientific Cooking.

5. Yellow Fever.—(*a*) The unprotected avenues through which
yellow fever is liable to be brought into the United States ; (*b*) the
sanitary requirements necessary to render a town or city proof against
an epidemic of yellow fever ; (*c*) the course to be taken by local health
authorities upon the outbreak of yellow fever.

6. The Prevention and Restriction of Tuberculosis in Man.

7. Methods of Prevention of Diphtheria, with Results of such
Methods.

8. How far should Health Authorities be permitted to apply known
Preventative Measures for the Control of Diphtheria.

9. Compulsory Vaccination.

10. Sanitation of Asylums, Prisons, Jails, and other Eleemosynary
Institutions.

THE

MONTREAL MEDICAL JOURNAL.

VOL. XVIII.   NOVEMBER, 1889.   No. 5.

Original Communications.

INTRODUCTORY ADDRESS

DELIVERED AT THE OPENING OF THE FIFTY-SEVENTH SESSION
OF THE MEDICAL FACULTY OF MCGILL UNIVERSITY,
OCTOBER 1ST, 1889.

BY R. L. MACDONNELL, B.A., M.D.,
Professor of Clinical Medicine.

At the beginning of a new session it has always been the custom in this college for the members of the Faculty to select one of their number to address words of welcome to the new-comers and to those who have already embarked upon their medical career. This year my turn has come. On such occasions it is customary for the lecturer to introduce himself with an apology for his general and special unworthiness, but it is not my intention to do anything of the kind. On the contrary, I think myself peculiarly well fitted to welcome and give advice to new students. Firstly because, not being yet stricken in years, though scarcely juvenile, I fancy I can still think and act as a young man and look upon the world from the stand-point of a medical student; and, secondly, because it has been my good fortune to have spent ten years of my professional life in daily companionship with students. And indeed it would be a strange thing if I did not, during that time, learn to know how students thought, how they lived and moved and had their being. It is for these reasons that I think my advice may be of some service to those who are about to begin the work of the 57th session.   21

It will be part of my object to show you that, although the
course of studies laid out for you is at first sight difficult, yet
that the means of overcoming the difficulties and obstacles of the
road are within your reach, and that to the industrious student
the journey to a degree is interesting and pleasant.   There are
long marches it is true, and sometimes temporary stoppages
(generally overcome by slight supplemental effort), but the road
lies through a pleasing country, with so much that is interesting
by the wayside that the traveller arrives at his destination sooner
than the length of time spent in the journey would lead him to
expect.

This is the problem to be solved by your faculty.
How to afford the best medical education possible in the short
space of four years ?   Our endeavour is to turn out as well educated a practitioner as we can—a practitioner I say, that is one
who can practise, a man able at once to earn his own living and
to make himself useful in the community.   I believe we do
turn out a practitioner, in the true sense of the word.   The
McGill graduate enters upon his career with a fair experience of
general medical and special work, and so far we have no good
reason to be dissatisfied with the result of our four years' work.
The question arises, though, ought we to be satisfied or ought
we be constantly endeavouring to effect improvements in the
course ?

The main difficulty in our way is the limited period of time at
our disposal, but this difficulty we could overcome were it not for
the attempts to regulate our teaching undertaken by the various
provincial licensing bodies.

You have, I dare say, read Æsop, and you remember how
the frogs, dissatisfied with the existing state of practice in the
somewhat malarious district in which they resided, fell to grum-
bling, and, after considerable deliberation, demanded of Jupiter
that some firm legislation should regulate the affairs of the profession.   The thunderer, accordingly, sent them a log which
met with contempt and disrespect.   Annoyed at their conduct,
he sent them a provincial board, and matters soon assumed such
a condition that the frogs bitterly regretted that they had not
et well alone.   And so with the Canadian medical profession.

Boards were established, at the instigation of the members of the profession themselves, by the provincial governments, with the good intention of regulating admission to practice and preventing quacks and charlatans from exercising their dangerous trade. So far so good. But the boards, like Jupiter's stork, were not satisfied. They have in some provinces assumed the *rôle* of educators, and dictate to teachers what they must teach and to learners what they must learn. They have injured the profession they were intended to protect, and they have hampered and impeded the progress of the medical schools. From their mischievous interference this school suffers to an extreme degree. In particular, the College of Physicians and Surgeons of Ontario imposes upon our students certain very vexatious regulations, and exacts of them pecuniary taxes, wholly out of proportion to the benefits they may ever expect to derive from becoming licentiates. It would seem that but two objects are aimed at by these regulations and impositions. Firstly, the establishment of a barrier to keep out of the field as many competitors as possible, the originators of the movement having affected an entrance before the fence was put up ; and, secondly, to render it more and more inconvenient and uncomfortable for an Ontario student to seek his education out of his own province. Failure will attend both these objects, for the fittest will survive in the battle of life by the law of nature, and no legislation will ever enable those unsuited by natural abilities and defective education to take a front rank in the fight. The struggle for existence in the profession must be a fair one from the start, and those who cannot live by their own talents and energies, will seek in vain for any benefit from legislative aid.

The claim is made, on the other hand, that provincial boards exclude quacks and charlatans, and so protect the practitioner from dishonest competitors. As I write there lies before me a Montreal paper in which at a glance I see the open advertisement of three notorious charlatans. The Ontario Board is active enough as regards the honest practitioner, yet no one can say that irregular practice does not exist in that province.

The system of examining by boards for admission to practice

is, in one instance, carried to a great length and to an absurd conclusion. The Province of British Columbia has secured the existence of a board. There are some fifty practitioners in that province (I counted 51 in the copy of the register for '87), and united they form the Medical Council of Physicians and Surgeons of British Columbia. " Now, we have got in, let us keep the others out," seems to be their motto. If they had contented themselves with examining diplomas and rejecting those that came from indifferent colleges, then, perhaps, a useful function would be fulfilled, but, as the law stands at present, there is not one of you who, after graduating, would not become liable to punishment if he dared to give advice in British Columbia. He would be obliged to pass before the members of the Council, or such of them as may be appointed for the purpose, a satisfactory examination touching his fitness and capacity to practice as a physician or surgeon. In other words, the Provincial Board of British Columbia would have to make it its duty to see for itself whether your teachers understood what they were about when they taught you, examined you and certified on your diploma that you were a fit and proper person to practise medicine.

Lastly, a money tax is exacted. The plea can be made by such boards that the public must be protected, and it would be unsafe to allow a legally qualified practitioner from another province to exercise his calling within their borders. But no one can defend the establishment of a money barrier. The $100 tax can have no other object than to limit competition.

If we wish the Canadian profession to gain the respect of the medical world, we must use every effort to rid ourselves of this provincial littleness, this parochial policy. Medicine is medicine everywhere, and a legally qualified Canadian practitioner ought to be able to practice in any part of his own country.

Another charge I bring against the provincial boards is, that they impede the progress of medical education by compelling teachers and students to devote an excessive proportion of their time to the giving and attending of didactic lectures.

The days have long since gone by when didactic lectures

were regarded as forming the principal part of a medical education. A century ago medical students were apprenticed to
practitioners, and everything they learnt was of a strictly practical character. Jenner was apprenticed to a country surgeon
near Bristol, and Sir Astley Cooper began professional life, at
the age of fifteen, as an apprentice at Yarmouth. In those days
the didactic lecture served a useful purpose in supplementing
the strictly practical instruction which the pupil received from
his master. The school system gradually replaced the apprentice system, and made the student, we wont say scientific, but
it made him a man of books and opinions, and cultivated his
memory to the neglect of his powers of observation.

A double course of lectures in all the more important branches
of study was thought to be necessary, and the number of lectures in each course was fixed at one hundred. Opinions have
changed, and improved methods are beginning to prevail. It
was found that lectures failed to replace practical instruction.
The professor has now to give way to the teacher. Students
were over-lectured and under-taught. Your faculty would wish
to replace a large proportion of the didactic lectures by practical laboratory work and instructive demonstrations, but the
boards will not let them. They exact the pound of flesh ; they
must have the one hundred lectures twice told.* For my part,
I see no hope of a change until such time as the affairs of our
profession are controlled by more enlightened men, and I look
to the time when you all shall be graduates, and I confidently
hope you will have the good sénse to vote with the party in
favor of letting the shoemaker stick to his last, and letting the
teaching be managed by the teachers. With no immediate hope
of a change, we try to do our best to mitigate the evil. Accordingly, a few years ago, a system of grading the course was
introduced, first in the classes in clinical medicine and clinical
surgery, and the plan has been extended to other courses.

The excessive time devoted to didactic lectures is the worst

---

* The Ontario Board have added to the course in anatomy fifty more lectures,
bringing the number of didactic lectures to the ridiculous figure of 250 ! !

feature in our Canadian system of medical education. There is no country in the world where so many lectures have to be attended. When your brain is weary with much listening, your fingers cramped with note taking, your ischial tuberosities worn away from much sitting, do not entertain hard feelings against the faculty, but remember the provincial boards.

And then when all is done and you stand before the world the possessor of a degree, the boards do not leave you. You have to make up your mind where you are to exercise your talents for the public good. As matters now stand you may register your degree and practise in any part or province of the Dominion—in Quebec, New Brunswick, Nova Scotia, Manitoba, anywhere except in Ontario and British Columbia. In a few months we shall be able to announce that reciprocal relations will be established between the College of Physicians and Surgeons of Quebec and the General Medical Council of Great Britain, as a result of which a McGill degree may be registered in Great Britain. Provided with such a guarantee of professional respectability, you may practice in any part of Her Majesty's dominion except the two provinces. In all the mighty empire of Great Britain there are only two provinces where the profession has attempted to protect itself from honest competition by calling in the aid of the legislature.

That examinations are uncertain we all know, but some are much more uncertain than others, and none so uncertain as those conducted by licensing bodies. The examiners are selected from the body of the profession, and no teacher is allowed to examine in the subject in which he teaches. It would seem as if unfitness were a special qualification. The would-be examiner must have shown no special aptitude for the subject. A professor of surgery, for instance, would be qualified for the post of examiner in chemistry, but he must not examine in surgery, because he knows too much about it. A good country practitioner, with a nice comfortable circle of midwifery patients, is, on this principle, made examiner in physiology or anatomy. And what are the results ? The examination is a scramble, sometimes the weak succeed while the strong succumb. " Quis custodiet ipsos custodes." Who shall examine the examiners ?

I have gone to some length to show how the licensing boards impede progress. Now it shall be my effort to prove to you that, in spite of all the obstacles thrown in our way, the number of our students has steadily increased with the imposition of fresh tests and annoying regulations.

We ourselves, during the last twelve years, have instituted changes in the curriculum which have made Jordan a very much harder road to travel than it was in my time, and it really seems that the more difficult the course the more there are who wish to take it. The class of 1875-6 was the smallest in the last twenty years. It was in the spring of 1877 that the first examination in practical anatomy was held. (The students have taken a very deep interest in it ever since.) Practical chemistry followed suit, and higher marks were awarded in these two important subjects. Practical courses in microscopy, histology and pathology were established about this period. Enlargement and extension of the course has taken place in other directions. The proportion of marks qualifying for a pass was considerably raised and the tests have been increased. New subjects have been added, such as hygiene and gynæcology. The whole course has been made longer by the addition of one compulsory summer session. Four complete years must be spent at college, and there are exemptions in favor of no one. But in spite of these changes, and there were not a few who thought our numbers would diminish, there has been a steadily increasing influx of students.

McGill was the first medical college on this continent to demand four complete years of study. She was the first to abolish the exemption in favour of the student who had spent his year of so-called study with a doctor, and that in favor of the bachelor of arts. And in this movement McGill is only doing what she has always done. She is leading. She did fifty years ago what some colleges are beginning to do to-day. She began her career with a matriculation examination. In the whole of the United States there is not a single college whose entrance examination is more severe than that which has always been demanded here. Very few colleges have any at all. Harvard University, which, owing to its great reputation and the extent of its endowment, can afford to introduce costly reform, insists on a matriculation examination of which Latin forms a part. Some other colleges, with less ambitious views in the matter of preliminary education, content themselves with the three R's; and, lastly, come the unholy army of colleges who demand no examination at all, and in its rank are included many so-called first-class colleges. Matriculation examinations do not pay. They cost too much. The popular voice in the great republic is against the severity shown in demanding that one who wishes to enter a learned profession should be made to prove that he can read and write.

Students always take an interest in examinations. You know that our standard has been raised. But bear in mind that the actual amount of work is really reduced because so much more practical teaching is done and so much more personal aid afforded to each student. Moreover, the examinations have been arranged with a view to encourage practical observation and to put a limit upon what is commonly called the cramming process.

In spite of all these changes, changes which have been attempted in some colleges and which have had to be abandoned, the class at McGill has steadily increased year by year. This is a thing of which every Canadian ought to be proud, that the greater the difficulties presented the greater the number of those who seek to overcome them.

Having pointed out the path that leads to a degree, and explained how difficult a struggle it is to get into the profession by that path, I am going now to tell you how this may be accomplished. Firstly, I address myself to those who are here for the first time. These are commonly called Freshmen. A silly notion prevails that there is some kind of opprobrium attached to the title Freshman. A Freshman is a fresh man. Observe the word man. It does not mean boy. A man must put away boyish things. He must think and act as a man. He must cease to depend upon others, act for and rely upon himself. Boys may be noisy, sing loudly in the streets and behave generally as boys, but men should not do such things.

There are members of other classes in the College who would like to make you believe that *fresh* means silly, idle, presumptuous, and a host of other bad things; but it means nothing of the kind. It means vigourous, active, intelligent, energetic. Freshman! you stand to-day in a position truly enviable, you have the world before you, and opportunities for study such as your fathers never possessed. See that you use them properly. The first year is the most important period in your professional career. It must not be spent in idle amusement. Be careful, then, how you form your habits, and be especially careful of the companionship you make. Friendships with senior students are of mutual advantage. The youngster derives help and support from the senior, and the senior in teaching his younger brother improves greatly his own knowledge. I would like to see the students here follow the example of their English brethren, and spend more of their time in asking each other questions and teaching one another.

Remember, Freshmen! that having once become medical students you must sustain the character of the school, and the reputation of the school is merely the sum of the reputations of each member of the school.

Do not be over-anxious about examinations. Any person of ordinary intelligence and common industry can pass. Don't deceive yourselves. There is no luck in examinations. The student who was plucked because his luck was bad was the man who provided himself with so little knowledge that an unexpected call upon his scanty store made him a bankrupt. There are a few students whose natural capabilities are such that the intellectual life is unsuited to them, but that number is very small. I believe that there are very few who cannot pass. And above all things, do not work with the idea that your only object in coming here is to pass examinations and get a degree. You are not so many cannons and your teachers are not gunners who ram home a charge of Anatomy, another of Physiology and Chemistry, and fire you off as a salute on convocation day.

The knowledge you gain here must be the nucleus of your

life studies, and, moreover, you must regard your studies as being undertaken not with the object of merely acquiring a store of facts, but as the means of training the powers of observation. "The habit of observation is the foundation of the art of medicine." And it is upon your own observations and experiences that you will have to depend, and not upon those of other people. Other people's experiences are like other people's clothes; they may keep off the cold, but they don't fit and are very unbecoming. All through life the primary subjects must be kept at your fingers ends. It is not an exaggeration to say that nearly all the errors in diagnosis commonly met with in practice can be traced to defective knowledge of anatomy and physiology. A good physiologist or a good anatomist does not necessarily make a good physician or a good surgeon, but no man can properly practice medicine without a sound working knowledge of the primary branches.

Do not be contented with a minimum of work, just enough to enable you to scrape through the examinations. In dealing out your share of work give good measure. Make it a rule to do always more than is asked. Don't stop working the minute the clock strikes. Remember the words George Eliot puts into the mouth of Adam Bede: "I hate to see a man's arms drop down as if he was shot before the clock's fairly struck, just as if he had never a bit of pride and delight in 's work. The very grindstone 'ill go on turning a bit after you loose it."

Use your text books more, and depend more upon them. Select a good one, and stick to it. Read over the subject of the lecture you have heard that day. Cultivate a spirit of enquiry. Think out the problems set before you, and try to find out the reason for everything. Do not be satisfied with what you hear your teachers say unless you perfectly understand what they mean· We are too apt to talk above the heads of our class, and a good deal of the subject matter of the lecture or demonstration is not quite taken in and understood. Always ask if you don't understand. We all like to have students point out to us their own difficulties, and thereby give a direction to our teaching.

Try to be careful, methodical, systematic. Make sure of one step before you take another. Give all your energies to facts and observations. Never mind the theories, they can take care of themselves. Waste no time. " Time is the stuff that life is made of." It is not the student who sits up late and burns most oil who succeeds best, any more than it is the person who eats most who becomes most healthy. Try to acquire the habit of utilizing odd moments. You cannot all take a prize, but you can all take a good degree.

Gentlemen! we begin our 57th session at a period in the history of the profession of unusual activity and progress, but with us in this college a period of sadness and mourning. This is the first introductory lecture for many a long year at which our late Dean is not present. Prof. Howard was in this room a year ago to welcome the new comer, but since our last meeting we have had to mourn his death.

It seems fit that I should speak of him to-day, but more in his relation to students than in his relation to the University and to the medical profession of Canada. I wish to point out to you how you may derive benefit from the example he set you. There is probably no student beginning his studies to-day who has before him greater difficulties to face than had our late Dean when his medical career began. He was a poor man. There were no powerful friends to advance his interests; there was nothing to depend upon but his own energy, his own perseverence and his wonderful capacity for hard work. His great love for his profession, and more particularly for the scientific part of it, showed itself in every day of his active life. His devotion to clinical studies made him a marked man in this University long before she honoured herself by granting him a degree. After his entry to practice his path was beset with many difficulties. The doors of the General Hospital were slow to open to him. He did not derive from that institution the fostering help it has afforded so many men who have since become eminent in the profession. The University herself at first overlooked his talents and energies, and he was not the first of his classmates to receive a teaching appointment. He had not been long in the school before he gained that loving respect and admiration from the students which he retained to the last day of his life. In the faculty his strong personal influence was always exerted in favour of reform and improvement. In all his relations with the students Dr. Howard showed towards them a fatherly affection and interest. Valuable as was his time, manifold his engagements, no student ever failed to gain audience with him, and with audience sympathy and good counsel. Those of you who had the benefit of attending his last course of lectures will remember, as do all his old pupils, the kindness and forbearance, and the patience with which he spent often more than his lecture hour over again in answering questions and showing the pathological specimens in which he was so much interested, to the knot of eager students gathered about him. I can only say of him as a lecturer, what Baillie said of William Hunter: " No one ever possessed more enthusiasm for his art, more persevering industry, more acuteness of investigation, more perspicuity of expression, or, indeed, a greater share of natural eloquence. He excelled very much any lecturer whom I have ever heard in the clearness of his arrangement, the aptness of his illustration, and the elegance of his diction."

Whatever may be the fortunes of this college, whatever may be the success to which it shall attain, the period during which the reins of government were held by Dr. Howard, must always be regarded as one of progress and enlightenment. The rise of the school which I have attempted to demonstrate to you, is mainly the result of his energy and labour. Though older in years than any of his colleagues, Dr. Howard was as young as the youngest in his ideas of medical practice and of medical education. Advancing years brought with them no diminished vigour nor flagging interest in the welfare of the college he so dearly loved. He was ever ready to accept new ideas and to carry out the improvements which the advance of education from time to time demanded. The late years of his useful life were mainly devoted to the advancement of projects directly affecting the welfare of the Canadian medical student, the establishment of the Campbell Endowment Fund, and the organiration of the Royal Victoria Hospital. By means of the revenue derived fron the former we were enabled to build, equip and carry on the magnificent laboratories in which you will learn in a practical manner the rudiments of your profession. In a few years too, the student will study disease in a hospital which will reflect credit on the noble benefactors and on the country in which they live. For these great benefits the student is indebted firstly to the generosity of the benefactors, but such gifts were largely the outcome of the life work and energies of our late Dean.

The new session we begin in sorrow, but our sorrow must not weaken our efforts. Let the death of our leader stimulate us to unwonted energy. *Let us do what we would like him to see us doing.* Let us prove ourselves worthy· pupils of Howard, and show the world that we can at least attempt to imitate the virtues of his character. Let us be as zealous, as honest, as upright, as conscientious as that noble example of all that constitutes the gentleman and the Christian who has been so recently taken from us.

VARICELLA.*

By James T. Whittaker, M.D., Cincinnati.

Varicella or varicellæ, diminutive of varus, pimple, pock; chicken (French, *chiche;* Latin, *crier,* insignificant) pox; water pock, wind pox, variole notha, spuria, false pox, a trivial acute infection of childhood, distinguished by a long period of incubation, absence of prodromata, slight fever, a vesicular eruption, varied in size and short in duration, without complications or sequelae. Chicken pox met its first description under the term crystalli, by the Itallian anatomists, Ignessias, 1575 and Guido Guidi (Latin, *Vidus Vidius,* as in the Vidian canal), 1585, and received its present unfortunate name from Vogel, 1764. Fuller, 1730, and Heberden, 1767, made the first attempts to separate it from variola (varioloid), with which it had been hitherto confounded, and

---

* Read at the meeting of the Canadian Medical Association. at Banff.

has been since by many authors (Hebra, Thompson) "with inconceivable persistence" (Thomas); a mistake which resulted in complete confusion regarding the nature of both affections, and in reproach and disrepute of vaccination in its early history.

The recognition of the fact that an attack of one secures future immunity from itself, but does not protect against the other, finally led to a distinct separation of the two diseases. Confirmation of this view was also obtained in the fact that vaccinia does not prevent varicella, nor varicella vaccinia. Czermak, after three failures in the ordinary way, succeeded in vaccinating a boy aged four, by introducing lymph into the interior of vesicles during an attack of varicella.

Varicella appears in sporadic and epidemic form, but epidemics never assume the range nor show the intervals of measles and smallpox. The disease does not die out entirely in large cities, but assumes something of an endemic proportion once or twice a year on the opening of schools and kindergartens. It is confined exclusively to childhood (exceptions by Heberden and Gregory) up to the age of twelve, and is rare after ten. The short-lived contagious principle, probably from the vesicles, is believed to be inhaled (contagium halituosum). Infants are never born with it.

Inoculation experiments fail oftener than succeed. Thus Hesse failed in 87, succeeded in causing a local eruption in 17 and a general eruption in nine cases. Steiner claims to have succeeded eight times in ten trials, but was unable to further propagate the disease from any case.

Tenholdt found in the contents of vesicles a micrococcus which, inoculated in man, produced light redness and swelling like that of spurious vaccinia, and in one case a vesicle smaller than a sudumen, the affection remaining local. Pfeiffer found in fresh vesicles of thirty cases, without exception, a parasite (proteid) showing an amoeboid stage, a cystic stage, spore formation, and, after the development of numerous spores, a return to the amoeboid stage. Inoculation with contents of vesicles showed, three times in five days, a localised, circumscribed varicellar exanthem, recurring scattered up to the 8th day. The parasite could not be cultivated upon any culture soil.

Incubation varies from eight to seventeen days.

Prodromata, in the forms of light malaise, occur only very exceptionally. The disease is announced by the eruption which shows itself in the form of spots of hyperæmia, in the centre of which appear, in the course of a few hours, distinct but slightly elevated vesicles, which attain their greatest circumference in the course of three to 24 hours. The vesicles contain a clear sticky serum, neutral or alkaline, never acid (as in sudamina) reaction, which fully distends the vesicle, and which exudes slowly, but not wholly, on puncture of the vesicle. The serum shows under a microscope a few pus cells which, when exceptionally present in greater quantity, may make the vesicle appear to resemble drops of wax. In lighter cases, without halo, the patient looks as if sprinkled with "drops of water" (Fagge).

The eruption shows itself first upon the neck and chest (face according to Thomas), to spread subsequently over the face and scalp, trunk and extremities, and shows itself always in successive crops, to the number of ten to fifty, or as many as 200 to 800 over the whole body, irregularly, never uniformly or at once.

Vesicles vary also in size, usually from a pin head to a pea, exceptionally from a dime even to a dollar. These large vesicles are, however, always lax, never full, as is the case in the blebs of burns, blisters and pemphigus. Distinct, isolate and irregular elsewhere, they may show aggregation like zoster upon the extremities, but are very rarely confluent anywhere. They are very superficial, lifting only the upper layers of the epidermis, and penetrate to the rete malpighi in only exceptional cases. Hence they but rarely show an umbilicus and seldom leave a scar.

The eruption may last two to five days when the residue dessicates to leave a light pigmentation, very exceptionally ulceration (Hesse), which gradually fades to leave no trace. Through premature rupture, air may enter a vesicle to produce the condition known as v. ventosa, emphysematosa, wind pock.

The eruption may also show itself on various mucosae, as in the eyes to produce conjunctivintis, keratitis; in the mouth and palate to cause a stomatitis; more or less dysphagia, swelling of the cervical glands.

A slight rise of temperature, maximum, 102° (exceptionally 106°, Heberden) with associate symptoms of fever, headache, insomnia, anorexia, nausea, etc., attends or may attend the eruption, to continue with it two to three, exceptionally five, days. Defervescence is by crisis, without subsequent elevation or eruption. Very light cases may show no fever at all. Recurrence is possible but not probable.

Inasmuch as varicella was so long, and is often yet, mistaken for variola (varioloid) the question of differential diagnosis assumes supreme importance. The diagnosis demands, first, a knowledge of the existence of either in the vicinity or community, and a definite history of the pre-existence or absence of either in the individual, together with the period of the last successful vaccination; second, the age of the patient, variola occurring at all ages, varicella being confined to childhood. Variola is preceded by prodromata, malaise, fever, headache, backache, sometimes initial rashes, and attended by a characteristic eruption on the third day. Varicella announces itself with its eruptions without prodromata.

Varicella appears first upon the neck and chest, or, if upon the face, irregularly over it, and irregularly over the body. Variola appears first upon the face, forehead, to extend over it regularly from above downward, thence to spread uniformly over the neck, chest, etc.

The superficial vesicles of varicella contain only serum, the deeper seated vesicles of variola, serum and, later, pus.

The eruption of variola is uniform in size, that of varicella varies greatly.

Varicella is very rarely confluent anywhere, and its vesicles are only exceptionally umbilicated. By the end of the third day spots of hyperæmia, fully developed vessicles and crusts may be perceived simultaneously and side by side in varicella, whereas the variations in the age of the eruption would be observed only at points distant from each other in variola.

Fever precedes by several days the eruption of variola to fall with its appearance; whereas fever occurs only with the eruption of varicella, to increase with its development. Variola shows in marked cases secondary fever, absent in varicella.

The mortality of varicella is practically *nil,* yet, inasmuch as complications, fatal hæmorrhages, catarrhal pneumonia, nephritis, has been recorded as coincidences or complications (Hutchinson), delicate children may be protected by removal from the area of infection, or isolation of patients insepar ate chambers.

Patients should remain indoors, if not in bed, during the existence of the eruption, and should not be permitted to re- turn to school untill all signs of it have disappeared. Treatment is superfluous.

HÆMATOMA OF THE VULVA AND VAGINA.

By A. H. Wright, M.D., Toronto.

Read at the Meeting of the Canadian Medical Association at Banff, August, 1889.

Thrombus, or hæmatoma of the vulva and vagina, from statistics which I have been able to gather, occurred fifty times in 103,424 cases where records were kept with this point in view, or about once in every 2,070 labors. The mortality is high, according to the reports of Deneux, Winckel, Barker, Scanzoni and others, which show in the aggregate about 90 deaths in 400 cases, or 18.5 per cent.

The following are two cases which have come under my observation :—

CASE I.—*Hæmatoma of the Vagina.*

Mrs. S., aged 22, primipara, attended in labor, May 27th, of last year, by Dr. MacCallum of Toronto. After the head had reached the middle of the pelvis, a lump was detected in the left wall of the vagina, immediately below the head. At this time labor had been in progress about twelve hours and the uterine contractions had been unusually strong. Shortly after this a copious hæmorrhage commenced. A message was sent for me, and, having but a short distance to go, I arrived in a few minutes. The patient showed the ordinary indications of severe hæmorrhage. On examination I found the hæmorrhage still continuing from a rent in the vagina on the left side, extending towards the posterior wall. The serious bleeding was evidently arterial, and I was fortunately able to control it by pressure with the thumb inside the vagina and the forefinger outside the vulva, using my right hand and leaving the left free. While I thus " held the fort," Dr. MacCallum had plenty of time to make the necessary arrangements for forceps delivery. After he had anæsthetized the patient, I applied the forceps very easily with my left hand, while I continued to control the bleeding, as I have described. I had found that the slightest relaxation of pressure allowed a recurrence of hæmorrhage, and the patient had already lost more blood than she could afford. I easily drew the head against the bleeding surface, when the substituted pressure completely controlled the hæmorrhage. The uterine contractions were still strong, and I removed the forceps, leaving the delivery to nature's efforts. No more chloroform was administered and the child was soon expelled, after which the hæmorrhage recurred, and I again controlled it by pressure. Dr. MacCallum expressed the placenta and the uterns remained well contracted. I then introduced a suture rather deeply through the left labium, and also through the upper edge of the vaginal rent. On tying this it tore through the vaginal wall above, but fortunately appeared to have caught the bleeding vessel, as there was no return of serious hæmorrhage. I used two other sutures, but think they did little or no good. A pad and T bandage were applied. Dr. MacCallum afterwards took charge of the case, and changed the dressings frequently with ordinary antiseptic precautions. There was some suppuration with high temperature for two weeks, after which the patient made a fair though rather tedious recovery.

CASE II.—*Hæmatoma of the Vulva.*

A. S., married, aged 31; primipara; confined in the Toronto Burnside Lying-in Hospital, December 12th, by Dr. Thompson, the resident accoucheur. Labor protracted, duration 24 hours; membranes ruptured two hours before delivery; uterine contractions unusually strong, especially during last three or four hours; head pressed on perineum for nearly two hours. Forceps not used; took several doses of chloral; no other anæsthetic. There was a slight rupture of the perinœum, for which one catgut suture was introduced. Condition of vulva apparently normal, when the parts were washed and the antiseptic pad applied. Child weighed 8 pounds, Swelling in right labium first noticed by nurse about 22 hours after delivery, at 4 a.m., December 13. I received a message to go to hospital during the morning, but was unable to reach there before 2 p.m., about 30 hours after delivery. I found a large hæmatoma of right labium majus extending backwards to the gluteal region, and pressing inwards on the vagina. The skin over the swelling was very dark in color—almost black. A large slough was evidently imminent. I decided on immediate incision. After ether was administered, I made the incision about 2½ to 3 inches long on inner side of labium, and removed clots amounting in the aggregate to the size of a child's head, leaving a very ragged, dark-looking surface within the cavity. I feared that a large portion of the skin and subcutaneous tissue had lost its vitality, and that considerable sloughing would occur. The cavity was washed out with a hot solution of mercury bichloride, 1 to 1,000. There was very little, or practically, no hemorrhage, and I therefore used no styptic, but introduced a plug of gauze dipped in the antiseptic solution and well dusted with iodoform, and applied a T bandage, leaving room for the lochial discharges to escape beside the dressings. I ordered the wound to be dressed in a similar manner every six hours, but directed that no force be used in introducing the gauze unless hæmorrhage occurred; and pads for lochial discharges to be changed every hour, at least until bedtime. On the following day I was surprised to find the cavity so much reduced in size—in fact quite insignificant when compared with the large opening which was left on the preceding day after the removal of the clots. Skin still dark colored, but there was less indication of sloughing. On the fourth day there was a healthy-looking granulating surface with scarcely any cavity. After this there was rapid progress; no sloughing occurred, there was no pus at any time, no rise of temperature, and the wound was completely healed on the 16th day, when the patient left the hospital.

These two cases are rather typical examples of the two most common varieties of hæmatoma of this region, caused by the rupture of vessels in the submucous tissue of the vagina or the subcutaneous tissue of the vulva. The vaginal thrombus may be formed at any point below the pelvic fascia, as happened in Case I., but in rare cases the bleeding may occur above the pelvic fascia, and the blood cannot then go towards the surface, but is forced upwards between the pelvic diaphragm and the peritoneum, as high, or even higher than the kidneys. Death in such cases may occur with the ordinary signs of concealed hæmorrhage. In Case II. the thrombus appeared to be between the superficial and middle fascia of the perineum—probably the most usual site.

In referring to the frequency of this accident, according to the evidence at our disposal, I, of course, referred to the gross cases which in the past have been discoverable, or, more correctly, discovered. Strictly speaking, it is far from correct to say that vaginal or vulvar thrombus is formed only once in two thousand labors. We are told by those who have investigated the subject carefully in post mortem examinations, especially Barnes and Matthews Duncan, that small submucous extravasations of blood along the genital tract during parturition are very common, if not practically universal. The more serious lesions which attract attention differ probably in degree rather than in kind. In a general way we may say they are all caused by pressure. Among the more definite explanations which have been offered I know of none which I consider at all satisfactory. One would naturally suppose that varicose veins would at least predispose towards the formation of these thrombi; but such is not the fact, as the majority of authorities agree. Winckel, however, is among the minority who think that this condition of varicosity does undoubtedly predispose towards such accidents. In both of my cases the veins were, as far as could be ascertained, entirely normal.

There is a variety of these cases which is more clearly described by Matthews Duncan than any other author so far as I know, i.e., vaginal submucous hœmatomata, generally, if not always, unrecognised, which are not absorbed, but subsequently suppurate, and form vaginal abscesses. At a meeting of the Obstetrical Society of London last month, Dr. Duncan related two cases of such abscesses, in which the finger could be introduced through a rounded opening of the vaginal mucous membrane into a cavity as big as a walnut. In the discussion which ensued, as reported in the *British Medical Journal*, various cases of vaginal abscesses were related which the speakers thought were of a similar nature. A number of these had resulted in death from septicæmia. It is quite likely that such cases are not uncommon, but are generally unrecognized or inperfectly understood; and it is unnecessary for me to dilate on the vast importance of a correct diagnosis and proper appreciation of the condition when it exists.

The statistics to which I have referred indicate a mortality that is almost startling, but I think modern antisepsis will show much better results. The great value of antiseptic methods is well shown by the results of the treatment of the large cavity left on the removal of the vulvar thrombus. The wound was kept perfectly healthy by the antiseptic dressings, and the natural elasticity of the parts appeared to have a remarkable effect in rapidly reducing the size of the cavity. The wonderful changes which took place within three or four days, by which a great ugly-looking hole had almost completely disappeared, seemed to me simply marvellous.

The treatment will, of course, depend upon various circumstances—whether the hæmatoma is large or small, whether it appears before or after the completion of labor, etc. I will make no effort to enter into details, but may simply say that we will probably all agree, in a general way, to leave alone these blood tumors which are small, do not obstruct labor, do not threaten to cause sloughs, and do not suppurate, with the hope that they will be absorbed. On the other hand, when such a tumor prevents delivery, is likely to slough, or becomes an abscess, we should freely incise, empty the cavity, check hæmorrhage if it occur, and afterwards wash out regularly, In my case of vaginal thrombus I think I should have made no effort to introduce sutures after the hæmorrhage was stopped. I think it scarcely possible to get such coaptation as to hope for primary union, and it is probably better in such a case to leave the wound in such a shape that it can be easily and frequently cleansed. In the case of vulvar thrombus, I think that, under the circumstances, there can scarcely be any doubt as to the propriety of making an immediate and free incision when I first saw it.

MINERAL SPRINGS.

By H. BEAUMONT SMALL, M.D., Ottawa, Ont.

Prepared for the meeting of the Canadian Medical Association at Banff, N.W.T.

It was my original intention to have prepared for this
meeting a thorough and exhaustive work on the mineral
springs of this country. In addition to a general review of the subject, I wished to prepare a handbook
for the practitioner, in which would be found all information
regarding the character of the water, how it compares with
other waters, where situated, the sanitary state of its surroundings, hotel accommodation, facilities for using the waters, and
such other points as are essential in the selection of a health
resort. The task, however, was greater than I anticipated,
and my work remains unfinished.

In the present paper I wish particularly to direct your
attention to the classification of mineral waters, and shall
glance at the geology and chemistry of the subject as far as is
required to make clear the divisions.

Anyone who has had occasion to refer to the literature of
the subject is aware of the meagreness of the information that
is to be found there. We have nothing whatever bearing on
the therapeutic value of Canadian springs, and such works as
there are on the springs of the United States possess very little
merit as scientific productions. All are very superficial, and
the analyses furnished are, many of them, old and unreliable,
in many instances the work of amateur chemists. Perhaps
the best and most scientific work on this continent was that
carried on by Professor Sterry Hunt, the result of which is to
be found among his contributions in the Reports of the Geological Survey of Canada, 1863-66. He treats the subject from
the chemist's point of view—giving the analysis of a large
number of Canadian springs, and explaining the origin of all
the constituents, in his well-known lucid and attractive style.
Anyone desirous to continue this study, should not fail to become familiar with these essays.

The classification of mineral springs is much the same the
world over, the divisions being based on the most marked

character of the water. The following will give some idea of the methods prevailing in the different countries as they are taken from standard works:—

TABLE I.

GERMAN.	FRENCH.	AMERICAN.
Alkaline	Sulphur.	Alkaline.
Glauber Salt.	Saline.	Saline.
Iron.	Bicarbonate.	Sulphur.
Salt.	Purgative.	Chalybeate.
Epsom Salt.	Ferruginous.	Purgative
		Calcic.
Earthy.		

All are purely arbitrary. The great difficulty is that in any of them a water containing soda salts with iron and sulphuretted hydrogen may be placed in any one of three classes—alkaline, iron, or sulphur—with perfect correctness. Another objection, and one which I think points to a very great defect in the classification, is that the name gives no indication of what the other constituents may be. When a chalybeate water is mentioned, we know it contains iron, but have no idea whether it contains neutral, alkaline or even acid salts. It is the same with sulphur waters, or the waters of any class.

In the classification I propose to overcome this difficulty, we form the three divisions according as the waters are neutral, alkaline or acid. No classes are provided for sulphur, iron, etc.; instead, when any of these constituents, which may be called "accidental," are present, the term will be used as a prefix, and we will then refer to waters as sulphuretted salines, sulphuretted alkalines, sulphuretted acids; or ferrated salines, ferrated alkalines or acids, as the case may be. The Banff springs are commonly known as *thermal sulphur* to the public, if we call it a *thermal sulphuretted alkaline water* it at once conveys an idea of its chemical character and therepeutic possibilities.

The advantage of this nomenclature must be apparent at once, and commend itself to members of our profession, not only on account of its scientific accuracy, but also on account of its being both simple and serviceable.

The salts which these waters contain are not dissolved at haphazard from the soil of the locality at which they emerge. They are of much deeper origin, arising from geological formations of a definite chemical composition—their source as Prof. Hunt points out, is the oldest sedimentary rocks termed the "Silurian," which were deposited from the earliest known sea, and are very generally distributed throughout the whole world. The constituents of which these formations are composed were at one time in solution in the waters of this primeval sea; from which, as a result of chemical reactions, they were deposited as carbonates of lime and magnesia, silicate of soda, sulphates of lime, alumina, and other insoluble salts.

At a later period, owing to terrestrial disturbances, parts of this sea became land-locked, forming great inland seas, one of which occupied the extent of country that is now the valley of the Ottawa, St. Lawrence and Upper Lakes. The conditions for evaporation being favorable, these bodies of water gradually diminished, leaving beds of chlorides of soda, lime, magnesium, sulphates of the same bases, and bromides and iodides of soda and magnesium. Towards the end of this process the concentrated solution that remained resembled the "bittern" of modern salt works, and filled the basins and fissures of the sediments already formed.

Since that period other geological formations have been deposited, convulsions of nature have disturbed their relations, and cracks and fissures have occurred that reach from the surface to this deep saliniferous strata. Water from the surface slowly penetrates these depths, following the fissures and percolating rocks, and in time again reaches the surface, bearing in solution the salts which for so many ages have remained buried.

In this rapid geological sketch, what I wish to point out is, that it is evident there are two distinct sources from which these springs may arise; one a sediment of soluble saline matter, the other an older and more stable formation upon which water acts more slowly.

Class 1.—In the first instance the salts of the concentrated

sea water are dissolved at once by the water in its passage
through the earth, the result being the simple saline
waters, such as St. Catherine and Borthwick springs, or the
stronger purgative waters, such as the (*Fredrichshall*).
They are neutral in reaction, contain no carbonates,
or only such small amounts as may be dissolved in
their course to the surface. They are never strongly carbon-
ated nor sulphuretted, and are rarely thermal.

Class 2.—From the second source the salts are the results
of chemical reaction, as when a solution of carbonate
of lime and magnesia comes in contact with a formation containing soda, carbonate of soda and magnesia is
formed, the lime being deposited as an insoluble salt. In other
instances carbonic acid gas, formed at great depths, may
be held in solution by the water by which it acquires
very decided solvent properties, and readily acts on the beds
of soda, magnesium and lime. They are alkaline in reaction;
they contain as the characteristic salts carbonates of soda
and of the alkaline earths with lithia, silica, and sulphates
of lime; they have no bromine or iodine; they contain varying amounts of carbonic acid gas; may be sulphuretted and
thermal. The great number of our springs are an admixture
of these two classes, as at Saratoga, Caledonia, &c.

Class 3.—Acid waters. Waters also rise to the surface
which are strongly acid in reaction, due to the sulphuric acid
which they contain; the salts they hold in solution are the
sulphates of soda, and of alumina and iron. The acid is probably
formed at a great depth by the influence of subterranean heat
on sulphates, in the presence of an organic matter; or, under the
same influences H_2S with water may produce the acid. In
Canada a spring of this character occurs at Tuscarora, near
Brantford, and another near Niagara.

All other ingredients commonly met with in mineral springs
—iron, sulphuretted hydrogen, arsenic, carbonic acid gas, &c.,
&c.—are what may be termed accidental, they are not derived
from any special geographical formation, they may or they
may not be present in any one of three classes.

Iron is derived from the soil, in which it is very generally
distributed, after the other salts had been obtained and the
character of the water determined. It is rendered soluble by

organic matter and carbonic acid, except in the acid waters where it is a sulphate.

Sulphuretted hydrogen may be generated at great depths in the same way as sulphuric acid, or it may form more closely near the surface from the decomposition of sulphate of lime by organic matter, which reduces it to a sulphide, and this is decomposed by carbonic acid into carbonate of lime and H_2S.

The temperature of the water is due to terrestrial heat. All our thermal springs of any importance are in the Rocky Mountains. In Eastern Canada there are two or three, the temperature of which is several degrees above that of the locality; one at Chambly, the other at the acid spring at Tuscarora. These are distinctly thermal, but in so slight a degree as to be of no service.

As the springs of Europe, as well as those of this country, arise from the same geological formations, it follows that they are alike in both countries; that is, the salines in Canada have their analogues in Europe, so also with the other classes. The only waters we have not got are the purgative salines such as the "Fredrichshall." In every other class we have waters equal to any of the European Spas. The Banff waters have their counterpart in the waters of the French Pyrrenees; a comparison of the two analyses will show them to be almost identical, not only in composition, but also in temperature. The waters of the United States are simply a continuation of those of this country. The most common in the east are the alkali-salines, a union of the first and second classes, examples of which are given in the accompanying table.

In this crude and hurried paper, I feel that I have not at all done justice to the subject which is of so much importance. I trust, however, that it will make clear the points I wish to raise, and it should sufficiently introduce the subject to elicit a discussion on all its phases, should no other paper treat on it more fully. What we want in this country is a proper scientific study of our springs, thorough analysis, not only of the solids, but also of the gases, a proper study of climatic influences, and, what is of the greatest importance, a careful observation, on the part of physicians, of the results of courses of treatment.

One Pint.	SALINE.			ALKALINE.		ACID			
	St. Catherine	Friedrichshall.	Borthwick.	Banff.	Idaho	Tuscarora.	Saratoga	Caledonia.	Chambly
Chloride Sodium	20.64	67.37	98.08	.09			50.05	46.93	7.12
" Potass:	2.30		1.30				1.	.21	.27
" Magn:	36.26	31.08	2.11						
" Calc:	148.58		1.83						
Sulphate Sodium		41.73		.28	3.67	.42			
" Magn:		39.55	2.45	1.03	2 34	1.29			
" Calc:	16.99	11.24	2.01	4.70	.43	6.20			
Carbonate Sodium				2.97	3.85		.94	1.93	9.01
" Mag:		3.53			.36		9 01	3.76	.65
" Calc:	.08	.11		1.30	1.19		12 44	.85	.30
Iron	.44				.52	3.09	.03		
Br. I	.07	.02	.35				1.08	1.33	
Alamina						3 74			
Sulphuric Acid						34.31			

𝕽etrospect 𝕯epartment.

QUARTERLY RETROSPECT OF MEDICINE.

By R. L. MacDonnell, M.D.,

Professor of Clinical Medicine in McGill University; Physician to Montreal General
Hospital.

Life Insurance.

Within the last few years there has been a change of opinion
regarding the import of certain conditions of the system and
of certain chronic morbid processes resulting in decided
modifications of the rules governing the selection of lives
for assurance. An absolute rule was enforced that the
presence of a heart murmur effectually excluded from all benefits, and so did the presence of albuminuria, even though unaccompanied by any other deviation from the normal condition
of health. And while it is becoming acknowledged that
albuminuria and chronic valvular affections may be consistent
with a fair expectation of life, other points formerly regarded
as being but of secondary importance are now looked upon as
being very dangerous to life, and consequently damaging to
the value of a life risk. These are intemperance, gout, obesity,
and syphilis. In the following pages an abstract will be presented of some of the more recent addition to the literature of
life insurance, in the hope that the practitioner may gain
aid in manag ng the cases that come to him for examination.

The Presence of a Heart Murmur.—At the Brighton meeting
of the British Medical Association in 1886, Sir Andrew Clark
read a paper on " Cases in which disease of the valves of the
heart had been known to exist for upwards of five years without causing serious symptoms." He noted 684 cases of valvular disease without symptoms, showing how many persons
must be going about with heart disease and yet not suffering
from it. Lesions of the heart produced in youth were noticed
to be greatly recovered from, if development were not complete.

In the ensuing discussion, Dr. Gairdner, of Glasgow, stated
that he had referred to this subject in print 25 years ago, and
that there was a tendency to overrate the importance of mur-

murs, to pay too much attention to sound rather than the circumstances, and to take too serious a view of cardiac murmurs and disease generally. In summing up, Sir Andrew Clark said that considering a case for life insurance he weighed these facts—the time the mitral disease must have existed; whether independently of disease of the heart-walls ; whether in existence for over two years; whether associated with attacks of negative congestion; whether the general health was good, and whether there was a fair radial pulse. Murmurs must be considered in their relation to the general health and the condition of the heart-wall.

Following up the evidence of so keen and accurate an observer as Sir Andrew Clark, the medical advisers of some of the life insurance companies arranged a series of questions, and indicated the direction of the special examination of those who had heart murmurs and wished to insure. One of these papers is before me. The home office wishes to have information on certain points, and puts the following questions, which I give in full, forming as they do a guide for the examination of cardiac cases, not only for insurance but for general purposes :—

Does the proposer suffer (1) from breathlessness or (2) from palpitation? Is there any pallor or congestion of the face? Is there, or has there recently been, any dropsy, and, if so, in what situations? Are the superficial veins enlarged, or the arteries thickened? Describe the state of the pulse, including (a) its rate per minute, (b) its characters, especially noting if it be regular or irregular in rhthym or quality? State the results of your examination of the heart, in respect especially to (a) position of the apex and the nature of its import on palpitation, (b) size of the heart, (c) character of the heart's sounds in the different areas—(1) Mitral, (2) aortic, (3) pulmonary, (4) tricuspid. Note if any murmur be heard; state where it is most distinct, and to where it is propagated. State the results of auscultation of the carotids, and of the veins at root of the neck. What are the characters of the urine? If any abnormality of the circulation be detected, what, in your opinion, is the nature of the abmormality? The influence now being produced by it upon health? The probability of its being recovered from or continuing indefinitely.

The question of the acceptance of heart cases affects merely those who are the subjects of mitral murmurs and those whose murmurs depend on blood causes. Aortic murmurs are a barrier to acceptance. "These cases of *aortic murmurs*, systolic, diastolic or double, are entirely uninsurable, the elements of durability being wanting. We have not to deal, as in mitral cases, with gradually accumulated alterations of structure, which imply a definite series of progressive morbid events, and so become somewhat calculable as to time ; but life may, and often does, end suddenly, owing to the failure of the systemic supply—especially of the brain. The ordinary results of cardiac dropsy, overgorged right cavities of the heart, pulmonary œdema, and hæmorrhage, are rarely seen in these aortic cases, and then only when the mitral valve and right chambers of the heart have yielded. But the sufferer rarely lives long enough to die in that mode." *

But the case is different with mitral murmurs. Numbers of persons may have a mitral murmur from childhood to old age without undergoing any symptoms, and therefore without the effects of heart disease recognized as injurious to life. All depends upon the maintenance of compensation. The dangers to such a life would probably arise after middle life, owing to the supervention of fatty changes in the heart muscle. The rule of insurance companies has been to unconditionally reject such cases. They are not insurable in any case at the ordinary rate.

Suppose that the applicant presents every good point, good personal and family history, that his occupation is such as not to require great muscular strain, and his habits are in every way desirable, and that the only objection to immediate acceptance is the presence of a murmur at the mitral area. "But, if such a case present with murmur only, and without great enlargement of the heart or any secondary disorder, and especially if the ventricular contraction be moderately strong, without the signs of much hypertrophy, and the murmur be well pronounced ; and if, in addition, it can be shown that such condition must have prevailed for a long time, say from the

* Medical Handbook of Life Assurance for the use of Medical and other Officers of Companies, by James Edward Pollock, M.D., F.R.C.P., and James Chisholm. London. 1889.

date of one attack of rheumatic fever many years previously, and if the proposer have unimpaired health, and does not exceed 35 years of age, it is our opinion that it is possible to accept such a life with a considerable addition to the premium. * * * * * We hold that such lives are insurable, and certainly if a sufficient number of them presented, so as to make the risks spread over a number of similar cases, we feel sure that offices would be safe in accepting them. But to take one or two only, which, by chance, might not verify the prognosis, might bring the practice into disrepute." The most dangerous are those indicating failure of power and muscular tone, and that the aortic cases are much more perilous than the mitral, the former being ineligible at the rate which may be assigned to them, while it may be possible to compensate the increase of risk in the latter by additions in some form to the premium.

Albumen in the Urine.—The insurance examiner will sometimes meet with a case of this kind. A person in good health, who has never had any previous illness and has no suspicion of the presence of any disease, presents himself for examination. The family history and the personal points are unexceptionable, but when the urine is examined a small amount is present. Ought that risk be entirely rejec ed, or can it be accepted at a rating? I have met with a few such cases, and they have not been taken by the company for which I was examining. There seems lately to have been a change of opinion on this important point, and it is an important question to consider —is albumen necessarily a sign of disease?—and not only from an insurance standpoint, but also as regards the welfare of our patients. Two valuable papers on this subject have recently appeared.

" We have still a number of cases, by no means insignificant, in which albumen is continuously present in the urine of persons of various ages, but beyond that of adolescence, or early youth, it is to be disregarded as of no importance, or it is to be looked upon as the early stage of nephritis. It is possible that in some of these a more m nute examination, such as is by no means easy on a large scale, would bring to light casts and

---

* Ibid., p. 77.

settle the question of some renal disturbance, the question then becoming—What is the prognosis in slight cases of chronic nephritis ?"

These cases should be regarded with grave suspicion. " Some of them seem to be instances of a real nephritis, running a very chronic course, and presenting at the time of their first examination no constitutional symptoms. Munn found that in a considerable number of cases, in which at first only albumen was noted, that casts were subsequently present. Four of sixty-nine had died within three years, and in the majority a general deterioration of appearance was noticed."

It may further be suggested that among them there were many over-weights, a class peculiarly liable to nephritis, and also that middle-aged business men, such as are the majority of those presenting themselves for life insurance, form a class especially liable to *interstitial* nephritis, a form attended with the least marked symptoms for a long time, perhaps for years." *

Dr. James Tyson, of Philadelphia, believes that a certain number of good risks are lost to companies by the indiscriminate rejection of all cases of albuminuria. Two cases are cited in his paper as illustrating a class in which, although there is albuminuria, its subjects have not renal disease, and are insurable risks. Could a set of rules be laid out for his guidance, the well-trained examiner might save his company a certain number of risks which are now lost to it.

" Unfortunately, from necessity perhaps, at the present day the majority of medical examiners are neither well educated nor well trained. Supposing, however, that these important desiderata are attained, as it is reasonable to believe they will, at no distant day, are there any conditions which, if observed, will enable the companies to secure these risks which are now rejected ? I believe there are, and I submit them to your consideration." †

1. The applicant must in all other respects present the signs of good health. 2. The albuminuria should be unaccompanied

---

* *Edes.*—On the absolute and relative value of albumen and casts, and of renal inadequacy in the diagnosis and prognosis of diseases of the kidney.—Transactions of the Association of American Physicians. Vol. iii.

† Tyson.—The Relation of Albuminuria to Life Insurance.—Ibid, p. 175.

by tube casts. However perfect may appear the health of an applicant with albuminuria, the presence of casts in his urine must effectually close the gates of life insurance against him. 3. If the quantity of the albumen is large, the applicant should be rejected irrespective of the presence of casts. 4. " A consideration which goes far toward establishing the functional character of an albuminuria, although not essential to this end, is the absence of albumen on rising in the morning. Nor dare it be said that such an albuminuria precludes the existence of organic disease. It must be taken in connection with the other considerations mentioned." 5. The specific gravity of the total amount for 24 hours must alone be taken into consideration. If we regard the specific gravity of a normal 24 hours urine (say 50 oz.) as 1020, the following may be laid down: Albuminuria is least significant when the specific gravity is high, throwing out, of course, the consideration of sugar." In all forms of renal disease the solids are diminished, and in all, except true nephritis and cyanotic induration, the specific gravity is lowered. In these two it is lowered, because in them the quantity of urine is also markedly less, and, in consequence, the specific gravity is increased to 1028 and even higher. In acute nephritis the presence of blood may also contribute to such specific gravity. Strictly speaking, acute nephritis may be ignored, because no one ill of it is ever likely to apply for life insurance. In functional albuminuria the specific gravity remains normal. When the real specific gravity is above 1020, another most important fact is in evidence against the presence of organic disease, and in favor of the view that the albuminuria is functional. On the other hand, if the real specific gravity of the urine be 1012, 1010, 1008, or even less, as it sometimes is, it would be hazardous to accept such a case of albuminuria. 6. The signs of hypertrophy of the left ventricle, and of high vascular tension asso ciated with albuminuria, are conclusive symptoms of renal disease, and should exclude the candidate. 7. The age. Albuminuria is much less apt to be functional after forty than between twenty-one and thirty-five. 8. " The presence of true gout in any shape precludes admission to life insurance, be cause gout is always, sooner or later, followed by nephritis." 9. Retinal symptoms are in some cases the earliest noted sign

of Bright's disease, and, whether or not conjoined with albuminuria, must effectually exclude the candidate.

These observations, Dr. Tyson considers, should be made
to extend over a considerable portion of time, and should be
made by competent persons, a class in which he does not
include the ordinary American practitioner.

The most recent paper on the subject is that of Dr. Pavy in
the *Lancet* of the 21st August of the present year,* and it con-
stituted an introduction of the subject for discussion,
at the last meeting of the ' British Medical Association. The cases in question are divided into three
groups—(1) Cases in which traces only of albumen
are observed ; (2) cases in which a notable amount of albumen
exists, and is always present, and (3) cases in which a notable
amount of albumen is found at one period of the twenty-four
hours and none at another, or, in other words, cases which
possess a cyclic character. Only those cases must be taken into
consideration in which all the other evidences of Bright's
disease are absent, and the albuminuria must constitute the
only factor.

A careful survey of all the collateral circumstances is therefore called for, and the points to which attention must be given
are mainly identical with those enumerated in Dr. Tyson's
paper. Dr. Pavy considers too, that the specific gravity of
the urine is important apart from the presence of albumen.
An occasional large quantity with low specific gravity is not
a matter of import, the permissible inference being that a nervous or some other temporary state has given rise to it. As
an habitual occurrence, however, it may possess great significance, and will suffice to excite suspicion of grave disease.
No opinion should be given without a microscopic examination.
Blood corpuscles will prompt delay and further enquiry. The
absence of casts does not imply the non-existence of renal
disease. Casts of the seminal tubules may be met with which
closely resembles renal casts, and they may or may not be
accompanied by spermatozoa. " With traces of albumen thus
found, and with everything else bearing upon the point to be

---

* "On the Prognosis of Cases of Albuminuria with Special Reference to Life
Insurance."

pronounced satisfactory, after a full and careful investigation of the case, I should not consider the cases invalidated. The granular kidney is the form of renal disease which is especially associated with small amounts of albumen, and what calls therefore for most consideration in the investigation of the collateral aspects of the case is attention to the main coincident conditions belonging to this affection, viz., increased quantity of urine, low specific gravity, and morbid changes in the cardio-vascular system."

The second group of cases is that in which a notable amount of albumen exists and is always present; no history of nephritis; no casts of tubules; none of the general symptoms of Bright's disease. "I do not consider that medical knowledge is at present in a position to enable us to differentiate these cases from those which may become developed into well marked Bright's disease. * * * * It would be only in a case that had been under distinct obvservation for a considerable time without anything wrong becoming developed, that I would venture to look favorably upon the prospects, and even then I should consider that a decidedly more than ordinary risk existed."

The third group comprises cases with a notable amount of urine appearing and disappearing in such a manner as to give the case a cyclic character. At the period of rising in the morning there is no albumen to be discovered. In an hour or two's time albumen shows itself, increases in quantity for a while, and then, as the day advances, declines and becomes usually entirely lost before bed-time is reached. Remaining absent during the night, it returns after rising the next day, and subsequently follows the same order that had been previously observed. "I feel it warrantable to state that with a sufficiently full and careful enquiry, it may be ascertained whether the case falls or not in the cyclic functional group, and that, if it does so, a favorable opinion of the future may be given." If insurance companies should decide to admit these cases as eligible for acceptance, it is not unreasonable that an additional premium should be demanded.

In the discussion of the paper, Dr. Gairdner stated that he was still unconvinced that we could talk of "functional albuminuria." The presence of albumen in the urine is a danger signal. The amount of the danger varied enormously. He thought the occurrence of albumen in healthy persons was a rare event. In insurance such cases should be postponed.

A communication was read from Dr. George Johnson, in which he gave it as his decided opinion that all albuminuria was pathological.

DISEASES OF THE HEART AND LUNGS.

Spontaneous Rupture of the Heart.—In connection with the history of a case of rupture of the cardiac wall, not very long ago discussed at the Medico-Chirurgical Society, the observations recorded by G. Meyer (Deutsch Archiv f. Klin. Medicin, XVIII., p. 378) may be found interesting. In the first case the following were the anatomico-pathological changes: Spontaneous rupture of the heart at the very apex of the left ventricle; sclerosis of the coronary arteries with foci of obliteration by thrombosis of the descending branch of the right coronary artery; fatty degeneration of the cardiac muscle in the neighborhood of the rupture, chronic fibrous endocarditis of the aortic valves, with marked stenosis and insufficiency; hypertrophy and dilatation of the heart. In the second case there was an incomplete rupture of the left ventricle, the result of a chronic aneurysm of the heart; obliterating thrombosis of the left coronary artery; fatty degeneration of the myocardium, limited to the neighborhood of the rupture.

Meyer also report seven other cases from the archives of the Pathological Institute at Munich.

Cerebral Abscess Following Empyema.—Dr. W. B. Hadden describes in detail, in the last volume of the St. Thomas' Reports, three cases of empyema in which the formation of a cerebral abscess occurred.

Case I.—Male, aged 27. Pleurisy of left side twelve months before admission, when empyema was diagnosed and resection of a rib practised. A few days after the operation vomiting was noted, and this symptom was more or less present, though not urgent, for months and was thought to be due to the troublesome cough from which the patient suffered. The progress of the case was unfavorable, the temperature remained high, and at the end of six months several epileptic fits occurred, followed by continued drowsiness and marked weakness of the left arm and leg and left side of the face. Left hemiplegia, more marked in the arm than in the leg, finally set in. No optic neuritis. Sensation in the left arm, and left side of the face was thought to be impaired. P. M.—An abscess, which measured two inches from before backwards by one inch from above downwards, was found to occupy the white matter, corresponding to the posterior two-thirds of the superior frontal convolution, and the adjoining part of the middle frontal convolution on the right side. The ascending frontal was not involved. There was also an abscess in the white matter corresponding to the fore part of the right occipital lobe.

Case II.—Male, aged 28. The patient was reported to have had tropical abscess of the liver, but the autopsy showed that this had probably been a pleurisy, because the liver presented no signs of suppuration at the autopsy. Resection of rib January 21st, 1884. Left the hospital in May, a small fistula being left at the site of the wound. Pus re-collected in 1886. Another operation was performed with a view to facilitate drainage. After this, vomiting was noted. Ten days after the operation the patient suddenly became very pale, but did not lose consciousness. He complained greatly of pains in his chest and became delirious. Fifteen days after the operation the left arm became weak; drowsiness; the eyes were continually turned to the left; paralysis on the left side of the mouth; left arm and leg completely paralysed; pain in the right side of the head in the situation of the right frontal eminence. Later on, there was total anæsthesia of the left forearm and hand, and partial anæsthesia over the left side of the face and neck and left upper arm. P. M.—Occupying the centrum ovale minus and majus of the right hemisphere, just behind the fissure of Rolando, was a globular abscess, 2½ inches in diameter, whose walls reached the deeper layers of the cortex.

Case III.—Male, aged 4. Scarlet fever four months before admission, which was followed by nephritis; empyema of the left side. Nine days after resection of the rib vomiting set in. There was evidently pain in the head, but no screaming, no paralysis, no unconsciousness.　P. M.—A globular abscess in the left frontal lobe.*

Pneumonic Paralysis.—Stephen (*Rev. de Med.*, January, 1889.) reports two cases of paralysis occurring in the course of pneumonia, and gives a review of the literature of the subject. He concludes by saying that paralysis may develop at the beginning of pneumonia, in its course, or during convalescence. The cause of these paralyses is in some cases a meningitis (cerebral, spinal, or cerebro-spinal), but in many others there is an entire absence of gross organic lesion. In cases of the first category it is admitted that there is an extrapulmonary localization of pneumococci in the meninges; and in those of the second category it seems most probable to the author that the pneumonic affection was determined either directly or indirectly by the medium of the cerebro-spinal disturbances of a dyscrasic, dynamic or functional nature in the nervous centres or in the nerves.

DISEASES OF THE STOMACH.

The Sensation of Hunger in Gastric Ulcer.—In a paper† on the treatment of gastric ulcer Dr. Wm. Ord observes that in cases where hunger is urgently present, and where the taking of food seems to relieve pain, there are usually adhesions of the walls of the stomach of such a nature as to prevent the narrowing of that cavity. A lay sister in a home presented for several years recurrently the ordinary signs of gastric ulcer. At length the pain became persistent, and had constant tenderness associated with it. Vomiting was frequent and there was often blood with it. Inordinate appetite. For several years she took nothing but mashed potatoes freely enriched with butter. After freely partaking, vomiting set in in about an hour and a half, followed by pain. Such symptoms he thought due to the prevention by adhesions of the collapse of the walls of the stomach. Sensations of extreme hunger arise when the walls of an empty

---

*See Montreal Medical Journal, Vol. xvii., p. 601. An abstract is given of a paper by Cérenville, "Des Manifestations Encéphaliques de la Pleurésie Purulente."

† American Journal of the Medical Sciences, June, 1889.

stomach are prevented from coming into contact. An elderly gentleman was under the care of Dr. Ord for several years. His appetite was enormous. He ate voraciously of whatever was set before him, with a special selection of the richest possible dishes, after partaking of which he vomited freely. The autopsy showed that an old abscess connected with the gall bladder had caused adhesions between the stomach and surrounding parts, so that it became no longer a movable viscus, but a large permanent cavity, as firmly bound to the adjacent organs as if a stomach had never existed.

Exaggerated Epigastric Reflex in Gastric Ulcer—In the Edinburgh periodical *Clinical Studies*, conducted by Dr. Byrom Bramwell, and in the first number, attention was directed to the presence of marked exaggeration of the epigastric reflex in a case of ulcer of the stomach. Dr. W. J. Clarke, of Birmingham, has also observed the same sign in a case of ulcer of the stomach in a woman aged 23, with severe attacks of profuse hæmatemesis. Was this association of the two conditions accidental ?

On the Diagnosis of Motor Insufficiency of the Stomach.—Brunner, at the Medical Clinic of Professor Riegel, in Giessen, undertook the task of putting to the test recent methods for estimating the motor power of the stomach. The salol method of Ewald and Seivers was tried in healthy as well as in diseased people, and as a result he found that there was great variation in healthy stomachs as in diseased ones. Even when there is great motor debility small quantities of salol sufficient for the establishment of the re-action readily find their way into the intestine. According to Brunner, therefore, the salol method for accuracy and practicability is not to be recommended.

The oil method of Klemperer was then put on trial. Brunner's results both in healthy and diseased stomachs failed to tally with those of Klemperer, and consequently he concludes that the method is not suitable for practical purposes, moreover, it is an uncertain test, since out of the number of oils present, one can scarcely come to any decision on the presence and still less on the degree of motor insufficiency present.

Finally, the author considers that the plan followed in Reigel's Clinic is the best, viz., that of determining the degree of motor disturbance in the stomach by the quantity and properties of the gastric contents after a test meal.

On the other hand, Ewald* asserts that he never founds the diagnosis of disturbed motor function of the stomach on the Salol method, but that he finds it useful when considered in conjunction with the other symptoms present. The degree of alkalinity necessary for the decomposition of salol is a factor quite beyond reach, and depends upon the secretion of the pancreas and the bile ducts. In fifty-eight trials of the salol method, the normal period for the appearance of the reaction was but twice exceeded. The reaction depends upon the quantity of salol used, the form in which it is administered. and the periods at which the estimates are made, facts which Brunner seems to have overlooked. Ewald sees no reason to depreciate the diagnostic value of the salol method, from which very useful information as to the motor functions of the stomach may in certain cases be derived.

---

* Deutsche Med. Wochenschrift, 1889. No. 7 and No. 11.

Hospital Reports.

MONTREAL GENERAL HOSPITAL.

GYNÆCOLOGICAL CASES UNDER CARE OF DR. ALLOWAY.

(Continued from page 300 –Reported by Dr. Low).

Laceration of Cervix—Trachelorrhaphy.

CASE XIV.—Aged 23 ; admitted July 30th, 1889 ; married five years ; two pregnancies ; menstruation regular ; leucorrhœal discharge profuse ; pain over epigastrium and sacrum ; dysmenorrhœa severe. These symptoms have lasted during the past two years, making serious inroads upon the patient's general health.

Examination.—Bilateral laceration of cervix ; ectropion and extensive glandular hypertrophy.

Treatment—After due rest in bed Dr. Alloway performed Schrœder's trachelorrhaphy on the 10th August. Patient discharged from hospital 28th August. Union good and patient much improved.

Laceration of Cervix—Hæmorrhagic Endometritis.

CASE XV.—Aged 45 ; admitted August 20th, 1889 ; married 24 years ; nine children ; two miscarriages. After the last miscarriage she was metrorrhagic for seven weeks, and dates her present illness from that event. She has been losing blood continuously for the last seven months, and the discharge is at present very offensive. She complains of pain in pelvis and lumbar regions. These pains have existed for the past two years, and have increased in severity.

Examination.—Bilateral laceration of cervix with marked hyperplassia and eversion, chronic endometritis, etc. After undergoing the usual preparatory treatment for three weeks, Dr. Alloway sharp-curretted the uterine cervix and performed Schrœder's operation. Patient had an uninterupted recovery, and left hospital on the 29th in good health.

XVI.—Age 24 ; admitted July 25th, 1889 ; married one year ago ; had one child at full term, (3 months ago), still born. Directly following labor she complained of some sharp pain in

left iliac region and back, which soon increased in severity up
to the present time. Profuse leucorrhœal discharge and painful menstruation. There is great prostration, and patient
incapacitated for work.

Examination.—Perineum lacerated to sphincter ani muscle.
Bilateral laceration of cervix with hyperplasia, retroversion of
uterus, chronic pelvic peritonitis and extreme tenderness of pelvic floor.

Treatment.—This patient was confined to bed for several
weeks on hot douches and iodine and glycerine treatment.
The uterus eventually became righted to its natural position
after absorption of the products of posterior parametritis, the
cause of the retroversion.

August 15th—Dr. Alloway performed Emmet's trachelorrhaphy and Tait's perineorrhaphy.

August 30th.—Patient left hospital in excellent condition of
health.

CASE XVII.—Aged 21 ; admitted July 21st, 1889 ; married
two years, never been pregnant ; menstruation regular, accompanied with little pain, but preceded by severe headache and
nausea. Duration of flow six days. Her sterile condition was
her chief complaint.

Examination.—Some vaginitis ; cervix elongated, conoid and
extensively eroded ; catarrhal endometritis ; uterus anteflexed,
mobile and not painful. No parametritis at present, but some
cicatricial shortening of utero-sacral ligaments from past existing posterior parametritis.

Treatment.—Confined to bed under iodine and glycerine
treatment for some weeks. Dr. Alloway dilated, sharp-curetted
the uterine cavity, and removed the elongated cervix after
Schrœder's method.

August 20th.—Patient left hospital free from uterine discharges and feeling well.

Alexander's Operation.

CASE XVIII.—Age 22 ; admitted August 5th, 1889 ; unmarried ; menstruation regular, but painful. She states that

some two yeas ago, after undergoing severe bodily exertion and strain, she was suddenly seized with agonizing pain in both iliac and lumbar regions ; that she became so ill she had to remain in bed for some days. She recovered somewhat, but has never been free from pain in these regions, more or less, since the accident. Her general health has been so much impaired that she has been quite unable to do even light house-work.

Examination.—In this case a very novel form of hymen was found. It consisted of a strong, thick membrane, perforated at three or four different places, (cribriform). This was completely dissected out with the scissors. The uterus could now be palpated and the vagina explored. The uterus was found in sharp retroflexion, but could be replaced. It would, however, quickly fall back again into retroflexion. The posterior wall of the vagina seemed much shortened and tense, as also did the broad and utero-sacral ligamemts. Ovaries normal and no parametritis present.

August 7.—Dr. Alloway performed Alexander's operation of shortening the round ligamonts.

September 1st.—Left hospital to-day entirely relieved of symptoms.

[This patient, (a housemaid of a city clergyman,) I had occasion to see on the 29th of October. I found the uterus in its normal position. She was in robust health, and declared she was absolutely free from any feeling approaching to that of pain in the pelvis. She had gained largely in weight, and was doing heavy general house work. This form of uterine displacement in young unmarried ladies is not uncommon, and is especially amenable to this operation. Good results invariably follow.—T. J. A.]

Trachelorrhaphy and Perineorrhaphy by Alexander's Operation.

CASE XIX.—Aged 38 ; admitted August 14th, 1889 ; married sixteen years ; five full-term pregnancies ; menstruation regular, though somewhat profuse. She complains of constant pelvic pain, accompanied with bearing-down sensation. Frequent and painful micturition. Patient states that shortly after her second confinement she noticed a mass protruding from the vulva which she had to replace with her hand in order to allow her to empty the bladder. This condition of prolapse continued during the following twelve or fourteen years to the present time. She has had four operations performed upon the perineum, with the object of obtaining relief, but all have been unsuccessful.

Examination.—Uterine and vaginal walls found in complete prolapse—*i.e.*, uterus completely outside vulva in retroflexion. Cervix has been lacerated bilaterally, and the perineum is completely so, and atrophied from pressure.

Treatment.—The patient was confined to bed, with hips elevated and vagina well packed with astringent tampons every day until the 23rd September, when Dr. Alloway performed Emmet's trachelorrhaphy on the cervix, a high colpoperineorrhaphy (Tait's) to restore the perineum, and Alexander's operation of shortening the round ligaments, at one sitting. Patient made an uninterrupted recovery, and was discharged on the 30th September. The uterus was found in good position and high up in the pelvis. The patient expressed herself as free from discomfort beyond some tenderness in inguinal wounds.

Reviews and Notices of Books.

A Cyclopædia of the Diseases of Children—Medical and Surgical, by American, British and Canadian authors. Edited by JOHN M. KEATING, M.D. Vol. I. Imp. Oct., p.p. 992. Illustrated with plates and charts. Philadelphia: J. B. Lippincott & Co.

In the preface the editor states that the work consists of a collection of monographs, not mere dictionary articles arranged in the form of a systematic treatise, and devoted to the consideration of the anatomy, physiology, medicine, surgery and hygiene of infancy, childhood and adolescence. As each contributor has been selected with special reference to his familiarity with the subject he writes upon, it is hoped that these articles will not only be of immediate practical utility, but will also serve as standards for future reference. This is the first work of the kind that has been published in the English language, and as Dr. Jacobi says, it marks an immense progress in the history of both general, medical and pediatric literature. On glancing over the list of authors, we notice an unusually large number of names widely and favorably known. The volume opens with an introductory article by Dr. Jacobi. "Pediatrics," he says, "is no speciality in the common acceptation of the term. It does not deal with an organ, but with the entire organism at the very period which presents the most interesting features to the student of biology and medicine. Infancy and childhood are the links between conception and death between the foetus and the adult. The latter has attained a certain degree of invariability. His physiological labor is reproduction; that of the young is both reproduction and growth. . . Pediatrics does not deal with miniature men and women with reduced doses, and the same class of diseases in smaller bodies, but has its own independent range and horizon, and gives as much to general medicine as it has received from it. . . There is hardly a chapter more interesting than that of the history of the relation of the bones of the cranium to its contents. The solid skull serves as a support to the brain and its blood vessels, but it may form an obstacle to their developement: an insufficient degree of ossification will enhance the possibility of enlargement of the blood vessels and the liability to effusion ; premature ossification, however, either partial or general, is a cause of asymmetry, epilepsy or idiotism, and influences the cause of inter-current diseases." In his article he calls attention to many of the peculiarities of infancy and childhood, and briefly touches on the therapeutics of these periods.   Finally, as a proof of the need of such a work on pediatrics, he refers to the fact that so little time is allotted to special instruction in this branch of medicine in many of the medical schools, both of this country and Great Britain, where few schools have more than a clinical chair on the diseases of children ; which, he adds, only means the authority given an enthusiastic worker to teach as much or as little as he can without recognition, thanks or reward, of a doctrine not officially recognized by examination.   The continent of Europe has made more progress.   Most of the large and small universities have their distinct chair on diseases of children, and their students know beforehand that they will have to prove, before being permitted to practice, their acquaintance with what they are *compelled* to learn of this subject.

Part I, General Subjects.   Beginning with an interesting article of forty pages *On the Anatomy of Children*, by Geo. McLellan of the Philadelphia School of Anatomy, wherein the author studies the body regionally, describing the anatomy of each, and discusses the features characteristic of children. His paper is freely illustrated both by engravings and photographs.   Angel Money of London writes on the Physiology of Infancy.   James Finlayson of Glasgow contributes fifty-nine pages on the Diagnosis of Disease in Infancy.   It is a most interesting article, and should be thoroughly read by every young practitioner.   William C. Dabney discusses very thoroughly in an article all that is known on the strange subject of *Maternal Impressions*.   He has collected from various sources ninety cases which seem to him worthy of credence ; these he classifies in a series of tables according to part of body involved.   Some of

these appear clearly as errors of development, but many are of
such as nature a can only be explained by admitting the power
of strong emotional impressions in a pregnant woman.   Barton
C. Hirst follows with an article on *Diseases of the Fœtus*.
The care of the Child at and immediately after Birth, by A. R.
F. Penrose; *The Closure of the Ductus Arteriosum and of the
umbilical Hypogastric Arteries* by J. Collins Warren; and
Injuries of the New Born, by Theophilus Parvin, are excellent
papers, freely discussing their several subjects.   They are
followed by one of the most interesting papers in the volume,
that of J. M. Rotch on *Infant Feeding*—who has managed to
give us much that is new and interesting.   Samuel S. Adams
writes on *Diet After Weaning*, and Miss Catherine Wood of
Great Ormond Sick Children's Hospital, contributes an article of
twelve pages *On the Nursing of Sick Children*, from which
much useful information may be gained, and which may be
specially commended to the physician who thinks he knows
always more than the nurse.   Articles on Nursery, Hygiene,
Dentition, Puberty, its Pathology and Hygiene, and the Influence
of Race and Nationality on Disease, complete Part I.

Part II is devoted to Fevers and Miasmatic Diseases, and contains articles by Wm. Pasteur, and Collie and Cheadle of London,
Lewis Smith, S. C. Busey, Forchheimer, and many others.   The
volume closes with an article on the General Therapeutics of
Children's Diseases, by Roberts Bartholow of Philadelphia.

The work as a whole is cordially recommended to our readers.
All the articles are good—not a few are masterly expositions of
their subjects—while their publishers have certainly lightened
the task of the reader by the more than usual excellence of the
type and binding.

A System of Obstetrics by American Authors. Vols.

I. and II.   Edited by BARTON COOKE HURST, M.D., Associate Professor of Obstetrics in the University of Pennsylvania, &c.   Illustrated with one colored plate and 309
wood engravings.   Philadelphia: Lea Bros. & Co   1888.

The first volume of this erudite work contains a special
treatise on the following subjects :   The History of Obstetrics,

by George J. Engelmann, M.D. The Histology and Physiology of Ovulation, Menstruation, and Fertilization. The Development of the Embrio, by H. Newell Martin, F.R.S., &c. The Fœtus, its Development, Anomalies, Monstrosities, Disease and Premature Expulsion, by Barton Cooke Hurst, M.D. Pregnancy: Its Physiology, Pathology, Signs and Differential Diagnosis, by W. W. Jaggard, A.M., M.D. The Conduct of Labor, and the Management of the Puerperal State, by Samuel C. Busey, M.D. On the Mechanism of Labor, and the Treatment of Labor based on the Mechanism, by R. A. F. Penrose, M.D., LL.D.

The second volume contains: Diseases and Accidents of Labor, by Theophilus Parvin, M.D., LL.D. The Forceps: Embriotomy, by Edward P. Davis, A.M., M.D. The Premature Induction of Labor, by James C. Cameron, M.D. Version, by James C. Cameron. The Cæsarean Operation, Symphysiotomy, Laparo-Elytrotomy, and Laparo-Cystectomy, by Robert P. Harris, A.M., M.D. Puerperal Infection, by Henry J. Garrigues, A.M., M.D. Inflammation of the Breast and Allied Diseases connected with Childbirth, by Henry J. Garrigues, A.M., M.D. The Etiology of Puerperal Fever, by Harold C. Ernst, M.D. Some Complications of the Puerperal State, Independent of Septic Infection, by Barton C. Hurst, M.D. Insanity and Diseases of the nervous system in the child-bearing woman, by James Hendrie Lloyd, A.M., M.D. The Management and the Diseases of the new-born infant, by J. Lewis Smith, M.D. The Surgical Diseases of Infancy and Early Childhood, by Stephen Smith, A.M., M.D. Congenital Anomalies of the Eye, by G. E. De Schweinitz, M.D.

The magnitude and importance of this truly great work can be surmised from a glance at the above list of subjects and eminent authors. It is a lasting exponent of the perseverance, toil and brilliant scientific attainments of those in whose charge the various subjects were intrusted. To make any special criticism would be difficult, and if made would invariably be of a favorable nature. It is so pleasing to feel that the old Churchill-Ramsbottom style of teaching has passed away like the dust of its authors, and that we have in " The System of Obstetrics " a method which no man can study without enthusiasm. The numerous illustrations are scale-drawn, and anatomically correct; they are a special feature of the work from their freshness and individuality.

We cannot conclude these remarks without paying a high tribute of admiration to the indefatigable editor. The very complete nature and scientific accuracy of the treatise shows how arduous the task must have been, and much credit must be given to Dr. Hurst in its successful accomplishment. We think no practitioner can afford to be without the work.—T. J. A.

An Introduction to Pathology and Morbid Anatomy. By T. HENRY GREEN, M.D., and STANLEY BOYD, M.B , F.R.C.S. Sixth American from Seventh English Edition. Philadelphia : Lea Bros. & Co. 1889.

In this new edition of "Green" great pains have been taken by the editor, Mr. Boyd, to bring the work up to date. To this end, a large amount of new matter has been added, and thus the individuality of the book has been to a great extent lost. If one were disposed to be critical, it might be said that these new portions greatly need boiling down, but even with its defects, the book is still probably the most useful one we possess for beginners in pathology. The publishers have done their work. quite as well as ever, though the plates in the English editions are clearer. A number of very ambiguous micro-photographs, which have been introduced, might very well have been spared.

Strathpeffer Spa : its Climate and Waters with Observations, Historical and General, Descriptive of the Community. By FORTESQUE FOX, M.D., (Lond.) London : H. K. Lewis, 136 Gower street. 1889.

This little book is all that its title announces, and nothing seems to have been left undone to make the virtues of the Spa and its surroundings known. It is, moreover, illustrated by a beautiful map. photographs, &c. The entire work has an air of thoroughness about it, and seems to have been inspired by a desire to make the qualities of a valuable spring within easy access known as they deserve. The book is creditable to both author and publisher.

Inebriety: its Etiology, Pathology, Treatment and Jurisprudence. By Norman Kerr, M.D., F.L.S. Second edition. London: H. K. Lewis, 186 Gower street. 1889.

Between the covers of this book of 450 pages is contained about all that there is to be said at present on the subject of inebriety. The key to the work is furnished by the author in the preface to the first edition, where he says: " The present volume has been written in the hope that it may aid, however feebly, through the medium of the attending practitioner, who, I trust, will be among my readers, in the enlightenment of the patient, his sorely-tried relatives, and the community, in the great truth that inebriety is a disease as curable as most other diseases, calling for medical, mental and moral treatment." We think no one can read this valuable work without agreeing with the author's main conclusion, and if the profession and the public once become convinced of the truth of this and what is implied therein, an enormous advance will have been made in knowledge, and the foundation thus laid for intelligent efforts in the improvement of the condition of a large class of unfortunates. And what is of equal importance. A host of evils, now apparently inevitable, may in time be prevented by that wisest recognition of the bearings of heredity and causation, which is alone the path by which a radical cure—if such is possible—will be found for the disease. The paragraphs of this work are so summarized in the marginal headings that a general idea of the scope and even the teaching of the book may be readily gained in a comparatively short period of time· This is a method not only desirable in text-books, but worthy of imitation in many others, and has as yet been too little employed. Apart from the establishment of the author's ideas, the book is valuable for the amount of information it conveys. It has nothing to do directly with advocating total abstinence; at the same time, if the temperance reformers could but see it, efforts in accordance with the principles set forth by the author, would probably be more effective than those in the direction at present, cunningly followed so exclusively. This work tends to advance real civilization.

Society Proceedings.
MEDICO-CHIRURGICAL SOCIETY OF MONTREAL.
Annual Meeting, October 4th, 1889.
WM. GARDNER, M.D., PRESIDENT, IN THE CHAIR.

The annual meeting of the Society was held this evening. There were present: Drs. Roddick, Shepherd, Blackadder, Johnston, J. A. MacDonald and others, 31 in all.

After the minutes of the preceding meeting and that of the last annual meeting had been read and confirmed, the President introduced Dr. E. A. McGannon, of Brockville, and invited him to take part in the discussions. The following were proposed for membership: Dr. J. M. Jack, proposed by Dr. Ruttan, seconded by Dr. G. T. Ross; Dr. E. A. McGannon, proposed by Dr. J. A. MacDonald, seconded by Dr, G. T. Ross.

Dr. JOHNSTON exhibited specimens from a case of gout where almost every joint throughout the body showed infiltration with urate of sodium. There was marked deformity of the fingers. The sheaths of the tendons were everywhere filled with similar deposit. The patient during life vomited chalk stones and passed them in great numbers; but at time of autopsy the alimentary canal was free from concretions. The cause of death was pleurisy with effusion.

D. DeCow exhibited a specimen of medullary cancer of the stomach, with secondary nodules in the liver. The disease had run a very rapid course. The onset dated from a period when the patient, a man aged 52, was much depressed, owing to the death of a near relative.

Dr. G. A. BROWN exhibited a specimen from a case of pyo-salpingitis. In brief, the history of the case was, that four weeks previous to admission to the General Hospital patient was seized with severe attacks of vomiting, no food being retained in the stomach. She also suffered from severe abdominal pain. This illness had been preceded by a drinking spree of about six weeks duration, and at the time of admission patient had symptoms of delirium tremens. Upon examination the abdomen was found to be much distended and so tender to the touch that an examination was rendered almost impossible. Examination of the other regions of the body was negative. Temperature, 101. The patient's general condition continued to grow worse, in spite of all treatment—the vomiting and abdominal pain not being alleviated—until, six days after admission, the patient died. Post mortem examination revealed a purulent peritonitis —one pint and a quarter of purulent fluid being found in the cavity, and a great deal of lymph on the parietal and visceral layers of the peritoneum, the intestines being matted together. The entrance of the fallopian tube into the uterus on the right side was found to be closed, but just beyond this the tube was found to be dilated, and which, on being opened, was found filled with pus. This sac was fount to have a communication with a portion of the small intestine. Examination of the remaining organs of the body was negative.

The treasurer reported : Receipts, $484.23 ; expenditure, $486.58, thus leaving a slight deficit in the funds of the Society.

The notice of motion regarding an amendment to the constitution, given by Drs. Trenholme and Shepherd, was then considered. The notice was that all members of the resident staff of the Montreal hospitals be ex-officio members of this Society. Carried.

The treasurer's accounts were then duly audited and found correct.

Upon motion of Dr. Roddick, seconded by Dr. Blackadder, the report was adopted.

Drs. G. T. Ross and E. Blackadder were appointed scrutineers, and the Society proceeded to elect officers for the ensuing year. The elections resulted as follows :—President, Dr. Geo. Armstrong ; 1st Vice-President, Dr. Shepherd ; 2nd Vice-President, Dr. W. Mills ; Secretary, Dr. H. S. Birkett ; Treasurer, Dr. J. A. Macdonald ; Librarian, Dr. T. D. Read ; council, Drs. W· Gardner, Ruttan and Roddick.

Moved by Dr. Proudfoot, seconded by Dr. Roddick, that a vote of thanks be tendered by the Society to Dr. Ruttan, the retiring secretary. Carried.

A general vote of thanks to the retiring officers was then moved by Dr. Roddick and seconded by Dr. J. Gardner. Carried,

The Society then adjourned, the President's address being postponed until the next meeting.

ASSOCIATION OF AMERICAN PHYSICIANS.

ANNUAL MEETING.—(*Continued from page* 315.)

Dr. JAMES J. PUTNAM, of Boston, remarked that the reported cases of tetany showed such a variety of infectious sources,
that it seemed hardly probable that they should act in such a
similar manner unless there were something else behind. Two
or three things are to be considered. First, the influence of
habit. The disease set up by a variety of causes may continue
as a result of habit. Second, the suggestion that in such cases
of disordered action we have to deal with an over-sensitive-
ness of physiological arrangement is important. In these conditions we have the disordered manifestation of what is really
a function, but one which we ordinarily recognize, as it has no
independent existence. It would seem that, in the absence of
further knowledge with regard to infection and the manner in
which this infection arising from various sources may act, we
should insist upon the possibilities of explanation which are
presented to us by what we know of the physiology and disordered physiology of the nervous system, in attempting to
explain conditions met with in this and similar diseases.

DR. JAMES STEWART, Montreal, said, in connection with the
influence of peripheral irritation, that in the cases of dilatation
of the stomach where tetany had caused death, the symptoms
came on a few hours after the stomach had been washed out.
This would point to irritation rather than decomposition as the
active cause in this class of cases. There are many other cases
where infection could not enter.

DR. JOHN T. CARPENTER, Pottsville, said, in regard to
anæmia as the cause of tetany, that we should have to go back
of the anæmia to the cause that produced it. He knew of no
cause that would produce anæmia so surely as septic absorption.

Afternoon Session.

Dr. A. B. BALL, New York, read a paper on *Thrombosis of
Cerebral Sinuses and Veins*. The author first referred to the
influence of the following factors in the production of thrombosis:—(1) blood stasis; (2) vessel lesion; (3) blood changes.
The anatomical conditions in the sinuses that favor thrombosis
were described at length. A number of cases of marantic

thrombosis of cerebral veins and sinuses in chlorotic girls were given. The symptoms were next considered. Much importance has been attached to distension of external veins collateral to the internal veins supposed to be affected, giving rise to hæmorrhages and œdema. These signs are frequently absent, and may be due to other conditions. The mobility of the symptoms have been considered of value. In these cases the cerebral symptoms undergo strange alterations not seen usually in other affections. Active delirium is exceptional. The depression continues, but alternates with a certain amount of improvement. Fever is absent at first, and, if present, is to be attributed to complicating conditions. Paralytic symptoms of varying extent are usually present. With the exception of the variation in degrees, the paralysis does not differ from paralysis from other causes.

Discussion.

Dr. WILLIAM OSLER, Baltimore, exhibited two specimens illustrating the conditions prescribed by Dr. Ball. The first specimen was one of extensive thrombosis of the lateral sinus occurring in a man who died from phlegmonous erysipelas of the cheek. There were no special symptoms in that case. The second specimen was from a woman dying of consumption. It was thought that gradually increasing coma and the onset of cerebral symptoms were supposed to be due to the basilar meningitis.

Dr. A. JACOBI, New York, enumerated certain additional aiding causes. The first was a disproportion between the white and red blood corpuscles. The second cause was the relative absence of muscular tissue in a number of the veins. A third cause was absence of water in the blood, often due to the withholding of sufficient fluid in the diet of patients. The last cause referred to was weakness of the heart. When in exhaustive diseases, the heart is allowed to become feeble, thrombosis with all its bad results must be expected. It is certainly a good therapeutic measure to stimulate and strengthen the heart in every disease that will last long or tends to terminate in exhaustion.

Dr. WILLIAM H. WELCH, Baltimore, said : There is one point of great force in explaining the production of thrombosis, that is the possibility that there is some form of intoxication analogous to that produced experimentally by various substances, such as the fibrin ferment. Under such circumstances there is almost instantaneously thrombosis wherever the ferment reaches. Pathologists are aware of the frequency with which thrombi, usually of a mixed character, are found in the cerebral sinuses, particularly the superior longitudinal, in cases that have presented no symptom during life.

Dr. SAMUEL C. BUSEY, of Washington, D.C., read a paper on *The Effusion of Chyle and of Chyle-like, Milky, Fatty Fluids into Serous Cavities.* The object of the paper was to present the subject of effusion of chyle, chyle-like and fatty fluids into serous cavities. It was limited to the effusion of such fluids into the cavities of the pleuræ, peritoneum and tunica vaginalis. The subject of traumatic injuries of the absorbent vessels seems to have been peculiarly attractive to many of the older writers; Ruysch, as early as 1665, drew attention to wounds of the lymphatic vessels. The reported cases of effusion of chyle and milk-like fluids into the pleural and peritoneal cavities, including the doubtful cases, do not exceed forty-three; and these cases cover a period of one hundred and ninety years. Nevertheless, twenty-three of the cases of effusion of chyle and chyle-like fluid into the abdominal cavity have been observed during the present century, fifteen since 1850, and thirteen during the last and present decades. The increasing frequency of the occurrence is thus clearly shown.

Effusion into the Pleural Cavities: Chyle-Thorax.—Of this, including the doubtful cases, there have been ten cases reported. In five of these the chyle poured directly from the thoracic duct. The diagnosis in these cases can only be made by evacuation and examination of the fluid. The prominent symptoms are dyspnœa and accumulation of fluid in one or both cavities. The prognosis is improvable, and the treatment expectant.

Effusion into the Tunica Vaginalis Testis.—The case of galactocele reported by Vidal (de Cassis) seems to have been the first observation of this class of effusions. In two of the reported cases the patulous orifices of the vessels from which the lymph exuded were found. Since 1885 there have been reported in this country thirteen cases in which filaria were found; and two of these were cases of lymphocele. It has not been shown, however, that filaria are present in every case of lymphocele. It is conceivable that adenitis, gonorrhœal lymphangitis or other conditions which obliterate the permeability of neighboring and connecting glands, might cause stasis of lymph and dilatation and rupture of lymph capillaries and plexuses with which the serous membranes are so richly supplied. The opinion of those who have had the best opportunity to study the relation of filaria to disease in general, seems to be that of Sir Joseph Fayre's, that " it has been shown that disorders of the lymphatic system are most frequently associated with, if not caused by, the filaria." The recent invasion of portions of the sub-tropical belt of this country by the filaria, and the reports of cases of disease with which the parasite has been so uniformly associated, together with the fact that the mosquito has been proven to be its intermediate host, present considerations of the highest importance to the profession and general public. Some of the cases have been cured by injection of iodine, others have been cured by dissecting back the vessels, and tying the bundle *en masse* with a silk ligature.

Chylous and Oily Ascites.—A tabulated statement, arranged chronologically, presenting a condensed summary of the reports of cases of chylous and oily ascites was given. The number of cases reported were thirty-three. Primary rupture occurred in but five cases. Chylous ascites may be the secondary result of a variety of morbid conditions which directly or remotely obstruct the flow of the chyle through the lacteals, receptaculum or thoracic duct, impede its exit into the left subclavian vein, or retard the current of blood in the left subclavian vein, right side of the heart or lessen circulation. The relation of puerperal conditions to the effusion of chyle are not susceptible of explanation. In five cases the fluid found in the peritoneal cavity was associated with tuberculosis, and in four it is stated that the peritoneum was more or less studded with tubercles. No perforation or rupture of chyle-conveying vessels was found in any of these cases.

The symptomatology of effusion of chyle into the peritoneal

cavity is not sufficiently distinctive to differentiate such cases from ordinary ascites, and a diagnosis is only possible after examination of the evacuated fluid. Of the thirty-three cases nineteen died, nine recovered, and in five the result is not stated. Of the twenty-two cases of chylous ascites proper, twelve died, five recovered, and in five the result is not stated. Meagre and unsatisfactory as are the clinical details of these cases, they point to two conclusions: (1) that a free and obstructed channel of communication between the venous system and the chyle-conveying vessels is esssential to the proper nutrition of the body and preservation of life; and (2) that death following the partial or complete obliteration of this communication is the result of inanition.

In seventeen of the thirty-three tabulated cases tapping was practised, and in most of the cases repeated several times. Six of these recovered. In two, laparotomy was resorted to with recovery of both patients. One was a case of intact retention cyst, and the other was probably a ruptured cyst. As a medical resource, paracentesis is of questionable value. The treatment is mainly directed to the prolongation of life. The causative condition may in some cases be amenable to medicinal treatment, but in most cases some surgical procedure might offer a prospect of cure. In filarial cases, the treatment applicable to such would be admissible. Sonsiua thinks that astringents such as gallic acid and tincture of the chloride of iron with rest, tonics and proper alimentation are useful. Lancereux thinks that the parasitic forms of lymphatic disease are curable. He has found mercurial inunction in the region of the affected gland in connection with hydropathy, of service. He suggests the injection of parasiticides into the affected glands for the purpose of destroying the female adult worm.

Discussion.

Dr. Wm. Osler, of Baltimore, said that in ordinary postmortem work it was not unfrequent to meet with varices of the chyle vessels of the mesentery covering the walls of the intestine. Sometimes there are extravasations which may form large chylous cysts. With reference to chyluria he was positive that there was a non-parasitic form. He had made thorough examinations in one such case and failed to find filaria. On post-mortem examination nothing was discovered. Also in a case of lymph scrotum, he had examined the fluid and the blood, and had found no embryos. He laid a great deal of stress upon these cases, as it is generally stated that these conditions are always parasitic.

Dr. WM. H. WELCH, of Baltimore, exhibited a specimen of chyle removed from the abdominal cavity of a boy twelve years of age. He described the chemical and microscopical characters of the fluid, and dwelt upon the importance of distinguishing between chylous and fatty hydrops.

Dr. J. F. ADAMS, of Pittsfield, Mass., read a paper on *Substitutes for Opium in chronic diseases.* The disadvantages attending the use of opium are: (1) in an overdose, it is poison; (2) in ordinary doses, its benefits are largely offset by various functional derangements; (3) its use involves the danger of the opium habit. Other remedies may be substituted for opium for the relief of pain. The antipyretics, antipyrine, acetanilide, phenacetine and exalgine have well-grounded claims to be regarded as rivals of opium. They are, however, less certain, and less prompt, particularly where pain is very violent. Antipyrine in five to ten grain doses, had been found vuluable as an analgesic, particularly in headache, neuralgia and rheumatism. Acetanilide he had found less active than antipyrine. Used in doses of seven or eight grains, he had found it particularly serviceable in lumbago and dysmenorrhœa. In the latter condition one or two doses had afforded prompt relief. Salicylic acid and its sodium salt for the relief of pain in rheumatism, is to be included.

Discussion.

Dr. G. M. GARLAND, of Boston, referred to the value of the fluid extract of gelseminum as a substitute for opium. In frontal headaches it has had an admirable effect. It is used also with advantage in difficult and painful menstruation, and certain forms of neuralgia. As a simple hypnotic, gelse-minum answers well in cases of temporary congestion with insomnia and headache. In hysterical conditions, this agent will often induce sleep in a short time. The drug is given in doses of five to ten drops every half-hour until the desired effect is obtained, or its physiological effect is produced in diplopia and ptosis. These appear sufficiently early to serve as a warning.

Dr. ISRAEL T. DANA, of Portland, reported two cases of opium habit occurring in a man and wife. The husband was a young man who had for some time given hypodermic injections of morphia to a patient dying of cancer. He subsequently broke his leg, and remembering the effect of the injections in the case of cancer, he tried them on himself. The result was so exhilarating that he "could not see why his wife should not have a little of the fun," and he began giving her the injections, although she was perfectly healthy. In this way the habit was induced, and when admitted to the hospital, each one was taking six grains of morphia daily.

Dr. M. G. DADIMAN, who had practised in Asia Minor and Constantinople, stated that he had never seen a case of opium habit in his practice in these places.

Dr. D. W. PRENTISS, of Washington, read a paper on *Remarkable Case of Slow Pulse.*

Second Day—Thursday, Sept. 19th.

Dr. FREDERICK P. HENRY, of Philadelphia, read a paper on the *Relation between Chlorosis, Simple Anæmia and Pernicious Anæmia.* The discussion of the relation between chlorosis, anæmia, pernicious anæmia, etc., may be divided into three heads :—(1) Are they separate diseases? (2) Are they of a kindred nature? (3) Are they different stages of one affection? Pernicious anæmia is first considered, because the determination of its status is of fundamental importance. It is admitted by all that the clinical features of this disease are common to a number of affections, especially cancer and atrophy of gastric glands; but those who argue most forcibly in favor of its independent nature exclude from the category of pernicious anæmia all cases in which an anatomical lesion of any organ is found. This appears to me unscientific, for an independent disease is one which rests upon a constant anatomical basis or is invariably produced by the same specific agent. Hunter has endeavored to establish pernicious anæmia

as an independent disease by the demonstration of an excess
of iron in the liver in cases of that affection. He regards this
as the essential anatomical feature of pernicious anæmia. The
work of Hunter is of great value, and certainly demonstrates
the existence of an excessive hæmolysis in that disease. In
my opinion, however, this excessive hæmolysis is a consequence of defective hæmogenesis, for certain facts show the
red corpuscles of pernicious anæmia to be abnormally weak and
perishable. Chlorosis is universally admitted to be due to
defective hæmogenesis, and therefore I regard it and pernicious anæmia as closely related affections. Transitions from
one affection to the other have also been observed by myself
and others.

Dr. F. Forcheimer, of Cincinnati, read a paper on *The Relation of Anæmia to Chlorosis.* The speaker first referred to the
confusion which existed in regard to the definition of the two
diseases. Immermann states that we are justified in stating
that anæmia is that condition in which there is a diminution of
red corpuscles as well as of the albumins of the plasma in the
blood (hypalbuminosis). Strumpell considered that " the essential element in anæmia is therefore a diminution i·· the number
of red corpuscles, or so-called oligocythæmia," and states further that "oligocythæmia is not invariably accompanied by a
diminution in the amount of serum-albumin (by which he
means plasma-hypalbuminosis)." Going on, it is found that
anæmia or oligæmia vera really means a diminution of the
whole quantity of the blood, and that this condition can be
divided into hydræmia, oligocythæmia, oligæmia sicca and
oligæmia hypalbuminosis. We have three representative
definitions : the one, broad and general, including a diminution of any one or all of the constituents of the blood ; a second
in which hypalbuminosis and oligocythæmia are the principal
if not the only factors ; and a third, which makes oligocythæmia alone the characteristic feature. From a purely practical
standpoint the latter seems the best. The same confusion in
regard to definition is met with in a consideration of chlorosis.
Duncan (1867) was, however, probably the first to make the
distinctive feature, oligochromæmia characteristic for chlorosis, that is, in chlorosis we find the individual red corpuscles

deficient in hæmoglobin. Unfortunately for this definition, the term chlorosis is to be looked upon as an essentially clinical one; it is not going too far to state that by far the great majority of reported cases of chlorosis are not chlorosis at all. Another difficulty is that both oligocythæmia and oligochromæmia may occur in the same individual, so that the term chloranæmia is justified by observation of existing conditions. It is more than probable that anæmia is a forerunner of chlorosis in a great many instances; and possibly a number of cases occur in which there is a combination of both conditions. Almost any cause put down for anæmia will hold good for chlorosis. Sex, age, a peculiar composition of the blood, and certain vascular anomalies are held to be especially characteristic of chlorosis. The two latter are the only ones to be found in chlorosis. The process of sexual development is looked to as the time of most common occurrence of chlorosis. This age also produces a great number of cases of anæmia; but children and old people are subject to anæmia, and practically excluded from chlorosis. The greatest number of cases occurs between the ages of fifteen and twenty-five years, decidedly after the time of first menstruation. Furthermore, an anæmic constitution is a strong predisposing cause for chlorosis. The clinical characteristic of chlorosis lies in the peculiar changes in the blood. In anæmia, the red corpuscles, as well as the albumin of the plasma, are reduced in quantity, and frequently there is production of a greater number of smaller corpuscles (microcytes). As a result of the reduction of the number of red corpuscles, the Hb. is correspondingly reduced in quantity. In pure chlorosis the number of red corpuscles is not diminished, and a tendency to the production of larger red corpuscles (megalocytes) is especially well marked. These changes are, however, not sufficiently characteristic to establish a diagnosis. It is also found that the amount of Hb. in each corpuscle is diminished. It has been said that in anæmia there is always hypalbuminosis, while in chlorosis this is absent; but this has not yet been positively proved. One respect in which chlorosis is said to differ materially, if not absolutely, from anæmia, consists in the pathological changes, first described by Virchow. These are narrowing of the lumen of the aorta and larger arteries, as well as thinning of their walls. The heart is sometimes small, somotimes hypertrophied. This view would permit us to state that chlorosis is always congenital, in some cases latent for years, while anæmia in most cases is acquired. Many objections have been urged against this view. The relation of the symptoms of anæmia to chlorosis depends upon the conditions of the blood and the anatomical sub-strata. Given a case of anæmia in which there is only a reduction of Hb. as a result of oligocythæmia, and a case of chlorosis, in which there is a reduction of Hb. as a result of oligochromæmia, and metabolism in both cases will be approximately the same; but if in anæmia we have oligocythæmia as well as hypalbuminosis, which is said to co-exist in the majority of cases, the metabolism must be different from that of a pure case of oligocythæmia. As a result of reduction of Hb. there is simply reduction in the process of oxidation; at the same time the waste products are carried off, and sufficient albuminous food is carried to the tissues by the plasma of the blood, which is unchanged. Hypalbuminosis and oligocythæmia produce an entirely different result. We have the same factor, suboxidation; but we have, in addition, deficiency of supply. In mild cases of anæmia there is produced a loss of weight; in severe cases the condition called marasmus. In chlorosis very little if any loss of weight occurs; very frequently the opposite condition is brought about by too great supply, and by the presence of too much CO_2 preventing decomposition of fats. When anæmia is associated with chlorosis, we have a very unfortunate combination, especially if there is a great amount of hypalbuminosis. Unless we believe that the anatomical lesions of Virchow belong to chlorosis, there exists no difference between the symptoms of chlorosis and anæmia. The therapeutic relations of the two diseases must be considered. While the indiscriminate use of iron in anæmia must be deprecated; yet, upon the whole, iron is just as much looked upon as a specific in anæmia as in chlorosis. Where in anæmia we try to remove the cause and institute causal treatment, we are satisfied in chlorosis with removing that symptom which is the essential of the disease. It has been repeatedly demonstrated that the removal of this essential symptom is followed temporarily by complete recovery. Whereas, in anæmia, treatment is followed by complete recovery or complete failure, iron in chlorosis will always result in amelioration, even if the tendency to relapse cannot be removed. There are few cases of chlorosis, even those with the lesions of Virchow, that are not benefited by the administration of iron in sufficient quantity. In a great many cases of anæmia, the use of iron would be followed by negative or by bad results.

Discussion.—Dr. WILLIAM OSLER, of Baltimore, took issue with Dr. Henry in regard to chlorosis. He held that chlorosis is absolutely distinct from pernicious anæmia, and for the following reasons: (1) The sex. He had never seen chlorosis in the male. (2) The pathological conditions. He regarded the hyperplasia of the heart and great vessels as a specific anatomical distinction of a certain number of cases. (3) The character of the blood. He considered the diminution of the percentage of hæmaglobin a distinctive feature of chlorosis. (4) Curability. Although in chlorosis there is a tendency to relapse, each given attack can be cured if sufficiently large doses of iron are employed.

Dr. FRANCIS P. KINNICUTT, New York, agreed as to the lack of relation between chlorosis and pernicious anæmia. He had never seen true chlorosis in the male. All his cases of pernicious anæmia on the other hand, with one or two exceptions, had occurred in males. He agreed with Dr. Henry in regard to the relationship between Hodgkins' disease and true leukæmia. He reported a case which came under his observation with typical symptoms of Hodgkins' disease. At this time the proportion of white corpuscles to red was normal. The spleen and liver gradually enlarged, and two years later, at the time of the patient's death, there was one white corpuscle to five or six red.

Dr. W. W. JOHNSTON, Washington, thought that a study of certain anæmias which are met with in women will throw light upon the association of anæmia with diseases of the intestinal glands and gastric tubules. The explanation of the chronic anæmias of parturition is probably the continual pressure upon the intestinal tube, causing a long starvation lasting nearly a year. This seems to produce an actual organic change in the intestinal glands. Several illustrative cases were cited.

Dr. WILLIAM PEPPER, Philadelphia, agreed with Dr. Osler in regard to the relation between true anæmia and chlorosis and progressive pernicious anæmia, so-called. He was not prepared to admit the analogy between true chlorosis and progressive pernicious anæmia. The conditions of the blood are widely antagonistic in these two affections. The clinical differences are also very marked. In the present state of knowledge, it is probably wiser to consider essential anæmia as an independent affection.

Dr. FREDERICK P. HENRY, Philadelphia, thought that the definition of chlorosis given by Dr. Osler could not be maintained, that is, that there is always a diminution of hæmoglobin with a nearly normal number of red corpuscles. The arguments that he had advanced were based entirely upon personal observations. While chlorosis is readily relieved by treatment in the early stages, yet, if it is neglected, the chlorosis may become more intense and may present the appearance of pernicious anæmia.

Dr. S. WEIR MITCHELL, Philadelphia, read a paper on the *Subjective False Sensation of Cold, Considered as a Symptom.* The speaker had met with many cases where a feeling of cold is complained of in members which do not present any objective changes in temperature. These may be placed in three classes : (1) Those due to a central cause ; (1) those due to neuritis ; (3) those whose origin is at present inexplicable or due to hysteria. A number of cases exhibiting this symptom to an extreme degree, were reported. In the first case, a marked sensation of cold, involving the left side of the body, followed an injury to the head. Three or four cases were referred to, coming in the second class. The sensation of cold involved the posterior part of the legs, the back or buttocks. In all these cases, there was either neuritis at the time or it developed subsequently. When this symptom is noted neuritis may be expected. Two cases belonging to the third group were described. One was an elderly individual with no sign of hysteria. The other was a case of a young woman with marked hysterical symptoms.

Discussion.—Dr. JAMES J. PUTNAM, of Boston, had frequently seen the coldness spoken of in chronic spinal disease and in neuritis, and described such a case in a man with chronic sensory neuritis.

Dr. F. T. MILLS, Baltimore, regarded this sensation of coldness as a very important symptom of neuritis, and reported a case associated with acute neuritis of the ulnar nerves.

Dr. G. M. GARLAND, of Boston, read a paper on *Gastric Neurasthenia.* The author first reviewed Leube's observations on dyspepsia nervosa, and presented a category of the gastric neuroses. A case of anorexia nervosa, occurring in a woman sixty-three years of age, was reported. The woman was of feeble constitution. She had digested her food without consciousness of the process, and her bodily functions were practically normal in every way except that she suffered from anorexia. Three cases of nervous vomiting were then reported. The conclusions drawn from the cases were that: (1) All the women have been of dark complexion. (2) They have not been of the so-called hysterical temperament. (3) Feeding by the mouth was abandoned in every case, and rectal enemata were necessary. (4) None of the drugs usually potent in soothing a nauseated stomach were of any avail. Morphia subcutaneously was the only remedy that was of benefit. (5) The vomitus caused great discomfort along the throat, and in one case caused severe glossitis. In connection with the hyperacidity, the reader referred to certain cases of acid vomiting described by Rossbach, and designated nervosa gastroxynosis. The acidity of these cases depends upon excessive secretion of hydrochloric acid, and is independent of the presence of food in the stomach.

Afternoon Session.—The discussion of Dr. Garland's paper was taken up.

Dr. S. WEIR MITCHELL, Philadelphia, said that in all cases of neurasthenia where there are great complaints of gastric and intestinal difficulty, the presence of hypochondriacal conditions must constantly be considered. It is rare for grave cases of neurasthenia to present themselves without some abdominal symptoms. In regard to anorexia nervosa he thought that in the majority of cases a background of hysteria would be found. It is suspicious that this condition is never seen in men.

Dr. WILLIAM PEPPER, Philadelphia, asked in what respects, other than the invariable and extreme acidity of the matters vomited, these cases differ from those that have been described under the head of cyclic and recurrent vomiting. He had seen many such cases, and some like the fatal case reported. In some of the cases the vomited matters were extremely acid. He had had these matters examined chemically, with the hope of finding some leucomaine, but so far with negative results. In regard to the treatment, the only remedy that had been of benefit, had been antipyrine. In one or two cases this had apparently stopped the attacks.

Dr. F. W. WHITNEY, of Boston, presented specimens from two cases of *Cretinism*.

Dr. JOHN H. MUSSER, of Philadelphia, read a paper on *Primary Cancer of the Gall-bladder and Ducts*. The speaker, after describing two cases of this affection that had come under his observation, reviewed the cases that had been reported and presented the following conclusions:—Primary cancer of the gall-bladder is not so rare as is generally believed. It occurs in the female nearly three times as often as in the male. A large number (fifty-seven per cent.) of the cases occur under the age of sixty. Gall-stones are an exciting cause, especially in persons predisposed to the affection. The organ is generally not much enlarged save as the result of secondary processes.

Dr. HENRY FORMAD, of Philadelphia, read a paper on *The Anatomical and Physiological Relations of Lesions of the Heart and Kidneys*. The paper was based upon the post-mortem study of three hundred cases observed in public and private practice.

Dr. P. G. ROBINSON, of St. Louis, read a paper on *The Contagium of Diphtheria*. The subject is one which merits our most earnest and continued study, because of the prominent place it occupies among the prevailing causes of annual mortality, and because of the diversity of opinion which is entertained in regard to its etiology, pathology and treatment. The disease has become familiar to the practitioner only within the last generation, although traced historically to a very remote period. It prevails very generally throughout this continent, and constitutes one of the chief and most constant causes of mortality, which amounts to nearly 125 per thousand of the population of the

United States, and of cases reported the percentage of deaths is from thirty to thirty-five. Diphtheria is an acute infectious disease, doubtless due to a living organism (microbe), the exact identity of which cannot yet be regarded as settled. Primarily a local affection, the system becomes secondarily and generally infected through absorption of a poison generated at the primary and localized seat of inoculation. The modes of infection are numerous, the contagium being directly transferred by contact in a dry state through the air for limited distances in foul clothing, in polluted food and drink, milk probably being a prolific source of infection. The most difficult problem to solve is that which relates to the conditions most favorable to the growth and development of the germs and the propagation of the disease. While, strictly speaking, diphtheria can hardly be called a filth-disease, since it prevails often to a very limited extent in those localities whose hygienic surroundings are apparently the worst, yet certain kinds of filthy accumulations, such as the ordure of animals, notably the refuse of cowsheds and dairies, seem to furnish the most favorable conditions for the culture of this particular germ. Until this problem can be solved and the life history and habitat of the diphtheritic germ is understood, no definite plan can be formulated for the arrest of the contagion nor for the hopeful treatment of the disease.

Third Day—Friday, Sept. 20th.

The following officers were elected :

President, Dr. S. C. Busey, Washington; 1st Vice-President, Dr. William Pepper, Philadelphia; 2nd Vice-President, Dr. Henry U. Lyman, Chicago; Recorder, Dr. I. Minis Hays, Philadelphia; Secretary, Dr. Henry Hun, Albany; Treasurer, Dr. W. W. Johnston, Washington; Member of Council, Dr. G. Baumgarten, St. Louis; Representative on Executive Committee of Congress of American Physicians and Surgeons, Dr. William Pepper, Philadelphia.

The following members were elected: Drs. William G. Thompson, William H. Thomson, J. West Roosevelt, New York; Drs. Charles Carey, Charles G. Stockton, Buffalo; Drs. Victor C. Vaughn, Heneage Gibbes, Ann Arbor; Dr. Charles W.

Purdy, Chicago; Dr. Starling Loving, Columbus, O.; Dr. W. H. Geddings, Aiken, S.C.; Dr. William C. Dabney, Charlottes-ville, Va.; Dr. B. F. Westbrook, Brooklyn; Dr. Henry P. Walcott, Cambridge, Mass.

The date of the next meeting to be between May 20th and June 15th, 1890.

Dr. JAMES J. PUTNAM, of Boston, read a paper on *A Supplementary Inquiry into the Frequency with which Lead is Found in the Urine.* The paper embodied further researches as to the frequency with which traces of lead are found in the urine of persons in good health, or not presenting the classical symptoms of lead poisoning; and discussed the propriety of enlarging our clini-cal conception of that disease. A table was shown in which the results of the present investigation were combined with those reported upon two years ago, which may be summarized as follows : The urines of sixty-eight persons, either presenting no symptoms (healthy medical students), or only symptoms of specific or local disease (phthisis, pleurisy, local injuries, etc.), were found by Dr. A. M. Comey and Dr. C. P. Worcester, to contain lead in the proportion of about seventeen per cent.; while those of another group of 125 persons, presenting various symptoms of disease such as it was thought might possibly be due in part to lead poisoning, contained lead in the proportion of fifty per cent. The largest sub-group of this latter class embraced thirty-six cases, not strictly homogeneous, but made up of chronic or sub-chronic affections of the spinal cord and peripheral nerves. One (typical) fatal case of this sub-group was analyzed at some length, and the results of the microscopic examination of the spinal cord and nerves were reported upon.

Dr. E. M. GREENE reported a number of observations made on Boston drinking water, showing the frequency with which lead is present, and the length of time required to wholly rid a pipe of its presence.

Dr. HAROLD C. ERNST, of Jamaica Plain, Mass., read a paper on *How Far a Cow may be Tuberculous before the Milk Becomes Dangerous as a Food-Supply.* The observations which he re-ported were made at the instance of the Massachusetts Society for the Promotion of Agriculture. The surroundings of the animals used were prepared in the most careful manner. One hundred and fourteen samples of milk were examined for the bacillus, and these were obtained from thirty-six cows suffering with tuberculosis of some organ other than the udder. Seventeen samples were found to contain tubercle bacilli. These specimens came from ten cows. The cream was found to contain bacilli as often as the milk. The bacilli were present with a fair degree of constancy. Well animals were then inoculated with the result of inducing the disease in 50 per cent. of the cases treated. Feeding experiments were also made with the result of inducing the disease in a number of calves and young pigs. The following conclusions were presented:—(1) Emphatically, milk from cows affected with tuberculosis in any part of the body may contain the virus of the disease. (2) The virus is present whether there is disease of the udder or not. (3) There is no ground for the assertion that there must be a lesion of the udder before the milk can contain the infection of tuberculosis. (4) On the contrary, the bacilli of tuberculosis are present and active in a very large proportion of cases in the milk of cows affected with tuberculosis, but with *no discoverable* lesion of the udder.

A paper on *Primary Cancer of the Duodenum*, by Dr. E. N. Whittier, of Boston, was read by title.

Dr. WM. OSLER, of Baltimore, exhibited a patient showing anæsthesia, the result of lesions of the cauda equina, from spina bifida which had healed.

Dr. E. L. TRUDEAU, of Saranac Lake, read a paper on *Hot Air Inhalations in Pulmonary Tuberculosis*. The paper presented a brief clinical history of four cases treated during periods varying from one to four months, by Weigert's method. This was considered as secondary and only as a basis for the bacteriological study which is left to answer the claim of specificity made for the method. The question to be answered is whether breathing of hot air can prevent the growth of the tubercle bacillus in the lungs of living individuals. The clinical evidence obtained brings out no positive proof in favor of the treatment. From the bacteriological research the following notes are made: In all the cases the bacillus which was present before the treatment remained in the sputum, and

no effect was produced upon that important element of the
disease. The claim of diminished virulence was tested by
inoculations made on rabbits before, during and after the treatment. The sputum of one of the patients who improved was
found fifteen weeks after the uninterrupted daily breathing of
hot air to produce tuberculosis in the animals injected, as
promptly and to a similar extent as that injected before the
treatment had been instituted. The author's conclusions were:
(1) The therepeutic value of hot air inhalations in phthisis is
doubtful; (2) the evidence obtained by bacteriological study of
the cases recorded does not confirm the assumption that inhalations of heated air can either prevent the growth of the
tubercle bacillus in the lungs of living individuals or diminish
the virulence of this microbe when it has gained access to
them.—*Boston Medical and Surgical Journal.*

Selections.

Pathological Affinities of Lead and Alcohol.

By Dr. Norman Porritt, Surgeon to the Huddersfield Infirmary.—To account for the prevalence of lead
poisoning in Huddersfield it is only necessary to be acquainted
with the character of the water supply. The water supply is
derived from several sources, and it is found that the water
from two reservoirs is not only abnormally acid, but has also
the dangerous property of dissolving lead, and when left standing in the lead service pipes attacks them and forms a plumbic
solution. As is well known, other towns have, or have had,
water supplies which act upon lead. Keighley and Sheffield
have each acquired some notoriety.

Noticing, in the first place, that both alcohol and the salts of
lead coagulate albumen, we may, for convenience sake, divide
their actions into two great groups—(1) the excretory group,
and (2) the nervous group. Turning first to the excretory
group of phenomena, we are at once confronted by the action
of these substances on the kidneys. Each is a recognized cause
of albuminuria, each can play a part in the causation of granular kidney, while the subtle power of each to initiate or develop
gout is well known. In short, each damages the kidneys, and

may set up not only temporary and functional disorder, but even ineradicable organic renal disease. On the other excretory organs, the chylopoietic viscera, the actions of alcohol and lead, though analogous in their ultimate results, are different in their *modus operandi*. Alcohol attacks the liver ; lead, the bowels. Alcohol encourages secretion from the mucous tracts : lead diminishes it. But the increased activity of the alcohol-stimulated mucous membrane is more than counterbalanced by the diminution of oxidation which is taking place in the rest of the body. This diminution of oxidation has a counterpart in the case of lead, for, according to Dr. Lauder Brunton, lead has the power of checking the elimination of uric acid.

Both lead and alcohol have a special, a peculiar, and a well-known action on the nervous system. Alcohol is eliminated from the system much more easily and more rapidly than lead, and we are not so familiar with its paralyzing effects as in the case of a poison which, like lead, slowly accumulates in the body. As is well-known, however, paralysis from alcohol, when given in a dose too large for the excretory organs to be got rid of, or when administered in smaller quantities over a long period, is not uncommon. The effects of alcohol are essentially paralytic, as are also those of lead, and there is not only nervous or muscular paralysis, but there are, if I may coin a phrase, excretory and metabolic paralysis.

Then alcohol and lead resemble each other in both being elective poisons. Some men are made tipsy by a quantity of drink which would do no more than serve as a thirst-quencher for others ; and, on the other hand, of two individuals imbibing a plumbic solution, the one may suffer the throes of colic, while the other escapes any unusual manifestation. Lead has little or no elective affinity for children, or the numerous children of our lead-poisoned patients would surely suffer. Of twenty-two cases of lead-poisoning which have been under my care, fourteen were males and eight females. Of the eight females three only suffered severely, and they were all above the age of sixty. The conclusions from these facts are that lead has a greater elective affinity for men than women, a greater elective affinity

for women than for children, and a greater elective affinity for
old than for young women.

Without denying that there is such a thing as elective action
I would suggest that by professing to explain the way in which
lead singles out one of several victims by the term of " elective
action," we are in many cases just glossing over our ignorance
by a plausible and pretty figure of speech. There must be
some causes for the elective action of lead, and, although in
many cases they may elude us, let us endeavor to search for
them, and not take refuge in such an empty phrase as " elective
action." I suggest, as one explanation of this elective action,
that whatever hinders metobolism or checks excretion will
enhance the susceptibility to lead poisoning. Children with
active metabolic processes and vigorous excretory organs rarely
suffer. Women, whose kidneys are less often afflicted with
Bright's disease than those of men, are less frequently the subjects of lead poisoning ; while my own cases suggest that young
women suffer much less severely than old ones. *A priori* there
is a strong presumption that men, from more frequent exposure
to sources of poisoning, should suffer more often than women.
But this presumption can only be held when the cases of workers
in lead are considered. In my twenty-two cases one man and
one woman were poisoned by lead other than that derived from
lead service pipes. Twenty cases remain—thirteen in males
and seven in females, or not quite two to one. In all these
cases the source of the lead, on chemical examination, was found
to be the drinking water.

Now, in cases of poisoning from a water-supply, it is the wife
and not the husband, who is the more exposed to the poison.
She spends her greater part of her time at home ; she takes all
her meals at home, and often takes supplementary meals or cups
of tea when her lord and master is at business. It is, therefore, much more likely that she and her little ones will imbibe
more of the toxic material than her frequently absent spouse.
The point was illustrated in the case of Milnes *v.* the Corpora-
tion of Huddersfield. The plaintiff, a solicitor of Huddersfield,
being lead-poisoned, sought for the lead, not in the domestic

water-supply, but at the water supply at his office in town. The lead was ultimately discovered in the domestic water-supply which was used by the whole family, but which Mr. Milnes did not suspect, as after breakfast he spent his whole day from home at his offices and business in the town. Notwithstanding, my cases show that more men are affected than women. What is the explanation of this unexpected disproportion? If the lessons of my twenty cases have been rightly understood, I have a clue to the explanation in the greater alcoholic consumption of the male sex.

Examining my thirteen cases more closely, I find that one died with all the symptoms of abdominal obstruction; two had wrist-drop, two had general convulsions, with more or less complete unconsciousness. The remaining eight cases suffered from nothing worse than colic, though that is bad enough. All the eight colic cases occurred in workingmen, and in every case but one there was no evidence to show that the patients were otherwise but steady and usually abstemious men; indeed, one was a total abstainer. Of the five severe cases, three were drunkards or " soakers ;" the fatal case was that of a man who worked as a cloth finisher in a very hot room, had the pot-belly of a drinker, and always drank beer, although his wife never knew him to be the worse for liquor more than three times. Of the two cases in which there was wrist-drop, one man is known to be unsteady, and, though preferring beer, never turns up his nose at spirits. The other wrist-drop case is employed at a hotel, where the opportunities for getting drink are many. Then we come to the two cases where general convulsions with unconsciousness occurred. One of them caused me much anxiety, and when the man's condition was at its worst, as I was leaving his house a neighbor stopped me. The neighbor, after enquiring after my patient, asked me where the lead came from that was poisoning him. I told him the drinking water. He shook his head doubtfully, and said he was sure it could come from nowhere else but the top of the patient's beer-barrel, the beer having taken it up as it ran from the barrel. The hint thus given was followed up, and I elicited that the patient had drunk beer to excess for some time before I saw him. In the other case with convulsions a similar history was discovered. These men were respectively twenty-eight and thirty-two years of age, and seemed vigorous, healthy men. One I have lost sight of, but the other occupied the same house for three years after his illness, became a teetotaller, and has had the best of health. In none of these five cases was any other inmate of the house affected, although at one house the drinking water contained as much as 1.8 grain of lead per gallon. Each patient was married and has a family, and their occupations did not bring them into contact with lead.

Alcohol, then, has a very powerful influence in intensifying the effects of lead. My friend, Mr. Abbott, late of Almondbury, tells me that the worst case of lead poisoning he has seen is that of an inebriate painter; while a practitioner in a neighboring township, where an epidemic of " water-supply lead poisoning" is occurring, asssures me that the case of the landlord of a beer-house is the most severe one he has had under his care.

Although Dr. Clifford Allbutt has observed the frequent concurrence of spirit drinking and lead poisoning, he thinks the increased ingestion of leaden water which is taken with the spirit explains what is evidently not a mere coincidence. Here I should join issue with Dr. Clifford Allbutt, and allot a considerable share of the toxic work to the alcohol. As we have seen, both alcohol and lead interfere with metobolism and check excretion. The result is : the alcohol locks in the lead ; the lead chains up the alcohol. A combination like this accentuates the action of lead, or produces a hybrid sort of affection partly alcoholic and partly plumbic, as in the two cases with general convulsions.

My cases justify, I think, the views I hold, but my contention is further strengthened by a knowledge of the remarkable way in which the kidneys excrete lead. In one of my cases I was uncertain whether the patient was suffering from plumbism or hidden malignant disease. To decide the question, I had, not only the drinking water, but the patient's urine, analysed by Mr. George Jarmain, F.I.C., the borough analyst. His report was that the drinking water contained 0.8 gr. of lead per gallon, the urine 0.28 gr. of lead per gallon· Thus the patient's urine contained such a proportion of lead as would have caused poisoning if present in drinking water. When we bear in mind the albuminuria of inebriety, fluctuating with each increase or diminution in the alcoholic consumption, and disappearing, perhaps, during the abstemious intervals, and when we remember that a great outlet for the excretion of lead in the kidneys, we must allow that there is *a priori* probability that the combination of lead and alcohol is not likely to be so readily got rid of as either substance singly. The question is important from a practical point of view, and I would suggest in all cases of lead poisoning, but more especially in the rarer cases where the higher nerve centres are affected, that a careful enquiry into the patient's habits be made.—*London Lancet,* January 26, 1889, p. 164.

On the Lobar Pneumonia of Children.

By DR, THURE HEKSTRÖM, in Stockholm.—In the children's clinic of Professor von Iaksch in Graz, thirty cases of croupous pneumonia came under observation in one year. Hekström publishes the histories and fever charts and adds some remarks thereon. The initial symptoms were always sudden, a special rigor but seldom occurred. The inflammation affected in a majority of the cases the upper lobe, (19 times in 30 cases) and the upper lobe of the right lung was twice as often attacked as that of the left lung. Pneumonia of the upper lobes is no more dangerous than that located elsewhere. The crisis follows in between four to ten days generally in twelve hours. In one case a relapse occurred—a rare event in childhood. All the cases ended favorably. Of the complications, pleurisy occurred four times in one of the cases—a dry pleurisy set itself up on the side opposite to that on which the disease existed. A little girl, six years old, became covered with an erythematous rash on her face and abdomen, which disappeared after some days. In the urine—whose quantity was always diminished and in some instances considerably—albumen was found in only five cases and traces of it in two others. Frequently, on the other hand, peptone, acetone and acetic acid were found. Whilst the latter in grown up persons indicate a severe course of the disease, a similar significance can be assigned to thèm in the case of children. Von Jaksch conjectures that certain nervous symptoms in the course of a pneumonia are in connection with the diaceturia. The therapensis was as simple as possible. Antipyrin and thallin were given in cases where the temperature was very high. For the severe pains dry cupping was found very serviceable. To relieve the severe cough urethan and antipyrin were of use; for the debility, which was rarely present, alcohol as a stimulant was prescribed.—*Schmidt's Jahrbücher*, Band 222. Jahrgang 1889, No. 4.

THE

Montreal Medical Journal.

| VOL. XVIII. | NOVEMBER, 1889. | No. 5. |

THE TRANSMISSION OF ACQUIRED PECULIARITIES.

The interesting discussion as to whether acquired peculiarities are capable of being transmitted seems as far from settled as ever. The assortment of recent literature is something appalling, and makes very dry reading. The difficulty is to find some crucial test. No sooner does some believer in the affirmative side suggest some case, supposed to be free from fallacies, than an opponent proceeds to shew it to be full of them, and to the ordinary reader both appear to be equally right.

Thus far it seems to be a drawn battle, if any advantage exists, it can scarcely be denied that the noes have it. The cases advanced by the upholders of a possible transmission of acquired peculiarities have depended largely upon a mass of hearsay evidence and on cases or experiments capable of two interpretations. Thus the fact that among animals whose tails or ears are docked, isolated cases occur in their offspring where these organs are stunted, was taken as a proof that the condition was capable of being transmitted. Bonnet, however, has shown that in the domesticated animals the tail was an organ shewing a gradual process of involution and reduction of the vertebræ, and liable to be stunted independent of any interference. Weismann has followed the matter up in the case of white mice, where he had through five generations docked the tails without any of the hundred individuals showing any tendency to inherit the defect.

Thus the inheritance of abnormalities of traumatic origin

appears to be very questionable. The question of the hereditary immunity from contagious diseases is even more interesting clinically. Prof. ———, of Budapest, who has experimented extensively in rabies, exhibited a dog born of parents who had each been subjected to prepared inoculations of modified rabic virus. This puppy on being inoculated with fixed virus (*i. e.,* virus of maximum intensity) was found to be perfectly immune. Of course this case is open to the objections that with the uncertain incubation period characteristic of rabies, the disease may have affected the animal in its modified form while still *in utero.* Then again some dogs are naturally immune.

On the whole, the solution of this problem appears to be far off, but even should acquired conditions be proved beyond cavail incapable of transmission, there is little doubt that their real or supposed transmission will continue for all time to form an important plank of the temperance platform.

A NEW ANTHRAX VACCINE.

Professor Hueppe, of Prague, has recently made an important contribution to the subject of the protective inoculation for anthrax. His method of investigation was extremely interesting. The present vaccine, an alternated anthrax virus, though very serviceable, is difficult to prepare and liable under certain conditions to regain its full virulence. Further, the person inoculating is always, after all, propagating genuine anthrax, though in a mild form.

In solving the problem of how to procure a protective vaccine, free from these objections, Hueppe resorted to the plan of investigating the chemical decomposition products of albnminoids (ptomaines) obtained by the action of various non-pathogenic bacteria in pure cultures. He finally in this way discovered a harmless organism found in garden earth whose ptomaines were almost identical chemically with those of anthrax. By previously inoculating cultures of this he succeeded in rendering white mice, the animals who, of all others, are most susceptible to even very attenuated anthrax, completely immune to inoculations by it, even in its most virulent form.

Thus far the results are most brilliant, and if it proves suited to practical purposes, this method will place anthrax vaccinations in a position comparable with those against smallpox as regards their freedom from untoward results.

MULTIPLE MYELOMA AND ALBUMINOSURIA.

Kahler, of Prague, reports a case of multiple myeloma affecting only the bones of the trunk. The ribs, spinal column, and the iliac bones were found to be extensively diseased. Spontaneous fractures had occurred in a number of the ribs. The patient, a man aged 43, succumbed after an eight years' illness.

A very interesting fact was that during the last six years of his illness the urine was constantly found to contain considerable quantities of albuminose. Kahler suggests that the presence of albuminose in the urine in considerable quantities in this disease may aid us to distinguish it from osteomalacia.

Albuminose is only exceptionally found in the urine in cases of osteomalacia, and then only in small quantities.

THE HARVEY CASE.

The man Harvey, who killed his wife and two children a few months ago in Guelph, has been tried, found guilty of murder, and is sentenced to be hanged in a few days.

Active steps are being taken to petition the Minister of Justice to commute the sentence of this unfortunate man, on the ground of insanity. For the sake of humanity it is to be hoped that this effort will be successful. Four of the leading experts in insanity in Ontario, testified at the trial, that in their opinion Harvey was insane at the time he killed his wife and children. The Jury, however, appear to have laid little stress on the opinions expressed by those best able to judge of the prisoner's mental state. They found him guilty. The Judge sentenced him to be hung, and unless proper representations are made to those in authority, the sentence will be carried out, and another case will be added to the long and cruel list of judicial murders.

Medical Items.

—Dr. R. W. Reid has been appointed Professor of Physiology in University College, Dundee.

—Prof. Neumann received, it is said, the sum of $20,000 for his professional visit to the late King of Portugal.

—Prof. von Krafft-Ebing is the successor of the late Prof. Leidesdorf in the Clinic for Mental Diseases in the Vienna Landes-Irrenanstalt.

—Dr. Robert W. Reid, Joint Lecturer on Anatomy at St. Thomas Hospital, London, has been appointed to the Chair of Anatomy in Aberdeen, rendered vacant by the retirement of Prof. Struthers.

—Dr. Hofman von Wellenhof, assistant to Professor Gruber, of the Vienna Hygiene Institute, died recently from glanders contracted from a coachman whom he was attending. The infection took place through the respiratory passages.

THE JOHNS HOPKINS HOSPITAL BULLETIN.

The Trustees of the Johns Hopkins Hospital have authorized the issue of a monthly publication to be known as the Hospital Bulletin. It will contain announcements of courses of lectures, programmes of clinical and pathological study, details of hospital and dispensary practice, abstracts of papers read and other proceedings of the Medical Society of the Hospital, reports of lectures and all other matters of general interest in connection with the work of the Hospital.

In size of page and general make-up the Bulletin will resemble closely the Johns Hopkins University Circulars. In fact it will attempt to fill in the Hospital the same place which the Circulars fill in the University. Nine numbers will be issued annually. The first number will appear in November, 1889.

The subscription price will be one dollar per year. Subscriptions may be sent to "The Publication Agency of the Johns Hopkins University, Baltimore, Md."

THE

MONTREAL MEDICAL JOURNAL.

| VOL. XVIII. | DECEMBER, 1889. | No. 6. |

Original Communications.

CURETTING THE UTERUS, AND THE METHODS OF TREATING THE CAVITY AFTERWARDS.

BY T. JOHNSON-ALLOWAY, M.D.,

Instructor in Gynæcology, McGill University; Assistant Surgeon to the Montreal General Hospital; Gynæcologist to the Montreal Dispensary.

Since specialists no longer regard curetting the uterine cavity with apprehension, when performed by an experienced operator, and under properly chosen circumstances, it is interesting to study the best methods of treating or dressing the wounded surface thus deprived of its endometrium. Included under this subject matter I place those cases of uterine disease which require the use of the sharp curette for the relief of abnormal hæmorrhages in all their protean forms, also in abortion cases where much manipulation has been necessitated, and the uterine contents have been removed with the curette and uterine forceps.

Before entering directly upon the subject it will be necessary to say a few words regarding the cases which generally require curetting, and the best kind of instrument to use.

Menorrhagia and metrorrhagia indicate local disease or change in the lining membrane of the uterine cavity. In certain zymotic diseases, when we have blood change, increased menstruation is not at all uncommon. This increase in the flow is due to increased stimulation of the sexual organs under the influence of these blood changes, and I have no doubt is often determined and made more pronounced by some pre-existing

26

... ...and metrium. Also such conditions as in-
... the cardiac valves or emphysema will cause an
... in another and different way. Metrostaxis
... does not come within the range of our
... ... gives a passing notice. If, however, a men-
... ... after the febrile attack has passed away,
... ... date from it, the condition should be recog-
... treatment. This is self-evident because
... conditions of the blood and disturbances
... never cause prolonged menorrhagia
... already diseased local condition.
... ... will often point to a statement made to
... menorrhagia began with some illness, and has
... ... ever since. In such a case we have un-
... disease which only wanted the opportunity to
... manifest in the organ involved.

... local conditions which cause menorrhagia
... may classify them as follows :—Those in-
... ovarian and parametral tissues, and those
... the uterine tissues proper. Metro-
... condition generally gives relief to
... return after the inflammatory lesion
... better not to check it; the
... will be all that is necessary. I-
... begins to manifest a tendency
... recurring to the curette.

... the uterus seldom give rise to hæmor-
... noticed that the endometrium under-
... in its vascularity. Tumors growing
... involving the outer uterine layers
... vascularity and hyperplasia of the en-
... tend to grow outwards and become
... vascular or nutritive changes in
... are therefore not accompanied
... cases of uterine myoma, accompanied
... it is advisable to curette the cavity
... instead of wasting time and reputation with

palliative methods.   A short time ago I removed a long finger-like mucous polyp from the uterine cavity of a patient the subject of a medium sized interstitial fibroid. The hæmorrhage ceased almost immediately, and gave no further trouble.   In another similar case I removed a so-called placental polypus some three inches long.   The patient in this instance expressed a desire to undergo the recent fashionable treatment by electricity to cure the hæmorrhage supposed to be due to the mural fibroid.   It, however, occurred to me to explore the uterine cavity with the curette first and obtain a knowledge of its contents, if any.   The result was sufficiently satisfactory to require no further treatment.

In cases of hæmorrhage from fibroids, I would advise in every case where it is possible, to explore the cavity and thoroughly curette the hyperplastic endometrium. I am of opinion that this should first be done before resorting to removal of the appendages or hysterectomy.   In every case of chronic hyperplastic endometritis following abortion, cervical lacerations with sub-involution, gonorrhœal imflammations, and displacement with exhaustive menorrhagia and leucorrhœa, the cavity should be curetted of every vestige of diseased endometrium and the wounded surface treated as will be pointed out further on. It is understood that uterine discharge due to malignant disease will not be considered.   I may however say in passing, that cancer is a common cause of metrorrhagia in women over thirty-five years of age, and I regret to acknowledge that there are still men high in the respect of their colleagues—especially in England—who regard menorrhagia at the time of the menopause as evidence of its normal approach.   To my mind there is no more iniquitous teaching, or one fraught with more disaster to our reputation with the public.   In my experience of such cases, I have never failed to find either malignant disease or fungus degeneration of the endometrium, and who can say but that the menorrhagia was, in fact, a warning note to remove the benign embryo that the destroying parent might not get vigorous life.   Clinical examples have occurred to most of us wherein the microscope could not discover evidence of malignancy and yet these patients died of undoubted cancer.   All physicians should therefore insist upon examination of their patient under such circumstances and advise them ac—cordingly.

A few words now about the kind of curette to be used. In cases of chronic endometritis there are three forms of curette from which we can take our choice—Martin's, Sims' and Hanks' (figured as below). Of these Martin's is the one

MARTIN'S CURETTE.

SIMS' CURETTE.

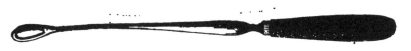

HANKS' CURETTE.

[CHAPMAN, Montreal, Instrument Dealer.]

I give the preference to and use most frequently. Sims' instrument is a good one, and Hanks' curette is also serviceable, though somewhat difficult to introduce should the cervix be not dilated sufficiently and the cavity not straight; also, the shank of the palliative methods. A short time ago I removed a long finger-like mucous polyp from the uterine cavity of a patient the subject of a medium sized interstitial fibroid. The hæmorrhage ceased almost immediately, and gave no further trouble. In another similar case I removed a so-called placental polypus some three inches long. The patient in this instance expressed a desire to undergo the recent fashionable treatment by electricity to cure the hæmorrhage supposed to be due to the mural fibroid. It, however, occurred to me to explore the uterine cavity with the curette first and obtain a knowledge of its contents, if any. The result was sufficiently satisfactory to require no further treatment.

In cases of hæmorrhage from fibroids, I would advise in every case where it is possible, to explore the cavity and thoroughly curette the hyperplastic endometrium. I am of opinion that this should first be done before resorting to removal of the appendages or hysterectomy. In every case of chronic hyperplastic endometritis following abortion, cervical lacerations with sub-involution, gonorrhœal imflammations, and displacement with exhaustive menorrhagia and leucorrhœa, the cavity should be curetted of every vestige of diseased endometrium and the wounded surface treated as will be pointed out further on. It is understood that uterine discharge due to malignant disease will not be considered. I may however say in passing, that cancer is a common cause of metrorrhagia in women over thirty-five years of age, and I regret to acknowledge that there are still men high in the respect of their colleagues—especially in England—who regard menorrhagia at the time of the menopause as evidence of its normal approach. To my mind there is no more iniquitous teaching, or one fraught with more disaster to our reputation with the public. In my experience of such cases, I have never failed to find either malignant disease or fungus degeneration of the endometrium, and who can say but that the menorrhagia was, in fact, a warning note to remove the benign embryo that the destroying parent might not get vigorous life. Clinical examples have occurred to most of us wherein the microscope could not discover evidence of malignancy and yet these patients died of undoubted cancer. All physicians should therefore insist upon examination

necrose, and the base of the shaving forms a little eddy for
retention of discharges to decompose and set up trouble. The
principal locality in which these spots of danger occur is just
above the internal os. When iodized phenol or other cautery is
applied, these jagged points are converted into little ulcerating
pits from which septic absorption takes place, culminating in a
sharp attack of pelvic inflammation. Every gynæcologist has
experienced such unpleasant results after curetting when there
previously existed no legitimate foundation for such a sequence,
and may be accounted for in the manner I have described. This
danger will always exist with the injection of fluid or the application of caustics to the interior of the uterus, and should not
therefore be made a routine practice.

Now that we are cognizant of these dangers, we can see the
great safety and therapeutic advantage of filling tightly the uterine cavity with a soft elastic and aseptic material prepared with
iodoform suspended in parafin. This material, prepared by
Dyer of Montreal, is in advance of every other for this purpose.
It can be left in for four or five days, if necessary, without the
least fear of having it undergo change. There is absolutely no
drain so good, and by its side pressure on the uterine walls all
remnants of undetached membrane re-unite, resulting in a perfectly smooth cavity surface. The cases which are generally
met with in which this dressing is applicable are :—Curetting
for hæmorrhagic endometritis ; with Schrœder's trachelorrhaphy;
in bleeding myomata ; for removal of retained products after
abortion, the method is especially satisfactory here. It arrests
all bleeding at once, secures good drainage and induces contraction of the uterus, thus favoring rapid involution. In a case
of this nature I saw recently in consultation with Dr. Gurd, I
removed a large adherent placental mass.Pregnancy had ceased
at about the fifth month,but the placenta continued to grow for
some time afterwards. It was so firmly adherent that it became
necessary to remove it in very small fragments with curette
and forceps. I packed this uterus to a fair degree of pressnre,
and on the second day I found the gauze had all been expelled
and the uterus reduced in size with firm contraction. The gauze

packing is often expelled, especially in abortion cases, but it can easily be removed on the third or fourth day by simply introducing the dressing forceps to the cervix along two fingers of left hand as a guide and gently withdrawing the gauze. No irrigations are required after its withdrawal as the vagina is still aseptic and will remain so if not interfered with.

A word in conclusion in regard to the use of the sharp curette. This instrument has been held in great awe for many years by a large section of practising physicians ; and these gentlemen have always urged the use of Thomas' dull wire curette when an operation of this nature was about to be performed. This general professional impression having prevailed it seems apparent that there must have been some good cause for this strange aversion to the instrument. Those who have had experience with it, and have necessarily become skilled in its use will see that the cause of the above impression rests with two facts—first, carelessness or neglect in making the field of operation absolutely aseptic ; second, unskillful use of the instrument due to want of constant experience. When we consider the important meaning of these facts, it is surprising the little harm the instrument has done.

A CASE OF NECROSIS FOLLOWING A COMPOUND FRACTURE.

OPERATION WITH ANTISEPTIC PRECAUTIONS—AN EXCELLENT RESULT.

BY JOHN CAMPBELL, M.D., SEAFORTH, ONT.

(Prepared for the late meeting of the Canadian Medical Association at Banff.)

Mr. President and Gentlemen—We humbly submit the following report of a surgical case in practice, which we hope may be of some interest to the members of this Association, meeting here by the health-giving waters of Banff, in the shadow of the world's crest—the far-famed " Rocky Mountains."

History.—The patient, D. M. R., is a native of Canada, and 35 years of age. In December, 1881, while working in the lumber woods of Michigan, he met with an accident, resulting in a compound fracture of the right tibia. He said that the bones protruded through the skin in *four* places, while the doctor affirmed that the bone was broken in no fewer than *six places.*

He was over 100 miles from surgical aid. He was conveyed by the following means. He was carried five miles, taken in a waggon ten miles, and rode the rest of the journey in the van of a lumber train.

He was treated in St. Mary's Hospital, Saginaw. Seventeen days after the accident the limb was put up in a plaster bandage, and he was sent home to Whitby, in Canada, where Dr. Fields took off the cast and put the leg in a fracture box.

He was able to walk with crutches in 12 weeks from date of fracture, and in 6¼ months resumed work. Nine months afterwards he was troubled with pain at seat of fracture, after which pus formed. In March, 1885, he was laid up four weeks with local pain accompanied with fever and formation of pus. In March, 1888, he jarred his leg, and was treated by Dr. Evans, who painted the part with collodion and wanted to lance it. In september, 1888, he suffered again, when the writer attended him. The part was painted with tr. iod. co., the limb was raised, and the part afterwards lanced down to the bone. After two weeks he partially recovered.

We proposed to make a long incision down to the bone, so as to enable us to examine it thoroughly, and, if necessary, remove the diseased bone. The patient at last consented to the operation, which he agreed should be performed on the 1st of October, with the assistance of Dr. MacKid.

Full antiseptic precautions were taken. The leg was washed with soap and water, with the aid of a brush. The instruments were steeped in a solution of acid carbolic, 1 to 20. Our hands were thoroughly disinfected. After Dr. MacKid had put the patient thoroughly under the influence of Squibb's ether, I made an incision eight inches in length down to the bone, on the anterior aspect of the tibia. We found the shaft denuded of the periosteum and rough. It was bare for six inches over the region of the old fracture. We chiselled off the necrosed bone until we reached bone which bled freely.

At the point of the old fracture we found a softened condition of the bone. This we trephined with Langenbeck's bone trephine, but after going through the substance, had to use a gouge to remove all the decayed portion of bone. We packed the wound along the whole tract with iodoform gauze, over this, corrosive sublimate cotton, and over all, carbolic acid bandages. The wound was not opened until the third day. During this time there was no pain or any bad symptoms whatever.

On the fourth day he got feverish and pulse became rapid, when we opened the wound and irrigated it with weak carbolic lotion, and gave quin. sulph. in gr. x. doses repeated at proper intervals. In 24 hours the temperature became normal again. He had transacted a lot of business during the day, and he blamed that for the rise of temperature which took place the same evening. The only other drawback which took place was an attack of acute eczema which yielded promptly to ung. zinci oxidi.

In four weeks the granulations filled up the wound so that the parts could be brought into apposition. The bone was nicely covered with granulations.

We had to go through from $\frac{1}{8}$ to $\frac{1}{4}$ of an inch of necrosed, before we reached the sound bone. The patient has applied for no treatment since the operation, and has frequently remarked that he considers the leg in question nearly as sound as the other. He is attending to business every day. I was taught in my college days that if we removed the periosteum the inevitable result would be death of the bone. In this case six or eight inches of the bone was denuded of its periosteum, and in a rough condition yet we had the most happy results, thanks to the recuperative powers of nature and the blessings of antiseptic surgery.

A RARE ANATOMICAL ABNORMALITY OF THE NASO-PHARYNX WITH REPORTS OF THREE OBSERVATIONS.

By GEORGE W. MAJOR, B.A., M.D., &c.,

Specialist to the Department for Diseases of the Nose and Throat, Montreal General Hospital; Instructor in Laryngology and Diseases of the Throat, McGill University, Montreal, Canada.

(Read before the Medico-Chirurical Society of Montreal, October 18th, 1889.)

The naso-pharynx varies greatly in contour and in capacity, and extreme anomalies may exist without giving rise to discomfort. So long as the function of this part is properly performed any departure 'from normal conditions is likely to escape observation.

The relation of the plane of the choanæ to the horizontal plane offers a diversity of angles. The choanæ may look almost directly downwards, as was observed in a case of adenoid disease operated upon this month, and at which Dr. John A. Macdonald assisted. The antero-posterior and lateral diameters show constantly marked differences amongst themselves when a comparison is instituted. The cavity occupies a position in the skull by no means constant. It is occasionally situated so far back as to be reached with difficulty when examining with the finger or when operating. The posterior pharyngeal wall also affords examples of varying degrees of inclination, the integrity of the naso-pharyngeal cavity being sometimes seriously trespassed upon, so great is the obliquity. Prominent cervical vertebræ also project into the cavity and render posterior rhinoscopy difficult of performance. There are a number of other departures from the normal state, of which perhaps atresia or a disposition thereto is most commonly met with. The abnormality, however, to which I shall call your attention, and of which I report two examples, which have come under my personal observation, is of very rare occurrence.

CASE No. I.—On May 6th, 1883, Miss B., aged 22 years, was referred to me by Dr. A. A. Browne. The young lady complained of difficult nasal respiration and its associated discomforts, as well as a temporary impairment of hearing. When suffering from an acute coryza she had occasionally been subject to similar attacks, but at other times, when in the enjoyment of her ordinary health, did not experience any great inconvenience or annoyance. On examination, the anterior nares were found free from any obstruction. I found in the naso-pharyngeal cavity, however, a well-developed septum running in an antero-posterior direction, continuous with the vomer, which divided the vault into two apparently equal and lateral halves.

On digital examination this partition gave to the finger the sensation of bone and was covered with soft, velvety mucous membrane. It was firmly adherent to the roof of the vault, and was fixed into the posterior superior wall at a point higher than its origin from the base of the vomer proper. The lower margin was sharply defined, and somewhat curved, presenting a slightly crescentic outline. A firm and steady pressure exerted in many directions failed to dislocate it, or, in fact, to produce any appreciable movement. The mucous lining of the region generally was much congested and swollen, accounting for the character of the symptoms. This case was reported in an article entitled "Buccal Breathing," read before the Canadian Medical Association on August 26th, 1884, and was subsequently published in the issue of the *New York Medical Record* of November 22nd, 1884.

CASE No. II.—On May 23rd, 1888, a boy aged five years, of feeble mind, was referred to me by Dr. George Ross. The child had previously been under the care of the late Dr. Howard, who had on several occasions communicated with me concerning the character of the case. The child was a confirmed mouth breather, and in the absence of a digital examination of the naso-pharynx, or, in fact, of any examination of the posterior nares, adenoid vegetations were considered to be the cause. The speech was " dead," but there was, in addition, an impediment that was of a central origin, and that no operation could in any way remove. In Dr. Ross' absence from the city, Dr. Browne administered æther. On passing my finger into the vault, I found a bony wall continuous with the vomer which divided the naso-pharyngeal space into two portions. This septum was covered with mucous membrane and was free from the vegetations which filled the spaces on either side. The width of the lateral halves was not more than a centimeter, and it was with difficulty that a very small ring knife could be introduced between the septum and the lateral naso-pharyngeal walls. After the removal of the growths a decided improvement took place in breathing, and the anæsthetic was notably much more easily administered.

Dr. Browne on examination was enabled to confirm the presence of the septum as described. In this case the septum was rather more dense and thicker through than in the case first referred to ; it was also less deep from above downwards.

To Dr. John N. Mackenzie, of Johns Hopkins Hospital, Baltimore, belongs the honor of having first described this malformation, in a paper read before the Clinical Society of Maryland, on February 16th, 1883, and published in the Archives of Laryngology in July of the same year. My first observation was made May 6th, 1883, communicated August 26th, 1884, and published in November of that year.

The only other observation on record is that of Dr. Ph. D. Photiades, of Constantinople, which appeared in a work on " Nasal Pharyngeal and Laryngeal Diseases," published at Athens in 1884, and a notice of which, translated from the Greek into German, occurs in the *Centralblatt für Laryngologie* for December, 1885. Whether Dr. Photiades' case antedated my first one or not I am unable to say. Dr. Photiades claims that Dr. Mackenzie's case was the only one published prior to his own.

In answer to a number of letters sent to leading teratologists inquiring as to the frequency of such a deformity, ·I have not been able to add a single instance to the four already communicated to you. Dr. Harrison Allen, of Philadelphia, who has devoted much time and attention to the study of the deformities of the skull, writes me that he has never met with such a case in practice or in museums. In over 3,500 skulls examined by him, he has never seen even a tendency to such prolongation of the septum.

Post scriptum:

CASE No. III.—On the 23rd of October, 1889, while operating on a child of 13 months for the removal of adenoid vegetations I encountered my third case of this abnormality. In this patient respiration had been most difficult from birth, in fact, nasal breathing was impossible. On examination I found the naso-pharynx divided as before described. There was also a marked narrowing of the choanæ. Dr. F. W. Campbell, Dean of the Faculty of Medicine of Bishops College, after examining satisfied himself of the correctness of my diagnosis. Under æther the adenoid vegetations were thoroughly removed and nasal breathing quite restored. The infant made a good and satisfactory recovery.

VERTIGO, AN EYE AND EAR SYMPTOM.

BY J. W. STIRLING, M.B., &c.

(Read by title before the Canadian Medical Association at Banff, August, 1889.)

Vertigo is that condition in which there is a tendency to lose, or a complete loss of equilibrium.

It is a feeling of uncertainty with regard to our position relatively to surrounding objects.

I will give a short resumé of our more recent knowledge and advances in the subject, especially from an ocular and labyrinthine standpoint, and append notes of a few cases which have come under my own observation.

For the maintenance of equilibrium, we have three factors to consider.

1.—The source of the afferent impulses to the brain, three in number, namely, visual, labyrinthine and tactile.

2.—The co-ordinating reflex centre in the cerebellum.

3.—The efferent motor impulses.

As to the centre, that it certainly exists in the cerebellum has been undoubtedly proven by Ferrier and others, in their operations on animals, for on excising the cerebrum, equilibrium was still maintained, but on excising the cerebellum it was lost, although the cerebrum was retained. From this also we see that consciousness is not necessary for equilibration.

Further experiments showed that in time cerebral activity could gradually, though imperfectly, assume the lost function,

although at a considerable expenditure of nerve energy,
fatigue rapidly ensuing. With this loss of motor co-ordination for the preservation ·of balance, there was, however, no
diminution of muscular power.

Ferrier found on stimulating certain areas of the monkey's
cerebellum with electricity, that movements of the eyes
and marked loss of equilibrium in definite directions followed.

1st.—Stimulating the pyamid, either on right or left side,
the eyes moved to the right or left.

2nd.—Stimulating the anterior part of the upper vermiform
lobe in the middle line, the eyes turned directly up; if the
electrode were placed to either side of the middle line, the eyes
turned to the same side as well as upwards, but without any
rotation.

3.—If electrode placed on posterior part of upper vermiform
lobe in the middle line, eyes were turned directly down, and
in addition to either side if electrode placed on one or other
side of middle line.

4.—If lateral lobes stimulated, the eyes looked up, and upper
end of vertical axis rotated towards side so stimulated.

5.—Stimulation of flocculus caused rotation on the antero-
posterior axis.

The *movements* of *the head, eyes and body* coincided.

It was also found that on stimulating the lateral lobes there
was a tendency to fall to the same side as that stimulated, associated with a rotation backwards. On stimulating the
anterior portion of middle lobe, a tendency to fall backwards;
on stimulating the posterior portion, a tendency to fall forwards.

On destruction of any of these areas, falling in the opposite
direction ensued, *e.g.*, if lateral lobe destroyed, animal fell to
opposite side, with a rotary movement backwards; if anterior
part middle lobe, animal fell forwards; if posterior, backwards.

The stimulation of the mastoid in man by electrodes placed
one on each mastoid, causes the head to be bent and the eyes
directed towards the side on which the anode is placed; objects
appear to be moving in the opposite direction, and there is a
sensation as of loss of support on the opposite side of the body;
hence the movement of the head and eyes to one side are compensatory to a feeling of falling to the opposite side.

Now, it is found that the movements of the head and eyes
thus engendered, by placing the electrodes on the mastoid in

man, are exactly similar to those caused by directly stimulating the corresponding side of the cerebellum in the monkey; hence it may be inferred very justly that the other movements of the head, eyes and body, set up by stimulating the other areas of the cerebellum, correspond to a sensation of falling in the opposite direction, and are all compensatory to preserve equilibrium.

Next as to the afferent factors concerned in the preservation of equilibrium.

That the eyes play an important part in the maintenance of equilibrium hardly requires iteration, as we are all aware of the uncertainty of gait following the sudden occlusion of vision, although that it is not absolutely necessary is certain, as evidenced by the movements of the blind.

Our movements are first learnt by observing and copying others, calling our consciousness into constant requisition, with the result of early fatigue, until after a while the act is performed reflexly.

That consciousness even yet plays a part, although subordinate, is evidenced by the rapidity and certainty with which attention is attracted by anything unusual in the conditions appertaining to any movement, e.g., movement of external objects, loss of sensation in limb, etc.

Hence, from our eyes, and by vision, by the muscular sense of accommodation or convergence, we gather experience of our position in space and relation to surroundings.

That all these assist in maintaining equilibrium is readily observed by the feeling of insecurity, giddiness and sometimes faintness which occurs if anything interferes with their normal action.

First, as to vision. We have referred to the sense of insecurity which follows its sudden suspension, this disappearing in time as the other two afferent factors, tactile and labyrinthine, partly take its place.

Let the whole field of vision be put in motion, as in watching a running stream, the eye in vain strives to fix our position in space, and take with this the very contradictoriness of impression of our stability, as obtained through the tactile and labyrinthine sources; then this disharmony of afferent impressions produces generally a feeling of insecurity, often of giddiness and faintness.

Secondly, let there be a lesion in the muscular sense, as occurs in paralysis of the ocular muscles. The field of vision is falsely projected, and the misinterpretation arising from the power of muscular impulse, and the small result obtained causes an apparent movement of objects looked at. This gives rise to uncertainty of gait, giddiness and even total loss of balance.

In certain paralyses this is more marked than in others viz.: in oculo motor paralysis, as in this form the visual fields of the two eyes nowhere coincide, in abducens, supratrochlear, and separate muscle paralysis it is not so marked, for, in certain directions, the fields coincide.

Cases are very common, but I may be permitted to mention the following typical oculo motor paralysis:

J. McK., aged 45; came to me on account of double vision, which had suddenly appeared three days before.

History of Syphilis.—There existed marked oculo motor paralysis of left eye, with ptosis upper lid; there was crossed diplopia, the field of vision of the left eye being projected to the right. On getting him to walk rapidly toward a given point he made a wide detour to the right, and on suddenly trying to correct himself became quite giddy and fell.

Acquired nystagmus is also accompanied by giddiness from the false impression as to the relation of surroundings.

Thirdly, as to the influence of accommodation.

This is seen sometimes in the strain of the accommodation muscle in hyperopia, giddiness occurring, although mainly in the neurasthenic and in hyperopia of high degree with sudden weakening of accommodation. The vertigo is mainly due to the apparent changing in position and shape of objects, arising from the varying focussing of the eye, caused by irregular actions of the ciliary muscle, the contradictoriness of muscular impulse and result confusing one. It is certain that the centering of the attention on any one of the three afferent factors specially, gives rise to a feeling of confusion, and this is likely partly the cause here of the feeling of insecurity. Examples are too numerous to make it obligatory to give any.

The connection of the optic nerves with the cerebellar centre has not been absolutely proved, but a case of Mendel's throws considerable light on this point.

In this case the post mortem examination revealed a hemorrhage in the pulvinar of the left optic thalamus; there was atrophy of the left red nucleus and a tract of secondary degeneration in the right superior cerebellar peduncle, traceable as far as the nucleus dentatus.

It would show that each lateral lobe rules over eye of same side, the decussation first occurring at the chiasma, then back again at the decussation of superior cerebellar peduncles. The pupil contracts mainly in eye of same side as that of the stimulated lobe.

Lesions in the course of superior cerebellar peduncles, of optic lobes, or of connection between optic and oculo-motor nerves must cause disturbances of equilibrium.

Before leaving the subject of ocular afferent impressions, I may just mention the curious condition of agoraphobia, where a man as long as he is in the street or between two walls maintains his equilibrium, but as soon as he is in a field or open space loses his balance. I am inclined to think this is partly due to psychical disturbances, as well as to contradictoriness of sensation.

I will now pass on to the consideration of the labyrinthine factor.

Beyond mentioning the semi-circular canals, it is hardly necessary to dilate on their well-known anatomy.

Three in number, a superior vertical, which has a direction forwards and slightly outwards, a posterior vertical, and a horizontal, each having its ampulla, with its crista, hairs, otoliths, endolymph and perilymph.

Proofs of their function are numerous, a good one being a case of Ferrier's of labyrinthine vertigo without deafness.

The ampullæ are supplied by the anterior or motor part of the auditory nerve. Tracing it backwards, it joins the acoustic division at the cribriform plate, then back through the meatus auditorius internus, to the medulla oblongata, where the motor fibres can be traced to the restiform bodies or inferior cerebellar peduncles, and thence into cerebellum. The further central connections are obscure.

The two theories as to mode of stimulation are well known. Crum Brown holds stimulation occurs through varying pressure of endolymph on ampullary dilatations. Cyon denies this as he could never experimentally prove it, but asserts stimulation arises from vibrations of otoliths, caused by variations in position of head and undulations of endolymph.

If it is pressure, inclination of the head to the right would cause endolymph to flow from the right to the left.

These symmetrical plus and minus variations would stimulate the ampullary nerves, and thereby excite the equilibration centres to set up muscular action appropriate to position of head and body.

Crum Brown has also shown that by the semicircular canals, independent of all other aid, we are able to detect any direction in which we may be rotated and the approximate rate of rotation.

This disappears after a time, and is due to the endolymph in virtue of its inertia not partaking of the same rate of rotation at first as the osseous canals.

Each canal has only one ampulla, hence the physical difference between rotation with ampulla first and ampulla last, and it is supposed that only one of these rotations, say with ampulla first, when endolymph flows into the canal, will stimulate nerve endings. On this supposition one canal can only give rise to sense of rotation in one direction, around one axis, and for sense of complete rotation in either direction, the canals must be in pairs parallel and with ampullæ at opposite ends, which is the case.

Vertigo could not be produced in pigeons with semicircular canals destroyed. In a large number of deaf mutes, and in cases where the labyrinth is destroyed by disease, vertigo could not be produced by rotation.

In lower animals of sluggish habits, as in reptilia, where equilibration is not called for specially, the semicircular canals are only slightly developed. However, as we occasionally see or hear of cases of necrosis of labyrinth, it is evident that the semicircular canals are not absolutely necessary for maintaining the upright position.

Now, as to the results of stimulation of the canals.

It frequently happens that from violent syringing or politzerizing, vertigo occurs. The stapes being violently driven in, alters the pressure of endolymph and stimulates ampullary nerve terminals; there is a feeling of loss of support on the opposite side, and as a result the heads and eyes are directed toward the stimulated side, objects appear moving to the opposite side.

Cyon, Högyes and others have found that stimulation of the separate canals causes the same motor disturbances as the stimulation of certain cerebellar areas.

For example, section of the superior vertical canal causes falling forwards and outwards, which corresponds to destruction of anterior part of middle lobe; section of posterior canal causes tendency to rotate backwards round a transverse axis, as occurs in section of posterior part of middle lobe; section of horizontal canal gives rise to lateral rotary displacements, as in section of lateral cerebellar lobes.

Rotation backwards, according to Crum Brown, would correspond to irritation in ampulæ of superior vertical canal, rotation forwards to that of posterior canal, while the rotary would correspond to irritation of ampullæ of horizontal canals; section of auditory nerve gives same result as destruction of semicircular canals; further yet, section of restiform bodies gives same result.

From these facts, the function of the canals, the course of the fibres backward and the location of the centres for the reflex co-ordination necessary for equilibrium in the cerebellum are clear.

Meynert asserts that fibres of the auditory nerve pass by channels as yet undetermined from the cerebellum to the pedunculus cerebri, and ultimately to the cerebral cortex.

We know that movements of the head and body are accompanied by corresponding movements of the eyes, which strive to maintain their primary passive position with relation to external objects. It is found that section of the aqueduct of sylvius at the level of the corpora quadrigeniam, or of the floor of the fourth ventricle, or of the auditory nucleus, both acustici as well as destruction of both membranous labyrinths causes disappearance of these movements, while conversely stimulation of these parts is followed by bilateral associated movements of both eyeballs, afferent impulses from the ear to centre, thence to nuclei of 3, 4, 6 nerves.

The motor fibres from the cerebellum cross in the middle cerebellar peduncles, join the opposite pyramidal tracts, then

cross again at lower part of medulla, so the relationship of
cerebellum is with the same side of body, while that of cerebrum is crossed, as proved by a very interesting case of Ferrier's of atrophy of the right lobe of the cerebellum, secondary
to destruction of anterior motor region of left cerebral hemisphere, the pyramidal tract had undergone secondary degeneration, and with it the right middle cerebellar peduncle and
right lateral lobe of cerebellum.

The blood supply of the labyrinth is from the basilar artery,
a branch of which enters the meatus auditorius internus with
the nerve. It thus can be easily seen how any variations of
blood pressure may influence functions of the nerve deletori-
ously. The venous outlet is into the petrosal sinus for the
vestibule, through the acqueductus vestibuli.

This acqueduct also contains the ductus endolymphaticus,
the walls of which are supposed to secrete the endolymph ;
hence any venous congestion in this osseous canal must act
injuriously by compressing the duct itself or hyper-exudation.

The perilymph escapes from the ear by the aqueductus
cochlea into the fossa jugularis along with the vein from the
cochlea which opens into the bulb of the jugular vein.

The endolymph reaches the subarachnoid space of the brain
through the sheath of the nervus acusticus. Hence an intro-
cranial tumour or other cause of increased intra-cranial pressure can injuriously affect hearing and equilibrium, although
no direct implication of the cerebellar centre exists, just as in
optic neuritis, either by descending inflammation or increase
of fluid in sheath.

A good example of the effects of hyperemia is the following :
J. B., aged 56. A few days before I saw him was going
off fishing ; it was a very hot day ; he had to run part of the
way to the station ; he bought his ticket, and on bending down
to pick up his basket he suddenly became very giddy and had
just time to grasp a seat to prevent himself from falling ;
immediately noted loud noises in left ear and marked deafness. He had been deaf in right ear for many years.

When I saw him the giddiness had disappeared, although it
had lasted for two days.

His hearing improved slightly under treatment and the tinnitus diminished.

Here the disturbance of hearing was not profound enough, nor the other symptoms severe enough for hemorrhage.

A very pretty example of the effect of anæmia on the middle ear came under my notice just before leaving England.

Hannah M., aged 40; married; was confined six weeks before I saw her; complained of giddiness, tinnitus and deafness whenever she is erect, these symptoms disappearing almost entirely on her assuming the horizontal posture. The woman was very anæmic, and gave a history of the same symptoms occurring with three previous labours.

Woakes considers that the inferior cervical ganglion of the sympathetic is at the bottom of much of the tinnitus, vertigo and nausea, as it controls the vertebral arteries and labyrinthine circulation, so determining aural symptoms, and by its connection with the vagus, causes the gastric symptoms. He bases his therapeutic treatment on the fact that this ganglion is functionally depressed by quinine and tobacco and stimulated by hydrobromic acid.

I might mention here that Ferrier holds there is direct communication between cerebellum and the viscera by the direct cerebellar tracts, which connect with Clarke's vesicular columns, and, as Gaskill has pointed out, Clarke's columns are confined to those regions of the central nervous system, which give origin to the rami viscerales.

Aural vertigo from middle ear lesions are frequent; in all there is ankylosis of the stapes or obliteration of the round windows. Now these fenestræ act as safety valves. Hence in ankylosis or obliteration of them any movement, even vibratory, of the labyrinth gives an injurious shock, and giddiness ensues.

We must also note the state of reflex hyper-excitability of the acoustic nerve, due to the repetition of local and functional irritations.

Vertigo is common from irritation, foreign bodies, wax, &c., in meatus, not generally excessive, and disappears with removal of cause.

Vertigo with the accompanying nausea tinnitus, deafness is more intense if cause is in middle ear. Syncope sometimes occurs if nausea is excessive, but loss of consciousness extremely rare, so differs from apoplexy and epilepsy.

Finally, just a word as to the abuse of the term Meniére's disease, which has been indiscriminately applied to all forms of aural vertigo.

Only vertigo of labyrinthine origin associated with profound deafness, which is permanent, the onset acute in a previously healthy ear, these and only these symptoms are characteristic of Meniére's disease.

All forms of aural vertigo, according to Burnett, are paroxysmal, excepting those due to a foreign body in the outer ear pressing on the drum, or to a tumour on or in acoustic nerve.

I will close by giving a few notes of a rare case which came under my charge during my last year at the Royal Edinburgh Infirmary.

J. McK., aged 63; three years before I saw him was at a volunteer review, slipped, fell and struck the back of his head; was unconscious for fifteen hours; had a nasty scalp wound on back of head, three inches by half an inch; just after accident blood escaped from both ears and the next day from the pharynx. On regaining consciousness was very deaf, his deafness becoming more profound until in ten days he was stone deaf. On attempting to rise he was so giddy that he had to give up the attempt. This symptom gradually diminished. When I saw him, three years later, he was stone deaf, his voice had the monotonous intonation peculiar to the absolutely deaf. He was very unsteady in his gait, with a tendency to fall backwards. His mind was clear and muscularity good; special senses normal, except hearing. On trying his sense of rotation it was found to be entirely gone. He could not detect the direction in which he was rotated, nor did it give rise to any sense of vertigo. He could not walk along a line foot over foot; his balance very easily lost, a slight push sending him over.

Here was a fracture of the base, involving both labyrinths. The eyes and sense of touch had assumed the duties of the semicircular canals, although imperfectly.

In this paper I have only referred to the tactile factor, having, as I mentioned at the beginning, dealt with vertigo, mainly from the ocular and labyrinthine standpoint.

As a last word, I may just mention the course of the sensory afferent fibres through the posterior column, through the olivary and restiform bodies to the cerebellum. Bechtereus section of the olivary bodies produced disturbances of equilibrium.

Retrospect Department.

QUARTERLY RETROSPECT OF SURGERY

By FRANCIS J. SHEPHERD, M.D., C.M., M.R.C.S., ENG.

Surgeon to the Montreal General Hospital; Professor of Anatomy and Lecturer on Operative Surgery, McGill University.

The Treatment of Scrofulous Glands.—With the advent of aseptic surgery and improved surgical methods, the treatment of scrofulous glands has undergone a great change. Where formerly glands were left to nature to effect a cure, they are now removed before they have broken down and before the surrounding tissues are infiltrated with inflammatory products. Formerly the disease lasted for years, ugly sinuses continued discharging, and the scars left were most unsightly. Now, even if sinuses exist, they are opened up, the remains of the altered glands tissue, which is their cause, scraped out with sharp spoons, and the result as a rule is most favorable. Still, in some cases, when the general health of the patient is poor, and where glands rapidly break down, favorable results do not always follow, the infection spreads from gland to gland, and unless the operation be most complete and radical, the last condition of the patient is worse than the first. Of late much attention has been directed to this subject.

There are still surgeons who support the let alone treatment, others favor erasion, while others again say that the knife is the only method whereby the disease may be entirely and permanently got rid of.

Mr. Fred Treves formerly advocated cautery puncture and rest by means of a stiff neck splint; now he has discarded the cautery puncture, and resorts entirely to the knife when practicable, using the short spoon for the treatment of old sinuses and cavities, which, of course, cannot be

excised. The cautery puncture he has entirely discarded, ex—
cept to open suppurating glands (*Lancet*, Sept. 21, 1889). I⁃
is most important to remember when speaking of the surgical
treatment of tuberculous glands of the neck, that so slight an
operation as erasion and scraping out of a gland may be followed
by a general infection. Not a few surgeons who have treated
scrofulous glands of the neck will be able to record cases of the
kind. It is also well to remember that some cases of tuberculous
disease of the glands cannot be treated to a successful conclusion
by surgical methods alone. In some cases the general system
must be improved by hygienic means, good food, sea air, &c.
Drugs seem to have but little effect, though many practitioners
seem to rely almost entirely on syrup of the iodide of iron.
Whilst treating the glands it is well to look at the original cause,
such as a tonsillitis, carious teeth, eczema, nasal trouble, &c.

In the *Lancet* for September 28th and October 5th, Mr. W.
Knight Treves has an excellent article on the " *Diagnosis and
Treatment of Scrofulous Glands*." After giving the diagnostic
points between simple adenitis, lymphadenoma and scrofulous
glands, he goes on to describe the various physical conditions in
which scrofulous glands may be found, such as soft elastic gland
growth without inflammatory action, hard glands with degenerated tissue, generally caseous ; suppurating glands, calcareous
degeneration, &c. They may be movable or attached ; in fact,
scrofulous glands afford infinite variety in their form, course and
duration, no two cases being alike. Two requirements are
necessary, viz., to establish the general health and to remove
thoroughly and completely the local disease. To establish the
general health, the patient should be out in all weathers, have
the benefit of the sea air, generous diet, wine, iron, cod liver
oil, quinine, no worry or fatigue, should sleep in large airy rooms,
and wear light warm woollen underclothing. Sea bathing is also
advised. As regards drugs, Mr. Treves has no faith in them ;
he has seen perchloride of mercury in small doses produce a
temporary improvement by reducing surrounding inflammatory
deposit and no other drug has done as much. He holds that the
local disease can only be got rid of in one way, and that is by

mechanical means. The first indication in local treatment is to remove all sources of local irritation, excise tonsils if enlarged, extract decayed teeth, etc.

Local treatment to be successful must be thorough. It is a mistake to meddle with scrofulous glands unless we can get the whole thing away. The knife is the only instrument with which diseased glands can be completely removed.

Mr. Treves says scooping is chiefly applicable to two conditions of disease, viz., limited superficial gland enlargements, which have uniformly softened, and old fistulous tracts kept open by withered caseated glands. It is also useful in scraping away rotten skin, old inflammatory deposits and cleaning up generally. In removing glands, the skin incisions should be free and generally over the mass. If glands are enlarged beneath the sterno mastoid, an anterior and posterior incision in the line of the muscle is needed, and sometimes two incisions, if the glands be adherent to the vessels. Nothing is more dangerous than trying to extract glands through an insufficient incision. By perseverance, masses of caseous glands can be separated from vessels to which they are adherent. The author does not advocate sewing up the incisions, he prefers to keep the flaps together by sponges or antiseptic wool. Absolute rest must follow the operation ; the head must be fixed by sand-bags, and there must be no mastication.

For years Mr. Treves has operated on scrofulous glands, sometimes removing as many as one hundred at a sitting, in others excising a mass of glands so large as to threaten suffocation, and yet he has never lost a case. He attributes this success to never having prematurely closed the wound.

The Treatment of Surgical Tuberculosis.—Since the discovery of the bacillus of tubercle by Koch, tuberculosis has been classed amongst the infective diseases. The fact that certain individuals are more predisposed to the attacks of bacillus than others does not alter the case, for under certain conditions persons not predisposed may yield to the attack of this microbe. At the Paris Congress of 1888, strong resolutions were passed relative to the destruction of all flesh belonging to tuberculous animals, and it expressed a wish that tuberculosis be includad in the sanitary laws of all countries in the world amongst the contagious diseases, requiring special prophylactic measures.

In the human being when tuberculosis exists, it is important to get rid of it, and so prevent a general infection of the body. In the recent lectures (*Lancet*, July 27, 1889), by Mr. Howard Marsh, he says that so long as tubercle was regarded as a constitutional affection with local munifestations, treatment was directed mainly to the constitution, as it was regarded as useless to remove a mere local manifestation if the essential disease were left behind. With the discovery of the infective nature of tuberculosis and the danger of a limited caseous deposit being a source of total infection for distant organs or for the whole body was impressed on surgeons, and the expediency of the removal of tubercular deposits was discussed. Now, everything was said to depend on micro-organisms, and perhaps this doctrine was carried to greater extent than was warranted by clinical experience. Mr. Howard Marsh, in speaking of hip joint disease, does not believe in the early removal of the tubercular focus, but would limit operative interference to the opening of abscesses, and trusts to prolonged rest with extension and fixation and general hygienic precautious. He gives statistics to show that the danger of general and distal tubercular affection from bone and joint disease has been exaggerated, and that it is known to occur in only about five per cent. of all cases of hip disease. Mr. Marsh thinks the tendency of tubercular disease of bone is to be self-limited and to undergo recovery, suppuration must not be regarded as destructive, but as nature's method of getting rid of dead tubercular matter. The mortality in the operation, he says, is twenty per cent., whereas if the joints are left alone it is only five per cent. I think Mr. Marsh has placed the mortality (20 p c.) rather too high. In the hands of skillful antiseptic men it is certainly not, as far as my experience goes, as great as one in five. If we hold these tubercular processes to be due to a distinct micro-organism and that they are infective, it seems to be more logical to remove the focus of infection than to wait for nature to effect a cure. The utility of operative interference in cases where patients cannot afford a prolonged treatment (such cases as those seen in hospital practice), in my opinion does not admit of a doubt. In knee joint affections and affections of the ankle, the results of operative interference have been brilliant. Of course, we must bear in mind that the later the case is left the more serious is the operation necessary for the removal of the disease and the greater the after deformity.

Immediate and Remote Results of Operations for Local Tubercular Disease.—At the recent Congress of French Surgeons, held in Paris during October last (*Le Semaine Médicale*), M. Guyon read a paper on the above subject. He recorded three cases of tubercular disease of the bladder on which he had operated. One patient had suffered from vesical tubercular disease for two years. After operation he made a good recovery, and has had no recurrence. The second case operated on in April, 1887, died two years after, in July, 1889, of suppurative nephritis ; at the autopsy the left kidney was completely destroyed and the right was deeply involved, but no tubercular growths could be found. The third case was operated on in 1888 for vesical mischief, dating back nine months ; his kidneys were evidently diseased, but, as the patient had painful micturition as many as 100 times during the night, he decided to operate. He operated by the supra-pubic method, scraped and cauterized the ulcer, and greatly relieved the symptoms, so that the patient lived in comfort for a year afterwards. At the autopsy there was not the slightest trace of any return of the tubercular matter. Dr. Guyon said he thought the supra-pubic operation was much the safer. The only case cured was the first, but he believes that he would have cured the others had not the kidney lesion existed. Tubercular disease of the bladder has a very superficial origin (in the mucous membrane) and scraping and application of cautery removes completely the disease.

The Treatment of Erysipelas.—According to the *Therapeutische Monatsch*, Sept. 1889, the treatment of erysipelas by germicides is growing in favor. Carbolic acid is too irritating.

Koch, of Vienna, uses creolin, his formula is one part of creolin, four of iodoform and ten of lanolin.   This is spread on the erysipelatous area, and an inch or two beyond its boundaries, and covered with gutta percha tissue.   The theory is that iodine is set free in the combination, and that it, as well as creolin, acts as a germicide ; the results appear to be good.—(*Vienna Klin. Woch.*, 1889, No. 27.)

Mechanical Treatment of Erysipelas.—Dr. Wölflers, in an article lately published (*Wiener Klin. Woch.*, June 6th, 1889) reports two cases in which the mechanical treatment was unsuccessful, and three in which it was successful.   His treatment is to outline the area of the disease with strips of sticking plaster. He has found that the disease will not pass over these limits. Care should be taken that the strips be closely applied to the skin and the hair should be shaven from the skin.   In facial erysipelas it is advisable to shave over the scalp.   In a case of erysipelas following ulcer of the arm 7 strips of plaster were placed about the wrist, and as the axillary glands seemed already affected, the second strip was placed over the shoulder and along the sides of the thorax, and the limits were completed by a third strip at the waist.   The disease progressed, accompanied by fever, until it reached the sticking plaster, but went no further, the fever ceased and rapid healing followed.   Another case of erysipelas following ulcer of the leg.   The bands of plaster were placed around the thigh.   The disease quickly extended to the first band, and a very slight inflammation extended beyond it, but did not reach the second band ; fever now disappeared, and the ulcer healed.   The third case was one of facial erysipelas.   A strip of plaster around the neck quickly checked the progress of the disease.   The two unsuccessful cases consisted of one of gangrenous erysipelas of the thigh and pelvis, death in twenty-four hours ; and a case of erysipelas of the chest, following an operation for empyema, death in three days.   In the same journal for June 14th, Wölflers records seven additional cases, all of which resulted favorably.

At a meeting of the Suffolk District Medical Society, Dr. J. C. White said that he could get control over erysipelas generally

in three days by simple treatment.   Of 100 cases of ordinary
facial erysipelas, perhaps three would not yield within three
days by simple antiseptic treatment.   Dr. White applies, during alternate hours of the day and evening, a mild
solution of carbolic acid and alcohol as an evaporating
lotion.   It is in only very exceptional circumstances that the
disease is not under control or has disappeared within forty-
eight hours, but it would astonish him if every vestige of the
disease had not disappeared in three days.   He has treated
erysipelas in this way for many years, and has never known it
to fail.   He speaks of ordinary cutaneous erysipelas only, not
the phlegmnaous variety.   He uses a formula of acid carbolic
crystals, 3p., alcohol and water ʒiv.—(*Boston Medical and
Surgical Journal*, June 13th, 1889.)

In an article on the "*Surgical Treatment of Erysipelas in
Children*," Dr. A Siebert (*N.Y. Medical Journal*, Oct. 19th,
1889), says that to open inflamed skin by numerous incisions
made all over the diseased surface, and then to cover the part
with antiseptic lotion, has been practised for some time with
·moderate success.   So has also the injection, hypodermically, of
a 2 per cent. solution of acid carbolic into the healthy skin surrounding the inflamed part.   Kraske's method was the first
step in the right direction.   He made regular incisions in the
border of the erysipelas extending into the healthy skin, and he
crossed these diagonally with others.   The object was to give a
good chance to the cocci to get to the surface and come in contact with the antiseptic fluid which was applied to the skin ; the
dressing was constantly moistened with the antiseptic fluid for a
few days.   The results were excellent.   Riedel and Lauenstein
(*Deutsch Med. Woch*, for Oct. 19th, 1889) proposed to improve
Kraske's method by locating the incisions entirely in the healthy
tissue, about one to two inches away from the border of the
erysipelas.   This was to avoid possible infection of the aseptic
tissue.   This modification has given better results than any
other method.   The patients were usually put under an anæsthetic, and the whole operation performed antiseptically.   Dr.
Siebert has used this method in three cases in children, with the

result of limiting the spread of the affection.   He does not put the patient under ether, but uses the " vaccination harrow," and so does away with objections parents have to the employment of anæsthetics.

Physiological Resistance of the Peritoneum to Infection.— During the past year Rinne (*Archiv für Klin. Chir.*, 1889) has made some most interesting experiments in surgical pathology.   Practically and clinically it has been demonstrated that the peritoneal cavity, under certain unknown circumstances, has the power of taking care of a vast amount of filth.   Rinne has found that large quantities of septic material and pure cultures of pyogenic bacteria were absorbed although injected daily into the peritoneal cavity of animals, provided the peritoneal surface was uninjured.   The injections produced only mild symptoms in direct proportion to the quantity of septic material used, and in no case was there more than a moderate rise of temperature. The results were very different when there were coincident defects in the peritoneum exposing the sub-peritoneal tissue to infection.   Then there invariably appeared progressive suppurative peritonitis going out from the infected connective tissue, which usually terminated fatally.   The practical import of these experiments can hardly be over-estimated.   They explain why the escape of pus into the peritoneal cavity, from the rupture of a pyosalpinx, is not necessarily fatal if the tube is promptly extirpated and the wound and stump properly treated.   They point out that the incision is the point of general danger in all abdominal operations, and they indicate that too great care cannot be exercised in bringing accurately together the peritoneal edges of the wound.   They explain why the removal of abdominal tumors is so much more dangerous after adhesions have taken place, because the resulting denuded spots offer less resistance to the invasion of septic bacteria.   They explain the success of those operators who disregard the dictation of scientific bacteriology, and also the recovery of patients after abdominal section by horned animals.   They teach us to consider cautiously the evidence presented by statistics of operators and await the demonstration of more exact methods as to the import of their results. They warn us that clinical evidence is inadequate to overthrow the deductions of experimental physiology and pathology, and that our time is provided with methods of precision which are yet imperfectly improved. The resisting and absorptive power of the peritoneum is beyond that of any other serous cavity (*Journal of the American Medical Association*, Oct. 17th, 1889).

Surgery of the Liver.—Mr. Lawson Tait has a very interesting paper on the above subject (*Edinburgh Medical Journal*, October and November, 1889), in which, in his characteristic and forcible way, he gives the history of this branch of surgery, and details his own experience, which consists in seventeen cases of exploratory incision with one death; seventeen cases of hepatotomy with two deaths, and fifty-five cases of cholecystotomy with three deaths—a remarkable record. Petit was the first to describe the operation of cholecystotomy as now performed, yet his description of the operation was unnoticed for 150 years until Marion Sims put it into actual practice in 1878. The result in this case was fatal. In 1879 Mr. Tait successfully performed the operation on a woman aged 40. The patient is still alive. Of the fifty-five cases performed by him, fifty-two were successful, one old woman died of a suffocative catarrh some weeks after the wound was healed, two others died of cancer of the liver, which was, in all probability, the cause of the. distended gall bladder, for no gall stones were found. In not a single instance did a patient die from the operation. All the other patients, with one exception, were in perfect health at the time the article was written. Mr. Tait's method of performing the operation of cholecystotomy is well known. He stitches the distended bladder to the abdominal wound and then incises it, evacuates the fluid, and removes the stones, leaving a drainage tube in the gall bladder. He condemns the practice advocated by Sir Spencer Wells, of opening the gall bladder, removing the calculi, and then closing the wound in the gall-bladder by continuous suture without attaching it to the abdominal wall. As far as Mr. Tait knows, the method has been fatal in every instance where it has been tried.

Mr. Tait says it is generally supposed that gall stones form in the gall bladder, but this is not true, for the nuclei of gall-stones are found in the streams of bile as they flow through the substance of the liver.   In fact he has cut gall-stones out of abscesses in the substance of the liver.   Gall–stone is not a disease of the gall-bladder at all.   Mr. Tait says that if this be true there is no justification for the removal of the gall-bladder, except in cases where it is greatly thickened and suppurating, and that these are the very cases where it is an impossible operation. The one argument against cholecystotomy, viz., that biliary fistulæ remain occasionally and permanently, is an argument of much greater force against the removal of the gall-bladder, and the so-called operation of cholecystectomy, for such a fistula, after cholecystotomy, must be due to the fact that the operation had been performed at a time when a gall-stone or gall-stones had become impacted in the common duct.   In several of such cases Mr. Tait has crushed this obstructing gall-stone, and has thus succeeded in clearing the common duct.   In one case (the exception alluded to above) he succeeded in crushing one stone. At the post-mortem held seven years after, both cystic and common ducts were found obstructed from one end to the other, and the result was the patient had a permanent fistula.   She lived comfortably four or five years, and finally died of phthisis. In such a case the removal of the gall-bladder would have been the very worst proceeding possible.

Mr. Mayo Robson has recently been successful in making a connection between the gall-bladder and adjacent coil of intestine, and in this way the trouble of a biliary fistula was avoided. However, most of these cases may be avoided by the operation of cholelithotrity, that is, make a fresh opening in the abdomen and crush the stone outside the walls of the duct by means of padded forceps.

Tait divides gall-stones into two varieties, viz , " solitary " gall stones and " numerous" gall stones.   The "solitary" is not always quite solitary, but it has rarely more than one companion. The "numerous" gall-stones are practically indefinite in number, are usually uniform and not of large size.   Several interesting cases are detailed. In one the abdomen was opened for a supposed par-ovarian cyst. The cyst was opened and found to be a distended gall-bladder ; the opening was enlarged, the hand introduced, and a large gall-stone, which was imparted in the neck of the bladder, removed ; the opening in the gall-bladder was stitched to the abdominal walls, and a drainage tube inserted ; bile began to flow on the morning of the third day. The woman made a perfect recovery.

Disappearance of Tumours after Exploratory Incision.—In the second article on the surgery of the liver, Mr. Tait begins by saying that there are certain diseases, in some instances unknown, which seem to yield to surgical treatment applied to them by accident. He says that he has, on more than one occasion, drawn attention to the astonishing disappearance of tumours, often of large size, after a mere exploratory incision. The absolute silence with which these statements have been received by the profession has surprised Mr. Tait. They are true enough, and the experience of others in the future will substantiate them. The cases in which he has seen tumours disappear in this way are chiefly cases of diseases of the liver, spleen and head of the pancreas. He has seen others where the exact site of the origin of the growths could not be accurately ascertained. Mr. Tait is satisfied, from the number of these cases seen by him, that the disappearance is not a mere co-incidence ; he is convinced that the mere opening of the peritoneal cavity has a direct influence in setting up the process of absorption of the tumour, and this conviction has increased his confidence in the principle of exploration. That some physiological change is at once set up by opening the peritoneal cavity is clearly indicated by the uniform onset of a most distressing thirst, which lasts for days, and is not seen so markedly after any other operation. In operations down to the serous cavity this thirst does not occur, but let the serous cavity be opened but a finger's breadth and the result is marked.

A number of remarkable cases of exploratory incision for tumours, &c., of the abdomen are narrated, in which the tumours disappeared, although apparently of a malignant nature. One very remarkable case was that of a lady aged 54, who was the subject of symptoms strongly pointing to the possibility of gall-stones ; Mr. Tait's own impression, however, was that she was suffering from cancer of the liver. An exploratory incision was made ; the liver was found scattered with large hard nodules, one of which closely imitated the lump which had led to the diagnosis of distended gall bladder· No doubt was expressed at the time of operation that this was a case of cancer of the liver. At all events, the patient was cured and is at the present time perfectly well.

Four times Mr. Tait has opened the abdomen for the purpose of removing enlarged spleens, and in every case he has been deterred from proceeding with the operation by reason of the hopelessness of the outlook for the patient. Strange to say, in three of the four cases the tumour has disappeared, and they are now in perfect health. The fourth succumbed to the explor-atory incision.

In another case he explored a tumour which appeared to be in the position of the head of the pancreas, in a lady who had become much emaciated, and was supposed to be suffering from cancer. The exploratory incision resulted in the complete dis-appearance of the tumour in five or six weeks, and restoration to former state of health.

Abscesses and Hydatids of the Liver.—Mr. Tait thinks modern surgery is to be congratulated upon the distinct advance it has made in the treatment of abscesses of the liver, and hydatid tumours of that organ. Mr. Tait has on seventeen occa-sions deliberately attacked these two diseases by abdominal section, and in fifteen cases he was completely successful. He was the first to remove hydatid tumour by opening the tissue of the liver, and reports his first case operated on in 1879. The patient recovered without a bad symptom. His method is to incise the liver and stitch its edges to the abdominal wound and put in a drainage tube.

Mr. Tait is perfectly sure that there are two varieties of hydatid cysts. The more common is the large single cyst, formed of gelatinous layers easily stripped from one another, the fluid is limpid and free ; these are the cysts that are sometimes cured by tapping. The other variety is the multiple variety, where the cysts are numerous, and vary in size from a pin's point to that of a cocoanut ; they lie packed together in a cavity of the liver, which is not lined by a sac, and in the wall of each of these cysts there are fastened to the base enormous numbers of scolices of another tape worm. In this class of cases the liver ruptures and the hydatids are poured out loose into the cavity of the peritoneum, and then they penetrate the tissues in all directions.

When the author first attacked the liver by surgical operation he was in terror of hemorrhage, for he thought that if an incision opened a large sinus, the arrest of hemorrhage would be a matter of considerable difficulty, but he once, while performing ovariotomy, accidentally tore the edge of the liver and free hemorrhage took place, which was immediately checked by the application of a small piece of solid perchloride of iron. In another case where he incised a large sinus in the liver, he passed a thread down one side of it and up the other, and tied the sinus, thus completely and easily arresting the hemorrhage.

In his operation upon abscesses of the liver all the cases have recovered, with one exception. He treats these cases of abscess like any other cyst. He sutures the edges of the liver to the abdominal wound and drains ; the stitches always hold well, and he thinks there is no need of procuring adhesion between the peritoneal surface of the abdominal wall and the wall surface of the liver, and that operations may be done at one sitting with as great readiness upon the liver as upon any other organ in the abdomen.

Lumbar Cholecystotomy.—In the last volume of *The Transactions of the American Surgical Association*, Dr. Mears, of Philadelphia, reports the case of a woman, aged 29, who was admitted to the hospital for the operation of nephrorraphy, or fixation of the kidney. She had a rounded tumor about the size of the kidney lying a little to the right of the median line at the junction of the hypogastric and umbilical regions. The tumor was freely movable in all directions. A vertical lumbar incision

Robson spoke of the difficulty of operation in those cases where the gall-bladder was shrunken, and where it could not be attached to the abdominal wall. In one case he sutured a piece of omentum, on the one hand to the gall-bladder, and on the other to the parietal peritoneum, thus shutting off the general peritoneal cavity. This method of omental grafting was suggested by the operations of Dr. Senn.

Mr. Robson said that, with due care, he thought the operation of cholecystotomy was attended with comparatively little danger, provided there was no malignant disease.

Mr. Knowsley Thornton said it was not always easy to distinguish between a distended gall-bladder and a tumor of the kidney, and cases where there were thick adhesions around the gall-bladder, with suppuration, were difficult to diagnose. If the gall-bladder was distinct, the operation was easy. If the stone had passed into the cystic duct, the operation was difficult. It was a good plan in such cases to break up the stone by needling it. In one case he had slit up the common duct, removed the stone, then stitched up the duct; the patient recovered. He considered artificial connection of the gall-bladder with the intestine a radically wrong procedure, inasmuch as the opening in the bowel wall was likely soon to close.

Mr. Thornton agrees with the German surgeons and, notwithstanding the opinion of Mr. Tait, thinks that cholecystectomy is the operation of the future. It causes no more risk to the patient and effectually prevents another stone from blocking up the cystic duct.

Mr. Barker mentioned a case where he had operated and had only found a distended gall-bladder with some hardening of the head of the pancreas ; he had closed the wound, and the patient was quickly better and recovered perfectly.

Sir Joseph Lister's New Antiseptic Dressing.—At a meeting of the Medical Society of London, held November 4th, 1889, Sir Joseph Lister delivered an important address on a new antiseptic dressing (*Lancet*, Nov. 9th and 16th, 1889). The author described his laborious and painstaking search for a new and more reliable surgical dressing. The address is characteristic

of the man, and the story it tells is a revelation of scientific
acumen, perseverance and minute attention to detail, which are
required for such work; it also displays a wide and practical
knowledge of chemistry. This subject has engaged the illustrious
surgeon during the last five years, the last report he made was
about his bi-chloride of mercury, when he showed that it formed
a compound with mercury, which was soluble in blood serum, and
he brought forward a serum sublimate gauze. This not proving
entirely satisfactory, Sir Joseph sought for new agents, and
experimented with the double chloride of ammonium and mercury, called sal alembroth. This was a good antiseptic, and less
irritating than bi-chloride, but again objections cropped up, for
the compound was soluble not only in water, but in serum, so
another series of experiments was made with cyanide of
mercury. This was found high as to inhibitory, but low in germicidal, power; it was also irritating and very soluble. The double
cyanides were next tried.   Mr. Martindale suggested one of
the insoluble double cyanides of mercury and zinc, and this
compound has proved superior to all substances hitherto used.
There are several of these double cyanides; there seems to be
some doubt as to the precise compound which exists in the preparation of cyanide of mercury and zinc, but it is certain that
the mercury in it is an important, though not in quantity a
large, factor.   The very ingenious method by which, after
many trials, the substance was incorporated with starch, with
which it forms a kind of combination whereby it can be affixed
to gauze so neatly that in the dry state it does not dust off and
in the wet state it does not wash away.   Sir Joseph looks upon
the gauze as a perfect success; it is antiseptic, porous, permanent
and non-irritating.   The double cyanide of zinc and mercury
was not at first successful, and some early difficulties caused it
to be abandoned.   Then iodide of mercury was tried, because
it was an antiseptic and sparingly soluble in water.   It is more
soluble in blood serum, but then it is very irritating, and
difficult to fix in the gauze; the latter objection was removed by
the starch, then used for the first time.   Here, as with the
double cyanide, a loose kind of molecular combination seems to

take place and the iodide does not dust off, but the experiment was not satisfactory so he went back to the double cyanides.

In wounds about the head or hairy parts, the cyanide moistened with a weak solution of corrosive sublimate may be rubbed into the hairy parts, when it will convert the hairs into an antiseptic dressing. In conclusion, the author says that there are those who still believe that the use of antiseptic substances in surgical practice is always useless, if not injurious. The germ theory of septic diseases is indeed now happily established incontrovertibly. All now admit that septic mischief in our wounds depends on the development of micro-organisms in them derived from without. But the gentlemen to whom Sir Joseph refers are disposed to trust everything to the antiseptic powers of human tissues. Sir Joseph was the first to direct attention to the antiseptic properties of living structures ; without it surgery in former days would have been absolutely impossible. Still he knows too well from experience that it cannot always be trusted, and that the use of antiseptic adjuncts is in the highest degree important. He again says, " I have the satisfaction of knowing that there is among you a constantly increasing number who, when they have operated on unbroken skin with a fair field around for the application of their dressings, if they see septic inflammation occurring in the wound with its attendant dangers, know that it is their fault or the fault of the antiseptic dressings at their disposal. To those among you who are impressed with this conviction, I offer the dressing which I have described as the most satisfactory that I have hitherto met with."

The Construction of a New Bladder after Excision.—At the Surgical Congress recently held at Bologna, Professor G. Tizzoni, of the University of Bologna, and A. Poggi, gave an account of some experiments they had made on dogs, with a view of ascertaining whether the bladder could be removed and an efficient substitute constructed by operation. First of all laparotomy was performed, and a loop of small intestine about 7 centimetres in length, with its mesentery attached, was isolated by two transverse cuts, washed out with a carbolized

solution and tied at both ends, one extremity being fixe
front of the neck of the bladder. The two ends of the divi
gut were then stitched accurately together by circular sutu
The dog soon recovered from the operation, and a month l
the second stage of the operation was performed. The uret
were separated from the bladder and the latter was complet
removed. The loop of intestine destined to be the new bladd
was then cut across at the lower end and then stitched to
neck of the bladder. The ureters were then turned into t
artificial bladder. A slender elastic drainage tube was plac
in the urethra to carry off the urine during the first few days. T
animal recovered perfectly, and gradually acquired control ov
its new bladder, and when shown to the congress two month
later showed no signs of incontinence. The operation has bee
repeated with success on several animals, and Drs. Tizzoni and
Poggi are hopeful it may be applicable to the human subject.—
(*London Medical Recorder*).

Trephining the Sacro-Iliac Joint.—Mr. Mayo Collier,
(*Lancet*, Oct. 19, 1889), reports a case of sacro-iliac disease
successfully treated by trephining. The case was a lady aged
34, who had suffered for some four years from pains in and
about the right hip and lameness. She was treated for ovarian
irritation by massage, etc. Mr. Collier diagnosed the affection;
the patient had a tuberculous family history; pain was complained of on walking or sitting on right tuber ischii, pain on
coughing, on deep iliac pressure, and when the ilia were pressed
together; pain was also marked on pressing immediately over
the joint behind. Thomas' splint did not relieve the case, so
Mr. Collier decided to trephine the joint from outside. A
curved incision eight inches long parallel with and an inch
below the posterior third of the crest of the ilium and descending vertically over the joint, exposed the bone sufficiently. The
bone was next denuded with the elevator, and now was seen to
be distinctly swollen and inflamed. A line being drawn from
the anterior superior spinous process to the posterior, two
inches were measured from this posteriorly. The pin of the
trephine was placed on the line so that the edge of the circle

should be on the two inch line. The joint was rapidly penetrated. It was found denuded of cartilage and the bone was eroded. The diseased structures were removed with gouge and mallet and the joint swabbed with chloride of zinc (40 grs. to the ounce) ; a large drain was introduced. The patient rapidly recovered and in six months was able to return to her home in South Africa.

Healing of Aseptic Bone Cavities.—Dr. N. Senn, (*American Journal of the Medical Sciences*, September, 1889), has a most interesting article on the healing of bone cavities. Neuber, of Kiel, some years ago introduced a method of implantation of skin flaps, after chiselling or gouging the bone sufficiently to allow the soft parts to be brought into contact with the floor of the cavity. These flaps were fastened securely into position with bone nails and in many cases primary union resulted. Schede and others also attempted to secure healing under aseptic moist bloodclot, and good results have been obtained, but also there have been many failures. Dr. Senn substitutes for the bloodclot aseptic decalcified bone chips ; they are absorbable, firm, and form a good scaffold upon which granulations can be supported. He made a number of experiments on dogs before applying the method to man. The results have been apparently satisfactory. In operations on the skull he fits an aseptic bone-disk into the trephine opening ; this arrests hemorrhage from the bone and prevents adhesions between the dura mater and external parts, it is gradually absorbed, a mass of granulations takes it place, and the defect is closed by dense cicatricial tissue or by bone. The disk is perforated for the purpose of drainage and to allow the granulations to penetrate easily. For the healing of bone cavities, chips of decalcified bone are used, after thorough disinfection of the cavity and dusting the bone chips and cavity with iodoform, the decalcified bone is rendered thoroughly aseptic and antiseptic by keeping it immersed in sublimate alchohol (1 500). The wound is completely closed with the exception of the lower angle where a capillary drain of a few threads of catgut is introduced. Rapid healing takes place in one or two dressings, with entire restoration of the continuity of the bone.

His conclusions are,—

(1). Antiseptic decalcified bone is the best substitute for living bone grafts in the restoration of a loss of substance in bone.

(2). Implantation of a bone disk into a trephine hole may be relied on as a hemostatic measure in arresting hemorrhage from the vessels of the diploe, and is a good temporary substitute for the lost portion of cranium.

(3). The packing of an aseptic bone cavity with antiseptic bone chips guards against unnecessary loss of blood and prevents infection by pus microbes.

(4). Capilliary drainage should be established after implantation to remove the accumulation of more blood in the wound than is necessary to form a temporary cement between the bone chips and surrounding tissues.

(5). Packing by bone chips acts as an antiseptic tampon.

6). Secondary implantation can be successfully carried out in treating a suppurating bone cavity after suppuration has ceased, and the cavity can be transformed into the same favourable conditions for healing as an aseptic wound.

Hospital Reports.

MONTREAL GENERAL HOSPITAL.

CONDENSED REPORTS OF CASES IN DR. MACDONNELL'S WARDS.*

October 4th.—The session has opened with an unusual number of instructive cases in the clinical wards. During the fortnight previous to the opening of the session, five of the beds were occupied by cases of pleurisy with effusion. In four, early aspiration was resorted to and with satisfactory results. One of the cases, that of a man of 30, was interesting from the fact of the fluid having escaped notice for a long time, and from the length of time the patient went about with one side of his chest completely full of fluid and his heart apex displaced to the right of the sternum. Another patient in a similar condition walked to the hospital from the end of St. Antoine street. In one case the fluid partially disappeared spontaneously.

On the 30th September a very interesting case of pleurisy was brought in. Here the cause was traumatic, the patient having had a large stone fall upon his chest some six weeks ago. The distension of the right pleural cavity was extreme. The heart beat two inches beyond the nipple line, and the liver could be felt two inches beyond the costal border. Dyspnœa was very urgent. The temperature was slightly raised. Aspiration showed the presence of pus, and, accordingly, resection of a rib was performed by Dr. James Bell.

The internal treatment of these cases of pleurisy with effusion has consisted of the administration of iodide of potash three times a day, and of concentrated doses of sulphate of magnesia in the morning.

TYPHOID FEVER.

The cases this year have been of much greater severity than those we have been accustomed to meet, and the mortality has been high. The following notes may prove interesting :—

High Temperature.—A very severe case, occurring in a strong, healthy servant maid, showed a tendency to hyperpyrexia. The thermometer registered 104½° to 105½° for the

---

* I am indebted for the reports from which the following are condensed to Drs. England and Campbell, house-physicians, and to my clinical clerks Messrs. Adams, Hamilton, Bowes, Murray, McKechnie and Inksetter.

first four days, and neither antipyrin nor antifebrin had any effect whatever. After the first week in hospital the fever abated. There were three distinct rigors on the twentieth day, for which no cause could be found. The patient eventually recovered.

Meteorism.—In the case of a strong man of thirty, who was brought to the hospital in about the middle of the fever, delirium having been very severe before admission, meteorism developed to an extraordinary degree. The abdomen became greatly distended, and brought such pressure upon the chest as to increase the respirations to 56 and to displace the heart and liver. The passage of a long rubber tube brought away a quantity of gas and gave temporary relief. We found it a good plan to leave the long tube in the bowel. However, we failed to avert the fatal result. The autopsy showed that death was the result of typhoid fever without any perforation or peritonitis.

Delirium Ferox.— A Hungarian, aged 35, was brought to hospital in a state of wild delirium, and became so unmanageable that it was necessary to lodge him in the padded room. The diagnosis was very doubtful, but after a few days the high temperature and the character of the evacuations enabled us to decide upon the nature of the case. Murchison mentions just such another case. He was called in to see a German gentleman, who was supposed to be mad. After four days of slight malaise, which had attracted little notice, he passed suddenly into a state of acute maniacal delirium, requiring two men to hold him down in bed. He was thought to be suffering from an attack of insanity, but with these symptoms there was pyrexia, quick pulse, temp. 102°, dry tongue, diarrhœa, but no spots.

Profuse Rash.—The case of a workman from Lachine is notable from the profuseness of the rash. Upon the chest and abdomen the general appearance reminds one of measles. The symptoms were very severe, the system being apparently overwhelmed by the intensity of the poison. There was deep stupor and incontinence of urine and fæces. At the time of death the rash was distributed over all the body.

Syncopal Attacks.—A female patient, one of those from Point St. Charles, suffered in the beginning of the fever from several attacks of fainting. Stimulants were freely used and recovery from the fever took place, though very slowly. I lost a patient some years ago from sudden and unexpected syncope in the course of typhoid fever. This mode of death has been reported as occurring in acute pneumonia, and in diphtheria it is a common occurrence.

ANTERIOR POLIOMYELITIS ACUTA.

An interesting case of this disease was that of Maggie L., aged 14, who was admitted on the 14th July with sudden loss of power in the left leg. The family history was somewhat neurotic, a sister having suffered greatly from chorea. Six days before admission she was obliged to give up work, owing to a great sense of fatigue. Twenty-four hours afterwards, after walking a short distance, her left leg became quite powerless. She had to be carried home, and has been unable to walk since. There was no loss of consciousness and no pain.

State on Admission.—Marked anæmia; slight pyrexia, the evening temperature running not higher than 100° for the first few nights; slight headache and loss of appetite. There was double vision on the day before the first attack. Pain was never present. All four limbs were enfeebled, as well as the muscles of the back, but in a different degree. The left leg was completely paralysed and its knee reflex abolished, but sensation was unimpaired. The right leg could be feebly moved, and its knee reflex was not quite absent. Superficial reflexes are absent in both lower extremities; no ankle clonus. At the time of admission the hospital batteries were undergoing repair, so that electrical tests could not be applied. However, shortly afterwards it was found that there was no response to the faradic current and a feeble one to the constant in all but the left leg. The weakness extended from the left leg to the right leg, to the left arm and hand, then to the right arm and hand. Lastly, the neck and back muscles became affected. The sphincters and muscles supplied by cranial nerves were never affected.

October 7th.—The patient has now been in hospital over two months, and there is considerable improvement. The anæmia has diminished, general nutrition is improved, and the paralysis has disappeared, the change for the better being most noticeable in the muscles of the back, which seem to have been the first to recover, but in the left leg there is no change. There is at present no muscular atrophy, but probably this may be deceptive, owing to the fatness of the patient.

URÆMIA.

October 9th.—There are three cases of uræmia in ward 11, each showing prominently a special feature of that condition. On the evening of the 7th of October a man, aged apparently about 50, was brought to the hospital by the police in a state of profound coma. The breath was not alcoholic. The small quantity of urine which was withdrawn by the catheter was heavily loaded with albumen. He was well purged with croton oil, and put into a hot air bath. Subsequently, pilocarpin was given by hypodermic injection (gr. 1-6) with a very good result. Convulsions had occurred also. In twenty-four hours the coma had disappeared, but he was still in a very stupid condition, unable to speak and breathing noisily, owing to the flapping of his lips. To-day, *i.e.*, 48 hours after admission, there is still great mental confusion, though he is able to say his name. At the clinic it was noticed that the respiration, which had previously been noted as slow, had now a rhthymic character, and was inclined to be of the Cheyne-Stokes variety.

October 10th.—The improvement was but transient, the convulsions recurred with increased violence and death ensued.

It was confidently expected that marked renal changes would be found at the autopsy, but such was not the case. No cause of death was found, unless the kidneys were diseased to an extent merely recognizable with the microscope. The symptoms present, the convulsions, the coma, the scanty urine loaded with albumen, rendered any other diagnosis than that of uræmia highly improbable. The body being unclaimed, it was injected with preservative fluid before the kidneys were removed, and consequently their finer structure could not be examined, but they were of normal size and appearance.

What was the cause of the convulsions and the coma? 1. There is a slight chance of its being due to early renal changes. 2. A poison, e. g., alcohol or opium,—against this interpretation is the fact of his complete recovery from the original coma and the recurrence of the convulsions.

The second case showed evidences of uræmia in a milder degree. The patient had had evidences of chronic Bright's disease for some years, dating from an acute nephritis nine years ago, which directly followed an attack of erysipelas. At present there are albuminuria, hyaline casts, and general dropsy, but the most important symptoms are the persistent frontal headache and the attacks of vomiting to which he is subject.

The third case, that of a baker, aged 34, was also one of chronic uræmia, and its principal manifestation was extreme dyspnœa. At first there was orthopnœa, but after a few days treatment this subsided. There was no dropsy. The patient for a long period had regarded himself as an asthmatic. It was difficult to determine whether these attacks were due to true asthma or were merely evidences of uræmia.

PROGRESSIVE MUSCULAR ATROPHY.

Two cases have been in hospital lately. The first case, that of a woman long past middle life, illustrates two points in connection with the etiology of the disease, its origin in fright, and its occurrence in members of the same family. The wasting began two years ago, immediately after she had experienced a shipwreck on the Atlantic. Eight years ago she had been under my treatment at the Montreal Dispensary for ulceration about the knee, which was thought to be syphilitic. The family history is interesting. The father died from the effects of an accident; the mother, an uncle and an aunt all died of "paralytic strokes." Two sisters of the patient died at the ages of 47 and 50, having suffered from a disease said to be exactly similar to that of the patient.

The occurrence of progressive muscular atrophy in families has been reported. Recently, the following notices of this point have fallen under my observation. In the last number of the *Revue des Sciences Médicales*, Lichtheim reports the history of a family of four brothers, three of whom suffered from progressive muscular atrophy; and in the same journal there are two other histories of families—in one two sisters developed the disease shortly after puberty. In a history reported by Herringham in *Brain*, the family tree, representing five generations, shows that 19 male members were atrophic; the remainder, to the number of forty-six, including all the women of the family, entirely escaped.

An interesting family tree will be found in a paper by Dr. Osler in *Seguin's Archives* for 1881.

The second case did not show such marked symptoms. The wasting and the loss of power began after an illness, which was characterized by pain in the stomach and vomiting. The wasting was very rapid. The patient was a street car driver, and suffered much hardship in the spring from the exposure to cold and wet incidental to his calling. He had been three months ill previously to admission. The right arm and shoulder first became weak, and there were such sensations as pricking, tingling and formication, and the symptoms extended to the forearm and hand. Within two days the left arm and hand became similarly affected. In two weeks the legs became affected, but to a much less degree. There was considerable pain and tenderness on pressure in the calves of the legs and the inner side of the thighs. The upper extremities are much wasted, the lower less so. There is dull pain in the arm and shoulder on both sides and exaggerated tenderness of the muscles of the arm and forearm. The extensors of the fingers and thumb are wasted, but there is no wrist drop. Patellar reflexes are normal. Fibrillar tremors are elicited by percussion over the shoulder muscles.

After a month's residence in hospital there was marked improvement.

Nov. 5th.--The progress of this case is such that a diagnosis of progressive muscular atrophy cannot be entertained. Improvement is distinct. Most probably it is a sub-acute poliomyelitis, and the sharpness of the attack at the outset rather favours that view.

Aortic Aneurism.—In the case of a man aged 50, a lumberman, there are well-marked evidences of the presence of an aneurysm of the ascending and transverse arch. The patient applied first to Dr. Major, the laryngologist, for the relief of his hoarseness, and was by him referred to me. The left vocal cord was paralysed. An interesting point in the case is the presence, in a very marked degree, of the sign on palpation of tracheal tugging, an evidence that the tumour is in contact with the trachea or one of the large bronchi, and also that consolidation of the contents of the sac has not far advanced. The clanging cough and the dyspnœa have been much relieved since he began the iodide of potassium treatment.

Acute Spinal Meningitis.—Bridget M., aged 10, caught a severe cold on the 11th of August, 1889. Hitherto she had been in very good health. The father is a drunkard, but there is no history of nervous disease in the family. Four days afterwards she had refused to eat her meals, had a severe attack of vomiting, which was followed by constipation and severe headache. For the next three or four days she was very feverish and was said to be delirious. She then seemed to improve slightly, but the gait was staggering and the articulation became thick and indistinct. The mother states that on one occasion she observed that the child was squinting. The patient was admitted to hospital on the 21st August, when she appeared to be in very great suffering. The body was held continually in one position on the side, with the back stiff and the head well retracted. The abdomen was hard and scaphoid. Meningeal streaks were readily obtained. Pressure on the legs caused great pain. Reflex action generally increased ; bowels very constipated, but there is no disturbance in the function of urination ; pulse, 120–140. Respiration (20–24) is somewhat irregular at times, but is not of the Cheyne-Stokes character ; no dyspnœa. During the 85 days of illness the symptoms varied slightly. Emaciation and debility increased. Pupils varied in size at different periods. The fundus, which at first was quite normal, showed optic neuritis a few weeks before death. There were no signs of paralysis. Death occurred before the irritative stage was passed. Patellar reflex disappeared as the disease advanced. There was no continuous vomiting, general headache or paralysis of cranial nerves, hence it was thought that the disease was seated in the spinal and not in the cerebral meninges.

Of the clinical features of the case, the most remarkable is the range of temperature, which appears in rhythmic waves. The first fifty-six days in hospital might, by the chart, be divided into sections of four days each, and on the evening of the first

day of each section the temperature ran to 101° or 102° ; then
on the three remaining days it went down to a lower degree,
until on the fourth night it was normal ; then a rise to 102° and
a gradual fall in the next three days. The pulse was frequent
(120) during the period of elevated temperature, but fell to 90
and 100 when the temperature fell to normal.

The following abstract of the post-mortem changes is furnished
by Dr. Wyatt Johnston, pathologist of the hospital : " Emaciation extreme.   Cerebral ventricles are distended and contain
seven ounces of fluid. Slight turbidity and œdema of pia at base
of brain, not extending along the sylvian fissure. No lymph.
No tubercles found in microscopic examination of the vessels of
the perforated spaces, arteria profunda cerebri, sylvian arteries,
or choroid plexus.   No cerebral pachymeningitis, or disease of
the bones of the skull. Slight optic neuritis. A severe and
extensive pachymeningitis throughout entire spinal canal, involving sheaths of spinal nerve roots.   Abundant fibrinous exudation
between dura and bones, which has partly organized.   Spinal
pia œdematous.   Spinal cord normal, except for slight grey degeneration in postero-internal tracts. Peripheral nerves (sciatic,
ant crural and brachial plexus) in both sides normal. No disease of bones of vertebral column. Localized emphysema of
left lung, with recent pneumothorax. No tubercle anywhere.
Cause of pachymeningitis not detected."

The pleumothorax, I take it, must have immediately brought
about the end, because it is unreasonable to suppose that in the
state of extreme debility in which she passed the last three
weeks of her life, she could have stood the shock of the sudden
entry of air into the pleura.

DISEASES OF THE STOMACH.

Gastric Ulcer (Oct. 31st).—A well defined case of gastric
ulcer, and two of cancer of the stomach, have lately been in the
wards.

The case of ulcer occurred in a young married woman,
aged 23, who entered on the 28th August, with epigastric
pain, aggravated to an intense degree by food, and relieved

by free vomiting. The ejected matter consists of partly digested food and a quantity of slimy mucus, with here and there streaks of blood. These symptoms have been present for the last seven months, and are thought to result from the debility which followed a difficult labour a year ago. There had been one sharp attack of hæmatemesis. In the middle of the epigastrium there is a spot of exquisite tenderness.

She left the hospital almost free from any gastric symptoms on the 3rd October. The treatment consisted of physical and physiological rest, a diet of milk with soda water exclusively, and at first a mixture of carbonate of bismuth, carbonate of soda and tincture of belladonna. When improvement had well set in, Fowler's solution in five minim doses was administered.

Cancer of the Liver (probably) Secondary to Cancer of the Stomach.—F. O., carpenter, aged 55, admitted August 29th, 1889 ; no distinct family history of cancer. For some years had been liable to slight attacks of dyspepsia, but with this exception had enjoyed good health until four months before admission, when he began to suffer from pain at the epigastrium and upper part of the abdomen, flatulent distension after food, and vomiting, the latter presenting the following characters : it was not present every day ; there were intervals of several days when he was entirely free from it ; the vomiting followed at a considerable interval after the taking of food, and the quantity ejected at a time was stated to be as much as several pints ; the vomited matter consisted of a sour smelling, sometimes watery, sometimes slimy fluid. On several occasions before admission it was noticed to be of a dark brown color with a sediment ("coffee ground"). The pain was never in any way affected by the vomiting. The bowels have been obstinately constipated. These symptoms increased rapidly in severity, and soon the patient lost appetite for food and became rapidly emaciated. In June last he first noticed that the upper part of the abdomen was prominent and hard. There has never been any jaundice nor have the legs been at any time swollen.

On admission patient was very thin ; weighed 129 lbs (former weight 167 lbs). The skin is somewhat lemon-coloured, but there is no jaundice. The liver is enlarged in the right mammary line, measuring eight inches, and extending quite inches beyond the margin of the ribs. In the middle line edge of the liver reaches to within two inches of the umbilic. There is marked tenderness on pressure over the liver, the face of which is smooth, but just in the upper line a small nodule can be felt. Percussion over the left hypochondrium gives unduly tympanitic note. The abdominal veins are not dilated. There is no ascites whatever. Splenic dulness is not increased. Tongue large, flabby and coated. Suffers continuously from pain, mainly in left hypogastrium, which is increased by food and not relieved by vomiting. The attacks of vomiting occur at intervals of two or three days, and are of the characters above mentioned. Since his admission there has not been any "coffee-ground" appearance of the vomited matters.

October 31st.—Since admsssion there has been very severe pain in the npper part of the abdomen and recurrent attacks of vomiting. There has not been any loss of weight. The ejected matter does not contain hydrochloric acid.

Salol Test.—Dr. England reports that he found the salicylic re-action in the urine two hours and a half after he had administered twenty grains of salol by the mouth.

Cancer of the Pylorus ; Very Rapid Progress ; Death ;
Autopsy.—Alexander E., a sailor, aged 57 ; admitted October 15th, complaining of severe abdominal pain, frequent vomiting and obstinate constipation. He states that he was in good health until about three weeks before admission, when the bowels became very constipated, and at that time he noticed that there was a painful lump in the epigastrium. A dose of castor oil freely moved the bowels, and after that the lump is said to have disappeared, but quickly to have returned. It was only fifteen days ago that he began to vomit, and he noticed that as soon as the vomiting set in the pain became very much worse. The bowels moved freely for about five days after the vomiting occurred, and then remained closed for the last ten days. Vomiting occurs usually about four hours after food. The ejected matter is liquid and the quantity got rid of is very great. He

states that his usual weight is 150 lbs. His present weight is 112½ lbs. No family history of cancer.

Emaciation is extreme ; no jaundice, but complexion is very sallow ; suffers extremely from pain in the epigastrium, which is markedly prominent and very tender on pressure, especially at a point about two inches from the umbilicus and one and a half inches from the middle line, where a hard nodule can be felt. The liver is of normal dimensions in the right lobe, but the left extends to within two inches of the umbilicus. The liver surface is smooth and its edge sharply defined.

October 30*th* (37th day of illness).—Vomiting has been continuously present and is very distressing. It occurs whenever anything is taken into the stomach, and consists of a large quantity of watery matter, which contains no hydrochloric acid. When salol (20 grains) is given by the mouth there is no evidence of the presence of salicylic acid in the urine for six hours, corroborating the evidence already stated as to the motor insufficiency of the stomach. The bowels are obstinately constipated, but can with great difficulty be made to move by castor oil and by enemata ; tongue coated ; constant desire to take food. Emaciation has been very rapid. In ten days he has lost fourteen pounds. Within the last twenty-four hours he has been in a moribund condition ; very delirious, evidently dying by starvation.

Autopsy.—" Great distension of stomach. A zone of ulceration extending around the entire circumference of the pylorus. On section the gastric wall in its entire structure is infiltrated with scirrhus, which has also extended into neighboring organs, the right kidney and supra renal capsule, the glands about the pylorus, the retro-peritoneal and retro-thoracic glands at the level of the diaphragm. The œsophagus at the cardia and bile ducts are slightly pressed upon by these enlarged glands. The growth has directly extended to the capsule of the liver beneath the left lobe, but no secondary nodules occur in the liver substance." (Dr. Johnston's report.)

Herpes Zoster in Connection with Disease of the Spine.—A

woman past middle life was admitted, complaining of pain in the
lower part of the lumbar region. No cause could be discovered
in the abdomen. but there was found a prominence of the spine
of the dorsal vertebræ, in the neighborhood of which there was
very marked tenderness upon percussion. After being two days
in hospital, there appeared an eruption of herpes zoster, which
began at the prominent spine and ran down the side of the chest
and abdomen in the direction of the umbilicus.

*Recurring Tonsillitis as an Evidence of the Rheumatic
Diathesis.*—In the case of a young man who had his first attack
of rheumatism (with endocarditis) there was a history of five
distinct attacks of acute suppurative tonsillitis.

Pneumonia.—Nov. 9th, 1889. Three cases have been in
my wards during the last week. The first of left apex pneumonia resolving rapidly, the second a more serious case, one of
right apex and left base, which ran a more protracted course,*
and in the third, a fatal case, the disease involved the whole of
the left lung except the apex, and the middle lobe of the right
lung as well. The respirations were very rapid, 80 and 90 on
the day after admission. Death occurred the day after the
crisis from œdema of the lungs. Loud mucous rales pervaded
both sides of the chest. There was throughout no expectoration.
The most interesting point in the autopsy, the discovery
that a fibrinous exudation, distinctly croupous, occupied the
trachea, in fact, a membraneous tracheitis existed. There was
commencing acute tubular nephritis on one side. There had
been albumen in the urine.

Cirrhosis of the Liver.—A woman aged 63 died in 24 ward
of the effects of portal obstruction. She had entered the hospital on July 26th. A history of spirit drinking ; venous stigmata ;
a moderate amount of fluid in the peritonæum ; extent of liver,
dulness in right mammary line, 2½ inches ; the splenic dulness
had increased to four inches in the axillary line. Had suffered
from bronchitis and shortness of breath upon exertion for the
last seven years, as well as from pain in the left inguinal region.

---

* Dec. 5th, 1889. The consolidation never underwent any resolution. The
patient, aged 44, an alcoholic, died in the fourth week, from the results, apparently,
of the concomitant bronchitis.

After some weeks residence in hospitals he went home, but returned in a fortnight much worse. It was now noticed that at about two inches below the costal margin a firm body could distinctly be made out upon palpation, and this was thought to be the edge of a large liver. Contact of the finger caused no pain. Appetite bad; much thirst, and latterly vomiting. Jaundice appeared about three weeks before death, but was transient. A week before death there was wandering, and at the end she was comatose.

Autopsy.—Peritonæum contained 330 ounces of fluid. The liver was typically cirrhotic (wt. 1100 grammes*). It is probable that a quantity of serum must have collected between diaphragm and upper surface of the liver.† There is no other explanation of the fact that the edge of the liver had been felt not only by me, but by many of the members of the class, extending a good three inches below the ribs. The spleen was enlarged (wt. 460 grammes*). Emphysema of the lungs and small spots of pulmonary hæmorrhage. A pedunculated ovarian cyst, as large as a foetal head, was found at the brim of the pelvis. Kidneys large; veins full.

Supposed Syphilitic Gumma on the Cortex of the Brain.—A man aged 25 was admitted with sore throat on 1st September, 1889, and it was found that he was just recovering from a chancre of the glans, and that a few weeks previously he had had a swelling in the groin. The primary sore made its first appearance in July, 1889, and on the 7th October he was seized with a "fit," which began with a twitching and up drawing of the left angle of the mouth, and afterwards he lost consciousness and was taken to the hospital in the ambulance, but soon discharged. On the following day, while resuming his occupation (an hotel servant), a similar seizure took place. Recovery was rapid, for I saw him a few minutes after the occurrence, and he had recovered himself completely. The bystanders told me that there was "working" of the face, that he had suddenly turned

---

* Normal weight of liver is 1400 to 1700 grammes, and that of the spleen is 140 to 200 grammes.

† Vide Murchison on Diseases of the Liver, third edition, p. 383.

round several times and had fallen to the ground.   There did
not appear to be any loss of consciousness.

On admission, on the 16th October, the tongue was found
recently bitten ; mental functions obtuse ; severe pain on right
side of head, from the centre of forehead to as far back as the
right ear, throbbing and hammerlike, and much worse at night ;
tenderness on pressure and great pain on percussion ; no optic
neuritis.   Ordered inunctions of blue ointment.   In three days
the pain in the head was nearly gone, and he was enabled to
sleep all night, but tenderness remained some days after the
pain had disappeared.   He remained in hospital until the 9th
November, and during that period there were clonic spasms of
the right arm on several occasions, and it was once noticed that
these slight clonic spasms affected the leg.   No twitching of
muscle was noticed after the 27th October.

Reviews and Notices of Books.

Chemistry, General, Medical and Pharmaceutical.
By JOHN ATTFIELD, F.R.S.   Twelfth Edition.   Philadelphia : Lea Brothers & Co.   1889.

Attfield's is probably the best reference book on chemistry for
the general practitioner and druggist that is written in English.
It is so well and favorably known that an extended notice is
scarcely necessary.   This twelfth edition contains briefly the
chemistry of the British and United States pharmacies arranged
so as, at the same time, to illustrate and teach the general principles of the science. · It excludes all reference to compounds
which are as yet of interest only to the scientific chemist, but
contains more or less of the chemistry of substances recognized
officially, or in general practice as remedial agents.   The present
edition contains such alterations and additions as the advances
in principles of chemistry and its application to pharmacy demand.   A new feature is a more extended section on organic
chemistry ; these compounds are classified on the modern system, and, like the rest of the book, are chiefly those of interest

to the followers of medicine and pharmacy. The volume closes with a very comprehensive index, containing no less than nine thousand references, which enhances greatly its value for consultation in the course of business or professional practice.

A Manual of Chemistry for the Use of Medical Students. By BROUDRETTE SYMONDS, A M., M.D. Philadelphia: P. Blakiston, Son & Co.

This little book is designed to contain, as the preface states, parts of general chemistry which it is necessary for medical students to know who are going up for the United States Government Medical Service or for their degrees in medicine. The whole subject of chemistry is briefly summarized, special chapters being devoted to water, air and urine, these being more fully dealt with. It is a book intended to float a slow student over the slight impediment offered by a badly conducted examination, or to be used by one who, having had a thorough training in chemistry, wishes to refresh his memory on the facts of chemistry.

Notwithstanding that every one of the 150 pages of this book is bristling with facts and figures, its utility as a manual for medical students is very questionable from the teacher's standpoint.

That there should be such a demand for text-books like Dr. Symond's manual, shows something radically wrong both in the requirements of the examiners and the method of imparting a knowledge of chemistry in medical schools.

Medical students should be required to show at an examination that they have a sufficiently broad grasp of the science to enable them to apply its principles and facts to the practice of medicine and surgery, and they should be taught those theories and useful facts in a way that tends to develop to the greatest possible extent their powers of accurate observation, and at the same time to give them scientific habits of thought. Chemistry, well taught, can do this far better than any other subject in the students' curriculum.

As a rule, however, medical students are badly taught and

equally badly examined in this subject, so it becomes what it never should be, viz., a severe tax on the memory ; the natural result follows—cram books and hard reading before examination and a lifelong blissful, ignorance of chemistry after.

Twentieth Annual Report of the State Board of Health of Massachusetts. Boston, 1889.

The State of Massachusetts has always taken the lead in sanitary matters. The past efforts of her Board of Health have yielded most valuable results. The present volume is quite up to the high standard of its predecessors. The work of the board seems to have been admirably carried out, and the papers contributed to the publication are of the highest scientific value.

During the year ending Sept. 30th, 1888, but thirty-two cases of small-pox came under the notice of the board. Several of these occurred in paper mill towns, and were probably connected with the importation of rags.

Some interesting investigations on food adulteration have been carried on under the auspices of the Board. The cruel analyst has made several of our old friends to appear under very different faces. " Pure" or " strictly pure" Vermont maple sugar is not produced in the maple groves of that lovely state, but has its principal origin in certain mixing houses in and about Boston. Of forty-six samples of honey, more than half were adulterated with corn glucose, twenty-one genuine and twenty-five adulterated. One specimen, which bore no label and was almost wholly glucose syrup, contained the dead body of a honey bee, inserted doubtless to lend an air of genuineness. In nineteen colored candies and four colored sugars no poisonous material was found.

The patent medicines come in for their share of criticism, and especially the kind of remedy advertised as tonic and nerve stimulant. When Artemus Ward, long ago, spoke of " a vegetable tonic on a broad whiskey basis," he was not far from the truth. " Whiskol," a non-alcoholic cure for the drink habit, contained on analysis 28·2 p.c., by volume, of alcohol. Harriet Hubbard Ayer's Vita Nuova consisted of a strongly fortified wine *plus* cocain, while the Recamier Cream Balm and Lotion, prepared by the same philanthropist, was found to contain mercury, probably in the form of corrosive sublimate.

Visitors to Boston who have been attracted by the shop of the seven Sutherland sisters, the hair of each of which reaches the ground, the extraordinary result of the use of the Seven Sutherland Sisters' Hair and Scalp Cleaner, also their Hair Grower, will be interested in knowing that the cleaner is simply a mixture of borax and soap, and the grower a diluted mixture of bay rum, and possibly some hamamelis and Spanish flies.

A very valuable paper on "The Micro-organisms in the Air of the Boston City Hospital," is the work of Mr. G. R. Tucker. In our limited space we cannot do more than commend to our readers its careful perusal.

A volume such as that of the Massachusetts Board reflects credit upon those who have accomplished the work no less than upon the Government who have carried out the undertaking.

A Treatise on the Science and Practise of Midwifery. By W. S. PLAYFAIR, M.D., L.L.D., F.R.C.P. Fifth American from the Seventh English Edition. Edited with Notes and Additions by Robert P. Harris, M.D. Philadelphia : Lea Brothers & Co. 1889.

Since the appearance of the fourth American edition, four years ago, a decided advance has been made in the practise of midwifery. Antisepsis is no longer on its trial, but the gospel of cleanliness has prevailed, and puerperal mortality has been considerably reduced. The improved Cesarian section operation is yielding magnificent results, and rapidly narrowing the field of craniotomy, so that it really seems as if some day the dream of Tyler Smith might come true and craniotomy be no more. Dr. Harris has rendered good service in bringing the statistical records of the various section operations down to the close of 1888. In four years the mortality of Porro's operation has fallen from fifty-eight per cent. to less than twenty per cent., and that of Cesarian section from forty-five per cent. to twenty per cent. In Germany Cesarian section shows a mortality of twelve per cent. The notes and additions by Dr. Harris are copious and enhance the value of the work, especially for American readers. In most English works the subject of abdominal palpation does not receive the attention it deserves; the same fault exists in Playfair's book, and it is to be hoped that in subsequent editions it will be remedied. On the whole, this edition is brought well up to date, and can be confidently recommended as a reliable text-book.

The Physicians' Visiting List (Lindsay & Blakiston's) for 1890. Thirty-ninth year of its publication. Philadelphia: P. Blakiston, Son & Co.

This well-known visiting list contains a large amount of useful information. Concise and accurate chapters are devoted to poisons and their antidotes, new remedies, aids to the diagnosis and treatment of diseases of the eye, disinfectants, incompatibles, examination of the urine, etc., etc. In addition, there are blank leaves for visits, consultations, obstetric and vaccination engagements.

The Medical News Visiting List. Philadelphia: Lea Bros. & Co. 1890.

This well known and much appreciated list comes to hand for the year 1890. It contains a great amount of useful information, in addition to the blank leaves for visits and previous engagements. There are tables of weights and comparative scales, lists of new remedies, table of doses, incompatibles, poisons and their antidotes, directions for the performance of artificial respiration, and for tying arteries, &c., &c.

Society Proceedings.

MEDICO-CHIRURGICAL SOCIETY OF MONTREAL.

Stated Meeting, November 1st, 1889.

DR. SHEPHERD, FIRST VICE-PRESIDENT, IN THE CHAIR.

Dr. JOHNSTON exhibited a pathological specimen from a case of chronic suppurative otitis media, in which there was, on the anterior surface of the right petrous bone, posterior to the edge of the semi-circular canal, and anterior to the region of the mastoid cells, a perforation a quarter of an inch in diameter, with thickened rounded edges. At the edges, slight adhesions exist between the petrous bone and the corresponding portion of the dura mater ; but the dura mater is readily removed, and is intact. The superior petrosal sinus is plugged with a recent thrombus ; the right lateral sinus is filled with greyish-brown, fetid fluid, extending half way up to the torcular herophyli. The inferior petrosal sinus and the internal jugular vein are filled with a similar material, their walls thickened, rough, and, in places, necrotic. On the external aspect of the inferior petrosal sinus the bone is exposed. On sawing into the temporal bone, the cavities of the middle and internal ear are found filled with a cheesy, fetid mass, which consists microscopically of leucocytes, crystalline fatty acids and bacteria ; the drum membrane represented only by a few fibrous bands holding the ossicles in place. The tympanic cavity, the Eustachian tube, obstructed by granulations, and its surfaces, in places, have become adherent. Near the mastoid process the soft parts are free from œdema and infiltration. The external auditory meatus shows no obstruction. The results of further examination of the organs of the body are as follows : Heart contains very little blood ; organ anæmic but muscular ; substance and valves normal ; right lung partially consolidated at lower lobe behind ; left lung crepitant throughout ; pulmonary vessels free, no infarcts ; spleen greatly enlarged, measures eight inches by four and a half ; weight, 520 grammes ; organ very soft ; the anterior border shows several infarcts each with thrombosed vessels at its apex; splenic artery and vein free from clot; kidneys in a state of parenchymatous nephritis; brain itself shows nothing beyond a single small white spot of infiltration, the size of a bean, in right optic thalamus, half an inch posterior to its anterior extremity. The rest of the P.M gave negative results.

The history of the case in brief is as follows: Patient, male, aged 28 years; admitted into the General Hospital 15th October, complaining of headache, pain in the back, and sore throat. These symptoms set in one week ago, and continued about the same until time of admission, when the headache seemed to increase, and at times so severe as to prevent sleep; no vomiting; temperature, 104; pulse, 110. Examination of heart: apex but one inch below and one inch inside the nipple line; superficial dulness from lower border of third rib downwards to extent of four inches; laterally, from mid-sternum to the left, to extent of three inches; slight blowing systolic murmur both at apex and pulmonary area; second sound slightly accentuated. Splenic dulness from eighth rib to extent of four inches downwards; swelling and redness of fauces, tenderness on pressure at angles of jaw. Examination of the rest of the organs negative. Ears not examined. Two days after admission patient became slightly delirious; had severe chill; temperature $101\frac{1}{2}°$ in the evening. Ten days after admission, examination of the heart showed a slight increase in the area of superficial dulness from that found on patient's admission; the murmurs at the base became louder and harsher. A few purpuric spots made their appearance on the extremities; delirium still continued; had chills each day; temperature fluctuating between 98° and $104\frac{1}{2}°$ in the morning, and 99° to 106° in the evening, and on the eleventh day after admission into the hospital, patient died.

Dr. MILLS inquired whether there was any P.M. appearances to explain the heart murmurs heard during life?

Dr. JOHNSTON replied negatively.

Dr. MILLS thought that the explanation of murmurs in such cases, especially as they increased towards death, was dilatation, with possibly weakness of action. The dilatation was due probably to defective nutrition, leading to a loss of elasticity. He had noticed this tendency to dilation in the hearts of dying animals on which he had experimented.

Dr. BELL mentioned an analogous case of septicæmia following perityphlitis, in which cardiac murmurs developed under observation, and became very marked before death. No valvular or other cardiac lesion being found on P.M. examination.

Dr. JAMES STEWART saw the patient 24 hours before death, and coincided with the view expressed by the physician in attendance that the case was one of ulcerative endocarditis. There was a loud systolic murmur at the base not propagated into the vessels of the neck. The heart's dulness was increased and the apex displaced downwards and outwards. All the signs pointed to dilatation of the heart. It appears to me highly probable that such dilatation can easily be accounted for by the fever and anæmia.

Dr. BULLER said: I notice the aperture leading from the antrum into the cranial cavity is a pretty large one, and has probably been formed quite gradually, as the edges are smooth and rounded. I would like to know what was the nature of the contents of the tympanic antrum and the aperture in question. I ask this question because it appears to me that this may have been a case of cholesteatoma, such as we sometimes meet with in chronic suppurative otitis media. This collection of epithelial scales, pus cells, cholesterine and fatty detritus, tends to cause erosion of the bone, and it occurs to me that the aperture might have been formed by the action of such an accumulation.

Dr. BROWN said the heart must have been dilated, from the fact that the beat was considerably displaced beyond the nipple line. The patient had never at any time complained of any symptom of ear disease.

Dr. JOHNSTON replied that the heart, at the autopsy, was not dilated nor displaced to the left. The displacement of the apex beat might have been caused by pressure of the enlarged spleen, which might possibly also have influenced the murmurs. The cheesy material filling the tympanic cavity contained no epithelial cells nor cholesterine crystals. There was no doubt of the bone disease being chronic.

Dr. ALLOWAY exhibited (1) a specimen of a large multilocular ovarian cystoma, weighing forty-five pounds, which he had removed some weeks ago from a patient forty-eight years old. The adhesions were extensive and the drainage tube used. Recovery was uninterrupted.

(2) Two cystic ovaries with their tubes. The case was one of recurrent pelvic imflammation. The chief symptoms caused by this condition were constant vomiting, headache and pelvic pain. All other methods of treatment had been tried unsuccessfully. It is now three months since the operation, and there has been no return of symptoms.

Dr. ENGLAND gave a history and exhibited specimens of a case in practice. The history is as follows: Patient aged 26 years; married; menstruated regularly until January, 1889, and from this time until three months later ceased to do so, when suddenly seized with a severe attack of metrorrhagia, which, under suitable treatment, soon ceased. Nothing unusual occurred until 18th October, when Dr. England was called to attend this patient, who thought herself about to give birth to a child. The patient was and had been for several hours suffering severe pains, apparently expulsive in their nature. Upon examination, Dr. England was surprised to find an empty vagina; a small, firm, fixed and retroverted uterus; the cervix very slightly dilated; no abdominal tumor or change in the breasts could be made out. The patient was only relieved of her pains some hours later by the removal of what proved to be an imperfectly developed ovum.

Dr. JOHNSTON said the specimen showed distinct traces of amnion and chorionic villi at an advanced stage. This would probably be recognized by microscopic examination. No fœtus was present. The intense pain might be accounted for by the supposition that if the case were one of missed abortion the condition of the uterine mucosa might be similar to that in membranous dysmenorrhœa.

Dr. ALLOWAY said that the case was most probably one of missed abortion; that pregnancy ceased about the third month, and that the uterus did not expel its contents for several months afterwards. The retroplaced uterus incarcerated in the pelvis might have accounted for the delay in expulsion. This would also account for the very severe pain experienced. He (Dr. Alloway) had reported a similar case to the society some three years ago, and he thought, under the circumstances, that Dr. England had adopted the proper treatment, but would advise in another similar case that every effort be made to replace the uterus before the induction was resorted to. As a rule, the uterus in such cases is not absolutely fixed by adhesions at the fundus; it is simply impacted in the pelvic cavity, otherwise sterility would more than likely have been absolute.

Dr. McCONNELL related a case of a somewhat similar nature. Mrs. S., aged 42, has large family; six months previous to my seeing her the menstrual flow had not come on, nor did it come the following month; but a week or so after, she had pains and a profuse flow, and she supposed she had had an abortion. She was regular at the next four periods, when I was again called to see her; pains and flowing had continued for some days and she became alarmed. I found, on examination, a membraneous sac projecting from os, which was easily removed; it was about the size of an egg; a bladder-like sac filled with fluid, and a small foetus floating in it. The foetus had perished at the time of supposed complete abortion, and although menstrual periods had come on regularly after (there had been more lost than usual) it had remained four months after.

Dr. RODDICK exhibited a mass of tuberculous glands removed from the neck of a young girl. Both sides of the neck were engaged in the disease, and were operated upon simultaneously, upwards of eighty glands being removed through the two incisions. The patient was discharged well on the eleventh day after the operation. There was no evidence of tubercular disease elsewhere. Her maternal uncle died of phthisis.

Dr. MILLS exhibited a dozen small calculi, of the size of very small peas, several like duck shot, taken from the urethra of a dog after death. They had been diagnosed during life by the catheter. Operation not being permitted, the dog died comatose. Bladder greatly distended.

Dr. RUTTAN here mentioned that the examination of Dr. Roddick's specimen of vesical calculus exhibited at the last meeting proved that it was purely cystine,

Selections.

The Moods of the Sane.—It has been said
" speaking scientifically, we cannot affirm that anybody is
fectly healthy." If the pathologist can detect the sympton
disease in the most apparently healthy body, no less cert
can the neurologist indicate subtle manifestations in the m
states of the sanest amongst us, which serve to warn us
perilously near we may all come at times to mental der
ment. Just as it is impossible to set up a standard of b
health of universal application, so is it with the mind ; one n
measure of mental health cannot be taken as that of ano
" Health" and " whole" are both derived from the Anglo-S
term, hál, and no one man has the completeness of either b
or mental soundness at any one time. We may be sane (
sound), but at best only relatively, and the varying moods
often be strangely like the true persistent phases of the acl
ledged alien. There are few of us who have not momei
depression or abnormal excitement, which, if unduly prolor
would make us the objects of unpleasant attentions at the l
of our friends, and not one of us can say at any time th:
shall never find those unhappy moods persist. Apart, how
from any such painful forebodings, it is an interesting subj
consider some of those mental attitudes of the perfectly sane
trace their causes to their actual source. There is a posthu
paper in the recent number of the *Neurologist*, by Dr. M
Fothergill, which deals—in the pleasant and instructive m:
for which its distinguished writer was so celebrated—with
interesting question. If we would rightly know the workii
the human mind in their varied conditions, we must study
as the brilliant author tells us, in the insane asylum.
angry man amongst us may not find food for reflection, and
the habits of self-control from the incoherent frenzy ?
garrulous, self-centred man may not be rebuked when h
his infirmity a little magnified in the flow of the tall
maniac ?

The delusions of the over-sanguine, the groundless fancies of the visionary, the baseless conceptions of the jealous, the morbid religiosity of the despondent man, all find their legitimate projections in some fixed condition common enough in the dread abode of the insane, and all have lessons for us. The asylum held up the mirror to the observant eye of Dr. Milner Fothergill, showing him our natural and healthy moods when perverted by disease, mismanagement or neglect, into forms of mental disorder. A bad habit or the dominance of an unfortunate predilection may disturb the balance of an otherwise healthy mind, as effectually as the touch of a magnet on the balance wheel of an exquisite watch will impede its regular motion.

How easily is our mental balance disturbed! A single serious reverse may blight a man's hopes for life, yet with another and a sterner habit of thought the advancing phthisis of a Richard Jeffreys will not have the least ill effect. What a variety of moods are caused by food alone! A hungry man can scarcely be termed quite sane in comparison with one who is comfortably digesting the dinner of one of the " city companies."

A cynic might turn upon us, and declare that the man who has just dined well evidences his cerebral disturbance by the ease with which a liberal subscription can be obtained from him, and that his less replete moments are his prudent and normal ones When the Church desired to reduce us to a proper sense of our deserts and shortcomings, she bade us fast, and as fasting has always been associated with penitence, it might be argued by a theologian that we are more truly our real selves when hungry than full. Andrew Boorde, the monk-physician, in his quaint book, *The Dyetary of Health*, rather inclines to the " city company" idea of sanity, when he advises his readers to " Fyrste lyne out of syn, and folowe Christes doctrine, and then vse honest myrth and honest company, and vse to eate good meate, and drynke moderatly."

Shakespeare thought that the "lean and hungry" looking Cassius must naturally be dangerous, and the general testimony of English writers at any rate is to the close connection between fat folk and good temper. Dr. Fothergill was a grand example in himself, and we can picture the relish with which he wrote, "When the brain is well fed it has a sense of well being; when it is ill-supplied with blood, it is irritable, miserable and despondent." But alas! the very process of feeding the brain and making general contentment in the body too often vitiates the blood, and, as the old writers would say, "disturb the humors." The good feeder gives a standing invitation to the gout, and the gouty material in the blood makes a man "choleric," that is to say, hasty and irritable. The over-fat, amiable man has fits of "the blues," he often descends to the melancholy mood, and then, as old Burton says, "he is the cream of human adversity, the quintessence, and upshot." A disordered liver has made many a one think he has sinned the unpardonable sin, and a good purge has often lifted a burden from the conscience as heavy as that of Bunyan's Pilgrim. Dr. Fothergill thought that the atmospheric conditions of Bath and Bournemouth are distinctly answerable for their religious tone, whilst the tonic effects of Clifton have much to do with its intellectual activity. It would be interesting to compare Margate and Brighton with the special moods of their visitors; but these theories may easily be pushed too far, and we might find ourselves inquiring what are the characteristics of Monte Carlo which foster the gambling spirit, and what makes the Neapolitans so light-hearted and frivolous. Perhaps the diet has even more to do with the moods of the sane than atmospheric conditions. An old adage says that, "he who drinks beer thinks beer," but there is beer and beer. The German philosopher stimulates his brain to the highest intellectual exercises on beer, while our working classes deaden their not over active cerebral organization on something called by the same name. Whether we are as sane as we might be in creating any sort of mood by alcohol, is extremely doubtful, for most competent observers agree that the best sorts of intellectual, as of other work, cannot be done under its influence. "The accursed hag dyspepsia," as Carlyle called it, has been answerable for a good deal of the gloomier theology of the past and present. What a victim must have been that monk who wrote *Hell Opened to Christians*, with its appalling pictures of demons driving bolts into men's sculls, and toasting them on great forks! The author of *The Imitation of Christ*, on the other hand, must have been blessed with a good digestion, and a liver which gave him no "moods." His biographers say he was " a placid, kindly, fresh-colored old man ;" and, indeed, his books reveal all that. Probably our best methods are always tinged with a shade of melancholy. Montaigne says, " the most profound joy has more of gravity than gaiety in it ;" and Dr. Fothergill wrote of the mental attitude of " feeling delightfully low-spirited." " The rainbow of our thought life," as the author of *Thorndale* so beautifully expresses it, " is made of joy and tears, the light and storm." The dark and the bright threads of our life are so interwoven, that our healthiest attitude cannot be called unalloyed joy. The highest music, painting and poetry most truly express the sanest moods of man when they exhibit joy chastened by the " sadness which is most akin to pain."

The lesson which we should endeavor to learn from a study of the moods which so easily possess us is the importance of a firm will-control acting like the inhibitory nerves. If our mental states are so often caused by pathological conditions, it is no less true that the mind can control the body ; and the man or woman who, in popular phraseology, " gives way" to his moods, runs imminent risk of becoming their slave.—Editorial in *Br. Med. Jour.*

The Hygienic Uses of the Imagination.

—In a recent editorial entitled "Considerate Judgment," we endeavored to emphasize the necessity of basing conclusions on well ascertained facts, and stated that only those theories which could be thus substantiated would be found enduring. But in the attainment of truth we are by no means debarred the full and free play of a well disciplined imagination; indeed, it often points the way to undiscovered truths; it is by no means infallible; its suggestions always need verification; but imaginations verified become with us accepted facts. Under the above heading, at the recent meeting of the British Medical Association, Sir James Crichton

Browne presented a very able address which is reported i
the *British Medical Journal* of August 24, and from which w
make the following abstract:

The cultivation of the imagination, then—and it can l
cultivated and disciplined to agility and steadiness of action-
is of high importance to us as medical men; for it can be se
viceable to us in collecting materials, in solving difficult pro
lems, and, by the analogies it suggests, in guiding us in ou
life-long search after truth. The precise character whic
medicine is happily assuming, as its several departmen
merge into the exact sciences, and which demands of its cu
tivators a physico-mathematical and chemical training of ev
increasing stringency, does not in any degree abrogate tl
necessity for the employment of the imagination. On tl
physical side of medicine that stillholds its own, and on i
psychical side it is indispensable in dealing with phenomei
that are beyond the province of physical and chemic
research. Medical men and medical students, then, ne
not fear that they are altogether wasting their time whe
they turn aside now and then from their professional tas.
to ramble for a little in the green pastures of literature,
climb the pinnacles of art. True, their imagination may i
fully trained for its professional duty, as it is exercised,
conjunction with observation and judgment, in the scientii
sphere; but it will be braced, invigorated, and have i
resources multiplied, by recreating occasionally in its nati
air. Even if imaginative pursuits did not strengthen t'
hands of medical men in grappling with disease, or quick
their scientific vision, these would still be commendab
because of the refreshment they bring to jaded brains. '
turn from the fatigue and anxieties of practice into reali
where rivalry is no more and night bells never ring is
plunge into one of the most soothing and depurative
"tired Nature's" baths. Members of our profession are,
suspect, generally aware of this, and resort to imaginati
literature, music, and art more than any other class of pi
fessional men, except, of course, artists and men of lette
and to an extent that is remarkable, considering the engro,
ing claims made on their time and the scant leisure th
enjoy.

The contributions of medical men to the departments of imaginative work have been far from insignificant. At least four eminent members of our profession now living might be named who have found leisure, amidst absorbing occupation, so to use the pencil and brush as to gratify not only their private circles but the public, and a list of medical poets would be a long and goodly one, including such names as Akenside (the gifted singer of the pleasures of that imagination whose usefulness I am attempting to extol), Garth, Blackmore, Goldsmith, Smollet, Armstrong, Erasmus Darwin, Crabbe, Moir (better known as Delta, John Brown, whose *Rab and His Friends* is idyllic), and Oliver Wendell Holmes. Nay, even one or two of the greatest names in poetical literature might not improperly be added to such a list. Keats was apprenticed to a surgeon at Edmonton, and afterwards attended St. Thomas' Hospital. It has been argued, I am afraid not very convincingly, that Shakespeare's extensive medical knowledge proves him to have been engaged in the study of medicine during one or two of those years that are unaccounted for, but it is indisputable that Dante was enrolled amongst the *medici è speziali* (leeches and druggists) of Florence, and that he attended their council meetings for several years. But it is not as producers but as consumers of poetry and imaginative literature that medical men derive from them their restorative influence, and as consumers they are, I feel sure, amongst the bookseller's best friends. Sydenham, when asked by Sir Richard Blackmore what course of study he would recommend for a medical student, replied, "Let him read *Don Quixote*, it is a very good book; I read it still." Connolly, the apostle of that non-restraint system to which we owe everything that is most excellent in the treatment of the insane in this country, and with which I trust professional opinion and public sentiment will permit no tampering—Connolly told me in his latter years that he took ever renewed delight in *Gulliver's Travels*. I know hard-working doctors in town and country who hold habitual converse with some of our great imaginative writers. Two of the most distinguished and busiest physicians of this day are, to my knowledge, inveterate novel readers. I have heard one of our great surgeons deliver an address betraying a deep study of the poetry

of Keats; and another of our great surgeons, present :
meeting, told me recently that on his way to and from
serious operation he dips into Shelley.

But it may be objected that the imagination, if som
stimulating and restorative in its influence, is often mo
its tendencies, and that its indulgence is to be guarded :
by those who desire to possess well regulated minds.
habit can be more opposed to a healthy condition
mental powers," says Abercrombie, "than that which]
the mind to wander in a mere vision or waking drean
scene to scene, unrestrained by reason, probability or t
and the answer to Abercrombie is supplied by Tynda
says that those who have denounced the imagination k
they have seen its disastrous effect on weak vessels, "
with equal justice point to exploded boilers as an arg
against the use of steam." But the weak vessels wrecl
imagination are really fewer than is commonly suj
Now and again some erratic genius, of highly strung n
temperament, gives himself up to pleasures of imaginat
he becomes intoxicated with them, and staggers ov
boundary of sanity. Now and again an intensely imag
child, like Jerome Cardan or Hartley Coleridge, so in
in day dreams that his fancies grow into phantoms that
him; but I do not hesitate to say that for one case of ir
caused by excess of imagination, there are a dozen cau
want of it. Apathetic dullness and torpor of mind are
deepen into dementia; and those entirely given up to
care of this life and the deceitfulness of riches" are
likely to be choked by them than those who can sur
them, and breathe the free and ample air of æsthetics
tion. A vulgar error as to the nature of insanity has p
conduced to exaggeration as to the dangers of imagi
Visitors to asylums invariably arrive expecting t
growths of morbid invention and belief, wild, tangle
luxuriant as a tropical forest, and leave much disappoin
the barrenness of the land, for the insane are the least
native of beings. At rare intervals a madman is encou
—a Blake or a Swedenborg—whom two intrepid docto1
certified, who dazzles all around him by the meteor
liancy of his conceptions; but, as a rule, the lunatic is

as a stone. He is the victim of a fixed idea, or his delusions pursue a treadmill round, or occur in groups so unvarying that, if you have ascertained one of them, you can predict all the rest. His mind is a blank or a blurred and unreadable page, or his fancies, if they come thick in the tumult of mania, are so disjointed or huddled together as to defy recognition. Idiocy is the absolute negation of imagination, and insanity undermines and destroys or enfeebles it more or less, and, when we try to drive out insanity, the first thing we do is to invoke imagination's aid, for moral treatment consists mainly in appeals to this faculty, and fully acknowledges its hygienic uses. The first recorded cure of melancholia was by the harp of David, and to-day in every lunatic hospital worth the name persistent efforts are being made by music, by pictures, by poetry and the drama to stimulate the imagination, and thus "cleanse the stuffed bosom of that perilous stuff that weighs upon the heart."

Imagination seems to have a trophic influence on the brain. When it is absent tardy growth goes on; when it is more or less in abeyance, weakness exists; when it is active, there is vigorous development; and the immediate effects of imagination in causing exhileration and preventing sleep when it is excessively indulged almost suggest that the states of the cortex which accompany it have some control over metabolic changes in the body. We now know that, besides alkaloids exercising a poisonous effect, which owe their formation to microbes, and are called ptomaines, there are others which are produced by the cells of the living organism themselves in breaking down albuminous matter, and which are called leucomaines. Now Bouchard has shown that the alkaloids of the latter kind formed during sleep have a stimulating action, so that, when they accumulate to a certain amount, they excite the nerve centres and cause awakeniug, while those formed during waking hours have a depressing action and tend to induce sleep. And it is just possible that in the formation of leucomaines of different classes, under varying conditions of the supreme nerve centres, a key may be found to the curious fact that certain emotional moods, after having persisted for a time, tend to induce their opposites—excitement, depression; appetite, disgust—and also to the influence of imagination, when very active, in causing exhileration and wakefulness. It is just possible that under such circumstances it may arrest the formation of those leucomaines, usually manufactured during waking hours, which are depressing and lead up to sleep, or so modify decomposition that other leucomaines of a stimulating character are produced. There can be no question that, in insanity, certain states of the highest nerve centres are accompanied by rapid disintegration of the tissues and emaciation, while in other states of these centres metabolism is reduced to a minimum, so that prolonged starvation may be sustained with comparatively little wasting.

But it is only an inordinate indulgence of the imagination that produces excitement and interferes with natural slumber; its reasonable and regulated use causing only a certain buoyancy of spirits with which a sense of soothing is associated. Imagination, indeed, legitimately used, combines to some extent the pleasureable effects of both morphine and caffeine, without any disagreeable after-consequences, such as headaches, despondency, or confusion of thought. On the one hand, it may heighten happiness, and on the other afford solace in suffering and sorrow. It may give zest to appetite and allay the pangs of hunger, brace to exertion, or lessen the sense of fatigue. It would not be wrong to speak of it, when rightly used, as a true physiological stimulant, and analgesic, capable in some degree of taking the place of those crude agents drawn from herbs and trees, with which in all quarters of the globe mankind has sought to mitigate the dullness or assuage the pains of life. Moreover, its massive pleasures have a distinctly sedative effect in connection with those petty but exasperating animosities and jealousies that are the thorns of social intercourse, and fret and fray fine-textured brains. Lifting us above the turmoils and worries of the moment and opening up wide and distant prospects, they promote altruistic feeling, lull to rest our wounded sensibilities, and allay feverish excitement.—*Journal of the Amer. Med. Association.*

THE

Montreal Medical Journal.

| VOL. XVIII. | DECEMBER, 1889. | No. 6. |

CLINICAL TEACHING IN ASYLUMS.

Asylums for the insane, located within easily accessible distances of medical schools, can and ought to be made of great use in clinical teaching. The great majority of graduates of English, American and Canadian medical schools have only a very superficial knowledge of insanity. This is a great misfortune, as they are not infrequently called upon to attend such cases in general practice, and not uncommonly the unfortunate patients have to suffer as the result of this ignorance. Clinical instruction in asylums would not only benefit the afflicted and the students, but also the physicians in charge of the asylum.

It is a well recognized fact that an hospital in which clinical instruction is carried on is greatly superior to an hospital in which no teaching is done. The clinical hospital confers its benefits on its patients, on its students, and on its physicians and surgeons. Such an hospital always attracts the best men, and, in consequence, in it the best temporary and permanent work is done. It is in clinical hospitals that, with very few exceptions, the great advances in modern medicine and surgery have been worked out.

What is true of general hospitals is also true of hospitals for the insane.

All the leading German universities have clinics for mental diseases connected with them, and under the direction of men whose names are household words in the scientific world. In Vienna the clinic for mental diseases is under the direction of Meynert, who mainly through taking advantage of his unrivalled opportunities for the study and teaching of insanity, is now recognized as one of the leading authorities in the world in this department.

The paucity of scientific work emanating from asylum physicians on this side of the Atlantic is, in part, attributable to the want of that stimulating influence which the presence of students infuses, and in part also to the fact that they are burdened with the multifarious duties pertaining to the necessary ways and means of their establishments.

Not until the time arrives when we will only require asylum physicians to attend the scientific part of their work, will we have attained that high level long ago reached by Germany.

As things are at present, let the asylum physician's scientific capacity and enthusiasm be of the highest order, he will be a non-producer, because he is required to attend to duties which are antagonistic to the highest mental work.

THE TREATMENT OF THE INSANE IN CANADA.

It is expected that within a few months the Protestant Hospital for the Insane in this city will be open for the reception and treatment of patients.

As yet no appointment has been made to the position of medical superintendent. The future success of this institution will, in a great measure, depend on the wisdom displayed by the governors in making this appointment. The first and essential requirement for this position is experience in the management and treatment of the insane. Unfortunately, in this country it is not the custom to appoint men to these positions because from experience and special education they are fitted for the work. In most of the provinces, the first, and, in fact, the only qualification is the reputation of being an energetic machine politician. The credentials of the candidates do not consist of what they know and what they have seen of insanity, but what they have done for their "party." To be a rejected parliamentary candidate is a qualification which rarely fails in securing the desired position.

The nature and treatment of the diseases of the mind is, beyond all doubt, the most profound and difficult department of medicine. In no specialty is it so necessary that there should be special training as in psychiatry, and yet we find men willing to undertake these very onerous duties without any special knowledge.

We believe that several eminently qualified physicians are ready to make application for the medical superintendency of the Protestant Hospital for the Insane, and we hear also that several physicians in no way qualified for the position are anxious for the appointment. It will be easy for wise and competent men to separate the eminently qualified from those entirely unfitted for the position. It will, however, be more difficult to decide who among the former will best fill the important position.

It does not appear to be generally known that the insane of the North-West Territories are housed, not in an asylum, but in the Manitoba Penitentiary. Formerly, by an agreement with the Provincial Government of Manitoba, the care of the insane from the territories was entrusted to the Superintendent of the Manitoba Asylum at Selkirk. This arrangement, which we believe worked satisfactorily, fell through from the inability of the Dominion and Provincial Governments to come to terms as to the price to be paid by the former.

If the treatment of the insane in this Province is highly unsatisfactory, it is due to causes beyond the reach of our profession, but the case is otherwise with the insane in the North-West. A representation from the Canadian Medical Association of the injury done to the insane by their retention in a convict establishment would, we have no doubt, induce the Dominion Government to build a proper asylum in the territories or continue the arrangement previously in force.

We have had occasion repeatedly to call attention to the pernicious system of dealing with the insane in the Province of Quebec. This state of matters still continues, and there is little hope that it will ever be different until the day comes when

the mass of the population will be educated, and until the time
comes when politicians will dare to do what is right.   As neither
of these events are likely to occur during the present generation
of men, the unrighteous method of hiring out the insane now
in force will be continued.

THE TREATMENT OF FUNCTIONAL NERVOUS DISEASES BY CORRECTION OF OCULAR DEFECTS.

The Commission appointed by the New York Neurological
Society to enquire into the results of the correction of ocular
defects, in the treatment of epilepsy and chorea, have reported,
on the whole, unfavorably towards this proceedure.   They
examined into fourteen cases, and report six improved but none
cured.   The result of this enquiry affords an additional proof of
the folly of rushing into print, and claiming at once for new
methods results which can only be determined by prolonged and
careful investigation.   That six cases were improved may be
considered as saying much in favor of this operation by some,
while by others it will be looked upon simply as a happy coincidence.   The latter can, no doubt, bring forward abundant proof
that almost any treatment would be followed by similar results.
That such a proceedure should be curative in any case of
essential epilepsy or chronic chorea, appears to us, on purely
physiological grounds, to be highly improbable.

Correspondence.

PROVINCIAL MEDICAL BOARDS.

To the Editors of THE MONTREAL MEDICAL JOURNAL.

SIRS:—In the admirable introductory address delivered by my friend Dr. MacDonnell, and published in your last issue, I subscribe to everything except to his remarks on the subject of "Provincial Medical Boards." I had hoped that the day of antagonism to them was past, but I regret to see that the spirit of opposition is not yet dead, and still more that it should be evinced by one of the younger generation. I am bold to say that if in the Provinces of Ontario and Quebec a higher standard of general medical education exists to-day, than on any other part of this Continent, it is because for forty years or more the medical boards have sought for uniformity in the qualification to practise—a uniformity which the public has a right to expect, but which it certainly cannot obtain from irresponsible medical schools. Unrestricted competition between the colleges without state supervision leads to the chaos which is seen on this side of the line; and that the same state does not exist in Canada, is not owing to any virtue on the part of the schools— far from it—but is due solely to the wisdom of the men who organized and have supported the medical boards. We must remember that it is a new thing for the university degree to carry with it the license to practise, and it has only crept in in the case of the Doctorate in Medicine. It is a function of the state to determine whether a man is fit to be entrusted with the lives and limbs of citizens; and to carry out this function through an organised profession, by its representatives, is a thoroughly Anglo-Saxon way, certainly preferable to the arbitrary Teutonic plan in which the *Staats-examen* is conducted by nominees of the Crown.

I freely concede the difficulty to which Dr. MacDonnell refers, in having to comply with regulations inconsistent with modern ideas of education; but we must have patience. The schools are not themselves quite ready for a thoroughly advanced system of teaching, though now with the compulsory four years and the addition of a summer session, the didactic and the practical work could easily be re-arranged. Certainly the time has come for dividing absolutely the work of the different years. Fewer didactic lectures ; increased laboratory instruction, particularly in the dissecting-room ; junior and senior classes in the Hospital, practical examinations in all departments—these are the changes to which boards and schools must alike look forward.

Yours, etc.,   WILLIAM OSLER.

JOHNS HOPKINS HOSPITAL.
    Baltimore, Dec. 2, 1889.

Medical Items.

—Dr. W. H. Gaskell has been awarded a medal by the Royal Society for his researches in the anatomy and physiology of the sympathetic nervous system.

—Prof. Eulenburg, of Berlin, the editor of the *Real-Encyclopædiae der Gesammten Heilkunde,* has recently celebrated his silver jubilee as a medical teacher.

—The late Professor Ricord has bequeathed the sum of 10,000 francs to the Academy of Medicine, the interest of which is to be devoted bi-annually for a prize in any subject the Academy may determine.

OBITUARY.—Through the death of Gaetano La Loggia, Italy has lost a distinguished citizen, and medicine one of her ablest students. For many years he held the chair of physiology in the University of Palermo, and for some time the chair of biology in the University of Turin. He, however, not only taught physiology with effect, but also taught the Italian youth the priceless value of civil and religious liberty. His part in the regeneration of Italy was a prominent one. For a number of years previous to his death he was director of the Palermo Asylum, and devoted his great energies to the elucidation of scientific questions relating to his special department.

PARIS EXHIBITION.—W. R. Warner & Co. have received a silver medal at the Paris World's Fair, being the highest of its kind, in recognition of the following claims : 1st. W. R. Warner & Co.'s Pills, quick solubility and accuracy. 2nd. Reliability and permanency unsurpassed. 3rd. Perfection in coating, thorough composition and accurate subdivision. 4th. Excellence in solubility of the finished product in from four to six minutes. 5th. Quinine Pills, for accuracy in weight and purity of material. Also for Warner & Co.'s Effervescent Salts. 1st. Superior effervescing properties. 2nd. General elegance and excellence. 3rd. Stability of the effervescing quality sustained by critical examination.

THE

Montreal Medical Journal.

| VOL. XVIII. | JANUARY, 1890. | No. 7. |

Original Communications.

THE PULMONITIS OF PARALYTICS AND DEGENE-RATION OF THE VAGI NERVES.

By Dr. Bianchi,

Director of the Psychiatric Clinique of the University of Palermo.

Translated and Abstracted by Dr. Joseph Workman, Toronto.

We are indebted to the illustrious author for a copy of the above very interesting brochure, containing 42 pages, and illustrated by three beautifully executed plates. Dr. Bianchi is well known as one of the most assiduous cultivators of experimental physiology and general pathology of the present day. It would be no unpleasing labor to turn into English the whole of his present valuable contributions to the rational practical study of the influence of nerve degeneracy in the etiology of a disease, which, up to the present, has continued to be a *quasi oppro-brium medicinæ*. We allude to that now too widely extending malady, known to alienistic physicians under the designation of *general paralysis*, or, more appropriately, *general paresis of the insane*. Italian psychiatrists name it *progressive paralysis*, which is an improvement on the misleading English title, yet not unobjectionable, for, as Dr. Christian has contended, actual *paralysis* has never been observed in its course, before the final supervention of lethal prostration, or absolute coma.

In prosecuting his study, Dr. Bianchi experimented pretty freely on rabbits and dogs, and he availed himself of the instructive clinical and pathological materials furnished by the Palermo

31

(*a*) In the first place, the grave disturbances of the respiration, after cutting the vagi in the neck, appear relatively too soon to be ascribed to the foreign substances, which, because of paralysis of the larynx and œsophagus, may enter into the air passages. After some seconds, or, at most, after a few minutes, that intense characteristic dyspnœa sets in, which accompanies the life of the animal operated on up to the last breath.

(*b*) The very same phenomena are provoked, and in the same succession, when, by means of ligaturing the trachea, and introducing a tube for the animal to breath through, alimentary substances and the buccal fluid are prevented entering the air passages, and the only difference between the rabbits spared from tracheotomy and those on which it is practised, is that the latter live longer, yet present the same morbid form, and no less grave anatomical alterations in the lungs. On this fact and the next one, we cannot at all agree with the assertions of Traube.

(*c*) The injection of one or two syringefulls of buccal liquid and fragments of food received by a rabbit having the vagi cut, does not usually provoke anything analogous in rabbits which have the vagi intact, and even less hurtful is the sole presence of a tube, when no obstruction in it is present.

The doctrine of Traube, which has been so vigorously defended by Frey,—that is, that the broncho-pulmonitis is provoked only by foreign substances (the buccal liquids and bits of food), entering into the air passages, in consequence of the conjunct paralysis of the larynx and œsophagus, does not withstand the evidence of the facts. We, in truth, hold that the entrance of foreign substances into the bronchi may be one of the factors which may co-operate in determining the pulmonary lesions mentioned; we would indeed say that it is the most efficient factor in determining a process which finds, in the altered physio-anatomical conditions of the pulmonary parenchyma, the most favourable conditions for its development.

We do not lean towards the doctrine of Fovelin, who ascribes to the altered chemistry of the respiration the chief importance, because he found the quantity of carbonic acid, emitted after section of the vagi, increased. In many other circumstances, even in man, the carbonic acid expired is augmented without those pulmonary lesions, found by us in paralytics, having been presented.

There is yet the mechanical theory, which has been maintained principally by Bernard and Boddaert. It furnishes a plausible, though a venturesome interpretation of the facts. Bernard holds that the respiration increases in intensity, because whilst a normal rabbit inspires 20 c.c. of air, after cutting the vagi, it emits 32 cc. of it, so that the pulmonary vesicles become distended beyond measure, and from this there results that traumatic emphysema, which is one of the most constant of the anatomical findings in animals subjected to these experiments, together with blood engorgement and finally rupture of the vessels and infiltration of blood in the air channels.

Boddaert, in his very interesting work, holds that by section of the vagi, not only is the sensibility of the air passages abolished down to the pulmonary vesicles, but also, and principally, the contractility of the bronchi, and hence the air is not all expired, and the respiration is diminished and aggravated by the consecutive repletion of the blood vessels, and by ecchymoses, hemoptysis, œdema, emphysema and atelectasis. On the other hand, because of the increased activity of the heart, increased blood pressure takes place in the pulmonary system, and in consequence, hemorrhage and serous exudation in the pulmonary alveoli. The atelectasis would in part result from the emphysema, and in part from the obstruction of the bronchi by serum, mucus, &c. True inflammatory processes, according to this author, are not verified ; he thus seconds the theory of Traube, which ascribes the morbid conditions to the entrance of particles of food and the buccal fluids into the air passages.

This is, within certain limits, true. The mechanism of respiration is notably changed by section of the vagi ; but whilst in rabbits the thoracic expansion becomes more extended than in normal conditions, and there is, therefore, as Bernard states, a more active exchange of gas, so that the the alveoli remain distended ; in dogs, on the contrary, the respiratory movements are slow, and they are deep only under the influence of emotions and strong muscular action ; the pauses are very long ; it is therefore more logical to admit collapse of the alveolar walls. In man with degenerate vagi the respiration is reduced to a minimum, apart from its disorder and arhythm, and these last characters much resemble the respiration of rabbits having the vagi cut.

Now it is very difficult to see how, with a mechanism so different that the exchange of gas may be exaggerated or diminished, pulmonary inflammatory processes may be developed similar in man to those in rabbits and dogs.

That the vagus influences the mechanism of respiration, the rhythm, the proportional duration of the inspiration and expiration, and the pause, cannot be doubted when we look at the tracings taken on both man and other animals ; but here we slide from the simple disturbance of the respiratory mechanism to an inflammatory process in the lung.

Nor does the pulmonary congestion, concomitant with the altered mechanism, fill up the great lacuna. If we should confine ourselves to the discussion of this disturbance only, we might find ourselves again facing the difficulties of the interpretation of the pulmonitis in the rabbits on which the canula was applied, with results contrary to the theory of Traube, and the pulmonitis in dogs which did not present laryngeal œsophageal paralysis.

Much value has been accorded to laryngeal paralysis, and we have observed it in rabbits and some paralytics ; but in dogs and some other paralytics we could not admit it. Yet the pulmonary processes in dogs with the vagi cut are similar, as well as in paralytics (? paretics) without distinction. In dogs the cutting of the vagi below the recurrent does not produce laryngeal paralysis, but it produces the special form of pulmonitis. We have observed many paralytics who did not present any disturbance of deglutition, nor any change in the timbre of the voice ; rather, indeed, were they often, up to a few days before death, loud scolders ; but the pulmonary lesions in these did not present the same characters as they did in others who had been mute in the last weeks of their existence, or had presented some slight

changes of voice.   On the other hand, it is known that section
of the recurrents in dogs (Arnsperger), just as paralysis of the
laryngeal muscles in man, from whatever cause, does not give
place to pulmonary diseases.   Laryngeal paralysis, like the
entrance of buccal fluids and fragments of food, is, *per se*,
inadequate to the explanation of the facts observed by Nasse
and Bernard ; the former having ascertained that the lung of the
side on which the vagus had been cut had been more diseased
than the other, the vagus of which was cut some time afterwards ;
the latter found pulmonary disease only on the side on which the
vagus had been cut.   A remarkable contribution to this subject
has been presented in the experiments of Genzmer, who observed
no pulmonary lesions in rabbits on which he cut one vagus only.

Recently a parasitic doctrine has entered the field.   Schow,
in three out of seven cases of pulmonitis in rabbits with both the
vagi cut, succeeded in discovering an elliptic coccus of medium
size, which was not colored by the method of Gram.   This coccus
he regards as pathogenetic of vagal pulmonitis.   When directly
injected across the thoracic cavity, or through the trachea, into
the lungs, in the form of a culture, it developed a typical vagal
pulmonitis.   But this coccus was found in only 1 out of 25 animals,
the buccal liquid of which was examined ; it could not from the
mouth pass into the air passages of the rabbits on which the
trachea had been cut and a canula inserted to continue their
respiration ; it could not be the cause of pulmonitis in dogs in
which the cutting of the vagus did not produce paralysis either
of the larynx or the œsophagus.   It might, at the most, be found
in the air inspired through the larynx or the canula ; but then,
even admitting its specificity, this would not explain why, after
cutting the vagi, that is to say, after preparing a soil suited to
its development and its pathogenetic action, or, in other words,
creating pathological, structural and functional conditions, without which, at least in dog and man, it proves ineffective.

The fact that the form of pulmonitis spoken of is frequently
associated with degeneration of the vagus, inclines us to regard
it, as does Vulpian, as a trophic disturbance, arising directly
or indirectly from the degeneration of the pneumogastric.

We do not desire to present here a sample of the old debated doctrine on the trophic nerves; but science now possesses a not despicable number of facts which demonstrate that the innervation of an organ presides over its nutrition, and guarantees resistance against disorganizing agents. The most acceptable form in which the question of trophism may be presented by anyone like ourselves in this case, is that which avoids going to the bottom of the question. We should now be engaging in a fruitless work did we affirm either the one or the other of the conceptions by which it has been sustained or upset, but never settled. It may be affirmed, on the basis of a large case history and experimental proofs, that the inflammation or the irritation of a nerve, or of certain centres, is followed by more or less notable trophic changes in the organs innervated by them. Thus zoster (herpes) in intercostal neuralgia; decubitus (bed-sore) in the neurites; lesions of the cornea from alterations and sections of the trigeminus; atrophies in different affections of the central nervous system; cutaneous affections in tabes: fatty degeneration of the testicle from section of the spermatic nerve, &c., &c.

On the other part, we have records of the existence of pulmonary affections from lesions of the central nervous system; the facts were well known long ago by Cruveilheir, and they have since been well studied by Ollivier, Navarre, Durand Fardel and Fabre.

Cases of pulmonitis from compression of the vagus nerve are known. Thus, e. g., a case of aneurism of the aorta recorded by Gull; the patient died of pulmonary gangrene with multiple foci; the aneurismal sac compressed the vagus. Three cases have been recorded by Dessenos, observed in patients with cancer of the œsophagus, which pressed the pneumogastric. Two others are recorded by Eichhorst.

We admit, with Arnozam, that Fabre has gone too far in forming a class of nervous pulmonitis, and that Fernet has erred in believing that frank, acute fibrinous pulmonitis is attributable to hyperæmia of the pneumogastric, merely because he succeeded in demonstrating its existence in three cases. We are unable to attach any very great importance to the coincidence of the pneumotic forms, studied by us in the insane, with degeneration, more or less advanced, of the pneumogastrics.

As a slight compression, from which the tissues in their normal conditions feel nothing, produces a bed-sore rapidly or slowly, when a neuritis, or an inflammatory process exists in the spinal centres, so also does a degenerative neuritis of the vagus changes the conditions of nutrition in the pulmonary parenchyma, and in these altered conditions stimuli, which previously were harmless, may become pathogenic, reaching the lungs through the larynx, the mouth, or the tracheal tube in the air inspired.

Hyperæmia, if it is present, the disturbed respiratory mechanism, increased endoalveolar tension, paralysis of the muscular fibres of the bronchi, insensibility of the mucosa of the deep respiratory passages, are but concomitants, so many factors, concurring to disturb the process of nutrition, which is so intimately connected with the function of all the anatomical elements that constitute an organ so complex as the lung ; but the inflammatory process with ready exit into necrobiosis, may spring from those stimuli—the buccal detritus or the coccus of Schow —which, in normal conditions, are ineffective. Even gangrene, which is so common a finding in the pulmonitis of paralytics, and in rabbits, simply indicates the frail vitality of the pulmonary tissues ; perhaps, too, preceding lesions in the vessel walls have contributed in determining the facile and prompt death of the tissue, however trivially more intense may have been the stimulus which it has been unable to resist.

SULPHONAL.*

By James Stewart, M.D.,
Professor of Pharmacology and Therapeutics, McGill University.

This paper† is based on observations made in 52 different cases, where sulphonal was administered to induce sleep. In nearly every case, before administering the drug, the precaution was taken to confirm the statements of the patient that there was actual insomnia. Such a precaution is especially necessary in hospital patients and those suffering from neurasthenia in its varied forms.

Where the drug induced a sleep of from seven to ten hours duration, the effect is described as a marked action. A three to five hours sleep is referred to as a moderate action, while a sleep of less duration than two hours is classed under the heading of negative results.

Out of the total of 52 cases, the drug had a marked action in 39 cases—i.e., in 75 per cent.,—a moderate action in 13 per cent. and a negative action in 11 per cent. of the cases.

In a large proportion it was administered on several different occasions with the almost invariable result that, if it induced sleep on its first administration, the same result followed subsequent doses.

The cause of its partial or entire failure in 26 per cent. is clear when we consider the cause of the sleeplessness.

The seven partial failures were in the following series of cases :—

1. In chronic interstitial nephritis with dyspnœa, and restlessness in an alcoholic subject.

2. In chronic interstitial nephritis with dyspnœa due to lead poisoning.

3. In acute parenchymatous nephritis with Cheyne-Stokes respiration.

4. In mitral incompetence with great dyspnœa.

5. In typhoid fever with peritonitis.

6. In chronic myelitis with distressing girdle feeling.

---

* Read at the Banff meeting of the Canadian Medical Association.
† The writer is greatly indebted to Drs. England, Brown and Low for the report of the cases on which this paper is founded.

7. In subacute rheumatism where pain was moderate **i**∋ severe.

The complete failures occurred in :—

1. Aortic aneurism where pain was a continuous symptom.
2. Lead poisoning where abdominal pain was severe.
3. In acute pneumonic phthisis with great dyspnœa.
4. Acute parenchymatous nephritis with dyspnœa.
5-6. Were in two of Dr. Gardner's cases (gynæcological), where pain was complained of.

The cause of the sleeplessness in seven of the above thirteen cases was pain of varying degrees of intensity. Where the pain was moderate the sulphonal had a slight action, but where it was severe the result was practically negative.

In the remaining six cases dyspnœa was the active factor in preventing sleep, and over which sulphonal was powerless.

In a case of aortic aneurism with great distress, the continuous use of morphine in doses of $\frac{1}{8}$ of a gr. two or three times during the day, and a xxx. gr. dose of sulphonal at night gave greater relief than much larger doses of morphia alone. This and the experience in many other cases show that sulphonal is not entirely destitute of analgesic powers.

The following case is a good illustration of the powerful hypnotic action of this drug, and also of its analgesic effects.

A highly neurotic subject was admitted to the Montreal General Hospital, complaining of pain in the abdomen, diarrhœa, headache and sleeplessness. These symptoms had been troublesome at intervals for years.

On July 14th he received 20 gr. of sulphonal, and fell asleep in an hour, which lasted till morning. He says it is the best sleep he has had since giving up morphia, three years ago. On the following night, no sulphonal—very little sleep. Next night, sulphonal gr. xx.—excellent sleep. Next night, no sulphonal—no sleep. The following night, sulphonal gr. xx.— within one hour he was asleep, and slept thoroughly well till the morning. The following night he had no sulphonal—no sleep. The next night 20 gr. of sulphonal was followed by a good night's sleep.

The following night he had sulphonal, gr. xxx., at 8.30 p.m. He kept awake as long as possible to notice the effects of the drug. He first experienced a general pricking sensation, soon his eyelids became heavy, and, in spite of all efforts to keep awake, he fell into profound slumber an hour after he had taken his dose. He volunteers the statement that he feels no disagreeable after effects from sulphonal, as with morphine, cocaine and caffeine, all of which he has used largely.

On the following night he complained severely of headache, for which antipyrine was prescribed with little benefit, 30 gr. of sulphonal apparently having more effect than 15 of antipyrine.

This patient was an unusually intelligent man for an hospital patient. He thoroughly entered into the spirit of the investigations, and being an old morphine, chloral, cocaine and caffeine eater, his observations were of considerable value and interest.

In the cases where sulphonal acted in inducing from seven to ten hours sleep, are included a great variety of both acute and chronic diseases. The essential disturbing element in the majority was a condition of restlessness, due usually to pyrexia, cardiac insufficiency or that general condition of erethism of the nervous system included under the term neurasthenia. It is in the latter class of cases that sulphonal acts with the greatest certainty. I question very much whether we have any drug to compare with it in these troublesome conditions. It is not the purpose in this paper to discuss to what extent hypnotics are useful or advisable in neurasthenic conditions.

Untoward Effects.—In estimating the value of any drug, the first and most important question to consider is, What are its untoward effects? Unfortunately many of our most highly prized hypnotics act at times so that any good effect that may be produced is more than counterbalanced by the subsequent evils.

How much more valuable opium would be were it not for the disagreeable symptoms that follow its use?

As regards the use of hypnotics in certain diseases we require to be especially guarded. Many a beginning neurasthenic has been converted into a hopeless incurable by the injudicious administration of hypnotics, especially opium.

So far as I have been able to make out from the use of sulphonal, there is no danger whatever in the acquirement of a habit. On the contrary, all to whom it was administered for any length of time were only too glad to give up its use, and felt no desire whatever to continue it after the cause for which it was employed had passed away.

This negative action on the higher centres I believe to be one of the most important advantages possessed by sulphonal over the more commonly employed members of this group of agents.

When sulphonal is given in doses of about 40 grains and upwards, there is occasionally a peculiar effect on the locomotion. It induces ataxia and giddiness. In the cases reported there is an account of these symptoms being present in three instances :

1. A woman received at 8 p.m. 30 grains of sulphonal. An hour afterwards she complained of nausea, but quickly fell into a deep slumber, which lasted ten hours. The following day she complained of giddiness and was so ataxic that she was unable to walk without support.

In another case, female, 20 gr. of sulphonal were administered in the evening. Was restless up to 1.20 o'clock, when she had a troubled sleep lasting two hours. On awakening she complained of nausea and dizziness, had sensations as if her bed was tumbling over her. She had to hold the sides of the bed to prevent her from falling out. When she closed her eyes, she had sensations of objects passing before them. These symptoms continued in a lesser degree during the two following days.

The night following the complete disappearance of these symptoms, another dose of gr. xx was administered with the effect of a good sleep and no untoward symptoms whatever.

The third case, also a female, received 20 gr. of sulphonal at 8 p.m. In three hours she awoke with a feeling as if her head would burst, complained of great nausea, dizziness, and felt as if she was falling through the bed. These symptoms continued for eighteen hours, and were followed by a deep dreamless sleep. A subsequent dose produced a deep sleep and no untoward effects.

The fourth case was in a male, of a highly neurotic temperament, suffering from neurasthenia from over-study.   25 gr. of sulphonal induced giddiness and ataxia almost invariably.   In one case of ataxia there was also loss of the knee-jerk.   It quickly re-appeared after the complete elimination of the drug.

Dr. Roddick had in his practice a case of very profound ataxia, following the administration of a 40 gr. dose of sulphonal.

It is an important point to decide, how is the sulphonal ataxia induced?   Is it a cerebral or spinal ataxia?   Judging from the loss of the knee jerk in the case referred to, it is probable that it is of spinal origin, and if so, we are brought face to face with an important problem—Is it possible for a permanent spinal degeneration to be caused by the long continued use of sulphonal.

We know that other hypnotics do, when long employed, induce changes—molecular and probably gross in the higher centres—and it is not at all unreasonable to believe that permanent organic change may be induced in one or other of the spinal systemic tracts.   At present I am conducting a series of experimental investigations, with the object of endeavoring to prove whether it is possible for sulphonal to bring about changes of a sub-acute or chronic degenerative character in any of the spinal systems.   At present it is well to be cautious in giving sulphonal for a long period, especially to patients who are apt to become ataxic from it.

Action of Sulphonal on the Circulation.—In not a single instance was there noticed any depressant action on the heart, even when given in the largest doses, and continuously for several nights.   It is very well adapted therefore in the delirium of broken-down drunkards, a state where choral is a dangerous remedy, owing to its powerful cardiac depressent action.   Chloral not only acts directly on the heart muscle as a depressant, but it lowers the blood pressure also.   A few cases have been reported where a depressant action on the heart has been observed to follow the use of sulphonal.

Action on the Stomach.—In only six cases was there any nausea or vomiting attendant on the administration of sulphonal, and in all these cases it was late in making its appearance and was attended by giddiness. This points to the probability that sulphonal does not act directly on the stomach in causing nausea and vomiting, but indirectly through its action on the nerve centres.

There is no record in any instance of an untoward action on the skin in the cases reported.

The Dose and Mode of Administration.—The adult dose of sulphonal varies from fifteen to fifty grains. Thirty grains may be considered an average dose, and in a first administration should not be exceeded.

Doses of fifty grains and upwards are apt to be followed by ataxic symptoms.

As the drug is not soluble in water at the ordinary temperature, it is best administered in a warm fluid, as beef tea or gruel. It is practically free from odor and taste.

As the salivary glands take part in its elimination, it is not uncommon to find patients complain of a peculiar, but not disagreeable taste 12 to 24 hours after its administration.

TWO INTERESTING QUESTIONS IN GYNÆCIC SURGERY, ILLUSTRATED BY CASES.

By T. Johnson-Alloway, M.D.,
Instructor in Gynæcology. McGill University.

First—The Relation of Schrœder's Hystero-trachelorrhaphy to future Parturition.

Second—The failure of Electrolysis, faithfully carried out for one and a half years, to influence a hard, slowly-growing Myofibroma Uteri. Removal of Appendages by Laparotomy, immediately followed by premature menopause and return to health.

Two years ago I read a short paper at the Ottawa meeting of the Canadian Medical Association on " *The Comparative Merits of Schrœder's and Emmet's Hystero-trachelorrhaphy.*" In this paper I embodied the results and experience obtained from fifteen hospital and twenty-two private cases. During the discussion which followed the reading of this paper, the question was asked,

" What effect would the operation have upon future pregnancy and parturition?" This question I could not satisfactorily answer from personal experience up to that time. I have since been informed by the attending physician of a few of the cases I had operated on, that they had confined their patients without any unusual complication. But I was anxious to have personal experience of this nature with a few of these cases. The opportunity presented itself to me some months ago. I was thus enabled to make some valuable observations during the progress of labor.

The first case of which I will speak had borne three children within the space of six years. She had been in very poor health for some time past, and was a subject of all the reflex neuroses which accompany a badly lacerated cervix complicated with chronic metritis and profuse purulent uterine leucorrhœa. A few months after the operation she regained her health and became again pregnant. She was carefully watched during the pregnancy, as she had suffered two miscarriages before the operation. It was interesting to observe the effects of the operation in this direction, whether it would have a tendency to favor the occurrence of the accident or otherwise. In this case no pregnancy ever progressed to the end more favorably. The observations made during the progress of labor were indeed interesting. Labor had just begun when I made the first examination. The pains were extremely light, and it seemed to me as if several hours might elapse before attendance would be required. On introducing my finger into the vagina I was surprised to find the bag of membranes distended to complete fullness occupying the vagina, and nothing else to be felt. There was no evidence of the usual resisting ring through which the membranes protrude; nothing, in fact, could be felt but this boundless bag of water containing, high up, the head. I ruptured the membranes, and before I could remove my coat the fœtus was expelled. The placenta presently followed, but the uterus remained a little soft. External manipulation was kept up for some time, still there seemed to be a want of reflex irritability about the organ. I introduced my hand into the cavity, but found no

clots to speak of. The uterus soon afterwards recovered its
tonic contractility and remained hard and small. During the
time my right hand was in the cavity of the uterus I could
distinctly feel what appeared to be the narrow, thin edge of
Bandl's ring. The convalescence of this patient was most
satisfactory. The cervical opening had the same appearance as
directly before impregnation, and involution of the pelvic organs
have been very perfect.

The second case of this nature occurred in a lady who had
borne eight children, but who had not been pregnant during
the past eight years. She suffered from incomplete uterine prolapse and general failure of health. One year after I had
repaired the cervical and perineal lacerations she became pregnant. Pregnancy followed a very even course ; but when labor
set in the pains were so violent that chloroform had to be given.
On making the vaginal examination the same condition presented
as in the first case—i.e., the bag of membranes completely filled
the vagina, no cervix being within reach. After the membranes
were ruptured the labor soon terminated. There appeared in
this case also a slight degree of inertia of the uterus. When,
however, the uterus once contracted firmly, it remained so.
This patient made a good convalescence, and the uterus involuted
well.

In regard to the changed condition of the uterus induced by
amputation of the cervix which was especially high in these
two cases, and to the course future pregnancies would follow, it
has been a matter of some question. Some have suggested that
the operation rendered pregnancy less likely to occur afterwards.
On this point my experience has pointed to the reverse, and it
is that which should be expected. An old hypertrophied, cystic
and bulbous stump discharging large quantities of muco-pus has
been converted into a hollow-shaped cone with a small opening
in the centre, absolutely free from abnormal secretion. There
is to me no condition of the parts in question so favorable to
impregnation, and in the last case recorded it proved an actual
cure for the relative sterility.

Further experience regarding this point, however, will be

required in order to enable me to speak more definitely. The question of the liability to early interruption of pregnancies can be answered, I think, negatively. I have not seen a case where early abortion could be attributed to the operation, and anatomically it would not be indicated.

In regard to the influence of the operation upon full-term labor, it certainly hastens it, renders it a much less painful and tedious process, and does away with all possibility to traumatism of the cervix, and therefore lessens the liability to infective disease. This latter is a most practical point, and in importance cannot be over-estimated. The relation which the cervix uteri bears to the whole female sexual system in the matter of septic infection is well recognized and needs no further comment. I do not mean by this that there has been a developmental error in the process of progressive evolution, but I certainly do mean that I have seen more evidence pointing to the cervix as an object of danger than I have to it being one of usefulness. And should experience prove that this operation will not involve any very serious drawback, I am afraid my convictions in this respect will rather gain than lose strength.

II.—*Case of Uterine Myoma treated by Electricity, and eventually by Laparotomy.*

This case was referred to me by the late Dr. R. P. Howard in April, 1888. History as follows: Married eight years; never been pregnant. For the past three years she has been losing blood very freely at each menstrual period; duration of flow from ten to twelve days, accompanied with a great deal of pain. Leucorrhœa very profuse. Extreme anæmia and general failure of health.

Examination.—Interstitial myoma apparently occupying the right anterior segment of uterus. Uterus mobile and not tender to manipulation. Sound enters 12 cm. and in a straight direction. Auscultation gives a distinct bruit over tumor. The tumor reached to within half an inch below the umbilicus, and could be freely moved in every direction.

After explaining to the patient the different methods of treat-

32

ment adopted for the relief of her condition, she selected electricity. From May 10th to August 18th, 1888, she received
thirty-one applications, chiefly of the positive pole, averaging
from 70 to 100 ma. for five to ten minutes each application.
During some of these sittings she suffered a good deal of pain,
and I had often difficulty in encouraging her to continue the
treatment. Towards the end of this course she became much
improved in her general health. She seemed to gain color, and
the blood condition was certainly much improved. She was
stronger, evidenced by her being able to walk longer distances.
She returned to her home, and spent August and September at
an inland summer resort. In October she began to fall a little
back in health, and the hemorrhages became again excessive,
also some pelvic pain. She returned to me for treatment on
October 11th, and remained until January 9th, 1889, receiving
thirty-four applications of positive pole of strength 70 to 100
ma., as in first series. I was under the impression that she
suffered more pain during this series, and I had greater difficulty
in encouraging her. The monthly hemorrhages lessened and
she again became stronger. During the six months of almost
constant treatment the tumor never diminished nor changed its
character permanently in any way. At times I would think it
was smaller, but it would regain its size without any accountable
reason.

She again returned home for a short time. In May, 1889,
she visited me and received ten applications as before. In
October she became discouraged, having received no lasting
benefit from the electrical treatment, and asked me to remove
the appendages. This was done on the 4th of October. I
found some difficulty in reaching the appendages on account of
the size of the tumor, but as there were no adhesions this did
not matter. This patient returned home on the 9th November.
She has, since the operation, passed two periods practically
without discharge. Her pains have all disappeared, and she is
as much improved in general health as could be expected in the
time.

During the electrical treatment of this case I had been most careful to take a record in detail of the effect of each application, and I am now convinced that my patient suffered more at each seance of over 70 ma. than she did during the whole of the period of convalescence following the operation. It therefore cannot be wondered at, although surgeons are straining every nerve at present to give the votaries of electricity in gynæcology as much rope as possible, that they break out sometimes in condemnation of the method, with what seems a feeling of just indignation.

NOTE ON PEROXIDE OF HYDROGEN AS A SOLVENT FOR THE MEMBRANE OF DIPHTHERIA.

By GEORGE W. MAJOR, B.A., M.D., &c.,

Late (1877) Clinical Assistant, Hospital for Diseases of the Throat and Chest, London, Eng.; Fellow of the American Laryngological Association: Specialist to the Department for Diseases of the Nose and Throat, Montreal General Hospital; and Instructor in Laryngology and Diseases of the Throat, McGill University, Montreal.

(*Read before the Medico-Chirurgical Society of Montreal.*)

Solution of peroxide of hydrogen, or hydroxyl in aqueous solution, has been used in France as a surgical dressing for ten years.

Its use as a solvent for the membrane of diphtheria is of much more recent origin. In so far as I have been able to ascertain, Dr. Love, of St. Louis, was among the first to call attention to hydroxyl as a valuable agent in the treatment of diphtheria. He employed it in a solution containing from 0.5 to 3 per cent., using most frequently, however, a strength of one per cent., diluting the medical "ten volume" peroxide with two or three times its bulk of water. Of its value in clearing away and effectually deodorizing the decomposing exudate in cases of diphtheria he speaks in the most emphatic terms.

Dr. Glasgow, of St. Louis, informs me that he has used hydroxyl for the past three years, and that it has given him very satisfactory results. He uses it locally as well as constitutionally in nasal, naso-pharyngeal, faucial and laryngeal diphtheria. He says it will do all that is claimed for it.

My individual experience of the remedy extends over a period of two years, and, though not as extensive as I would wish, still it may prove of sufficient interest to occupy a few minutes.

I have used hydroxyl in aqueous solution (formula H_2O_2) in 22 cases of diphtheria in my own private and in consulting practice. The cases were all of more than average severity with decided septic tendency. The nasal chambers were invaded in fourteen. To sum up—

Hydroxyl possesses the following advantages :—It offends neither the sense of taste nor smell—being tasteless and odorless.

When applied locally it causes no irritation and occasions no pain.

When swallowed it is harmless, as it is not poisonous.

It is a powerful antiseptic and deodorizer.

It in no way precludes the simultaneous use of any other local remedy.

It is a perfect solvent for the exudate of diphtheria.

When used locally the membrane seems to corrode and comes away in fragments of a more or less porous character.

I have seen it remove membrane as quickly as it could form. In nasal cases it keeps the nose free from membrane and gives the bichloride or other solution a chance to act. In the most offensive cases it deprives the discharges of their unpleasant odor. In the larynx it occasions a little alarm by the escape of gas as it comes into contact with the membrane, but it does not in any way interfere with respiration. I generally commence its use as a 60 per cent. solution, increasing to the full strength of the so-called "ten volume" peroxide of hydrogen. When used internally the dose is $\frac{1}{2}$ to 2 drams.

IODOFORM IN CHRONIC CYSTITIS.

By C. J. Edgar, M.D., Sherbrooke, Que.

A few weeks since there appeared in some of the medical journals a notice of the treatment of chronic cystitis, by Dr. V. Moestig-Moorhof, of Vienna, with iodoform injections. Having on hand at the time several cases of decidedly chronic cystitis, which did not show satisfactory signs of improvement under ordinary treatment, I decided to treat one-half the cases (3) with the iodoform injections. The bladder was first washed out with moderately hot water, as usual, and then an injection of the following emulsion made :—

> Iodoform, ʒx.
> Glycerine, ʒi.
> Tragacanth gum, gr. i.
> Distilled water, ʒii.

Sig. One tablespoonful to a pint of lukewarm water, well stirred, for one injection—injection made every second day. The first part of the mixture was injected and held about half a minute, until the iodoform had settled, and was then allowed to come away clear. The latter part was ordered to be retained as long as possible without pain.

The day after the first injection, the patients all agreed in finding micturition, less difficult, less painful, and much less frequent. They had all noticed also that the urine had deposited a yellow sediment—the iodoform. The effect of the second injection was still more marked, and the third injection completed the cure, leaving them perfectly free from any symptoms whatever of their old trouble. The remaining three cases were then put on the same treatment, with the same result, excepting that the two worst cases required five injections before they confessed themselves quite cured. Of these cases three were gonorrhœal, one from cold and two, cause unknown, and had all been under medical treatment for periods ranging from six months to three years. The treatment in these cases was alike for all, independent of their causation, and was followed by a

uniformly good result.   In one case treated last week, the iodoform was simply mixed with warm water and injected, but the
patient—a male—complained that the gritty powder hurt him in
coming away, and was stuck in masses like little calculi.   The
effect on the disease, however, was identical with those mentioned
before.   I have not had the opportunity of testing the use of this
drug as an injection in other affections of the bladder, but certainly in the cases mentioned, and occurring in both sexes, its
action was most satisfactory.

MISSED ABORTION.

By Geo. T. Ross, M.D.,

Professor of Physiology, Bishop's College, Montreal.

Mrs. A. B., æt. 40, the mother of six children, became pregnant with the seventh in September of last year.   Her former
history was good, having been ill only from diseases incident to
child-bearing.   She has evidence of a strumous constitution, the
irritable mucous membranes showing not only in herself but
plainly in her living children.   She is of thin, spare habit of
body and an active nervous temperament.   Several years ago
the husband was treated for specific trouble.   Before this the
mother had miscarried three or four times, the fœtus in every
case being discharged without unusual features.

The patient's condition was as follows :—Up till the end of the
fourth month of this pregnancy no symptom of a remarkable
character was presented.   The ordinary signs of the patient's
state in January last were to her unmistakable.   The fœtal
movements were very distinct during some three weeks, after
which they ceased entirely.   There seemed no reasonable ground
to doubt the nature of the uterine contents from the exact history given regarding all the indications.   The mother, an intelligent woman, had experienced the usual phenomena too often
to be mistaken in their nature this time, and the well-defined
fœtal movements, if the history were credited, seemed to place
the case beyond a doubt.   A short time subsequent to the
change noticed by the mother I was consulted regarding it.   On

examination 1 was unable to discover the fœtal heart-beat, and found that the breasts, from being enlarged and turgid, according to patient's statement, were soft and flaccid ; other indications also pointed to cessation of uterine activity. The general rule being that two weeks after the death of a fœtus it is aborted, and finding the patient in good health, with nothing existing to justify interference, I advised waiting for further indications. An interval of several months now elapsed and I was again consulted regarding the non-progress of gestation. It was quite evident now that since last interview no growth had occurred in the uterine contents, the size of the tumor being about the same, if anything it was smaller. Vaginal examination showed the os to be undilated, although somewhat patulous. Uterus was uniformly enlarged, such as would still be not inconsistent with a four months fœtal growth. At this time, say seven months after what was believed to be conception, there did not exist a single symptom calling for interference beyond this, that if conception had taken place, and the patient was right regarding the fœtal movements, it was certain growth had ceased during the past three months, and consequently a dead fœtus existed in utero. 1 was naturally surprised at not hearing from the patient long before this with evidence of the onset of a miscarriage, but the only symptom at all attributable to her condition was an occasional hardening of the uterus, which was readily noticed, the hard, round tumor being very plainly shown through the thin abdominal walls. No hemorrhages had ever shown themselves at any time. General health continued unimpaired, and still adhering to the expectant treatment, I advised further delay. As long as nothing existed calling for action on my part I felt that, notwithstanding the time that had elapsed, any day might bring evidence of uterine expulsive efforts. The risks attending the artificial emptying of the uterine cavity being greater than what attended the present condition and the expected natural expulsion, I inclined to wait further, warning her that at the first appearance of any unfavorable sign to at once notify me. During the next few months and in my absence from town I heard nothing further from her, but in September

she again called upon me, this being one year after the supposed
conception, and eight months after cessation of fœtal life. The
same general condition of good health existed now, with the
difference of slight tenderness on pressure over uterus. I felt
that now much longer time had elapsed than I had intended
should before interfering, and in consultation with Dr. Gardner
I arranged to remove the uterine contents the following day.
In the evening I inserted a faggot of four laminaria tents covered
with iodoform, retaining them with a tampon of absorbent cotton,
and gave a mild opiate. Next day I found the os fairly dilated
and proceeded to extract the fœtus. The patient declined to
take an anæsthetic, and assisted me throughout the operation.
Through the membranes I felt the child's feet presenting. On
rupturing the membranes, which were so strong and fibrous that
a steel hook was required to penetrate them, about half a pint
of a chocolate-brown semi-viscid fluid escaped. Using my nose
as the instrument of diagnosis, I found no putridity existing,
the fluid being odorless. By conjoined manipulation I extracted
the fœtus all but the head, which the os held firmly. Taking a
medium-sized Barnes dilator I passed it through the os alongside
the fœtal neck; then gradually filling the dilator, uterine contractions set in vigorously and quickly. The head being thus
delivered I had now the fœtus complete with the umbilical cord
intact, still united to the retained placenta. After some difficulty, owing to cessation of uterine contractions, the placenta
was extracted, considerable hemorrhage resulting. I now gave
an intrauterine sublimate injection, inserted a gr. x iodoform
suppository, and ordered vaginal douches every six hours. Pain
across abdomen was complained of greatly, but an occasional
opiate gave comfort. After seeing patient every other day for
a week, without a bad sign, I ceased attending. On the twelfth
day I was requested to call, and now for the first time since
emptying the uterus I found the patient sick. Temperature
104°; pulse 120; anxious look; coated tongue; loss of appetite; some marked abdominal tenderness and lochia arrested.
On examination the os was plugged with whitish, thick tenacious
mucus. No bad odor evident. The parts being cleaned I gave

another intrauterine sublimate injection, inserted a suppository, and ordered the latter every six hours. Hot poultices were put on abdomen and antipyrine gr. viii every four hours given. Next morning the temperature was normal and general condition much improved. Substituted quin. sulph. gr. v morning and evening for antipyrine. On the evening of this day the temperature rose again to 103°, with pulse 80, but on following day—viz., the third day after onset of fever—the temperature was normal and remained so, with a continuing progressive convalescence.

After being dead eight months in the uterus, I looked for a mummified condition of the foetus, but quite the contrary was the case as far as appearances went. Even the umbilical cord was about the natural size and fairly well preserved, not tearing easily on being dragged upon. The flesh, however, had assumed a brownish color, and was easily torn. The placenta had the appearance of a mass of very firm fat, dull white in color everywhere except the surface of its attachment to the uterine wall, where the circulation apparently had been recently interrupted. The decidual membranes were very thick and tough, and could not be ruptured by the finger-nail.

Matthews Duncan says that missed abortion is a subject lying between obstetrics and gynæcology, but inclines to include it more under diseases of women than obstetrical diseases. A missed abortion is not a threatened abortion, nor is it an imperfect abortion A threatened abortion is a very common occurrence. When a woman has a threatened abortion she suffers pain, has a bloody discharge, and the mouth of the womb may be found open. An abortion may only get the length of being threatened; that is to say, it may be averted and pregnancy may go on healthily, even when you have been able to feel, through the neck of the womb, the ovum as it hangs in the uterus. Cases have been known of the separation of considerable decidua and its discharge without abortion taking place. Among these cases of threatened abortion may be included cases of extreme rarity, viz., the abortion of one of twins while the other remains in utero and goes on in its development. This abortion of one of twins may be a missed abortion, or the miscarriage of one of twins may be a missed miscarriage. Again, missed abortion is neither a threatened abortion or miscarriage, nor an imperfect miscarriage. What is a perfect or complete miscarriage? If the fœtus alone, or the entire ovum alone, comes away, the woman has miscarried or aborted, as the case may be; but the coming away of the ovum does not involve a complete miscarriage, and an imperfect miscarriage is often a very disastrous thing. The ovum sometimes comes away alone without any of its uterine or maternal membranes. The fœtus also may come away alone without even the ovuline membranes. Again, sometimes the ovum comes away and the maternal membranes or decidua imperfectly. Sometimes only a bit of placenta is left. Imperfect miscarriage is a dangerous thing owing to the frequently recurring bleedings that result from it. It not very rarely leads to death from mere putrid intoxication, or septicæmia, or pyæmia, just as happens after full-term delivery. This is especially liable to occur if the miscarriage has come on in consequence of extensive endometritis, such as is found in pregnancies occurring during typhoid fever. Imperfect miscarriage is also often disastrous by inducing endometritis, generally purulent in nature, and this frequently in connection with putrefaction of the parts left behind. In some respects missed miscarriage or missed abortion is even more important than missed labor: for in a case of missed abortion the history of the woman and her size may have led either to no suspicion of pregnancy having commenced, or to suspicion which may have been dissipated by the further history of the case. In a case of missed abortion or missed miscarriage, the important element of suspicion as to the real condition may not have come into the mind either of the patient or her physician. Mistake is then extremely liable to occur. This is not so likely in missed labor; for in that condition the woman's size will almost certainly have made her aware that she is in an advanced state of pregnancy, and her friends will know it also. Missed labor may be a subject of great medico-legal importance; the same is true, and even more so, of missed abortion or missed miscarriage. If, for instance, a woman passed a two months fœtus at the end of a five months so-called pregnancy, and were to tell the husband, who had been away from home during the five months, that his wife had had a two months child, rather unpleasant consequences might ensue. The importance can be appreciated by the practitioner, therefore, of counting a woman's pregnancy not up to the time when the foetus was discharged, but back to the time when it died, if any evidence of death can be adduced.

When a woman has a missed miscarriage or missed abortion the foetus dies, the symptoms of pregnancy are arrested, milk signs appear at the breasts, and hemorrhages may or may not occur. If the liquor amnii is not discharged it is absorbed, and the contents of the uterus either macerate or become mummified. If the membranes remain entire, the process is that of mummification. It is only when germs are admitted, and generally after rupture of the bag of membranes, that putrefaction and maceration take place and the more or less complete dissolution of the ovum. If the uterus has been felt, the remarkable observation may be made that while a woman is apparently going on in pregnancy the organ is becoming smaller instead of bigger, and at last the ovum may be at any time unexpectedly expelled. When expelled, you have a mass nearly dry, of a dirty brown color ; the foetus and membranes may be concealed, being rolled up in the placenta, which is too firm to be compressed, and embraces the whole ovum. The remarkable freshness, if it may be so called, of the foetus in the case which I bring to your notice, after remaining eight months in utero, does not correspond to the usual appearance of such cases, as above defined, and is my apology, if any be necessary, for bringing the subject before your attention to-night.

Retrospect Department.

QUARTERLY RETROSPECT OF OBSTETRICS.

Prepared by J. Chalmers Cameron, M.D.,

Professor of Obstetrics, McGill University ; Physician-Accoucheur to the Montreal
Maternity, &c.

The Uncontrollable Vomiting of Pregnancy.—M. Guéniot, Chirurgien en chef de la Maternité de Paris, has recently made a lengthy communication on this subject to the Academy of Medicine (*Archives de Tocologie*). Every year, as the result of prolonged vomiting during pregnancy, a large number of women perish or have their health seriously impaired, while in many cases the life of the fœtus is destroyed and abortion produced. The waste of life is serious, yet, notwithstanding the numerous therapeutic and operative measures commonly in use, the treatment of this affection does not seem to be established upon a rational basis or to yield satisfactory results. Guéniot suggests a rational basis and recommends a plan of treatment which he claims to be effectual in most cases of so-called uncontrollable vomiting, saving the life of both mother and child.

The first essential of success is to find out the pathogenic cause of the vomiting ; this may usually be referred to

(1) *Uterus*, which is not only the organ which contains and nourishes the fœtus. but is also the source of special excitation of other organs ;

(2) *Nervous system* (spinal and ganglionic), which by means of its reflex powers transmits excitement to distant organs ;

(3) *Stomach*, which suffers excessively from the effect of uterine stimuli, and is the organ chiefly involved in this affection.

Between ordinary benign vomiting and the graver forms, the difference seems to be one of degree rather than of cause. If the ordinary pathogenic causes happen in any case to be reinforced by some pathological state, their action is intensified and vomiting becomes more persistent and severe ; if the attacks are very frequent and do not yield to treatment, the patient becomes exhausted and the vomiting uncontrollable. The cause of vomiting can seldom be referred solely to either the uterus, nervous system, or stomach ; usually all three factors cooperate, but not to an equal extent,—one generally predominates. While the treatment must manifestly therefore be complex, its general character should be determined mainly by the nature of the predominating pathogenic factor ; and success in any given case will depend very largely upon the ability of the practitioner to determine the relative value of the causative factors. In all cases the stomach is weak and irritable, and should be spared as much as possible by administering food and medicine by the rectum or skin, or hypodermically, whenever practicable. A cheerful, hopeful frame of mind should be encouraged ; a gloomy prognosis, despondency, fear and anxiety have a very detrimental effect. Distressing thirst is a common symptom, and unless the patient is under the charge of a responsible attendant who is intelligent, discreet and firm, liquids are apt to be taken in improper quantity or of improper quality. The fundamental indications for treatment are :

1. To allay morbid or abnormal *uterine excitability* by removing the various pathological conditions which produce it. Flexions or displacements interfering with uterine circulation may be relieved by posturing, the Gariel pessary, etc. Tumors must receive appropriate treatment, operative if necessary. Abrasions or ulcerations of the os and cervix must be treated by local applications. Hyperæsthesia of the passages with more or less inflammation yields generally to emollient or narcotic vaginal injections, pomades or vaginal suppositories. Belladonna, cocaine and morphia are the most efficient local sedatives. When the exciting cause of exaggerated uterine reflex is chronic or subacute inflammation of the appendages, rest in bed in the horizontal position is essential, with poultices and emollient sedative vaginal applicatons. If all other measures fail, dilatation of the cervix according to Copeman's method may be tried.

2. To diminish the activity or suppress the exaggeration of reflex excitability. The bromide of potassium or sodium (grs. xv–xxx) with chloral (grs. x–xxv) in warm milk (2–4 oz.) by the rectum usually allay irritability and produce sleep. Chapman's ice-bag applied to the dorso-lumbar region for several days

consecutively sometimes gives relief; ether spray to the same
region produces similar effects. Galvanism has been recently
much extolled. Mental tranquility must be secured.

3. To overcome the irritability of the digestive apparatus,
particularly the stomach. Morbid conditions liable to provoke
or increase vomiting must be cured, such as gastritis, hyperacidity of secretions, etc. The diet must be carefully regulated,
both as regards quality and quantity of food, and the frequency
with which it is to be taken. Milk and light broths are the best
foods, given alternately (day about) to prevent disgust, beginning with small doses—a tablespoonful every half hour or hour.
Ice and alkaline waters may be sparingly used—five or six small
lumps of ice and two or three tablespoonfuls of Vichy in the
twenty-four hours will be enough at first. In a few days, as the
stomach becomes stronger, the liquid nourishment may be cautiously increased and the ice stopped.

During the first few days of treatment no drink must be allowed
other than Vals or Vichy water and ice in the quantities prescribed. Lemonade, wine, alcohol, orange and lemon juice, and
all fruits should be absolutely prohibited. Thirst is so urgent,
and acid drinks so grateful, that it is difficult to prevent the
patient breaking through rules ; but strict abstinence from such
things is essential to success. The intolerable thirst is relieved
by alkaline waters, but aggravated by acids and wines. Frequent gargling with Vichy water generally affords relief more
promptly than anything else. Rigid observance of the treatment
is essential. Flying blisters to the epigastrium, followed by
morphia applications, sometimes have a prompt effect ; ether
spray to the same region acts in a similar manner. If constipation exists, laxative enemata or suppositories should be used ; if
diarrhœa occurs, narcotics or astringents may be administered
per rectum.

There is no specific treatment or drug ; each case must be
treated upon its own merits. In the great majority of cases
judicious management will carry the patient safely through without serious damage either to herself or her child. The artificial
induction of labor is the "*remedy of despair,*" rarely to be
invoked.

External Cephalic Version in Breech Cases.—In France a sharp controversy has been going on respecting the value of external cephalic version as a prophylactic when presentation of the breech is diagnosed during the last month of gestation. Pinard is perhaps the strongest advocate of the operation, and certainly his results in the Lariboisière hospital have been brilliant. His methods have been severely criticised by some of the older members of the Academy of Medicine, and as warmly supported by some of the younger members. Dr. Gaulard of Lille (*Archives de Tocologie*), as the result of his observations, is inclined to take a middle course and circumscribe the field of this operation within somewhat narrow limits. According to Pinard, all pelvic presentations may be divided into *permanent* (*franches*) and *accidental* or *temporary*. In the former the breech is always to be found at the superior strait, while in the latter the breech may present at one time and the head or some other part at another. The former is mostly caused by exaggerated volume of the fœtal head (hydrocephalus), excessive development of the lower uterine segment, or the accidental premature engagement of the half-breech or feet. The latter is due to globular form of the uterus, hydramnios, or certain conditions of the fœtus, such as undue mobility, death, or maceration. Gaulard thinks that version is contraindicated in the permanent variety—that it is then very apt to fail, or, even if successful, the life of the child may be imperilled by undue traction upon the cord (which may be naturally very short or may be coiled around the neck), or by partial separation of the placenta. This controversy is not one of recent date. Hippocrates taught that only head presentations are natural, and that all others should be converted thereto if possible. Ambrose Paré, on the other hand, maintained that presentation of the breech is as natural as that of the vertex, and with care may be conducted to as favorable a termination. The modern controversy is, after all, only a renewal of the old warfare between the pupils of Mauriceau and Levret, who followed Hippocrates, and those of Bandelocque and Boer, who followed Paré. Gaulard thinks that the infantile mortality in breech cases has been placed far too high. Mme. Lachapelle

estimated it at 10 per cent., Hegar at 35–40 per cent., Heck[...]er
at 22 per cent., and Pinard at 10–15 per cent. Gaulard co[...]n-
siders a high infantile mortality quite unnecessary, and attribut[...]es
it to anxiety, impatience, or undue interference on the part o[...]
the attendant. Premature, precipitate, or violent traction [...]o[...]
the trunk, the undue use of ergot, etc, are often responsible fo[...]c
still-birth, whereas when the case is left to nature the child rarel[...]l
perishes. He urges strongly the claims of a cautious, expecta[...]
treatment.

Curetting in Puerperal Septicæmia.—The treatment of pue[...]
peral septicæmia does not yet seem to be settled down to an[...]
thing like uniformity. Most authorities approve of local trea[...]
ment, but differ widely as to what constitutes a safe and at th[...]
same time efficient local treatment. Some content themselve[...]
with simple vaginal injections, and rely mostly upon supportin[...]
constitutional treatment and the elimination of waste products b[...]
means of skin and kidneys. Others employ uterine douche[...]
plain or medicated, at more or less frequent intervals; whi[...]
others prefer a prompt and radical treatment, scraping or brus[...]
ing away from the internal surface of the uterus any shred[...]
clots, etc., which may prove a nidus for infection. Against th[...]
radical treatment it has been urged that brushing or curettin[...]
serve to intensify the risk of infection by denuding large portio[...]
of uterine surface, through which absorption of septic matter[...]
readily takes place. In reply, it is claimed that there need b[...]
very little risk of re-infection after curetting if a strict antisept[...]
treatment is maintained for some days after the operation. D[...]
Chartier of Paris (*Nouvelles Archives d' Obstetrique et de Gyn[...]cologie*) has published the records of twenty-six cases of curettin[...]
gathered from various sources, and summarises his conclusio[...]
as follows :—

1. Curetting the uterus is an easy and harmless operatio[...]n,
yielding excellent results in the treatment of puerperal sep[...]ti-
cæmia.

2. Anæsthesia is useless and dilatation of the cervix general[...]ly
unncessary.

3. Antiseptic precautions must be insisted on for several da[...]s

after the operation, otherwise there may be phenomena of re-infection.

4. Curetting is indicated whenever intrauterine injections are insufficient to lower the temperature rapidly, especially if some placental debris remains in utero.

5. Complications involving the uterine appendages or even the peritoneum do not necessarily contraindicate the operation.

Measles in Pregnancy.—Dr. *Lomer* of Hamburg (*Central. f. Gyn.*) reports the following curious case. A healthy young woman, 22 years of age, who had never had measles, began her first pregnancy in the beginning of October, 1887, and expected to be confined about the middle of July, 1888. A severe epidemic of measles broke out in the suburb where she lived, and on June 7th she was seized with chills, cough, hoarseness, smarting of the eyes, and diarrhœa. On the evening of the 8th labor pains began, and during the night she was delivered spontaneously of a living child. In the morning both mother and child were seen to be covered with a distinct measle-rash. On the fifth day the mother developed pneumonia, from which she made a slow recovery. The child died in four weeks from diarrhœa and debility.

Cases of pregnancy complicated with measles are rare, and receive but slight mention in the text-books. *Gantier* (*Annales de Gynécologie*, 1879) mentions eleven cases which he had found in looking up the literature of the subject. Of these eleven cases, six became infected during the last month of pregnancy, and the children were all born with measle rash or developed it shortly after birth. In Gantier's case, the child was born without rash, and though nursed by its mother did not subsequently develop it. In the remaining four cases, the course of gestation was interrupted by the attack of measles and abortion produced. In this series of eleven cases two mothers died. In Lomer's case labor pains began within thirty hours of the initial rigor, and the child was born five weeks before time. The attack had no ill effect upon the course of the puerperium except such as resulted from the pneumonia, and no special ill effect upon the child except such as was consequent to its premature birth.

The Umbilical Souffle and Uterine Souffle.—In Breisky's klinic, Vienna, a series of observations has been made by *Ettinger* (*Centralblatt f. Gyn.*). He examined the *Umbilical* souffle carefully in twelve cases and came to the conclusion that it is only exceptionally attributable to the fœtal heart, being in most cases produced in the cord itself by compression of its vessels from knotting, coiling around the neck or body, or from congenital shortness and consequent over-stretching. The *Uterine* souffle was looked for in 100 consecutive cases. It was present in 88 of them, 63 times on the left side, 12 times on the right, 10 times on both sides, and 3 times all over the abdomen. He attributes its frequent occurrence on the left side to the normal rotation of the pregnant uterus to the right ; and it is remarkable that in the 12 cases where the souffle was heard on the right side, the uterus was not in its usual physiological position. It was heard post-partum in 60 cases ; post-partum souffle is more frequently heard in multiparæ than primiparæ.

Plugging with Iodoform Gauze in Post-partum Hemorrhage. (*Lancet.*)—Dührssen has strongly recommended plugging the uterus with iodoform gauze in post-partum hemorrhage from atony, where ordinary measures have failed. He directs the bladder to be emptied, the uterus vigorously kneaded and rubbed, hot and cold intrauterine irrigation, and hypodermic injections of ergot tried ; if these measures fail, he directs a speculum to be introduced and the uterus to be filled with iodoform gauze. Active and permanent contraction is thereby set up. He claims that the operation is not only certain but harmless, and easily performed. Olshausen, Veit and Fehling, however, affirm that it is not always free from danger and that contraction is not always permanent. Dr. Piering, assistant in Prof. Schauta's klinic in Prague, after carefully testing the method, praises it highly. In his hands it has always succeeded, and in no case has it yet done any harm. He thinks that its use should not be delayed too long.

Glycosuria in the Pregnant, Parturient and Puerperal state.—In the Basel klinik *J. Ney* has been investigating this subject and has recently published his results (*Archiv f. Gyn.*).

After reviewing the work of previous observers he proposes the following questions :

1. Does sugar appear in the urine only before labor, or afterward also ? Does the act of labor influence glycosuria ?

2. Does sugar appear only during the puerperium and is its appearance in any way connected with febrile processes ?

3. Is the appearance of sugar in the urine, either before or after labor, physiological or pathological ?

4. How do the children develop where, in a normal puerperium, sugar is present or absent ?

He tabulates his observations on 172 women, 148 confined and 24 pregnant, the results of which may be summarised as follows : In the urine of the 24 pregnant women, sugar was found in 4 (16.6 per cent.) The act of labor of itself does not seem to induce glycosuria. When sugar appears in the urine of pregnant women, the breasts are usually well developed and milk can be squeezed from them. In women recently confined, sugar was found 115 times out of 148 (77.7 per cent.) Glycosuria bears no relation to febrile processes. Glycosuria is a normal physiological process in good nursing mothers, but may also be pathological as the result of milk stasis, since engorgement of the breasts (from cracks, fissures or inflammation) is immediately followed by the appearance of sugar in the urine. When glycosuria is abundant and prolonged, the breast milk is usually sufficient for the nourishment of the child. He concludes that when the breasts are well developed and the puerperium normal, the quantity of sugar in the urine and the length of time it persists are a direct measure of the quality of the milk and the excellence of the nurse. The more abundant the sugar and the longer it persists, the better the nurse. When the patients return to their own homes, resume their household duties, and live on a less generous diet, the glycosuria diminishes or disappears. The kind of sugar present in normal physiological glycosuria is always sugar of milk, thereby differing from those pathological conditions where glucose* is found in the urine.

See report of case of Glycosuria from nervous influences where the form of sugar was glucose, MONTREAL MEDICAL JOURNAL, Jan. 1889, p. 481.

The Alcohol Treatment of Puerperal Fever.—*Dr. A. Martin*
read an important paper before the Berlin Obstetrical and Gynæcological Society, giving his results with this treatment. (*Zeitschrift f. Geburts und Gyn.*, Bd. xvii, Hft. 2.)   Since 1876,
when Breisky and Conrad introduced the treatment, he had used
it 18 times, in 3 of pyæmia and 15 of septicæmia. These were
all severe cases with unfavorable prognosis, and had been treated
more or less locally and with antipyretics before they were seen
by him.   Alcohol was administered in the form of brandy, rum,
champagne, Burgundy or Bordeaux.   Out of 18 cases 13 recovered ; some very slowly.   Of the 5 deaths, 3 were caused
by puerperal infection, 2 by phthisis and pulmonary œdema
after the puerperal infection had been overcome.   The good
effect of the alcohol is not in the reduction of temperature, as
Breisky affirmed, but in the stimulation of the heart and increase
of general resisting power as pointed out by Runge.   He tried
baths, as recommended by Runge, in only one case, but they
were not well borne.   In most of his cases he could not do altogether without local treatment and antipyretics.   The alcohol
acts as a powerful stimulant in such cases, and even when given
in large doses ($\frac{1}{3}$ to $\frac{1}{2}$ bottle Cognac, $\frac{1}{2}$ to 1 bottle champagne,
1 bottle Burgundy per diem, along with milk, eggs and beef-tea),
produced no signs of intoxication.   It is not a specific, but in
these desperate cases can do nothing but good.   In the discussion
which followed, Gottschalk reported five cases of puerperal fever
treated by this method, four of the severest forms of puerperal
septicæmia and one of pyæmia, all complicated with general peritonitis.   Four recovered.   Sixteen to thirty fluid ounces of
cognac were administered daily.   Cocaine was found useful in
allaying vomiting.   Signs of alcoholism were observed in one
case.   From his experience he strongly recommends the treatment.   Olshausen has not had the same good results from it in
puerperal septicæmia.

Placenta Prœvia.—At the Leeds meeting of the B. M. Asso
ciation held in August last, a general discussion on Placenta
Prævia was introduced by *Dr. Braxton Hicks (British Medical
Journal).*   He remarked that within the last thirty years the

mortality from placenta prævia has been reduced from 30 per cent. to somewhere near 5 per cent., a result attributable in large measure to the early handling of these cases and the adoption of more rigid antiseptic precautions during and after delivery. He submitted the following propositions :—

1. When the placenta is inserted somewhere within the lower third of the uterus, there is generally a liability to hemorrhage, which may be expected before or upon the supervention of labor, whether premature or at full time.

2. When once hemorrhage has declared itself, there is no security for the patient, but her life is in imminent danger from liability to recurrent bleedings.

3. The relative position of the placenta to the os has no influence on the frequency or quantity of the blood loss. Whether it be marginal insertion or central, the risk is the same.

From these propositions he deduced the following rules of practice :

1. After the diagnosis of placenta prævia is made, pregnancy must be terminated as soon as possible.

2. When once we have begun to act, we are to remain by the patient.

3. If the os is fully dilated and the placenta marginal, we rupture the membranes and wait to see if the head is soon pushed by the pains into the os.

4. If there be any slowness or hesitation in this respect, then we employ forceps or version.

5. If the os be small and the placenta more or less over it, the placenta is to be carefully detached from around the os ; if no further bleeding occur, we may elect to wait an hour or two. Should the os not expand, and if dilating bags are at hand, the os may be dilated. If it appear that the forceps can be admitted easily, they may be used, but if not, version by the combined external and internal method should be employed and the os plugged by the leg or breech of the fœtus ; after this is done the case may be left to nature, with gentle assistance, as in footling and breech cases.

6. If the os be small, and if we have neither forceps nor

dilating bags, then combined version should be resorted to, leaving the rest to nature, gently assisted.

7. If during any of the above manœuvres sharp bleeding should come, it is best to turn by the combined method in order to plug by the breech.

8. Where the fœtus is dead, or labor occurs before the end of the seventh month, combined version is the best method, no force following.

9. After-treatment must be conducted on modern principles. Should oozing occur after the expulsion of the placenta, the swabbing of the lower uterus with styptics will be easy. Inasmuch as the outlet of the uterus is liable more especially to be blocked by adherent clots, it will be wise to irrigate the uterus daily with some antiseptic solution, or insert iodoform pessaries in the vagina, particularly if irrigation cannot be done.

Hospital Reports.

MONTREAL GENERAL HOSPITAL.

CONDENSED REPORTS OF CASES IN DR. MACDONNELL'S WARDS.

A True Relapse in Typhoid Fever.—Genuine relapses are not very commonly met with. Murchison puts their frequency at 3 per cent., Maclagan at 13 per cent. The true figure lies between these extremes. John A., one of the cases of typhoid fever sent to us from Lachine, was admitted on the 4th October. The original disease was very severe, very tedious in its course, and it was not until he had been thirty-nine days in hospital that a normal night temperature was registered. The fever was high, the bowels had been somewhat loose, and the eruption was scanty. Convalescence was fairly established when the temperature began slowly and steadily to rise, until in four days it reached 104°, where it remained for about nine days with very slight lowering in the morning. At the outset of the relapse there was very severe frontal headache and pain in the right iliac fossa. On the sixth day of the relapse a rash appeared on the chest and abdomen, and remained for about a week. This rash was very profuse, better marked and of a darker color than the common typhoid rash, and almost was dark enough to classify among the " taches bleuâtres." Convalescence was gradual, but quite satisfactory.

Cheyne-Stokes Breathing with Hypertrophy and Dilatation of the Heart.—In the Hospital Reports already published (MONTREAL MEDICAL JOURNAL, Vol. xviii., p. 296), mention is made of the case of a French-Canadian farmer, 60 years of age, who presented the physical signs of a large heart, and whose breathing was of the Cheyne-Stokes character. There was a history of rheumatism in recurring attacks, but no evidence whatever of valvular disease. The apex beat was one inch outside the nipple line, but there was no enlargement to the right of the middle line of the chest clearly made out during life. The heart's action was weak, diffuse and laboured, and the sounds distant. Pulsation was visible but not forcible in the external jugulars. The exact duration of the whole cycle, 1 minute 40 seconds; respirations, 44; period of dyspnœa, 40 seconds; period of apnœa, 40 seconds. No sphygmographic tracings could be obtained. At the end the symptoms seemed to undergo some improvement under treatment (tincture of digitalis, 20 minims, every four hours), but on the 19th day of his stay in hospital he dropped dead in crossing the ward (against orders). There were no evidences whatever of renal disease.

The autopsy, which was made by Dr. Finley, showed that the heart was greatly enlarged, with its left border lying an inch and a half outside the mammary line, and it weighed three and a half times the normal weight ; the walls of both ventricles were somewhat thickened and firm, and the cavities were much dilated, the right containing loosely adherent ante-mortem clots ; the tricuspid orifice was dilated to almost double its natural size, whilst the mitral was normal ; the aortic valves, though slightly atheromatous, were perfectly competent, and the coronary arteries were healthy : the lungs were somewhat œdematous, but there was no pleurisy ; the liver was of the nutmeg kind, and the kidneys had undergone cyanotic induration ; there was hyperæmia of the stomach with eight or ten hæmorrhagic erosions, and œdema of the upper part of the small intestine. Microscopic examination showed that the muscular fibres of the heart were healthy, and that there was no material increase of connective tissue.

The sequence of events appears to have been hypertrophy of the heart, dilatation of cavities, especially of the right side, which permitted tricuspid regurgitation and subsequent changes in the various organs, We have no cause to assign for the Cheyne-Stokes breathing except that of disturbed circulation in the respiratory centres.

Another interesting case in which Cheyne-Stokes breathing is marked is at present (Dec. 7th) in Dr. Molson's wards. In this case, as well as in both those which I have reported, mental derangement is a marked feature of the case, and in all three a similar unrestful state of mind is present. They could not be kept quiet, they must be continually getting in and out of bed, and although they did what they were told, yet they immediately repeated the offence the moment the attendant's back was turned.

Hœmoptysis from Mitral Stenosis.—On Nov. 18th one of our old patients reported himself for examination. He was pale and thin, and said he had suffered from slight cough and shortness of breath on exertion for the last three years. He had twice lately been in hospital with severe attacks of hœmoptysis, and he had somewhat the appearance of a phthisical patient, but further enquiry established the fact that the hœmoptysis depended upon quite a different cause. He had had acute rheumatism on several occasions, and again last winter in hospital, and, moreover, there had existed a systolic thrill, and at the time of examination a pre-systolic murmur which many of the students had an opportunity of hearing. The lungs were in a perfectly healthy condition.

Thoracic Aneurism.—*Nov. 22nd*—At to-day's clinic, D. J., aged 64, came for examination. This was the man who spent the winter of '85-'86 in the hospital with an aneurism of the descending arch, which projected in the back. There was localized sweating. (For full report see *American Journal of the*

Medical Sciences for March 1888.) The symptoms are by no means as severe as they were four years ago. He has been taking ten grains of iodide of potassium every day since. Improvement was noted in the degree of dyspnœa and pain ; the tumor was apparently smaller. The pulse was noted formerly as being collapsing, but now it certainly has not that character. The improvement after the administration of the iodide showed itself at best for two years ; during the last year he has felt feeble, and has suffered from paroxysms of very severe coughing.

Locomotor Ataxy : Symptoms suddenly developed after an Injury.—A man, æt 44, three months ago fell into a hole about six feet deep, coming down upon his feet. He did not feel at all injured, but two days afterwards he felt a severe pain in the back, which lasted two days, and was immediately followed by severe vomiting at short intervals for six days ; then the gait became unsteady, and numbness in his feet and fingers was perceived ; no pain nor interference with sphincters of rectum or bladder ; no history of syphilis. On admission, three months after the accident, the patellar reflex was found to be absent, and there was great wavering of the limbs on an attempt to stand upright with the eyes shut ; gait is decidedly ataxic ; never had any lightning pains. After a month's stay in hospital there was considerable improvement showing itself by an almost loss of the numbness and by a much improved gait, but after spending three weeks at his home, the numb sensations returned and the unsteadiness increased. On readmision, it was found that the gait was steadier than when he left, but there was no change in the knee reflex phenomenon. Neuro-retinitis present in both eyes.

Cancer of Stomach with secondary Cancer of the Liver and secondary deposits in the Peritoneum.—The patient whose symptoms are reported on page 451 in the last issue of this JOURNAL died on the 3rd of December. As was expected, the symptoms became more urgent, emaciation was rapid, and the pain very severe. Death appeared to have been caused by exhaustion. Three weeks before death ascites made its appearance, and this was the result of a recent peritonitis of cancerous origin, for the membrane was reddened and the inflammation appeared to originate in a mass of jelly-like foreign material in the pelvis between the rectum and the bladder. The stomach was not dilated. There was an ulcer at the pylorus and the tissues about were thickened, but a little finger could be passed through the opening. This was in accord with the symptoms, for although there had been a history of copious vomitings, we had not observed any while he was in hospital. The salol passed through the stomach within the normal time limits (2½ hours). There was no hydrochloric acid in the vomit. The nodule we had felt through the abdominal parietes in the right mammary line was present, and there were very many more, but being situated flatly in the surface of the liver failed to make themselves perceptible. The liver weighed very nearly twice its natural size; spleen small.

The Co-existence of Cirrhosis of the Liver and Tubercular Peritonitis.—In the MONTREAL MEDICAL JOURNAL of May, 1889, p 317, there will be found some reference to the coincidence of these two affections. On the 4th December, 1889, Dr. Johnston made an autopsy on a case which Dr. Molson had had in his ward, and which he had very kindly allowed my class to examine. The liver was very small and hobnailed, and the peritoneum studded with tubercle. There was also a deposit of the same material in both lungs.

The clinical history was briefly as follows : The patient, aged 49, was admitted on the 15th November with jaundice, ascites and œdema of the legs. History of spirit drinking. Present illness was said to have begun eight weeks ago with jaundice and pain at the pit of the stomach, which was followed in a fortnight by dropsy of the belly and afterwards swelling of the feet and legs. A brother died of dropsy and jaundice after an illness lasting five months. There were on admission, evidences of fluid in the peritoneum, enlarged abdominal veins, deep jaundice, subcutaneous ecchymoses, which were especially extensive over the inner side of the right thigh.

Reviews and Notices of Books.

Report on the Sanitary State of Montreal for the Year 1888. By Louis Laberge, Medical Health Officer.

We are willing to acknowledge that in the city of Montreal there are many natural obstacles to the progress of sanitary reform, and, moreover, that our population is made up of so many kinds of men professing so many different kinds of faiths, religious and political, that the sanitary reformer has a task before him of more than ordinary difficulty. We have not space to say all we think about the sanitary state of Montreal, but we shall merely point out some of what may charitably be called, the peculiarities of the City Health Office.

To begin with, the salary of the medical health officer is absurdly small, and were the office to become vacant to-morrow, no medical man of any ability or professional standing would accept the duties at the price. The city doctor receives about half the salary of the city lawyer. Next, in the pamphlet before us we perceive that there is no assistant medical officer on the permanent staff, and that the only professional gentlemen connected with the office are the vaccinators, who, we believe, do not give up their whole time to the public service.

That there is no sanitary engineer connected with the Health Department accounts for much of the drain disease in the city. There is one drain inspector (who is not a qualified engineer) for the whole city. We are willing to admit that this gentleman performs his duty as well as the demands upon his time will allow, but the fact remains that, beyond this one unqualified sanitary inspector, there is no one in connection with the office whose experience and education enable him to lay claim to that knowledge of sanitary engineering which would render him useful to the citizens.

The statistics relating to the distribution of disease in the city are absolutely worthless, owing to the fact that but a small percentage of infectious cases are reported. This is not the fault of the health officials, but of the medical men in charge of the patients.

We turn with eagerness to the section relating to vaccination. That the epidemic of 1885–86 came to a full stop because it had consumed all the unvaccinated is, we take it, universally conceded. We ourselves feel confident that there is being accumulated an abundance of fuel for the next epidemic in the shape of a continually increasing unvaccinated infantile population, and that in the course of some five or six years, when people begin to forget about 1885–86, then there will be another epidemic and another 5,000 victims of ignorance and official incompetency will be laid in their graves.

Let us see what the city is doing. There are but three public vaccinators in the employ of the Board of Health. What can one expect in a population of 200,000 from the efforts of three vaccinators, whose time is but partially given up to the service. During the year, the sanitary police collected the names of 3,022 unvaccinated children, and during the months of July and August the vaccinators prepared an index containing the names of over 6,000 children. Altogether, about 6,000 children are born in Montreal every year, and if the city can only secure the vaccination of 2,802 every year, it is easy to see, even taking into account the proportion of children vaccinated by their own medical men, that we are rapidly accumulating a mass of inflammable material, and we only need a spark to set up a blaze.

Montreal owns up to a mortality in 1888 of 28.86 per 1,000 and the population is officially stated to be 201,743. Compare the death rate of other places. The death rate of twenty-six of the principal cities of America with a gross population of 9,873,448 is 20 per 1,000. (We take our figures from the president's address delivered at the meeting of the American Public Health Association, at Brooklyn, on Oct. 22nd, 1889.) The death rate for London for the year 1888 was 18.5 per 1,000. Now if we could reduce our high death rate to a figure as low as that of London it is easy to calculate that we should lose but 3,732 lives per annum instead of the 5,824 we put into their graves last year. In other words, sanitary supervision could save every year 2,092 lives in this city of Montreal.

But we are constantly being told that a high birth-rate com-

pensates for this great loss. Those who give the subject attention, know that high death rate is the cause of high birth rate,
and that high birth rate in no way, except by the most ignorant
or by those who seek to deceive the most ignorant, can be regarded as compensatory.

There is no analysis done in the Board of Health, because the
city will not pay for an analyst. Consequently poisoned food is
sold in many a shop in this city. We have already called the
attention of the public to the large number of cases of lead
poisoning. During the last summer a great deal of the ginger
ale sold in the city contained lead in poisonous quantities, and
we have every day patients in the General Hospital who have
been poisoned in factories. We do not believe the civic board
have ever taken a single step in this matter.

How can we expect a reasonable rate of mortality when we
allow the land on which the city is built to be riddled by some
thousands of privy pits, and when we allow streets to be made and
houses put up on them without the necessary drains to conduct
away the excreta of the inhabitants.

The Insane in Foreign Countries. By Wm. P. Letch-
    worth, President of the New York Board of Charities.
    New York and London : G. Putnam's Sons, the Knicker-
    bocker Press. Montreal : Wm. Foster Brown & Co.

This beautifully printed and well illustrated volume is the
outcome of a visit made by the author to ascertain " from a
practical point of view what are the most advanced, the most
humane, and the most economical methods of caring for the
insane."

In the introductory chapters a sketch is given of the treatment of insanity as conducted in the early decades of the present
century. Looking back from the present on these dark days,
what is surprising is the slowness with which the modern humane
methods found acceptance. In many instances this cruel apathy
was not owing to the want of desire on the part of the medical
superintendents to change for the better, but rather to the lay
governors. A notable instance is recorded where an able and

enlightened medical superintendent was compelled to resign because he attempted to introduce mild means of dealing with his patients. The prejudices against reforms in the treatment of insanity have now well nigh completely disappeared, except in places where ignorance is more than usually prevalent. Good accounts are given in these pages of the more important asylums in England, Scotland and Ireland, and also of the leading continental asylums. The work is a valuable one, as it is the result of a careful enquiry into an important subject.

Gedenkrede auf Ludwig Türck. Vorgetragen Am 22. März 1889. In Der Feierlichen Jahressitzung der K. K. Gesellschaft der Arzte in Wien. Von Dr. M. HEITLER, Docent an der Universität. Wien und Leipzig : Urban & Schwarzenberg. 1889.

Dr. Heitler in this pamphlet gives a graphic account of the life and work of Ludwig Türck, a name that will go forever down into medical posterity. Few men of the present century have such a record of indefatigable and productive work. Türck's most important contribution to medicine is the explanation of the secondary contractures that occur in cases of cerebral paralysis. This, as was first pointed out by Türck, is due to secondary spinal degenerations. The methods through which he demonstrated these secondary changes is a brilliant example of keen foresight coupled with profound patience in working out details. Türck worked in many different fields, many of which he notably enriched ; he will, however, be known mainly by the observations already referred to and the prominent part he took in introducing and perfecting the laryngoscope.

J. J. Rousseau's Krankheitsgeschischte. Von P. J. MÖBIUS. (The History of J. J. Rousseau's Malady, by P. J. Möbius.) F. C. W. Vogel, Leipzig. 1889.

Dr. Möbius has come to the conclusion that the famous Rousseau was insane, and maintains this through almost two hundred pages with characteristic German tenacity.

Rousseau that has puzzled almost every serious student of his character is clearly enough understood by this writer.

It is easy enough for the average man to pass judgment on an individual of Rousseau's type, but for most men really to understand in a true sense the nature of the Rousseaus of this world is we believe impossible. After all, we can understand others only through our own experiences—transient and feeble in most cases they must be,—but still from this source comes the only true light.

If this be so, what probability is there that a man of a healthy body and only mediocre intellectual and moral endowments can ever properly understand (realize the nature of) either the genius or the lunatic of a certain class? Perhaps those who have studied Rousseau most have been the slowest to decide as to the man's real character. That he was gifted with genius none can deny ; that he was erratic in the extreme is equally plain. But was he insane ? Dr. Möbius says he was of a "neuropathic" nature, and without doubt such he *ultimately* became. But that men of the Rousseau type are bound to become insane, no matter what the circumstances of their lives, is just an open question. Genius is " to madness close allied " was the verdict of a great man—one with a capacity for understanding his fellows that has probably never been equalled.

The perils of genius in a world of mediocrities is very great— *i.e.*, genius of a certain kind. That so many poets have made shipwreck of life in the ordinary sense of being unsuccessful in the struggle for existence is worthy of serious thought. That the great mass of men can in any adequate degree understand a Byron, Shelley or Burns is not probable. The really profitable thing is to see the relation of such organizations to the environment. A human being of ordinary development has much to be thankful for ; he is in reality best adjusted to the environment ; best fitted for the struggle for existence, though he can and will do little to modify the surroundings and make them more suitable to those of a finer, *more delicately balanced* organization.

Now and then, as with a Shakespeare, a Goethe, and, still oftener, with the genius whose special insights are into things rather than man and men, do we find great strength and penetration united with very stable mental and moral balance. But is this the rule or the exception with the genius? We think the work of Dr. Möbius interesting, but for ourselves we still prefer to believe there are more things in heaven and earth than are dreamt of in this writer's philosophy. **W.M.**

Society Proceedings.

MEDICO-CHIRURGICAL SOCIETY OF MONTREAL.

Stated Meeting, 15th *November*, 1889.

G. E. ARMSTRONG, M.D., PRESIDENT, IN THE CHAIR.

Dr. JAMES BELL presented a patient suffering from "multiple fibroma of the skin and nerves," whose right leg he had amputated in the upper third of the thigh for a recurrent sarcoma of the popliteal nerve. The patient, a man aged 37, a French-Canadian, had had a number of fibromatous growths in the skin ever since he could remember. For four or five years past a great many new growths had been constantly appearing, and in 1886 he noticed a growth about the size of a pigeon's egg in the right popliteal space. He also began to suffer from pain in the leg and foot. The tumor increased in size, and in a few months the pain ceased and complete paralysis of the anterior leg muscles supervened. The tumor continued to increase in size until August 6th, 1889, when it was removed by Dr. Fenwick, who found it to be an encapsuled (apparently) fibrous growth of firm consistence, about the size of a man's closed fist, and growing from the sheath of the popliteal nerve, which had produced a deep sulcus along its posterior surface. The wound had scarcely healed when the whole boundaries of the popliteal space were invaded by a rapidly growing and infiltrating nerve growth. Microscopical examination of the removed tumor demonstrated that it consisted largely of fibrous stroma, but contained in some parts nerve elements and in others sarcomatous tissue. The thigh was amputated on the 22nd of October, when the recurrent growth proved to be a spindle-celled sarcoma. The stump healed without trouble, and the patient was shown to the members of the society on the 23rd day after the operation.

Dr. BELL considered this case a typical example of a rare and interesting disease, the clinical and pathological history of which was somewhat obscure. It was described by dermatologists as *molluscum fibrosum*, and although it had been carefully studied by American dermatologists lately, and a number of cases had been reported, it seemed to be looked upon as evidently a skin disease, sometimes attacking the large veins at a late period of its course, and sometimes (apparently accidentally) ending in sarcoma (just as other persons were attacked by sarcoma). Reeklinghausen had investigated this subject, and in 1882 had published a work in which he showed that these skin tumors were generally, if not always, outgrowths from nerves. Other German and Continental observers had noted the special tendency to development of sarcoma in cases of this disease. Dr. Bell also mentioned two similar cases which had come under his observation some years ago, and expressed his opinion that probably the disease described as multiple sarcoma was an allied condition and not in reality a sarcoma at all.

Dr. SHEPHERD did not think there was so much obscurity about the case as Dr. Bell thought. He considered the case one of fibroma molluscum, and where several tumors ran together, a condition of dermatolosis resulted. The difference between multiple sarcoma and fibroma is distinct. In sarcoma the tumors are never pedunculated, and are of a rose red color. The subject has been worked out by Heintzman and others. It is not very strange that these tumors should take on a malignant and sarcomatous action, for instance even in warty growths. The prognosis of such cases is always unfavorable, usually ending eventually in death. Their connection with the nerves has long been recognized.

Dr. BELL, in reply, regretted that he had been misunderstood. He did not claim that there was anything mysterious about the disease, but that the same disease was described by American dermatologists and European surgeons and pathologists from entirely different standpoints, and in such a way as to confuse readers, and lead to the impression that two distinct diseases existed instead of one. He had no personal knowledge of mul-

tiple sarcoma, never having seen a case, but could not reconcile
it as described with the well and generally known disease sarcoma, which possessed such definite and distinct clinical and
anatomical characters. He reiterated the opinion that a more
careful study of such growths and on broader grounds would result in placing them all in one group—essentially "neurofibro-
mata, tending to a termination in sarcoma"—although, perhaps,
differing in detail.

Dr. SMITH then read a paper on a case of *Fibro Cystic
Tumor of the Ovary*, as follows :—

I have to bring before your notice this evening a somewhat
interesting case, a very brief history of which is as follows : D.
S., æt. 39, was sent to me on the 19th March, 1888, by the
kindness of Dr. Reddy, who was the first to discover that a large
tumor filled the entrance to the superior strait, extending two
inches above the umbilicus, and which had apparently been
growing for several years He had already sent her to the
Women's Hospital for consultation, when the opinion of the majority was that it was a fibroid of the uterus. This opinion was
based upon the following points :—1st, the uterus moving with
it ; 2nd, its very solid feeling, there being only a suspicion of
fluctuation ; 3rd, the sound could not be passed ; 4th, there was
great pain in it all the time, especially at the menstrual periods,
which lasted fifteen days, the abdomen was so tender that she
could not bear to be touched and walking was almost impossible ;
5th, great difficulty in micturition and defecation ; 6th, the fact
of the patient being 39 years of age and single.

In view of her very helpless condition, which was getting
worse, and that she had to earn her own living as a domestic,
combined with the gravity of the prognosis of operative interference if the tumor turned out to be a fibroid of the uterus, Dr.
Reddy decided to give her the benefit of the galvanic treatment,
which I carried out for him.

She began treatment on 17th March, 1888, from which date
till the 25th May, 1889, I gave her 70 uterine galvanic cau-
terizations, mostly negative, and varying from 100 to 250 ma.
in strength. At the end of a month she was able to resume her

duties as cook, and to walk long distances, and to micturate and defecate with perfect ease. At the end of two months she had decreased six inches in size around the largest part of the tumor. At this stage her progress was so satisfactory that I showed her to the Society, when the members were able to see the reduction in size by the length of the loops she had had to put on her clothes, and which were no longer necessary. Soon after beginning treatment I was able to introduce the sound a distance of two and a half inches by bending it sharply forward to to the right.

After four months the patient felt so well and the tumor was apparently so much reduced in size, its upper margin having come down midway between umbilicus and pubis, that she left off treatment with my sanction.

A year later, while she was at her home in the country, the tumor rapidly increased in size again, and I reported her as a failure in one of my recent papers. But why electricity failed we shall presently see.

In the meantime the mortality having diminished considerably since the adoption of the extra peritoneal or outside treatment of the stump and the use of Kœberle's *serre nœud*, I strongly advised abdominal section, to which she consented. On placing the case before my esteemed colleague, Dr. Perrigo, whose term of service it was at the Women's Hospital, he kindly agreed to take her into his wards. Another consultation was held, at which Dr. Marcy, of Boston, was present, and the advisability of operating was concurred in, although the majority were of the opinion that it was either a fibroid or a fibro cystic tumor of the uterus. The operation was undertaken with considerable anxiety by Dr. Perrigo, assisted by myself and Dr. Reddy.

On opening the abdomen, the tumor was at once seen, and presented distinctly the appearance of a cyst, but on plunging the trocar into it no fluid escaped. The abdominal incision was therefore rapidly extended several inches above the umbilicus, and there being no adhesions of consequence, the tumor was gradually delivered without any great exposure of the intestines.

It weighed about 26 pounds before the blood drained out of it. The pedicle was broad and was tied in two segments, the left Fallopian tube, which was elongated and stretched out over its anterior surface, was tied and removed. The abdominal incision was united with deep silver wire sutures, which brought the peritoneal surfaces accurately in apposition, with superficial silk ones for the skin. There being no oozing, no drainage tube was used. The operation took 39 minutes. Neither was any opium required. Flatus was passed on second day, and the bowels were moved by enema on the fourth day. The patient made an uninterrupted recovery, was up on the thirteenth day, and returned to her home in the country on the nineteenth day. I have since heard from her, and she was so far in the enjoyment of perfect health.

Comments.—This case is of interest to the gynecologist, as well as to the general practitioner, for several reasons. First, the difficulty in diagnosing. It is no disparagement, however, to admit that it is sometimes impossible to say positively what the exact nature of hard or semi-solid abdominal tumors may be, until the abdomen has been opened. Many of the ablest diagnostician have told me that they have frequently been deceived, in spite of the greatest care. In case of doubt, I think it is wisest to give the patient a short course of galvanism, and if she does not greatly improve, to make an exploratory incision, at the same time being prepared for either ovariotomy or hysterectomy. I felt so sure, from the hardness of the tumor and other symptoms, that this was a fibroid of the uterus that I reported her case as a failure of electricity to cure a uterine fibroid, but in so doing I did Apostoli's method an injustice. It is highly probable that many others fail for the same reason, viz., error in diagnosis.

I might mention in this connection that I wrote to Apostoli to ask him if he had ever failed to benefit a fibroid of the uterus, to which he promptly replied that he had failed in several cases of fibro-cystic tumors of the uterus, but never in a case of pure fibroid.

The next question is how are we to explain the marked diminution in size.   I think, as was pointed out by Dr. Trenholme, at the meeting at which I showed her, that it is due in part to the tonic effect on the walls of the intestines, which thus expel their gaseous contents, and of the blood-vessels, which are diminished in calibre.   This makes the tumour a little smaller, but not enough to take off the pressure from the iliac and ovarian veins, the obstruction of which is, I am sure, responsible for a great deal of the œdema of the tumor.   For in this, as in other cases, I have noticed a pasty swelling, which could be indented by firm and prolonged pressure with the finger, which has invariably disappeared soon after the patient has come under treatment.

The application of the negative current had the effect of dilating the cervical canal so that the finger could be inserted into it, but after treatment had been left off for a few months, it had retracted again to almost a pinhole.   This is a general result when very high currents are employed, but it can be avoided by insulating the cervical portion of the electrode.

The sudden increase in size, after she had become so much smaller, was in all probability due to hemorrhage into the cyst, for the part of the tumor that was cystic was filled with a semi-solid material, having the consistency of clotted blood.   The uterus was almost imbedded in the anterior wall of the tumor, which explains its moving with the uterus ; the latter was normal in size but not adherent.

Discussion.—In discussing this paper, Dr. Alloway said that from the title on the notice card of Dr. Smith's specimen, he understood it to mean a fibroma of the ovary, in which cystic change had taken place.   Under these circumstances it was a remarkable specimen on account of the extreme rarity of such growths and of the large size of the specimens.   He would, therefore, suggest to Dr. Smith the advisability of having the specimen examined by the pathologist to the society, and a re-port submitted at a future meeting.   In regard to the error made in diagnosis, and to the electrical treatment, which was carried out for so long a period, he thought it a severe blow to the reliability of the so-called relief claimed for the treatment of these conditions by electricity.   He thought the society should feel grateful to Dr. Smith for having, in so straightforward a way, placed before it, side by side, the relative merits of electrolysis and section in the treatment of abdominal tumors. He said the method spoken of by Dr. Gurd was different to that applied by Dr. Smith to his patient. The former had reference to passing grooved directors through the abdominal wall—one on each side—into the cyst contents. This method was introduced by Dr. E. Cutler, of New York, and is still practiced by him, but by no one else at present, on account of the high mortality connected with it.

Dr. LAPTHORN SMITH, in reply to Dr. Alloway, said that it was only by faithfully reporting failures as well as successes that the truth could be found out about the electrical treatment of fibroids. This he was determined to do. He had no other object in employing this treatment than to give it a fair and impartial trial, and if it were found to be useless, he would willingly discard it. Many cases of failure were, like the one he had shown this evening, due to error in diagnosis, and so employing the treatment for cases in which it was not suitable. He admitted that fibro-cystic tumors of the ovary were somewhat rare, but not so much so as to prevent one turning up once in a great while in Montreal. He was willing to hand it over to the pathologist of the society for a report.

Dr. ALLOWAY related a case of distressing incontinence of urine in an old lady (aged 60). There was no pain, but a constant desire to pass a few drachms of urine. On examination he found an old cicatricial stricture completely surrounding the upper part of the vagina, about on a level with the external os uteri. This stricture had in some way involved the walls of the bladder by traction upon them, so that the latter became divided into two portions, a very long one above and a very small one below. It appeared that the upper larger reservoir received the urine from the ureters and emptied itself only by overflow into the smaller one below, which, in its turn, quickly voided its contents, to be rapidly filled again from the upper reservoir. It was quite evident that there had been a myopothic process established, in so far as the upper portion of the bladder was concerned, and that there was a true senile paresis of the detrusor complicating this peculiar sort of structure.

The treatment adopted consisted in breaking down the vaginal stricture by digital dilatation. This was followed by complete relief to the symptoms, but unfortunately, as the stricture again contracted on cessation of dilatation, the symptoms returned. Dr. Alloway said that he intended shortly to resect the cicatricial vaginal ring, with the portions of the vagina above and below. He showed a crayon drawing of the condition and spoke of its rarity as a cause of bladder trouble. He said it was caused primarily by an injury to the vagina during parturition.

Dr. LAPTHORNE SMITH said that these cases of traumatic atresia of the vagina were becoming very rare, in fact could only be found in women who had been confined many years ago, because no medical man of the present day would leave the head long enough in the pelvis to cause death of the tissues. A cause which is still somewhat common is scrofulous vaginitis with destruction of mucous membrane and even adhesion of the anterior and posterior walls.

He thought that Dr. Alloway was mistaken in thinking that he had only a stricture of the vagina to deal with, for the reason that no stricture of the vagina could constrict the bladder so as to form an upper and a lower chamber. Such a condition never followed upon Lefort's operation, in which the surgeon artificially caused an atresia of the vagina. He thought that no amount of traction on the posterior wall of the bladder could cause a stricture; in fact it would be much more likely to cause dilatation. The true condition in Dr. Alloway's case was probably a stricture of the bladder, caused by destruction of the mucous membrane at the same time that the injury was taking place to the mucous membrane of the vagina.

NEW YORK ACADEMY OF MEDICINE.

At the meeting of the New York Academy of Medicine, held on November 7th, 1889, the President, Dr. Alfred L. Loomis, in the chair,

DR. SIMON BARUCH read a paper entitled " *A Plea for the Practical Utilization of Hydrotherapy.*" The fact that water in the treatment of disease had been chiefly employed by empirics seemed to have prevented in some degree general recognition of its virtues by the medical profession. The author justified his appeal for its more general utilization by physiological laws and clinical results, both ancient and modern. The literature showing the value of hydro-therapeutics was very extensive, yet modern text-books dismissed the subject with a few words. There were at present but three cities in which it was much used in the general hospitals, Vienna taking the lead. In spite of professional and lay prejudice, the remedy had stood the test of time better than any other. A review of the experience of those whose names had become prominently associated with hydrotherapy was given, and brief quotations were made from such modern therapeutists as Niemeyer, Dujardin-Beaumetz, Hoffmann, etc., testifying to the value of the method. But proof of its value did not rest alone on clinical experience; it was fully supported by ascertained physiological laws. What other agent than water could produce such a variety of results, according to its mode of application? Its stimulating or depressing effects could be made to manifest themselves either directly upon the skin where applied, or upon internal or remote organs, through reflex influence. One example of reflex influence was seen in the response of the blood-vessels of the pia-mater to a stream applied to the surface; if the stream were cold, they become dilated; if warm, they become contracted. The hand immersed in cold water increased in size, showing that by the use of water the blood could be driven from one part of the body to another. Water applied to the feet exerted an influence upon the cranial circulation; applied to the back, it influenced the circulation in mucous surfaces, etc. The heart also responded to temperature impressions upon the periphery. A low temperature briefly applied accelerated the heart's action ; prolongation of it diminished the action. Evanescent application of a high temperature to the skin caused a decrease of the pulse-rate, quickly followed by an increase. By cooling the blood in fevers, the heart's action could be slowed, and an invigorating effect thus brought about. Having stated that the vascular tension could be modified by hydropathic procedures, he said that this influence upon the circulation was so decided, indeed, that hydrotherapy became in reality a hydraulic problem. It was a most perfect means of influencing the vascular system. He said it was to be remembered also, in discussing the value of hydrotherapy, that the vital process by which the system sought to protect itself against thermic changes had also been ascertained. Vascular spasm protected the internal organs against too rapid cooling of the surface, while the secondary effect was reaction and vigorous dilatation of the cutaneous vessels. It had been shown that by hydropathic treatment the blood-cells could be increased in number, and also improved in quality. This, and the influence upon the nervous system, produced a healthy change in the functions of nutrition, secretion, and excretion. In this country, Dr. Putnam-Jacobi was one quoted as having added to our knowledge of the physiological and therapeutic action of water. In discussing the clinical aspect of the subject, he said he agreed with Dr. F. A. Hoffmann in the statement that he did not deal with the disease, but with the sick man. He approved of Hoffman's classification of the treatment as direct (removing the cause) and indirect, but he would add a third method, that by which he could so impress the various functions of the body, chiefly innervation, as to enhance the resisting powers of the patient, and thus enable him to pass over danger-points. He claimed for hydrotherapy only the position of being a valuable but indispensable auxiliary to other treatment. By hydrotherapy he meant water at any temperature, in any form, used internally or externally in the treatment of disease. Of the three therapeutic methods mentioned, the removal of the cause of the disease directly was not always practical because of our ignorance of the etiology. In the case of gastric and intestinal diseases, we seemed to be on the threshold of discovering the cause through bacteriology. In the removal of this and restoring gastric function, water had been used with great success. Intestinal irrigation, by means of the fountain syringe and Nélaton catheter, was the most efficient method of treating several types of summer diarrhœa. The value of sipping hot water in gastric troubles had been demonstrated. Other cases in which he had found the method of marked benefit were those of neurasthenia and other nervous diseases, rheumatism, gout, scrofula, etc. The neurasthenic cases were treated differently according to whether they were of an erethitic or an asthenic nature. Two cases were cited to show that much depended in the treatment upon the temperature of the water and the uniformity and frequency of its repetition. He said that hysteria was among the affections which would almost certainly yield to the water treatment when aided by other measures. They had discharged three cases from the Montefiore Home as cured, notwithstanding they had been sent there as incurables. No patients of any kind were admitted to this institution, except those who had been considered incurable ; yet by hydropathic measures they had sent out a number as cured, who had had gout, rheumatism, sciatica, hysteria, etc. Chorea often yielded to this treatment ; the active impact of very cold water by the douche was necessary here. Many cases of neuralgia were connected with anæmia and chlorosis, and were cured by hydropathic treatment ; indeed, he said that if there was any condition in which the tonic effects of hydropathy were pronounced, it was functional anæmia. During the winter it was often sufficient for the patient to stand with the feet in warm water, and splash cold water on the body, the duration being only until the entire body had been wet. The result of hydropathy in the treatment of phthisis had been also satisfactory at the Montefiore Home, and one pronounced case of the morphine habit was cured. Statistics had demonstrated that the mortality of typhoid fever could be reduced from twenty-five per cent. to two per cent. by this treatment. The fact should not be overlooked that the object was not to reduce the temperature, but to refresh the nervous system, that the body might be enabled to withstand the disease. The bath should be adapted to each particular case.

DR. GEORGE L. PEABODY, having been asked to open the discussion, said he would speak only of the application of water to the treatment of a form of acute disease which was of common occurrence here, and in the treatment of which our results had been almost uniformly discreditable to medical practice. He referred to typhoid fever. It was a matter of surprise that in this city, where physicians sought to introduce into their practice all that was good and new from all parts of the world, it was necessary for one to urge the desirability of trying this procedure. He thought that the sooner we rid our minds of the fallacy that it was likely to do patients with a high temperature harm to expose them to a considerably lower temperature, the sooner would we get at the rational treatment of this grave malady. It was almost impossible to give a patient cold who had a temperature much above the normal ; it was not likely that a patient with a temperature of 104°F. would take cold, even if he kicked the bedclothes off and lay entirely exposed. He thought the mortality from typhoid fever in our hospitals was quite unjustifiable ; it ranged anywhere from twenty-five to thirty per cent., and, here and there, it rose to fifty per cent. In the German army, where this treatment had been carried out in a large number of cases, the mortality had been reduced to below four per cent. Perhaps one reason why it had not been applied, except in a few instances, in our hospitals, was that it required two attendants and a portable bath-tub. Regarding the method of applying it, he thought there could be no question but what the full bath, of a temperature of between 65° and 80°F., was best ; the patient should be put into the bath at as frequent intervals as the temperature indicated. The temperature should be kept at or below 102°F. throughout the entire course of the disease. How much more rational was this treatment than that which he had often observed, of administering antipyretic drugs, bringing the temperature down from 105° or 106°F. to normal or below, allowing it to rise again equally high, and again bring-

ing down with the drug.   A good many patients were brought
to the hospital in a very unfavorable state, and in that case, instead of plunging them into a cold bath, he would apply the wet
pack.   Personally, he did not like the graduated bath ; it was
far more troublesome, and was less comfortable to the patient.
Cold affusions on the Kibbee cot produced rather too much
shock.   He thought it was folly to apply cold to the surface of
the body when it was already cool.   We often found profound
depression in typhoid fever in which the surface was cool and
the internal temperature high.   It was certain that no routine
habit of applying cold to the surface would apply in these cases.
He could conceive of no other direct object in applying cold than
to increase surface radiation, and if the heart was too feeble and
could not be stimulated to pump the blood to the surface, there
was no reason in cooling the surface further.

Dr. A. A. Smith hardly knew where to begin to discuss so
extensive a subject.   In Bellevue Hospital he had continued the
treatment of four cases of typhoid fever, begun during the service of Dr. Flint, and all recovered ; since then he had had five
cases, in none of which the use of the cold bath seemed to be
justified, since the temperature did not rise above 108.6°F.
They all recovered without such treatment.   This, he supposed,
would be the experience of others.   Unless the bath was used
in a large number of cases, it would be difficult to draw any.
conclusions regarding its superiority over other methods of treatment.   He was, however, a warm advocate of hydro-therapeutics.
He said that if there was any class of cases which made him very
unhappy, and which he failed to make very happy, it was that
of the neurasthenics.   If Dr. Baruch could teach us how to cure
these patients by hydrotherapy, he would put us under great
obligations.   Regarding the cure of hysteria by this method, he
must admit to some scepticism, yet he hoped others would try it
and have equal success.   Patients with hysteria deserved our
earnest attention, for he believed that underlying almost every
case there was some cause in irritation, or disturbance, which
should not be ignored.   He was a great believer in the wet pack,
and he thought that its only benefit did not consist in reducing

the temperature; he had felt that the soothing of the nervous system was as great an object to attain as the reduction of the temperature. Warm water had been of great service in reducing the temperature. He had known the temperature in scarlatina to fall a degree and a half from no other treatment than wrapping the patient in a sheet wrung out of warm water, repeated several times during the twenty-four hours. It often banished delirium and muscular disturbance, caused sleep, and reduced the temperature.

Dr. M. Putnam-Jacobi gave the details of a case of typhoid fever treated in the New York Infirmary by cold-baths. She differed from Dr. Peabody in the view that the benefit was alone from the reduction of the temperature. She saw no reason for pushing it further than to produce the desired reduction of the temperature and beneficial influence on the circulation and nervous system. She did not think, therefore, that hard and fixed rules for its use in typhoid fever should be necessary.

Dr. G. B. Fowler thought the physical properties of water commended its use in the treatment of disease to all physicians, and he was rather surprised to hear that the bath was as little used as Dr. Baruch had stated. He certainly had used it ever since he began practice, in all cases of hyperpyrexia. In the angina of scarlet fever, diphtheria, etc., he kept the throat almost frozen, using ice, and certainly with very good results. He expected it to do more than reduce the temperature. Its results were less violent than those of the therapeutic measures usually employed. The author had only hinted at one method of using water, namely, by drinking. Dr. Fowler regarded this as important in the treatment of fever as the external use of water. He gave his patients an excess to drink, and in the sickness of children gave it to them in the nursing-bottle. He saw a great many cases sometimes called neurasthenia; women with constipation, loss of appetite, catarrh of the alimentary tract, etc., the blood-corpuscles on the glass sticking to one another, crumpled, the urine scanty, want of free perspiration. Here the clinical facts pointed to a deficiency of water in the system. One might as well try to raise a crop without rain as to nourish an individual properly without water.

Dr. Baruch closed the discussion.—*N. Y. Medical Record.*

Correspondence.

PROVINCIAL MEDICAL BOARDS.

To the Editors of THE MONTREAL MEDICAL JOURNAL.

SIRS,—In the Introductory Address by Dr. MacDonnell, printed on page 321 of the MONTREAL MEDICAL JOURNAL for this year, the lecturer inveighs against provincial medical boards in general, and that of British Columbia in particular. The " some fifty practitioners in that province" do not constitute the Medical Council of Physicians and Surgeons of British Columbia, nor is their motto, " Now, we have got in, let us keep others out." The British Columbia Medical Council was incorporated in April 1886, and since that time twenty-two men have presented themselves for registration. Of these twenty-two, all have now their licences except one, who, if the Council had " contented themselves with examining diplomas and rejecting those that came from indifferent colleges," would probably have had a license also. However, by going through the formality of an examination it was found that although this candidate came from a reputable medical college in the United States his " fitness and capacity to practice as a physician or surgeon" was very doubtful. In reply to the question " Define caput succedaneum," this candidate stated that " caput succedaneum was an eruption which appeared upon the chests of patients suffering from typhoid fever." If Dr. MacDonnell thinks that an examination of this gentleman's diploma would have determined his fitness or unfitness to practice, I must beg to disagree with him. Rather than make my letter too long I purposely refrain from noticing many other points in the lecture where Dr. MacDonnell might be corrected, just pausing to mention the fact that the Medical Council of British Columbia at least has made no pretence of regulating the course of study pursued by those who apply for its license beyond the regulation that they must come with a diploma from a school which exacts at least three years of professional study. The profession in this province is not in the least afraid of honest competition, and McGill men in particular have nothing to fear from the examination here. Out of sixty-three men registered in the province eleven come from McGill—more than from any other one school—and I have never heard any of them complain of the severity of the examinations.

Hoping that Dr. MacDonnell, as well as others in the east, may at least give us credit for fairness both as regards our professional examination and fees,

I remain, very sincerely yours,

W. A. DeWolf Smith.

New Westminster, B.C., Dec. 9th, 1889.

Selections.

The Operative Treatment of Perityphlitis.

(By Prof. Sonnenburg, Berlin.)—At the meeting of the Association of Surgeons of Berlin, Prof. Sonnenburg demonstrated two patients upon whom he had successfully operated for perityphlitis. He thought that operative treatment in this disease was confined to those cases in which there were encapsulated exudations or abscesses, and that if general suppurative peritonitis had already developed an operation could be of little service. There are a number of cases of perityphlitis in which, as early as the first day, resistance and dullness, without fluctuation, can be made out, while on the next day these signs are obscured by commencing meteorism, and palpation is impossible on account of the great tenderness of the abdomen. It is well known that most deaths from perityphlitis occur during the first week ; and in order not to lose a favorable opportunity the author recommends that the abdomen be opened down to the peritoneum by a curved incision similar to that used in ligation of the iliac artery, or by an incision at the outer margin of the rectus abdominis. Palpation may now be practiced through the peritoneum, and it will often be found possible to detect resistance again and discover the abscess, which should then be opened. But there are cases in which, owing to protrusion of loops of intestine or the deep situation of the abscess, palpation through the peritoneum affords no positive data, and in these an expectant plan of treatment should be pursued. The abdominal wound should be tamponed with iodoform gauze, care being taken not to injure

incision is that in non-suppurating cases in which the pe
incision is not required, no harm results from the divisio
skin and abdominal muscles. In one of the patients the
which could be distinctly made out through the peritone
not go on to suppuration, and the peritoneal incision ·
pensed with, the abdominal wound healing promptly, a
patient making a good recovery.

In the discussion which followed, Prof. Küster expre
objections to the double incision. In extra-peritoneal p
litic abscess no incision of the peritoneum is required,
intra-peritoneal suppuration he regarded Sonnenburg's pr
as not wholly free from danger, since under this expecta
ment the abscess might rupture into the abdominal cav
has always been his practice to incise the peritoneum if
tion could be detected, and even if no abscess is found
cision is of value for diagnostic purposes.

Dr. Hahn reported a case of peri-cœcal abscess in wl
peritoneum was opened, but immediately sutured. In
all antiseptic precautions, however, a general peritonitis
veloped which terminated fatally. He thought that if tl
ation had been completed in two stages, the abscess wou
ruptured into the wound and a general peritonitis cou
been avoided. Since this unfavorable experience he ha
it a point, after cutting down to the peritoneum, not to ¡
any further unless distinct fluctuation was present. Al

the importance of examining the pulse, and then the joint alone, in making the diagnosis. He was inclined to believe in the existence of some yet unknown function of the skin connected with the respiration in the widest sense ; and he thought failure of skin-action of some sort was a means of causing the accumu· lation in the body of matters which were morbific of rheumatism. A chilling of the skin was usually present in the genesis of rheumatism, so the warm bath naturally acts as an anæsthetic as well as rendering urine alkaline. Flannel and oily inunction —especially with cod-liver oil—were useful. He agreed with Dr. Jacobi as to the liability of endocarditis, and has seen it develop when the joint trouble was very slight. To prevent this injury we must be on the lookout for the first symptoms of rheumatism, and especially for chorea. He dreaded " growing pains," and always immediately put the child on cod-liver oil and advised the use of flannel, etc. He believed salicylic acid only useful for the joint troubles and not for endocarditis ; for the latter he prefers antipyrine or phenacetine. He thought the reason why the heart lesions were so much more apt to remain permanent than the joint trouble lay in the fact that the heart was in constant motion and could not be given entire rest as a joint can, and since the heart-beat is more rapid in children than in adults, therefore heart lesions are more apt to be devel· oped. For this reason he advises aconite and not digitalis. Alkalies are also to be given and the skin well protected, especially that of the chest.

Dr. J. Lewis Smith said he had kept a record of all cases of rheumatism in children under 15 years of age which he had met with in the outdoor department at Bellevue. In 78 there had been a cardiac bruit, and in only one case had the patient been under one year old, and very few under two. In three cases in young children there had been very little swelling, but some tenderness in the joints. Generally the disease began in the lower extremities and tended to travel upward. The local manifestations were much less than in adults. He had often found a cardiac bruit in cases which gave the history of former " growing pains," and he thought the laity should be taught the

as " dentition," " malaria," " worms," or " colds"; this being
due partly to the difficulty of diagnosis and partly to the common idea among practitioners that they are of rare occurrence.
Fever in rheumatism might be slight and irregular, and, moreover, it is a common symptom due to slight distension. Swelling
of the joints is apt to be trifling in amount and easily overlooked;
and the pain might be much less than pain due to fatigue, rickets,
syphilis, etc.   The heart and joints should always be examined
when the child shows discomfort and the diagnosis is obscure.
Diagnosis is especially hard when only a single joint is affected.
Only too often is the pain called " growing pains," and in the
majority of cases the " growing pains " indicate the presence of
rheumatism and the liability to irreparable heart injuries.   As
regards treatment, a change of residence from localities in which
rheumatism is apparently epidemic is often desirable.   Alkalies
are often indicated.   The systematic use of cold water often
modifies, sometimes removes, the tendency to rheumatism of
children born of rheumatic parents.   A cold wash, sponge, wet
sheet, shower-bath, or bath (according to the child's strength or
power of reaction) should be given daily; then warm clothing
should be worn the rest of the day.   As local measures he advised swathing the swollen and painful joint in cotton and flannel,
or the application twice a day of a solution of iodoform in collo
dion.   For endocarditis he recommends absolute rest, cold applications over the heart, and salicylate of sodium.   The best preventive for muscular rheumatism, when a tendency to the affection
had appeared, is the regular and systematic use of cold water.
When real inflammation is present in the muscle, a mild continued current and small doses of bichloride of mercury do good.

Dr. W. H. Thomson said that his attention had been called
to the etiology of rheumatism years ago, and that he had heard
that it was as common among the Arabs of the desert as among
the fishermen of Norway and Scotland.   He had sought the
reason why it should appear under exactly opposite conditions
of soil and climate, and he was convinced that the cause must
be a common one, namely, chilling of the skin when moist.   This
could happen equally well in either extreme.   He emphasized

the importance of examining the pulse, and then the joint alone, in making the diagnosis. He was inclined to believe in the existence of some yet unknown function of the skin connected with the respiration in the widest sense ; and he thought failure of skin-action of some sort was a means of causing the accumu- lation in the body of matters which were morbific of rheumatism. A chilling of the skin was usually present in the genesis of rheumatism, so the warm bath naturally acts as an anæsthetic as well as rendering urine alkaline. Flannel and oily inunction —especially with cod-liver oil—were useful. He agreed with Dr. Jacobi as to the liability of endocarditis, and has seen it develop when the joint trouble was very slight. To prevent this injury we must be on the lookout for the first symptoms of rheumatism, and especially for chorea. He dreaded " growing pains," and always immediately put the child on cod-liver oil and advised the use of flannel, etc. He believed salicylic acid only useful for the joint troubles and not for endocarditis ; for the latter he prefers antipyrine or phenacetine. He thought the reason why the heart lesions were so much more apt to remain permanent than the joint trouble lay in the fact that the heart was in constant motion and could not be given entire rest as a joint can, and since the heart-beat is more rapid in children than in adults, therefore heart lesions are more apt to be devel- oped. For this reason he advises aconite and not digitalis. Alkalies are also to be given and the skin well protected, espe- cially that of the chest.

Dr. J. Lewis Smith said he had kept a record of all cases of rheumatism in children under 15 years of age which he had met with in the outdoor department at Bellevue. In 78 there had been a cardiac bruit, and in only one case had the patient been under one year old, and very few under two. In three cases in young children there had been very little swelling, but some tenderness in the joints. Generally the disease began in the lower extremities and tended to travel upward. The local manifestations were much less than in adults. He had often found a cardiac bruit in cases which gave the history of former " growing pains," and he thought the laity should be taught the

dren's underwear, and he had often been obliged to order better
underclothes. He had found lithia (as distinguished from lithia
water) of considerable value in treatment.

Dr. A. Caillé took much the same view as Dr. Seibert, and
believed the disease to be infectious.—(*Gaillard's Med. Jour.*

The Influence of Insanity on History.—
A complete study of the effects of insanity and the various Protean forms of mental weakness and disorder, on history, could
not fail to be of extreme interest both to the historian and the
psychologist. A paper on this subject in its general bearings,
by Dr. Grissom of Carolina, published some time since in the
New England Medical Monthly, is highly suggestive, and throws
a new light upon the psychological conditions underlying the
conduct of the great, the renowned, the gifted, the artistic, and
the crowned heads of the world, from the earliest dawn of history down to the present day. What control over the lives and
fortunes of their fellow-mortals has rested in the hands of men
who, in the light of modern knowledge, cannot be regarded as
other than "inspired" lunatics! How often, the author asks,
has a paroxysm of mania, an epileptic spasm, or a fit of melancholia, cast the die of war, broken treaties, elevated one gilded
puppet or dethroned another, and laid whole nations in tears
and their homes in ashes? When one looks back with trembling
horror on the scenes in the past which have made this earth a
hell, of people constructing and then destroying, greeting and
then killing, kingdoms rising on the ruins of kingdoms, and ever
the fierce play of individual human passions in tho foreground
of the action, the question naturally arises, what part did madness play in this kaleidoscope of events? It is not necessary to
go very far back to see that formerly only the more salient and
obvious forms of mental aberration were recognized. Wild fury
and dreary melancholy could be seen and feared by all, but
could we apply the torch of modern science, lighting up the
obscure places in the physiology and psychology of man, to the
great leaders whose influence has directed the lines of history,
we should doubtless find many of the mighty movements of men

monarch of Brazil, who for years vainly sought relief in travel from the cares of State. The revolution which has swept him from his throne may perchance restore to him that equanimity of mind to which he had long been a stranger. Who can resist the conclusion that the abnormal life of him who lives alone, elevated on an artificial pedestal above his fellows, is surrounded with precipices and pitfalls dangerous both to body and reason!——*Med. Press and Circular.* (*Cincinnati Lancet-Clinic.*)

The Need of Nourishment in Diphtheria.—(Dr. J. A. De Armond, in *Weekly Med. Review*, Oct. 26, 1889.)—Feed the patient. He is sick at the stomach and won't eat? Dissolve the membrane two to four times a day and he won't be so sick. He does not want to eat? Then give him liquid food, and milk easily stands at the head of the list. But he won't drink it? Then direct powders of pepsin to be given in two to four or six tablespoonfuls of milk every half hour. Alternate this with your internal medicament and you have a treatment that keeps step with good judgment, and it is strictly in accord with all that is known of the therapeutics of the disease. There is no cure for the disease. It is a self-limited disease, and being that, you cannot fail in preserving the strength of the patient. It is much more rational to help the system from the start than to jump in and fight the disease as an entity, striking right and left, hitting friend and foe alike, only to find in the end that the battle was all too large for the small battle-ground to stand. Of course milk, and by milk I mean the very best of milk, and the more cream the better, if not too hard to digest, will become very tiresome as a regular diet. It can be varied by giving beef broth, malted milk, and any of the prepared foods whose value has met the demands of investigation. Food may be given cold or warm, as best pleases the patient. Many times the allowance will be lost by emesis, but the same thing will occur if simple water is swallowed. I am very sure that by simply directing a powder of pepsin with the nourishment the attendants will not be likely to listen to the pleadings of the patient as when the food is given alone. It may be said that by giving nourishment so frequently you interfere with the giving of needed medicine. I know of no drug that is likely to be given that will in any way interfere with this system of nourishing the patient. The various forms of iron might, but if it comes to a question of supremacy between tincture of iron and nourishment, you will have no reason to regret the rejection of iron. Indeed there can be no question that in order that enough iron to be of any avail is given, providing it is of any avail—a matter I seriously question—the stomach must be kept in a state of great irritability continuously. After all, nothing has been found to equal good food in the fabrication of good blood. In diphtheria surely the blood suffers soonest. I am well satisfied that if nourishment were given with the same free hand that many drugs of doubtful utility are handed out there would not be so urgent need of battling a desperate foe at the end of the fight with stimulants. After all, stimulants are only valuable because they help to tide over a bad spot. When you come to enumerate the things you can do in diphtheria you find the number is not large. Control fever, dissolve the membrane, keep the nostrils clean and feed the patient. These you can do. Don't neglect their accomplishment in the questionable task of curing a disease which, after all, is only strong in weakness.—*The Epitome.*

THE

Montreal Medical Journal.

| VOL. XVIII. | JANUARY, 1890. | No. 7. |

THE Educational Committtee of the General Council of Medical Education and Registration of Great Britain have unanimously reported that it is desirable that steps should be taken by the Council to extend the period of medical study to five years. The Committee, while strongly of the opinion that the number of systematic lectures in certain subjects of medical education should be reduced, are not prepared to recommend the method of effecting such reduction till the Medical Council has expressed its mind on the suggestion for an extension of the period of study to five years. The committee's report will be the first business dealt with at the May meeting of the Council, and there appears no doubt but what its suggestions will be carried into effect. A very significant suggestion is the recommendation for lessening the number of systematic lectures given on the great majority of subjects. This is strongly recommended even should the course be extended to five years.

For the credit of the Canadian profession we sincerely hope that the members of our different Provincial Medical Boards will soon see the necessity of placing their houses in order. There is an urgent necessity for every board in Canada to diminish the number of systematic lectures required. Owing to the present faulty system of requiring attendance on so many didactic lectures, the students in this country are placed at a serious disadvantage as compared with their brethren in England and elsewhere. There is no country in the world at the present time that demands of its medical students so much attendance on didactic work. If this extraordinary attendance meant the turning out of men better prepared for their life work, the result might justify the means employed, but it is well known the contrary is the effect. Canadian graduates, no doubt, as a rule, take a fairly high place, but we feel confident that their position would be still higher if the requirements of our boards were brought more into line with European countries. In Canada we are in many respects keeping pace with the general progress of medical education, but in the matter of attendance on didactic lectures we are several decades behind the times.

At the meeting of the British Medical Council in May last general astonishment was expressed that students were required by some of the degree-granting bodies to attend as many as 1200 systematic lectures during their course. The Quebec Medical Board, which is the greatest sinner in this respect, demands an attendance on upwards of 1800 lectures during the four years course. The other Provincial Boards demand about 1700.

THE FACULTY OF COMPARATIVE MEDICINE AND VETERINARY SCIENCE OF McGILL UNIVERSITY.

A very interesting and important meeting was held in the library of the Medical College, McGill University, on Dec. 6th, being no less than the official inauguration and installation of the Faculty of Comparative Medicine and Veterinary Science.

Sir William Dawson, Principal and Vice-Chancellor of the University, assisted by Professor Craik, Dean of the Medical Faculty, inducted the members of the new faculty. After reading their appointments, and the amended statutes affecting the faculty, the Principal formally handed over the responsibility and direction of the faculty to the newly-appointed Dean.

The faculty consists of the following :—

D. McEachran, F.R.C.V.S., V.S. Edin. J.P., etc., appointed Professor of Veterinary Medicine and Surgery and also Dean of the Faculty.

Malcolm C. Baker, V.S., appointed Professor of Veterinary Anatomy.

Charles McEachran, V.S., appointed Professor of Veterinary Obstetrics and Diseases of Cattle.

And the following Professors in the Faculty of Medicine appointed associate professors of the new faculty, viz., Gilbert P. Girdwood, M.D., Professor of Chemistry ; Wesley Mills, M.A., M.D., Professor of Physiology ; George Wilkins, M.D., Professor of Histology ; D. P. Penhallow, B.Sc , Professor of Botany ; James Stewart, M.D., Professor of Materia Medica ; and W. G. Johnston, M.D., Demonstrator of Pathology and Curator of the Museum.

The history of veterinary teaching in the province of Quebec is of a comparatively recent date. In 1866, a few months after the arrival of Mr. D. McEachran in Montreal, he commenced to deliver a course of lectures on veterinary science in connection with the medical faculty in their lecture room on Cotte street. In this course he received the sympathy and support of the Board of Agriculture, of which the late Major Campbell was president, Sir William Dawson, the Principal of McGill University, the late Dr. George Campbell, who was Dean of the Medical Faculty, as well as the Professors of the Institutes of Medicine, Chemistry, and Botany. In 1875 the growth of the school was such as to necessitate a special establishment, and the present buildings were erected on Union Avenue at the expense of Mr. McEachran. It may truly be said of this school that it has all along been conducted solely in the interests of veterinary science, and at considerable expenditure of both time and money to its head and founder, as well as those associated with him. From its inauguration, students were required to pass a matriculation examination, and to attend three full sessions of six months, whereas, even to the present time, the majority of veterinary schools on this continent admit students merely on payment of fees and require only two short sessions of attendance. However, the high standing attained by this school both at home and abroad, and the success of its graduates wherever they have gone, many of them being teachers in the numerous veterinary colleges both in Canada and the United States (most of which are off-shoots of the Montreal school), and in agricultural colleges of both countries, besides having furnished most active members of the expert scientific staffs of the Bureau of Annual Industries in the United States and the stock quarantine service of Canada. It must be very gratifying, indeed, to the teachers of the school to receive such high appreciation of their earnest and successful labors as has just been made by a university occupying such a high position in the scientific world, and, withal, one so conservative. McGill, too, is to be congratulated on her efforts to encourage and promote a branch of medical science which is daily becoming more and more important, not only on account of the direct bearing it has on the great agricultural industries of nations, but also on account of the close and inseparable relations it bears to public health in dealing with and preventing those animal diseases which recent investigations have proven to be communicable from animal to man. The new faculty is to be wished every success, and there is little doubt but the same influences which have maintained it for the past twenty-three years will continue to improve the greater facilities and advantages which it must enjoy as a faculty of McGill, and it is to be hoped, too, that the friends of the new faculty will see that its progress and usefulness will not be hindered for want of means to carry out improvements and extensions incident to its new connection. Other cities and countries have done much to alleviate the sufferings of poor dumb animals by the establishment and endowment of homes for homeless dogs and hospitals for the treatment of the animals of the poor, in which connection the new faculty could be of great service in carrying out the wishes of the humane and charitable. Montreal has reason to be proud of her noble liberality in connection with hospital work, but, as is well known by every member of the Society for Prevention of Cruelty, there is much mute but unalleviated suffering among the animals of the poor. This faculty have already advertised free treatment on two days a week for animals belonging to poor people, and it is to be trusted that their usefulness in this direction will be extended.

EDITORIAL NOTES.

—The medical department of the University of Maryland has decided to extend its course to three years. When contemplating such changes, it would have been wise to have made the course four in place of three years. Before many years a five years' course will be the rule with those medical schools on this continent who really aim at turning out good men.

—Richard von Volkmann, the distinguished German surgeon, is dead. He was among the first to recognize and put into practice the teachings of Lister in relation to the treatment of wounds. Among his favorite studies was the investigation of cancerous and tuberculous formations. Volkmann will be remembered by many in his fatherland by his poetical effusions, especially his " Reveries at French Firesides."

—Dr. Burgess, of the Hamilton Insane Asylum, has been appointed medical superintendent of the Protestant Hospital for the Insane in this city. Dr. Burgess is in every way highly qualified for the position, and the friends of the institution are to be congratulated on the choice made by the governors. Dr. Burgess has had an extensive experience in the treatment of the insane, having filled important positions in several of the leading asylums of Ontario.

—The *Journal of Comparative Medicine and Surgery* will appear in future monthly instead of quarterly, and under the name of *The Journal of Comparative Medicine and Veterinary Archives*. Dr. R. S. Huide-Koper has undertaken the active management of the editorial department. In the past this ably conducted journal has filled a very important place in medical literature, and we have no doubt that in the future the same high standard will be maintained.

—A recent correspondent in the *Lancet* deplores the prevalence of the "sweating system" in the profession in England. Hard work and any quantity of it, with little remuneration, is, unfortunately, not confined to the medical practitioners of England.   It is the lot of hundreds of practitioners in Canada and the United States.   While we have so many men in our ranks who estimate their services as worth from 50 cents to a dollar per year, we are not likely to have anything better.

—We are pleased to hear that it is the intention of the University of Pennsylvania to establish and thoroughly equip a laboratory for hygiene.   The recent great extension of hygienic laboratories is one of the most important and hopeful advances ever made by medical schools.   With hardly an exception, all the medical faculties of the German universities have complete hygienic laboratories attached to them.   The University of Pennsylvania is to be greatly commended for its spirit and enterprise in being the first to establish a laboratory for hygiene on this continent.

NEW YORK POST-GRADUATE MEDICAL SCHOOL AND HOSPITAL. —The executive committee of this institution have established a clinic for diseases of the rectum, to be under the care of Dr. Charles B. Kelsey, for the treatment of poor persons suffering from these diseases.   Dr. Kelsey will also give clinical instruction in the Post-Graduate School on this subject.   It is believed that this is the first institution in New York city to organize such a clinic, which has been long needed.   The high and wide reputation of Dr. Kelsey, founded upon years of special work, will afford a guarantee that the cases will be skillfully treated.   Dr. J. Blair Gibbs will assist Dr. Kelsey in this new departure.

Medical Items.

-The College of Physicians and Surgeons, New York, have decided to raise their tuition fee to $200 per annum.

PERSONAL.—Dr. T. Johnson-Alloway has retired from the general practice of medicine, and will devote himself absolutely to the practice of his specialty.

—The number of students attending the Medical Faculty of McGill University during the present session considerably exceeds that of any previous year.

—The next meeting of the Congress of American Physicians and Surgeons will be held in Washington, in September, 1891, under the presidency of Dr. Weir Mitchell of Philadelphia.

—We are pleased to learn that active steps are being taken to establish a Maritime Medical Society, to be composed of the members of the profession in Nova Scotia, New Brunswick and Prince Edward Island.

—Prof. William Pepper of Philadelphia has accepted the invitation to deliver the Middleton-Goldsmith lecture before the New York Pathological Society. The subject of the lecture will be " Hepatic Fever."

—A recent number of the *Medical News* contains an account of a will made by an eccentric physician living in Pesth. He left a fortune of $250,000, with instructions that it should be allowed to accumulate until it reached the sum of $1,000,000,000, when it is to be devoted to the abolition of poverty throughout the world. It is no wonder that the trustees declined to serve.

—The American Academy of Medicine is endeavoring to make as complete a list as possible of the alumni of literary colleges in the United States and Canada who have received the degree of M.D. All recipients of both degrees, literary and medical, are requested to forward their names, at once, to

Dr. R. J. Dunglison, secretary, 814 North 14th street, Philadelphia, Pa.

—The *Ophthalmic Review* begins its new volume with an American editor. Dr. Edward Jackson of Philadelphia, who succeeds Dr. James Anderson of London. It will, hereafter, contain original papers from American as well as English ophthalmic surgeons, with a list of all papers on ophthalmological subjects published in this country or in Europe, and full reviews of the most important of them.

—The eighth yearly issue of the *International Medical Annual for* 1890 is announced for early delivery. The prospectus gives promise of excellencies surpassing all former editions. Its thirty-seven editors in the several departments are to give a summary of new remedies alphabetically arranged, also a resume of new treatment in dictionary form ; with references to the medical literature of the world pertaining to the year's progress of medicine. Such a practical and helpful volume is of inestimable value to the medical profession. In one volume of about 600 octavo pages; price, $2.75, post free. E. B. Treat, publisher, 5 Cooper Union, New York.

THE

MONTREAL MEDICAL JOURNAL.

| VOL. XVIII. | FEBRUARY, 1890. | No. 8. |

Original Communications.

APPENDICITIS—LAPAROTOMY—RECOVERY.

By FRANCIS J. SHEPHERD, M.D.,
Surgeon to the Montreal General Hospital.

WITH REMARKS ON CASE BY DR. R. L. MACDONNELL.

The following notes of the case have been furnished me by
Dr. R. L. MacDonnell, under whose care the patient was up to
the time of operation :—

" Julia B., æt. 20, was admitted into the medical wards of the
Montreal General Hospital on September 13th, 1889, complaining of severe pain in the abdomen. For the last twelve months
she has frequently suffered from occasional pain and tenderness
in the right iliac region, but the first really severe attack which
resembled the present one occurred five months ago, and was
very severe. She remained in bed for three weeks, and thought
that recovery was complete, but after being up three weeks a
second attack occurred, which was more severe than the first.
She was taken to the Notre Dame Hospital, where she remained
some three or four weeks, leaving the institution some time in
June. Since then she has never been free from some degree of
pain in the right iliac fossa. The present attack began nine
days ago. She awoke in the night with a very severe pain in
the right side of the abdomen, which was almost immediately
followed by vomiting. The pain next day was more intense.
Five days before entering hospital she had a severe rigor. She
was under treatment evidently by opium until day of admission.

36

At the time of visit she presented the following appearance:
A strong, muscular girl, with bright complexion; dorsal decubitus; legs drawn up; face pinched and expressive of the greatest suffering; great tenderness and pain over right iliac fossa, which extends towards the right breast and up the back of the chest; pulse 120, small and hard; respirations hurried and shallow (30); temperature, morning 99 4°, evening 100.8°. The bowels have not moved for several days. On admission an enema had been administered, opium was given, and fomentations applied.

Next day the condition was much worse. Pain and tenderness general over the whole abdomen. Dr. Shepherd was now called in."

I saw the patient, at Dr. MacDonnell's request, at mid-day, September 14th, 1889. She was suffering from well-marked symptoms of appendicitis. We both decided it was a case for operation, and without further loss of time the patient was put under ether. On examination, no tumor could be made out in the right iliac fossa, but there was a distinct sense of resistance. After thoroughly cleansing the abdominal walls, an incision was made in the right iliac region some four inches in length. The incision made was the usual curved one, the centre being a little internal to the anterior superior spinous process of the ilium. After cutting through the abdominal wall, the peritoneum could not be distinguished, but a mass of inflammatory tissue and omentum appeared; this was carefully pulled aside, and in doing so a small stinking abscess containing a few drachms of pus was evacuated. The appendix was now searched for, and was somewhat difficult to find. The first structures that came into view were some coils of small intestine and the right Fallopian tube. After some little search, which was complicated by the condition of the parts, the appendix was found, somewhat larger than normal, coiled up beneath the cæcum and imbedded in a mass of inflammatory tissue. Cautiously separating it preparatory to applying a ligature, an abscess behind the cæcum containing several ounces of stinking pus was evacuated, a portion of which escaped into the general peritoneal cavity. On examining the appendix, quite close to its junction with the cæcum a gangrenous ulcer was seen, which almost severed the appendix from the bowel. The appendix was with difficulty ligated above the ulcer, a piece of the cæcum being pinched up to make the ligature hold ; it was then removed at the site of the ulcer. The cavity of the peritoneum was now washed out with boiled water and the wound closed, except at the lower end, through which was introduced a large rubber tube to the bottom of the abscess cavity. Dressing consisted of iodoform and cotton wool, held in place by a couple of strips of rubber plaster.

After the operation the patient had a very restless night, with considerable vomiting and pain. Next day the dressings were changed, being soaked through with the oozing of a bloody serum, and also some bloody serum was withdrawn from the wound by means of a syringe having a piece of tubing attached. Two days after the operation the bowels moved freely. At the end of a week patient was doing well, had very little pain, and no rise of temperature. The discharge from the wound had a distinctly fœcal odor, and was yet in some quantity. The stitches were taken out, and near where the drainage tube was the wound gaped considerably, so it was packed with sticky iodoform gauze from the bottom.

From this time the case progressed favorably, a slough the size of a five-cent piece coming away at the end of the second week. The patient was placed on plain full diet at the end of the fourth week, and was then seized with severe colicky pains without rise of temperature. On enquiry it was found that she was constipated, so salines were ordered, but these not relieving the pain she was placed on milk diet, which in a couple of days restored her to her normal condition. Patient was discharged from hospital on the 4th of November ; she still had a small sinus at the site of the drainage-tube. I saw her on Wednesday, December 18th, and she had then been back to her work for three weeks ; she looked strong and fat, and said she had not the slightest pain. There was still a small shallow sinus at the lower end of the abdominal wound.

In laparotomy for appendicitis the lateral incision is much the most convenient, especially in cases where the diagnosis is as plain as in the one just related ; besides being the most suitable for examining the condition of the cæcum and appendix, the lateral incision is much the most favorable for after drainage. Some surgeons advise that in excision of the appendix the peritoneum should be dissected away and sewed over the end of the cut tube. I see no special advantage in this procedure, and, besides, it is only practicable in a few cases ; when the peritoneum is so altered by inflammatory action, as is usually the case, no such plan could be carried out. In this case the appendix was removed so close up to the cæcum that even if the peritoneum had been normal a flap of it could not have been removed. Omental grafting, as recommended by Dr. Senn in wounds of the intestines, might be a useful and practicable proceeding. The situation of the ulcer in this case was unusual ; it is generally situated at some distance from the cæcal junction, most frequently near the apex. No concretion was found.

This case was successful because early operation was performed and symptoms of general peritonitis were not waited for. In fact, to treat such cases on the expectant plan is obsolete and bad surgery ; a very few may get well, but the great majority will perish, and perish rapidly. Again, this case, from its history of repeated previous attacks and its not very rapid course, was one which was eminently favorable to operation. Where the appendix is curled up beneath the cæcum, the diseased area is usually separated from the general peritoneal cavity by a boundary of inflammatory tissue, and this is the time operation should be undertaken. Should the disease go on, the abscess may either present in the iliac fossa, rupture into the peritoneal cavity, or, if the pus be pent up, it may cause death by septicæmia. The cases which have a previous history of attacks of appendicitis should be operated on without hesitation early ; the danger of early operation is not great, and the patient is permanently relieved from a condition which will, sooner or later, cause his death. Such cases are advised to be operated on between the attacks and the appendix removed. Mr. Treves of London and Dr. McBurney of New York have successfully operated in such cases. These cases differ much from those others where the appendix hangs freely over the brim of the pelvis and perforation occurs almost without previous warning, and is not preceded by a limiting inflammation. In such cases there is a sudden lighting up of a general peritonitis of a most virulent type, which in spite of any operation rapidly proceeds to a fatal termination. I have operated on several such cases always with the same result. Death has not been averted by the operation, but pain and vomiting have been relieved.

There is no doubt in my mind that the degree and virulence of the inflammation of the peritoneum caused by perforation of the appendix varies considerably in different cases, depending on the condition of the individual and the quality of the poisonous matter extruded from the perforated appendix. I believe in some cases operation, even if performed at a very early stage, would be of no avail. Those cases where an abscess has burst into the peritoneal cavity, unless operation be *immediately* performed, are always fatal. A general suppurative peritonitis is lighted up—no amount of washing will cleanse the many nooks and corners of the peritoneal cavity from its infective material.

Remarks by Dr. MacDonnell.—Did the prognosis warrant an operation so formidable as laparotomy? (1) There were three distinct attacks of pain in the right iliac region, each worse than the preceding one. (2) The suddenness of the onset is characteristic of disease of the appendix. Sudden, severe abdominal pain was present in 216 out of 287 cases collected by Dr. Fitz of Boston (84½ per cent.) (3) In the intervals between the attacks of acute pain the patient still suffered, though not severely. It would therefore be unlikely that even if the present acute symptoms were to pass off she would regain her health. (4) The symptoms pointed to a change from a local to a general peritonitis, though after operation there were no indications of general peritonitis observed. Appendicular peritonitis has a special tendency to become general, and when general the result is almost invariably fatal. I therefore felt that in handing my patient over to the surgeons I was giving her the best chance for life which circumstances afforded.

Retrospect Department.

QUARTERLY RETROSPECT OF MEDICINE.

BY R. L. MacDONNELL, M.D.,

Professor of Clinical Medicine in McGill University; Physician to Montreal General Hospital.

DISEASES OF THE LUNGS.

On the Treatment of Pneumonia by the Ice bag.—Dr. Lees in a paper read before the Harveian Society on 17th October claims beneficial results from this mode of treatment, and cites the history of eighteen cases of pneumonia in which he had given the method full trial. When a treatment for a disease so self-limiting as pneumonia is advocated, one cannot help feeling critical and called upon to look closely into the evidence in favor of the new agent. There are eighteen cases cited. Two of these can be dismissed at once, since the writer of the paper acknow-ledges that the icebag was not beneficial. In two other cases the diagnosis is doubtful. A child aged 3 years (son of Dr. Lees) has " catarrh for two or three days, when he rapidly became acutely ill ; the temperature ran up to 104°, the breathing was very rapid, and his lips began to look a little dusky. Just the faintest impairment of resonance was to be detected at the base of one lung." This is very slight evidence on which to base a diagnosis of pneumonia, but the next case is even more doubtful. " A boy, aged 4, has a week's catarrh and a sudden tempera-ture of 104.5° ; pulse 140 ; respiration 50, occasionally inter-rupted by a short cough ; a shade of loss of resonance at the left base below the angle of the scapula. At this spot, and also at the corresponding spot on the other side of the chest, inspiration was a little harsh and attended by a little râle, and expiration was too plain." They may have been pneumonias, but when a plan of treatment is advocated, the first and most important question is whether the patient really had the disease which was said to be cured. Of the other fourteen patients none were old and none of them had an alcoholic history, and with the excep-tion of cases 11, 14 and 15, all were of the kind that would do well under any kind of treatment. Take, for example case 3, a schoolboy aged 16. On the fourth day the temperature was 104° with "moderate consolidation at the right base. On the fifth day the temperature fell. Certainly it has fallen to the lot of many practitioners to have witnessed a crisis on the fifth day even without icebag treatment.

Granting that the application of the icebag lowers temperature it is yet an open question whether it is beneficial to lower temperature. In pneumonia it is not the fever that kills, and if the patient be young and free from depressing influences, and if the extent of lung involved be not extensive, then certainly the depression of the temperature by cold will not lower the mortality rate.

Dr. Goodhart had also used the icebag in eighteen cases. A good result was obtained in eight. In seven it was doubtful if the treatment had had any effect whatever, while in three cases symptoms of collapse were produced of a new temporary nature. He thought that there was no danger in the treatment, such collapse as might occur being easily detected.

Dr. Sturges pointed out that Dr. Lees cases were all young, and the mortality in these was very small. He doubted if the evidence was yet sufficient for us to say that we arrested pneumonia, and recalled the brilliant statistics of Hughes Bennett, who had reported over one hundred cases, some of them in elderly persons, with but five deaths. He doubted also if it was, as a rule, a great good to shorten the pneumonia.

The Non-tubercular and Non-cardiac Hæmoptysis of Elderly Persons.—Sir Andrew Clark read a most instructive paper at the Medical Society of London on the 21st October, selecting as his subject the occurrence of hœmoptysis in elderly persons who were at the time and who remained afterwards free from signs either of pulmonary tuberculosis or of structural disease of the heart. A case which occurred in the London Hospital drew Sir Andrew's attention to a form of hœmoptysis which was probably due to a condition of the arteries. The autopsy revealed no cause for the hœmoptysis, but by means of the microscope two important facts were brought to light. The first that the seat of the hemorrhage was in the neighborhood of certain em-

physematous patches, the second that the minute vessels in those
which were for the most part terminal arteries were always diseased.   And, finally, it appeared in the highest degree probable
that there existed a direct casual relationship between the condition of the blood-vessel, the emphysema, and the hemorrhage.
For wherever there was an emphysematous patch there was a
diseased artery ; wherever the artery was much diseased the
capillaries and venous radicles were also affected ; and generally,
though not always, where the terminal artery was obstructed
and degenerating, there was adjacent hemorrhage.   " I inferred
that the initial visible movement in the malady had been some
minute structural change in a terminal branch of the pulmonary
or of the bronchial artery, and in consequence of this there had
been brought about a more or less complete obstruction of the
supply of blood through the territory involved ; that following
this there arose degeneration of the capillaries and venous
radicles determining a true atrophic emphysema, and that the
integrity of the blood-vessels being thus impaired, the formation
of thrombi or recurrent condition of pressure had brought about
the hemorrhage which ended in death."

What was the intimate nature of the structural vascular
changes ?   The importance of the case lies in the primitive
dynamic changes which gave the structural alterations form and
meaning.   " When I endeavored to determine the significance
of these changes, and for this purpose studied the life history of
the case—when I saw that the patient had been for years an
arthritic, that he had suffered on many occasions from many of
the constitutional manifestations of this diathesis, and that the
structural changes in the pulmonary blood-vessels were akin in
character to those which are found in the diseased articulations,
I permitted myself to conclude that the malady was of an arthritic nature, and that I had seen and dealt with a case of what
might be called, without serious scientific impropriety, ' arthritic
hœmoptysis.' "

The second case occurred in a stout man of 50, who was
rheumatic, fat, short-breathed, eczematous and indolent.   There
was bronchial catarrh, but no circulatory derangement.   Death

from hœmoptysis. Here, again, were found the emphysematous patches, the diseased blood-vessels, and the extravasated blood. The source of the fatal hemorrhage lay in the diseased blood-vessels. Probably the disease was of an arthritic nature, and pardonably enough one might say, here is another case of arthritic hœmoptysis. " Since 1875 I have seen in persons over 50 some twenty cases of hœmoptysis of the kind which I have now described." The cases thus related have led Sir Andrew Clark to substitute for the treatment, commonly thought orthodox, a light and rather dry diet, a sparing use of liquids, the discontinuanʒe of the use of ice, a calomel pill at bedtime, followed by a saline cathartic, and an alkaline mixture between meals twice in the day. The propositions framed from the results of Sir Andrew Clark's enquiries are as follows :

1. That there occurs in elderly persons free from ordinary disease of the heart and lungs a form of hœmoptysis arising out of minute structural alterations in the terminal blood-vessels of the lung.

2. That these vascular alterations occur in persons of the arthritic diathesis, resemble the vascular alterations found in osteo-arthritic articulations, and are themselves of an arthritic nature.

3. That although sometimes leading to a fatal issue, this variety of hœmoptysis usually subsides without the supervention of any coarse anatomical lesion of either the heart or the lungs.

4. That when present, this variety of hemorrhage is aggravated or maintained by the frequent administration of large doses of strong astringents, and by an unrestricted indulgence in liquids to allay the thirst which the astringents create.

5. That the treatment which appears at present to be most successful in this variety of hœmoptysis consists in diet and quiet, in the restricted use of liquids, and the stilling of cough ; in calomel and salines, in the use of alkalies, with iodide of potassium, and in frequently renewed counter-irritation.

ANEURYSM OF THE AORTA.

An interesting discussion of this important subject took place

at the meeting of the Medical Society of London, on the 9th
December, 1889, Dr. Theodore Williams in the chair.

Dr. Douglas Powell introduced the discussion and said that
the object of the meeting was to elicit the experience of the
Fellows in the diagnosis and treatment of aneurysm. It was
specially urged that the true clinical features of aneurysm were
alone—with very rare exceptions—yielded by the sacculated
form of the disease, and that both in regard to prognosis and
treatment the so-called fusiform aneurysm was totally different.
The aneurysmal sac was necessarily an enlarging tumor, producing (1) pressure phenomena, and (2) cardio-vascular phenomena.
In enlargement of the vessel without sacculation pressure phenomena were insignificant or absent, the cardio-vascular phenomena very marked. Pressure signs were of the first importance in the diagnosis of aneurysm, and to imperfect recognition
of this fact and the attachment of too great a value to circulatory
phenomena were attributable most errors in diagnosis, and illustrative cases were related. The value of the laryngoscope as
an aid to diagnosis and of the sphygmograph as a recording
instrument were emphasized.

Dr. Broadbent agreed that the pressure signs were more important for diagnostic purposes than the disturbances of the circulation, with this qualification that the pressure signs depended
upon the situation of the aneurysm. In aneurysm of the ascending aorta, the tumor might attain a considerable size and yet
produce very little pressure upon neighboring parts, owing to the
natural mobility of the vessels. To hear a murmur was rather
the exception than the rule. The " diastolic shock," either
audible or perceptible to the hand, was one of the most valuable
of signs. Fusiform aneurysm is not amenable to any treatment ;
the only thing was to lower the pressure, enjoining rest, but not
with the idea of promoting anything like a cure. He had nothing
to add to the Tuffnell treatment, but his own experience with the
iodide of potash was that it very strikingly promoted consolidation within the sac. He had many times found that consolidation
had followed the administration of the iodide, which virtually had
the same effect as the Tuffnell treatment, running off the fluid

by the kidneys and so inspissating the blood. He only resorted to bleeding when there was pain, but the relief was then very striking. Dr. Sibson's plan of treatment by the use of ergot unquestionably diminished the size of the tumor, though this was certainly not due to any specific action on muscular fibre in the sac wall, since he had never been able to discover any there.

Dr. Bristowe confined his remarks to treatment, in which he said that he was somewhat of a pessimist. Post-mortem appearances pointed to the fact that the permanently cured cases— *i.e.*, thoroughly filled up with clot—were cases in which aneurysm had not been suspected, and in which the patient had been bed-ridden and dying for weeks of something else. He was rather in favor of the Tuffnell treatment, but he had no faith in the treatment by wire or by galvano puncture. He had never witnessed any benefit from the iodide of potash treatment.

INFLAMMATION OF THE VERMIFORM APPENDIX.

The subject of operative interference in appendix disease was under discussion at the Surgical Society of New York on the 13th November last. Dr. McBurney, who read the paper of the evening, began by stating that his belief that inflammatory affections of the vermiform appendix gave rise to a considerable number of the so-called pericæcal inflammations is now accepted in every part of the medical and surgical worlds, although one still reads of perityphlitis and paratyphlitis, and of intra-peritoneal and extra-peritoneal abscesses. Every case of inflammation of the appendix is sooner or later accompanied by inflammation of the neighboring peritoneum, either on the cæcum, or mesentery, or ileum, etc., but if from the whole list of acute inflammatory affections occurring in the right iliac fossa we set aside those originating in the appendix, how many shall we have left ? Very rarely will occur a perforation of the cæcum by ulcer or foreign body, giving rise to a local peritonitis at this point, and traumatisms from without may accomplish the same result. For all of such causes as compared with inflammations of the appendix, the proportion is as one in one hundred. The observations of the operation table and of the dead-house do not support the idea, by a single instance, that localized peritonitis or perityphlitis arise from impaction of fæces in the cæcum. " I must therefore prefer to use the term inflammation of the appendix or appendicitis, and give up, once and for all, the terms perityphlitis, paratyphlitis, extra-peritoneal abscess, etc., as misleading, and not valuable except in explanation of secondary pathological processes. All abscesses originating in inflammation of the appendix are intra-peritoneal. Inflammatory adhesions which glue together the adjacent coils of intestine prevent the contents of the abscess from flowing into the pelvis or among the intestinal folds. At every point the pus is bounded by peritoneum.

When the operation is done at an early stage of the disease there is no difficulty in demonstrating that the collection of pus is intra-peritoneal. In all the cases observed there was acute peritonitis—usually a plastic peritonitis of greater or less extent —always involving the cæcum and generally the adjacent intestinal coils and abdominal walls. In one case the omentum was quite extensively involved, partly enveloping the appendix. In no case was the appendix more than lightly attached by adhesion to the peritoneum, covering the iliac muscles, and in none was extra-peritoneal inflammation observed, excepting sometimes in the anterior abdominal wall. In most cases some pus was found more or less confined by adhesions within a limited area, and one absolutely no adhesion of any kind existed, though the appendix was perforated by concretion, and very foul pus filled the pelvis and ran freely upwards beside the colon.

The pathological conditions of the appendix, as compared with the symptoms, most positively show that one cannot with accuracy determine from the symptoms the extent and severity of the disease.

Pain to a greater or less extent is always present in all cases of appendicitis, but many a mistake has been made, and a golden opportunity lost by looking for pain in the iliac fossa, and an absence of pain in other parts of the abdomen. In the first few hours of the attack the abdominal pain is general, but after that period it becomes more and more evident that the chief seat of pain is in the right iliac fossa, and the general pain then usually subsides.

The epigastric region is frequently the point first complained of. One patient, who died on the third day from violent septic peritonitis from perforation, complained of comparatively little pain even when the iliac fossa was firmly compressed. The exact locality of the greatest sensitiveness to pressure has seemed to me to be usually one of importance. " Whatever may be the position of the healthy appendix as found in the dead-house—and I am well aware that its position, when uninflamed, varies greatly—I have found in all of my operations that it lay either thickened, shortened or adherent, very close to its point of attach·ment to the cæcum. This must in early stages of the disease determine the seat of greatest pain on pressure. And I believe that in every case the seat of greatest pain, determined by the pressure of one finger, has been very exactly between an inch and a half and two inches from the anterior spinous process of the ilium on a straight line drawn from that process to the um-bilicus. This may appear to be an affectation of accuracy, but so far as my experience goes the observation is correct."

Chill and vomiting are frequent, but so often absent as to be in no sense of much diagnostic value. Fever is always present, but in a different degree, and is of value in diagnosis as exclud-ing non-inflammatory pains. Rigidity of the abdominal muscles, generally much more marked on the affected side than on the other, is a constant and valuable sign.

Tympanites varies greatly, and its degree measures the severity of the diseased process. When the gut has been found during the operation to be over-distended, the portion so affected has been the large intestine.

Tumor has been detected in most instances at an early stage, but the composition of this tumor, as shown during operation, has varied greatly. In one case the tumor consisted of the dis-tended unruptured appendix, which was partly wrapped in an inflamed and thickened omentum. In another it was formed of a mass of intestinal coils, swollen and glued together by recent plastic exudation. Ether constitutes a valuable aid to diagnosis, for with it some tumor can invariably be detected. The pulse during the onset of appendicitis is usually rapid and irritable.

The patient prefers to have the right thigh elevated, and objects to its over-extension.

The diagnosis of the seat of the disease is not so difficult to make as that of the stage to which the morbid process has gone.

There is much misapprehension as to the symptoms produced by perforation of the appendix. In the early stage no accurate diagnosis can be made as to whether the appendix is perforated or not, excepting in those cases where comparatively mild cases *suddenly* become much aggravated. Perforation often occurs with but few symptoms at the very beginning of the disease, but being preceded by the formation of more or less plastic adhesion of the appendix. No sudden increase in the severity of the disease occurs at all.

The histories of eleven cases of operation, seven of which resulted in recovery, are reported.

QUARTERLY RETROSPECT OF GYNÆCOLOGY.

By T. Johnson-Alloway, M.D.,
Instructor in Gynæcology, McGill University; Assistant Surgeon to the Montreal General Hospital; Gynæcologist to the Montreal Dispensary.

At a recent meeting of the British Gynæcological Society, Dr. Bantock showed a specimen of a soft fibroid which had developed in the anterior segment of the uterus, between it and the bladder. On exposing the tumor it was seen to be loosely covered with peritoneum, and he at once proceeded to shell it out. That was easily done until he got quite close to the base, and there he had some difficulty in separating it from the bladder. Before proceeding further he applied an elastic ligature around the base of the tumor. When he had completed the separation he found he had opened into a cavity which was lined with mucous membrane. He was rather puzzled at first to know what this cavity was, but he got his assistant to put his finger into the vagina, and then he discovered that they communicated. Before beginning the operation he had introduced a silver catheter into the bladder, and found that it went below the loop of the elastic ligature, showing that it was very intimately connected with the base of the tumor. When he had separated it he came upon the body of the uterus, which was connected with the lower and back part of the mass. The great difficulty was to avoid the bladder, and it was only by putting in the catheter and putting the pins almost through the raw surface and pulling it back that he managed to escape injuring that organ.

During a recent discussion on uterine fibroids, Mr. Tait said that a discussion had been opened for eighteen months past on the subject, yet no one had shown a single case cured by elec. trolysis. He had by chance seen a lady lately who had returned from Paris, where she had been under this treatment for a term of three months, had had 35 applications, of which 31 were done under anæsthesia, at a cost of £300, yet to-day, Mr. Tait said, she was in a worse plight than ever, and was anxious to be relieved by some other method.

Dr. A. V. Macan (President) said, during the discussion on fibroids, that the question really seemed to be, What are the indications for operation in cases of fibroid ? It was a complicated question, and one not very easy to settle. The great thing was to be as guarded as possible. He thought therefore that the possibility of enucleating these tumors ought to be more borne in mind. One's judgment, of course, depended largely upon what one's success had been in the past. He himself had tried the intra-peritoneal method, and he had lost nearly all his patients, but the extra-peritoneal method was much simpler. He said that if they could remove a tumor from the uterus and sew up the cavity from which the tumor was taken, and then return it all to the abdomen, the wound would not be greater than in an ordinary cæsarian section. He thought that this would be a great improvement. He thought that the tumor between the uterus and the bladder might have been enucleated and the uterus saved, and also without removal of the appendages.

Dr. R. T. Smith said he had removed a large fibroid a fortnight ago. In that case electrolysis had been tried during a period of three months without the slightest benefit. He said he was quite willing to give new methods a trial, but his experience of electrolysis was that it did not yield good results.

Dr. Edis showed a so-called mole. It looked like a polypus

protruding from the os.   The clinical history was interesting.
The patient was a married woman, 35 years of age, who had
been suffering from severe menorrhagia on and off since January
last, flooding for ten days or a fortnight towards the latter end
of June, when the loss was profuse.   In July, all sanguineous
discharge ceased until the first week in September ; then she
began to flood again.   She went on flooding until she was quite
blanched and anæmic, when she was sent to the Chelsea Hospital
for Women.   He had examined her, and he found the mass protruding from the external os.   He removed it by means of a pair
of forceps, taking care that there was nothing left behind.   Since
then the patient had been well, and there had been no return of
the hemorrhage.   He observed that there was no doubt as to its
being the product of conception.   There had been a certain
amount of hemorrhage into the tissues, and it was a very good
specimen of what used to be called a mole.   Had the patient
been examined in the first instance this might have been removed, and she would have been relieved at once.   The patient
had a miscarriage early in the year, and that was the starting-
point of the hemorrhage.   Then the bleeding ceased in the first
week in July and there was no return until the first week in
September, an interval of two months.   The question in his mind
was as to whether this was not the ovum which should have been
extruded at the beginning of the year.   He suggested that the
temporary cessation of the hemorrhage might have been due to
the partial extrusion of the mass from the cavity of the uterus
into the cervix.

The reviewer has had to operate upon many occasions in a
similar manner for the relief of such cases as described by Dr.
Edis.   And it proves the necessity of making a vaginal examination in every case showing a history of such nature.   The
principle of administering drugs to control the hemorrhage cannot be too strongly condemned.   Prolonged invalidism is insured,
loss of health on the part of the patient, and reputation on the
part of the attending physician.   The question invariably asked
by the patient, Why could not this operation have been done
before ? has to be met evasively.   It is therefore a good rule to

follow, that in recurrent uterine hemorrhage following a suspected abortion, an examination should be made and the uterine cavity properly explored.

Gynæcological Specialism.—An interesting paper read by Dr. Thomas M. Dolan before the British Gynæcological Society recently on the above subject excited some discussion. The part Dr. Bantock took in the discussion was certainly interesting.

Dr. Bantock said he could not agree with Dr. Dolan in his condemnation of the treatment of displacements of the uterus by pessaries, although Dr. Dolan was supported in his opinion by some of the ablest gynæcologists in England and America. Dr. Bantock admitted that he had not written in his book much about the dynamics of pessaries. Such a statement is also an admission that Dr. Bantock's knowledge of the dynamics of pessaries is somewhat imperfect, and renders his opinion on such matters therefore of little value. He observed that Dr. Dolan seemed to favor some of the more risky operations, such as shortening of the round ligaments (Alexander's operation). He said he had never yet seen a case in which he felt justified in performing so serious an operation, and that it was very evident the round ligaments had nothing whatever to do with the position of the uterus. Expressions of this kind coming from Dr. Bantock only cause us on this side of the water to gently smile. Dr. Bantock has written a book on pessaries and he fears the round ligament operation will render this work one of " labor lost." This is very English and we must therefore overlook it. It must be acknowledged that of all methods of treatment to which a woman with uterine disease is subjected, the wearing of a pessary is probably the most distasteful to her. She is ever alluding to the " unpleasant thing" and asking how long she will have to wear it. The quiet, silent and submissive bearing of the husband when he is informed that his wife has had an instrument inserted to support her displaced womb must not be lost sight of in its moral bearing. From my experience in Alexander's operation (now some twenty-five cases) the method is going to be eminently successful and the pessary must cease to be applied as a permanent support. To illustrate further the absurd length to which the application of pessaries are carried in England, Dr. W. H. Fenton of London relates the case of a large fibro-cystic myoma of the uterus, reaching to the umbilicus and filling completely the false pelvis, which he removed by hysterectomy.   Dr. Fenton states that at the consultation of his hospital colleagues prior to the operation, among other palliative measures suggested, one gentleman strongly urged the application of a pessary,—*shades of the immortal Hodge!*

Dr. Bantock gave, at a recent meeting of the British Gynæcological Society, a table of 238 cases of completed ovariotomy with 163 cases already reported, making a total of 400 cases. These operations were performed without the aid of antiseptics in about half the number.   He says that for his hands, instruments and sponges he uses plain water.   He takes no precaution to sterilize it by boiling.   He regards water considered fit for household purposes also fit to be used in any surgical operation.   He washes his hands with soap and water, using nail-brush and pen-knife to clean his nails.   He has no belief in the hurtfulness of " germs," and were it not for other inconveniences he would leave his wounds exposed to the air without dressing as he does breast and perineum cases. His results have been as follows:—First hundred ovariotomies under Listerian method he lost nineteen cases ; second hundred, gradually abandoning Listerian method, he lost fourteen cases ; third hundred, all performed with plain water, he lost eight cases ; fourth hundred, mortality reduced to four cases.   Dr. Bantock goes exhaustively into details, considering (1) washing out the peritoneum, (2) treatment of the pedicle, (3) opium, (4) general after treatment, and (5) peritonitis.   He mentions Dr. Polaillon's case of death following washing out of the peritoneum with a weak solution of carbolic acid in warm water, and without doubt shows that death was due to carbolic acid poisoning.   He points out that during the first minutes of flushing there is a large quantity of fluid absorbed, and that this is especially the case when the water is mixed with common salt in about the proportion of seven parts to one thousand,—the process then becomes " a true indirect transfusion."

Gill Wylie of New York has taken advantage of this process and found that large quantities of hot water in the peritoneal cavity had the tendency to lessen shock due to loss of blood.

Dr. Bantock states that he has washed out the peritoneum in more than one-half of his last one hundred cases. He uses plain hot water cooled down to the proper temperature by adding water from the tap. In speaking of the treatment of the pedicle, he says that since 1875 he has used the ligature exclusively. He, however, soon found a difficulty in its application. He lost his nineteenth case by the slipping of the outer edge of the pedicle—that edge which consists of two folds of peritoneum with its contained vessels. He now secures this outer fold by a separate ligature before transfixing for the main ligatures. Dr. Bantock chiefly uses the figure of eight knot. But when the pedicle is very thick he uses several double ligatures, as many sometimes as eight or nine. In such cases as these, however, he devised the method of first compressing the pedicle with powerful pairs of forceps. He thus succeeded in reducing the size of the pedicle to one half its size at the place where the ligature was applied.

(3) *Opium.*—Dr. Bantock says that it was about the same time that he resorted to flushing the peritoneum that he discontinued the use of opium. He relates the case of one of his patients who, ten minutes after receiving a hypodermic injection of one-sixth of a grain of marphia, died. He was so impressed with the unfortunate occurrence that he gradually reduced the dose until within a very short time he gave up the use of opium in any form after operations. He found that without opium there was less discomfort and sickness the next day and the condition of the patient altogether better. So that from the beginning of 1885 he had been obliged to give opium only in three cases. And he makes the remark that coincident with his giving up the use of opium his mortality has fallen to 4 per cent. Dr. Bantock draws attention to the admitted fact that opium is a poison in cases of chronic Bright's disease, and that it may have been the cause of death in many unsuspected cases. Opium not only diminishes the peristaltic action of the intestines, but it also diminishes the secretion. It is in this way that injury takes

place, and it is here where saline purgatives do good. Opium locks up the secretion; salines increase it and drain the peritoneal cavity.

General After-treatment — Vomiting.—He finds from experience that the best way to arrest sickness is to keep the stomach quiet by not putting anything into it. On this account he prefers operating in the morning when the stomach is empty after the long fast. If there should be vomiting, a few ounces of hot water will generally suffice to clear out the stomach, and there will be no more trouble. When, however, the stomach contains bile decomposed by its acid contents, then a few grains of carbonate of soda added to the hot water will be an advantage. It may be mentioned here that Dr. Bantock thinks, after an experience of thirty years, that chloroform is the best anæsthetic we possess. This sentiment we can understand in an Englishman who is prejudiced against ether and does not mind a death or two from the anæsthetic. Dr. Bantock may say that he has not had a death from chloroform, but we know that it is a matter of common occurrence to see recorded deaths from its administration in the London hospitals. And we doubt much if we could, in this country, find a coroner who would be willing to tolerate any such unpardonable waste of life.

Thirst.—Dr. Bantock strongly opposes the giving of ice to patients to allay the thirst following an operation, and mentions the fact that all Arctic explorers avoid ice if they wish to avoid suffering from thirst. Rinsing the mouth with hot water gives great relief, and instances the fact that a cup of hot tea is more lasting in its refreshing effects in hot weather than a cold drink. It is because of its warmth and consequent absence of reaction.

Peritonitis.—Dr. Bantock says peritonitis originates from causes originating within the cavity and without. The drainage tube has done much to obviate the former, and as the latter is due to irritating matters in the digestive tract, he stops all food by the mouth and gives rectal enemata of beef-tea. He is opposed to saline purgatives, the method of Tait and Greig Smith, and says that where they say it does good they cannot prove their case.

In conclusion, Dr. Bantock gives an epitomy table of the 238 cases, which is very interesting to study. .

Peritonitis due to the Passage of the Constant Current in a Patient with Double Salpingitis. (By M. TERRIER, in *Bull. Med.*)—A year since the author was called to a woman in whom the presence of abdominal tumors could be made out, which, after some hesitation, were diagnosed to be uterine fibromata. M. Terrier, however, doubted the accuracy of this diagnosis, and, acting in the belief that it was a case of double salpingitis, warned the patient that only an operation would relieve her. Disregarding his advice she resorted to the electrical treatment, which promptly determined a severe attack of acute peritonitis. The patient, however, survived, but the salpingitis had obviously increased in size, and the matting of the intestines could be felt in one spot through the abdominal parietes.

Vaginal Hysterectomy.—Dr. R. C. Dudley of Chicago recommends that the grooves in the forceps blades should run parallel with the blade and not across it. In this way the forceps will be less likely to slip. He has never left the forceps on the broad ligaments longer than seventy-two hours, and often removes them in twenty-four hours. He advises that the forceps hold the ligament in the vagina so that the peritoneal cavity will rapidly close and obviate the danger of infection from necrosed tissue. Vaginal injections should be begun on removal of the forceps or about the fourth day.

In regard to injections, the reviewer used creolin ($\frac{1}{2}$ per cent.) solution recently after a case of vaginal hysterectomy with most satisfactory results. It is a powerful deodorizer and perfectly harmless.

Dr. Dudley relates an interesting case of *Removal of a Uterine Myoma by a combined Vaginal and Abdominal Operation.* He began in the vagina by dividing the capsule of the tumor and removing piecemeal as much of the growth as possible for the period of an hour. He then opened the abdomen and removed the remainder of the tumor, also by enucleation. He then stitched the capsule to the abdominal wound and passed a glass drainage tube into the empty capsule through the abdominal wound.

Drainage went on very well until the vaginal end of the capsule closed, when the temperature rose to 103.5°. The closed end of capsule was opened by forcing a flexible sound through it. Perfect drainage was now instituted between the abdominal wound and the vagina by means of a rubber tube. The patient recovered. This operation must have been a somewhat interesting one to the surgeon, but it seems odd that he did not see the necessity of carrying a *through* drainage between the vagina and abdominal wound.

Non-retention of Urine in Infancy, Girls and Women.— Dr. H. Marion Sims of New York writes an interesting article in the *Amer. Jour of Obstet.*, giving his experience of the treatment of cases of this nature by the gradual dilatation of the bladder with water pressure. Dr. Sims says the disease he alludes to is the gradual contraction of the walls of the bladder due to a hypertrophy of the muscular coat and the consequent reduction of its holding capacity to little or nothing. He uses an ordinary Davidson's syringe and silver catheter. The injections are continued every day, each day getting a little more than the day before. He carries out this practice daily until the bladder can retain from eight to thirteen ounces of fluid without pain. And he generally accomplishes this in two or three months. The treatment is somewhat tedious and painful, but is certainly effective. The reviewer has had some experience in the method, and is pleased with the results obtained, so far, in some very intractable cases to other methods of treatment.

Dr. Hall of Cincinnati, O., read a paper before the American Association of Obstetrics and Gynæcology upon *Some Points in the Diagnosis of Pyosalpinx.* The author believes the importance played in the production of suffering by this disease has not received the attention which it merits. The general practitioner sees and treats the great majority of these cases before they are seen by the operator, and if it is hoped or expected to afford relief to a great number of suffering women all over the land the subject of diagnosis must be better understood than at present. The importance of septic infection in the production of inflammatory disease of the uterine appendages is the cause of this disease in a large percentage of cases. Repeated attacks of acute exacerbations from perhaps trivial causes finally produce complete closure of the ends of the tubes. As a consequence, the normal secretions of the tubes soon become pathological, and by repeated attacks of inflammation may become changed into pus, producing the typical pyosalpinx. The speaker is convinced that this affection frequently follows puerperal diseases and gonorrhœal infection, but does not consider these the most common causes of the disease. He believes pyosalpinx to be contracted in two different ways : (a) By a chronic process, causing dropsy of the tube, which, by repeated attacks of inflammation, is changed to pus ; (b) it may be rapidly produced by an acute process following gonorrhœa and puerperal diseases. A history of almost constant suffering for years, directed to a certain locality, perhaps originating in an attack of pelvic or abdominal inflammation, connected or not with parturition. To this may be added sterility, and we have a most important aid to a correct diagnosis in the history of the case. Diseased appendages can usually be recognized by a vaginal examination, yet this is not always possible. In most cases it is difficult, and in many impossible, to make out the exact disease of the appendages except in cases of pyosalpinx. We usually have an irregular ovoid tumor, showing swellings and contractions not found in any other pelvic tumor but tubal collections. This tumor is generally of small size ; it may be in the retro-uterine space extending toward the pelvic brim on the one side, with a second tumor on the other side higher up ; or it may be distinctly felt as a narrow furrow, which is occasioned by a portion of the uterine end of the tube remaining undistended by pus, while the distal end of the tube is enlarged to form the tumor. This furrow is not so plainly felt in those cases where there is a periodical discharge of the pus through the tube into the uterine cavity. This is a very valuable sign to help in making a diagnosis. If we have all the other symptoms of pyosalpinx with a history to confirm them, where we can feel the enlarged tube before a discharge of pus from the uterus, and immediately after the discharge has occurred we find that the tube has collapsed, then we have proof

positive of the existence of pyosalpinx. If the previous history
of the case be carefully learned and given due weight and consideration, the author believes the diagnosis is not so difficult as
usually thought. The uterus is more or less fixed and misplaced.
In the majority of cases seen by him there has been pain during
defecation—particularly where the tumor occupied the retro-
uterine space. Most cases gave a history of dyspareunia. If
pain has long been a prominent symptom and it is evident the
tube contains pus, the case must be looked upon as serious and
demanding prompt relief. Delays are dangerous, as the bursting of the tube may cause fatal peritonitis, and escape should
be afforded the offending pus by removal of the tube.

Ruptured Pyosalpinx.—At a meeting of the New York
State Medical Association Dr. C. S. Wood of New York related an interesting case. The case well illustrated the difficulties
sometimes encountered in diagnosis. The patient was an unmarried woman, aged 28, who had been in good health, except
at times pains were present in the lower part of the abdomen.
In May last Dr. Wood was called, and found her suffering from
abdominal pain, slight fever, and gastric disturbance. A cathartic
was administered, which acted the following day. The pain became greater in the pelvic region, especially in the region of the
cæcum, where was present indistinct hardness. The tumor in
this region increased in size, and Dr. Wood became convinced
the case was one of perityphlitic abscess. She was getting along
well until after some days she was awakened in the night by
" sickness of the stomach," had a severe chill, and partial collapse. The induration in the iliac region was found to be softer
and less prominent. Projective vomiting of watery fluid took
place when she was turned on her side for examination. The
temperature was 103.5F., pulse 140. Being satisfied of rupture
of a perityphlitic abscess, Dr. Wylie was called in consultation,
laparatomy was performed, and they were surprised to find no
evidence of inflammation or tumor in the immediate region of the
cæcum ; instead, there was an effusion of lymph over a large
surface, matting together of pelvic viscera, and rupture of a
pyosalpinx on the right side, which had been mistaken for a peri-

typhlitic abscess. The sac and ovary were removed. The ovary on the left side being cystic, it was also removed. The patient recovered within four weeks. He afterwards learned that she had, five years previously, brought on an abortion, which might account for the attacks of pelvic pain.

Ligatures and Sutures : what material shall be used.—Dr. Cushing of San Francisco read a paper before the American Association of Obstetrics and Gynæcology, Sept. 1889, on ligatures and sutures. Dr. Cushing seems favorably impressed with the use of catgut for tying the pedicles in ovariotomy and oöphorectomy. The reviewer has never used this material for such a purpose and never will. It must be unreliable from the difficulty of its being made sufficiently tight, and from the fact that the knot will open when moistened. The necessity for absolute security in the matter of pedicles is of too great importance to play with catgut. The material is rapidly disappearing from surgery altogether, as it cannot be made aseptic—boiling being inadmissable in its case,—and from the fact that we do not want any better material than properly prepared silk or silkworm gut. We need have no fear of the pedicle becoming infected if we take proper precautions in the preparation of the material. The method the reviewer adopts is as follows : First wash in warm running water with soap, then place in sulphuric ether for two days, then boil for three hours in filtered water ; the silk is then carefully wound on glass bobbins according to size and put away wrapped in towelling carefully made aseptic previously. When required for use it is again boiled just before the operation and carried directly from the gas-jet into the operating room and used from the vessel. The silkworm gut is prepared in the same way. It is the best ligature in cervix and perineum operations and for closing the abdomen after section. When a patient requires to return to her home in two or three weeks, it is advisable to use catgut in the cervix and silkworm gut in the perineum when the double operation is done at the same sitting. But if time is of no object to her, the silkworm gut can be removed from the cervix months after the removal of the perineal. And it has this advantage, that when the husband knows there are more stitches there which have yet to be removed, he will not be likely to interfere with the perineum until it has become strong and lost its sensitiveness. The employment of shot to fasten the silkworm gut is very objectionable. The method unnecessarily prolongs the operation and the shot always cut into the tissues and interfere materially with union. The plain, rapidly-tied double knot is by far the best, and if the ends of the gut are not cut too short they give no trouble. Dr. Cushing speaks of fistulæ being caused by silk ligatures and the drainage tube. Suppuration at the pedicle and a fistulous tract being established is more likely to be due to unclean ligatures and the employment of too large a tube ; also omitting to thoroughly wash out the peritoneal cavity with warm water in such cases where pus or large quantity of blood escaped ; also a surgically unclean and careless nurse may infect the tube-fluid and give rise to trouble. Homan's smallest sized tube is large enough for the majority of cases. It fits in easily between the sutures, and a few hours after its removal the wound is closed.

Physical and Mental Changes after Removal of Ovaries or Uterus.—Dr. Glævecke of Kiel has lately published a paper in the *Archiv fur Gynækologie* on this subject. According to this author the changes usually met with were those observed at the menopause (*Berlin Cor. Medical Press*). Menstruation permanently ceased immediately or shortly after the operation of removal in 88 per cent. of the cases. In the remainder it was less frequent and more scanty. Practically, no vicarious menstruation was observed. Menstrual molimina were observed in 30 per cent. In the time between the periods the familiar characteristic disturbances were observed—hot flushes, perspiration and faintness. He looks upon them as disturbances of the vasomotor system, in consequence of the cessation of the ovarian function ; an observation, by the bye, that does not throw much light on the subject. He does not remark the very long continuance of this most uncomfortable condition in many of the cases—four and five years. In four cases out of a total of forty-three, palpitation and headache came on : in one, nausea coming on several times a day ; in another, vomiting ; in one, diarrhœa ;

in one, acne of the face lasting over a year, and in two, increasing weakness of intellect. Atrophy of the internal genitals was a consequence of the operation. In twenty-three cases in which the operation was performed for myoma uteri, distinct shrinking took place in the tumors in 90 per cent. In 42 per cent. of the cases a distinct increase in weight, due to deposit of fat, was observed.

Dr. Lusk of New York reports in the *New York Medical Journal*, Oct. 19th, 1889, two very interesting cases of *Ruptured Tubal Pregnancy*, in which he performed laparotomy. One recovered, and one died on the eighth day of Bright's disease. The first case was 19 years of age ; had passed two periods, then a metrostaxis. Next day was seized with cramp, faintness, nausea and vomiting. Similar attacks occurred daily during the following ten days. On the tenth day the pains became very severe, the patient suddenly became exsanguinated, and syncope ensued, lasting about twenty ₊minutes. She now became chilly, nausea and vomiting constant, pulse 140, and abdominal pains ceased. She was removed to hospital, but allowed twenty-four hours to obtain reaction before operation. When the abdomen was opened two quarts of blood-clot were turned out. The left tube opening into a sac, was brought to the surface, ligatured and removed, and the pedicle dropped. The right tube and ovary being healthy, were left untouched. Abdominal cavity irrigated with Thiersch's solution, drainage tube, and closed. The patient left hospital in the fourth week quite well.

The second case was 36 years of age ; had not menstruated for six weeks, and without warning was seized with a violent attack of pain, followed by blanching of the surface and syncope, from which she did not recover for some hours. In this case there were no antecedent symptoms—*i.e.*, no colic, no sanguinolent discharge, nor expulsion of decidua. The day following the attack she was removed to hospital, and laparotomy performed that afternoon. The cavity was found filled with clots, and the tube found ruptured on its posterior surface above the folds broad ligament. The rupture was caused by a four weeks ovum, and the villi were beautifully apparent through the rent. The patient had persistent albuminuria up to the operation, and died of uræmia on the eighth day.

These two cases illustrate the ordinary history of tubal pregnancy. In both, without antecedent symptoms, at an early period of gestation rupture with hemorrhage takes place ; in the one instance the blood primarily making its way between the folds of the broad ligament, in the other pouring suddenly, without check, directly into the peritoneal cavity. They are simply additions to the long list already furnished by Mr. Lawson Tait upon which he has based his scheme of ectopic gestations. In Mr. Tait's belief, all cases of extra-uterine pregnancy are *ab initio* of tubal origin. When the ovum develops in the free part of the tube, rupture, he holds, occurs at or before the fourteenth week. If rupture occurs at once into the abdominal cavity, death ensues from hemorrhage, or, later, from suppuration of the sac and peritonitis ; if rupture takes place in the lower portion of the tube between the folds of the broad ligament, the ovum may develop to full term ; may die and be absorbed as an extra-peritoneal hæmatocele ; may suppurate and be discharged at or near the navel, or through the bladder, the vagina, or intestinal tract ; may remain quiescent as a lithopædion ; or may become an abdominal pregnancy by secondary rupture. In the tubo uterine form death occurs from intra-peritoneal rupture before the fifth month. Mr. Tait denies the possibility of a primary abdominal pregnancy. The ovarian form he regards as possible but not proved. There is no question as to the utility of Mr. Tait's scheme. It is based upon his exceptional personal experience and has received substantial support from the observations of others. It has stimulated active inquiry, and has given proper direction to pathological study ; but the subject of ectopic pregnancy is still too new to make it possible for any scheme to be regarded as a finality.

Rupture of the Uterus ; Supra-Vaginal Amputation ; Recovery.—Dr. Henry C. Coe of New York reports a remarkable case of this desperate accident followed by laparotomy and recovery. (*New York Medical Record*, Nov. 2, 1889.) The patient was 23 years of age, and lived in a dirty, small tenement house. She had been under an anæsthetic for three hours, and over two hours had elapsed since the rupture had taken place. The head of the child occupied the left iliac fossa, and the body of the uterus, in tetanic contraction, lay over to the right side of the abdomen. The patient was in a state of collapse, with rapid, feeble pulse. Prolonged attempts with the forceps had been tried, and eventually version, to extract the child. Dr. Coe performed laparotomy at once. After turning out a quantity of blood-clots he found a rent extending upward from the cervix through the left broad ligament and the lower uterine segment. The head of the child lay in the left iliac fossa, outside of the uterus, being grasped by the edges of the tear. The uterus was turned out of the cavity, the cervix constricted by a piece of rubber tubing from a fountain syringe, and the child extracted through the rent. The uterus, ovaries and tubes were excised and the bleeding vessels secured. The torn peritoneum was sewn with continuous catgut suture, the cavity washed out with warm water, and the stump secured in the wound with knitting needles. No drainage-tube was used. From the second day after the operation free catharsis was maintained and the ice-bag to avert peritonitis. On the fourth day Dr. Coe replaced the rubber tubing by the *serre-nœud*, and removed the entire mass at the end of a week, packing the cavity with iodoform gauze. The patient during her convalescence evidently became septicæmic, judging from the subsequent history of the case, and the reviewer thinks that this condition might probably have been avoided had Dr. Coe employed drainage. The suppurating hæmatocele in the left broad ligament which Dr. Coe speaks of obtained an outlet through the rent which fortunately existed in the cervix at that side, or by some other route. And we would advise Dr. Coe in future cases to, above all things, secure good drainage before closing up the abdomen. In cases of this nature drainage is of vital importance on account of the severe injury to tissue which must be followed by extensive necrotic areas. The carrying out of details of the operation, the distressing disadvantages under which it was performed, the fertility of thought and decisive action displayed under such circumstances by Dr. Coe reflects much credit upon that gentleman, and he well deserved the successful result of his endeavors.

This operation has now been performed fourteen times, with nine deaths and five recoveries. It is known as Prevôt's operation, being first performed by Prevôt of Moscow.

Iodoform Gauze in Post-partum Hemorrhage.—Dr. O. Piering, assistant in Prof. Schauta's obstetric clinic in Prague, has published his experience in the employment of Dührssen's plan of plugging the uterus with iodoform gauze for post-partum hemorrhage due to an atonic condition of the organ. Dührssen recommends that, when post-partum hemorrhage comes on, the bladder should be emptied and forcible friction, intra-uterine irrigation with hot or cold water, and hypodermatics of ergotin employed: that if the hemorrhage still continues, the cavity of the uterus should be filled with iodoform gauze, the irritation produced by this setting up active and permanent contraction. The method has, according to Dührssen, the advantages of great certainty, complete harmlessness and facility in its performance. Olshausen, Veit and Fehling, however, say that the contraction [illegible] is not always permanent, and that the method is not so free from danger as Dührssen believes. In consequence of these conflicting views, Dr. Piering resolved to give the method a trial, and he has recently published several cases in which it was employed with complete success. In no case was harm done by it. He advises that resort to the plug should not be too long delayed, and considers it an important feature of iodoform gauze in post-partum hemorrhage.—*Lancet*, Nov. 4, [illegible].

[illegible] against the method of treatment [illegible] after-consequences might [illegible] danger from the hemorrhage.

[illegible] *[illegible] Uterine Hemorrhage.*—[illegible]

though so terribly common in the human female, was scarcely known in other mammals, and was hardly known to veterinary surgeons. This induced them to commence the investigation by a study of the cervix uteri in monkeys in order to ascertain if any anatomical conditions existed favoring the development of cancer in the human female. A few years ago one of them exhibited before the Society a series of specimens, which demonstrated that monkeys (macaques and baboons) which were living in confinement in this country were liable to uterine flexions. Subsequently evidence was given before the Gynæcological Society that macàques and baboons menstruated after the same fashion as human females. The inquiry was followed up, and it was found that the menstrual period in these monkeys was very variable. In some it lasted a longer time than in others, whilst now and then a monkey appeared in an almost chronic state of menstruation. In many the menstrual period was followed by profuse leucorrhœa. Normally, the discharge of blood would last from one to two days, but the redness of the less hairy parts persisted as long as a week. The average interval between each menstrual period was difficult to fix with accuracy, as it varied from a month to six weeks, or even longer. It was a safe inference when a monkey menstruated two, three, or even four times a month, each attack lasting three or more days, followed by leucorrhœa, that it was a case of metrorrhagia. During the past summer a macaque was particularly watched. The metrorrhagia and leucorrhœa became so profuse as to render it unfit for exhibition, and, being of small money value, the monkey was killed. The uterus was removed before the parts had lost their tissue life. The uterus was acutely retroflexed, the cervix greatly enlarged, the os patulous, and a florid-looking mass projected from it, identical in appearance with what it was the fashion to call in gynæcology an erosion. After hardening the parts, sections were prepared for the microscope in such a way as to include the parts about the os externum, the cervical canal, and portio vaginalis. Under a low power the mass protruding from the os, as well as a polypoid mass some distance up the canal, resembled a cervical adenoma, and was in structure identical with the glandular tissue held to be characteristic of erosions in women, the acini being apparently lined by columnar epithelium.   Many of the most typical acini were filled with a singular apparently homogeneous material.   Under higher powers and with careful illumination tne supposed columnar cells were seen to be club-shaped, and, in favorable sections, the supposed glandular crypts turned out to be rosettes fringed with clubs characteristic of actinomyces. The clubs varied somewhat in shape ; many of them fringed the rosettes with the greatest regularity.   In other places they appeared in " banana-like bunches," especially when stained with fuchsin.   The clubs which surrounded the rosettes stained with difficulty.   In some places a cluster of clubs had been cut transversely ; in such, a characteristic mosaic was produced.   They could not detect the filaments, but this was owing to their want of skill in staining methods ; but numbers of granular bodies presented themselves in various parts of the section.   Thus far the microscopic characters were consonant with actinomycosis.   On critically examining the centre of the rosettes some rounded bodies were seen, mostly in association with clumps of epithelioid-looking cells.   These, when examined, turned out to be cysticerci with heads and necks retracted.   Whether their presence in the midst of the rosettes was accidental or otherwise would require further elucidation.   As far as they had examined the sections these cysticerci appeared to stand in some causative relation to the rosettes.   Although they wished at first to limit this preliminary statement to facts connected with monkeys, they could not refrain from observing that they had detected similar appearances in erosions from the human cervix uteri, and in a case of cancer of the cervix.   They mentioned that Dr. John Williams, in his *Lectures on Cancer of the Uterus*, plate xiv, fig. 1, had depicted as appearing, under a high power, cancer cells ; but they thought that these columnar cells were identical with their clubs, and that the peculiar clump of cells in his drawing was identical with that seen in their monkeys in association with the cysticerci.   Again, in Mr. Harrison Cripps's beautiful drawings, which illustrated his paper on " Adenoid Cancer of t′   xii of their *Transactions*, they found -

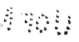

of great beauty. Many of these exquisite drawings, representing the microscopic character of rectal cancer, represented equally the lesions found in monkeys and the erosions of women. They thought it right to mention these things to show how wide a field was opened up in regard to cancer of the uterus and alimentary canal, and hoped thus to incite the Society to help in the investigation by appointing a committee to carry it out.—*B. M. Jour.*

The Abuse of Uterine Treatment through Mistaken Diagnosis, by Wm. Goodell, M.D., is the title of a lengthy paper appearing in the *Medical News* of Dec. 7th, 1889. All hail to the Gladstone of medical politics! ! ! One patriarch *when in power* puts all the landlord-killing rascals of Ireland in jail on bread and water. When out of power he pats them on the head, saying, " My poor fellows, I was altogether wrong; take some bon-bons now and I'll cry out against your being punished any more." This is bad enough in politics, but we have now arisen a veritable Gladstone in medicine. During his active lifetime he incised, split and sewed up more cervices than any man living. He taught us how and under what circumstances to do such operations. Quoted hundreds of cases without mortality (116 cases of trachelorrhaphy without a death). Set us all agoing with scissors, tenaculum and divulsor, like Henry Bennet and the speculum—caustic romance. When, lo ! and behold, presto——! ! Father Time appears upon the scene. Give me, sir, that scissors, tenaculum and divulsor, they do not become you now. Tell the poor cervix you have been wrong all this time—(do not be particular as regards time, say a quarter of a century)—and say that you will henceforth cry out against its being punished any more. " Oh my prophetic soul !'' What a theme for Hamlet to soliloquize upon. To attempt to discuss in detail Dr. Goodell's paper in this criticism is out of the question. We do not require to look at the title page to recognize the author. It is the same theme which has occupied his attention so much of late years. Everything that female flesh is heir to comes from over-education or nerve exhaustion, ... er his private hospital to be cured. Dr. ... us how these nerve exhaustion patients,

38

and what percentage of those who come under his care, are cured. We have heard of some who returned to their homes in the same condition as when they entered the doctor's sanitarium plus the disappointment. Probably these were a part of the seven Dr. Goodell speaks of as being under treatment in his private hospital.

Dr. Goodell's paper will undoubtedly command a wide acceptance. It will relieve the physician's mind. He can now cure his nerve-exhausted lady patients without any trouble, and his young ladies with pale faces, by taking them from school. We must remark however here, that Dr. Goodell stands alone when associated in opinion with such men as Thomas, Chadwick, Mitchell, Starr, and Putnam upon the subject of the influence of higher education upon the sexual system and general nutrition of females. All of these authorities are, without exception, agreed that advanced education improves the health of young females working at colleges, and the reasoning upon which they base their opinion is certainly more logical and more in accordance with our experience.*

Dr. Goodell is a most elegant writer and an easy and fluent speaker. He has done exceptionally good service in the ranks of his specialty. He has built up a noble edifice of scientific gynæcology, and all we ask of him now is, that, since it has been decreed that he build no more, he will not ignobly attempt to pull the whole structure down in anger, lest some one else to come, should occupy and continue to add to it. *Pax vobiscum*.

The Physiological Resistance of the Peritoneum to Infection. —In the past year hardly a more interesting series of experiments has been made in the interest of surgical pathology than those of Rinne (*Archiv für klinische Chirurgie*). Practically and clinically it has been demonstrated that the peritoneal cavity under certain unknown circumstances has the power of taking care of a vast amount of filth. It remained for Rinne to harmonize observed clinical facts with *à priori* deductions. He found that large quantities of septic material and pure cultures of pyogenic bacteria were absorbed, although injected daily into

* Medical News, Dec. 14, 1889.

the peritoneal cavity of animals, provided that the peritoneal surfaces were uninjured. The injections produced only mild symptoms in direct proportion to the quantity of septic material used,
and in no case was there more than a moderate rise of' temperature. The results were very different when there were coincident defects in the peritoneum, exposing the subperitoneal connective tissue to infection. Then there invariably appeared
progressive suppurative peritonitis going out from the infected
connective tissue, which usually terminated fatally. The practical import of these experiments can hardly be overestimated.
They explain why the escape of pus into the peritoneal cavity
from the rupture of a pyosalpinx is not necessarily fatal if the
tube is promptly extirpated and the wound and stump properly
treated. They point out that the incision is the point of greatest
danger in all abdominal operations, and they would indicate that
too much care cannot be taken in coaptating the peritoneal edges
of the wound. They explain why the removal of abdominal
tumors is so much more dangerous after adhesions have taken
place, because the resulting denuded places offer less resistance
to the invasion of septic bacteria. They explain the success of
those operators who disregard the dictations of scientific bacteriology, and also the recovery of patients after abdominal section
by horned animals. They teach us to consider cautiously the
evidence presented by the statistics of operators, and await the
demonstration of more exact methods as to the import of their
results. They warn us that clinical evidence is inadequate to
overthrow the deductions of experimental physiology and pathology, and that our time is provided with methods of precision
which are yet imperfectly improved. They beckon the ambitious
into fields of activity and thought far less crowded, though more
promising than the operating room and the dead-house. The
resisting and absorptive power of the peritoneum is beyond that
of any other serous cavity. This is as we should expect. The
peritoneal surfaces are only a line distant from the most filthy
and prolific culture-medium about the body. It is connected
with this seething and turbulent mass by the most active absorbent lymph-channels. Doubtless it is frequently invaded by

septic bacteria from the intestinal contents. From these frequent invasions an immunity has been developed which has been perpetuated and transmitted by the working of the ordinarily recognized laws of evolution. Again, we are taught to consider the causes which determine the localization of infection as more important than the quantity and quality of infective material. Doubtless traumatism is one of the most important of these causes, but we must not forget that the depression of the general temperature of the body, the interference with nutrition, and general *malaise*, frequently observed after operations, are factors which may speak for the life or death of our patient. Not only should the abdominal section be made with the greatest attention to cleanliness, but the peritoneal edges must be accurately coaptated, the operation must be done with the greatest celerity and delicacy, and depressing influences of starvation, over-medication, and deprivations of every kind must be avoided if we would eliminate all those causes which determine the localization of that infection, which is still the greatest danger the operator has to meet.

Surgical Operations for the Repair of Ruptured Perineums, by A. B. Carpenter, M.D., Cleveland, O.—The above is the title of a paper appearing in the *N. Y. Medical Record* of Nov. 16, 1889. Dr. Carpenter says he is an advocate of the old denudation methods, and protests against Dr. Barnes of London for declaring in favor of Tait's flap-splitting operations. Dr. Carpenter argues that if Dr. Barnes failed to obtain good results from the denudation plan of operating it must have been the fault of the operator and not the method. This line of argument is simply absurd; every surgeon knows about the failure, difficulty and danger to which the denudation method is liable. The reviewer has seen too many cases go the round of the New York hospitals in order to obtain a successful closure of a ruptured perineum, and be abandoned in the end as incurable. He has seen such men as Thomas, Emmet and others declare that they did not hope for success in such and such a case, as they had operated several times before, and each attempt became more difficult and less hopeful. The late Dr. Jas. B. Hunter assured the reviewer, upon the occasion of a visit to him, that two (or three) cases died in the New York State Woman's Hospital within a few weeks, and that the autopsy showed extensive purulent infiltration of the connective tissue of the pelvis. Many other American surgeons have lost cases after the denudation operation, and it was not at all uncommon for the Germans also to meet with disaster. It may be asked, Why should the denudation method be so uncertain and dangerous? The principal reasons are : The uncertainty of freshening and the frequency in which "islands" are left containing pus in their folds; the length of time taken for the performance of the operation, which means prolonged exposure of the wound; and the utter impossibility of closing the wound so as to completely exclude the discharges coming from above and thereby infecting it. Let us on all of these points compare the flap-splitting method, and it will not require much intelligence to see the great advantage of this latter operation. Dr. Carpenter speaks of having an assistant on each side of him with retractors, another to thread the needle, another to administer the anæsthetic, supplemented by a nurse. This army is certainly a formidable array to carry out so simple a procedure.

Dr. Carpenter allows his suture (silk) to remain *in situ* twelve to eighteen days. Why not a year? They cannot possibly perform any fixation function after the sixth or eighth day, and if left longer will only cause suppuration and cutting, followed by scar tissue—the very condition we wish to avoid. Let us now look at Tait's flap-splitting method. There cannot possibly be left any "islands" to infect the wound. The freshening of the tissue can be carried just as high as in any of the denudation methods. No assistant is required but the anæsthetiser and nurse. Time, from drawing of blood until patient is comfortably placed in bed again about two minutes and a half, at outside, three minutes. Here we have *comparatively* no exposure of wound. It is impossible for discharges from above to enter the wound and infect it. There is no pain from the sutures, and the results have been better in the experience of men who have tried all methods. We have not heard of a single case of *accident* resulting from the flap-splitting method, and its great advantages, safety and superiority over all other methods will be maintained by all impartial observers. We are afraid Dr. Carpenter has been advancing somewhat after the fashion of the crab, when we consider that he still remains partial to silk ligatures, vaginal injections and denudation methods in perineal operations.

RETROSPECT ON THE PROPHYLAXIS OF TUBERCULOSIS.

By WYATT JOHNSTON, M.D.,
Demonstrator of Pathology, McGill University.

During the last two or three years the question of preventing tuberculosis has received much attention from various government and local sanitary boards throughout the world. For the most part the numerous committees which have reported on the subject seem to regard the flesh and milk of tuberculous animals as a very common cause of tuberculosis in man, and the measures they advise chiefly refer to eliminating this source of danger. The literature of the subject has become so extensive as to prevent its being given here in any detail : but the action taken in regard to preventive measures is of great practical interest. A special committee of the Dominion Parliament appointed in 1888 to examine the question have published a small blue-book bearing the title of April 17th, 1889. Report of the Sub-committee of the Senate of Canada on its Communicability to Man. (Ottawa, Government Printing Bureau, 1889.)

The committee sent circulars addressed to physicians, veterinary surgeons and dairymen, using printed forms of questions to obtain information as to the actual experience as to the frequency of tuberculosis among men and animals, and as to the possession of personal knowledge of any cases of the disease having been communicated from animals to human beings. Answers were received from 210 physicians, 42 veterinary surgeons and numerous others, most of which were affirmative. Numerous answers to these questions with actual cases being given, and this showed that there was in the minds of the profession at large little doubt as to cases of infection caused by defective information as to its contagious nature. They think it desirable that information on this head should be widely circulated, and hope that during the present session such special legislation as is expedient may be enacted. They recommend that any imported cattle showing signs of tuberculosis be refused admission to the country, and advocate the establishment of a system of observing and recording vital statistics throughout the Dominion. Summaries of reports on the same subject by the Privy Council of Great Britain, a special committee of the Legislature of the State of Maine, and by the Hatch Experimental Station of Massachusetts are appended.

With regard to the prevention of tuberculosis in cattle, the measures now being carried out in France (on the recommendation of the Congress on Tuberculosis of 1888), Germany, Great Britain, etc., viz., the confiscation of meat of tuberculous animals, the sanitary supervision of dairies, and the prevention of breeding from tuberculous stock, will no doubt diminish the prevalence of tuberculosis among the domesticated animals very considerably in the course of the next few years.

With regard to the prevention of tuberculosis in man, however, the case is more complicated, the simple and effective measures of segregation, slaughtering, etc., not being admissable.

There seems to be a general impression that the lessening of tuberculosis among animals, and the regulations dealing with the food and milk of animals affected with tuberculosis even in a slight degree, will be followed by a corresponding reduction in human tuberculosis. The probability of human tuberculosis being derived chiefly through infection from tuberculous meat and milk seems to be very largely accepted. The fact that animals can be experimentally infected in this manner has been proved over and over again. The conditions, however, do not appear to be similar to those attending human tuberculosis. The latency of the disease in man, its prevalency at a period of life when milk is not extensively used as a food, is not in accordance with the theory of infection by food.

Dr. George Cornet of Berlin published, in November 1888 (*Zeitschrift für Hygiene*, Bd. 5), an extensive series of experiments covering two years, and dealing with the distribution of the tubercle bacillus outside the body. The methods he adopted consisted of intra-peritoneal inoculations in guinea pigs.

Dr. Cornet investigated two sets of localities. First, those which were presumably constantly contaminated by the virus, viz., the dwelling-houses of phthisical persons, the phthisical wards of general hospitals, insane asylums, and a room in which inhalation experiments in tuberculosis were being constantly made upon animals. Secondly, the localities which were presumably only occasionally exposed to contamination by the presence of tuberculous persons, such as prisons, polyclinics and public buildings, streets, etc.

The air of these localities was first investigated. A number of experiments in which large volumes of air were filtered through sand, and an emulsion made from this was tested with regard to its infectiousness, gave entirely negative results, even in the localities most likely to contain contaminated air, e.g., in phthisical wards, which had just been swept and the bed linen shaken. It was inferred that the danger of infection in this manner was not very great. The dust collected from these localities similarly tested gave very positive and uniform results. Of a total of 39 animals tested by 147 samples of dust, 59 animals became tuberculous (of 196 which died of septicæmia we may infer that a like proportion would have become tuberculous had they lived).

The experiments were so carefully performed as to preclude the possibility of any cases of spontaneous tuberculosis being included among the positive results. These positive results were all obtained with the dust from the phthisical wards, insane asylums, and the houses of private patients suffering from tuberculosis. In the prisons, though the dust was taken from the immediate neighborhood of prisoners suffering from tuberculosis, the results were negative.

Dr. Cornet was led to regard the sputum as the direct source since recent investigators have failed to find bacteria of any kind in expired air. A special inquiry as to the habits of the private patient with regard to the disposal of sputum showed that all the positive results of inoculations were obtained where the patient expectorated either in a handkerchief or upon the floor. In the cases where these practices were excluded, the dust in no case produced tuberculosis in the animals.

Experiments in disinfecting sputum showed this to be extremely difficult, and in experiments with instruments employed in laryngeal examinations the particles of mucus adhering to the mirror still remained infectious, even after being left in 2 per 1000 sublimate solution or 5 per cent. carbolic acid. The bed linen was also proved highly infectious. A number of bed feathers infected with sputum were marked, mixed with other feathers, and sent to factories where bed feathers were supposed to be disinfected and cleaned. These feathers, after the disinfection had been performed, were found to be capable of infecting guineapigs.

Dr. Cornet concludes by recommending a system of prophylaxis based on his observations. He contends that the infection is to be dreaded from the sputum, as well as from the consumption of tuberculous meat and milk. He regards the sputum of living patients, and the linen, etc., of those just dead, as the chief source of contamination. While indoors, the patient shall, under no circumstances, expectorate anywhere except in a proper spittoon capable of being readily cleansed, and preferably provided with a cover. The handkerchief should not be used for receiving the sputum, except in case of a sudden attack of coughing where it is unavoidable. In all cases the handkerchief or any other linen possibly contaminated should be disinfected by boiling, and washed apart from that of any of the other members of the family. The table utensils used by patients should be washed with hot water before being employed by others.

The bed linen in fatal cases should be disinfected as thoroughly as in cases of smallpox. The patient should be instructed not to put to his mouth anything such as pipes, toys, etc., likely to be put into the mouths of others. The operation of kissing (when necessary) is to be performed antiseptically, so to speak, and upon some portion of the physiognomy (forehead or cheek) where infection is not likely.

Considering the difficulty attending the disinfection of sputum, he does not consider it practicable to insist on its disinfection, but prefers to insist on scrupulous regularity in its removal, and in the frequent emptying of the spittoons. In fact, the essential element of his prophylaxis might be summed up in the four words occasionally seen across the line—

PLEASE USE THE SPITTOONS !

The possibilities of avoiding infection by care in disposing of the infecting material may be judged from the fact that the dust beside the bench where Dr. Cornet had been working continuously for two years with tuberculous material was found incapable of producing tuberculosis.

Dr. Cornet has, at the request of the Prussian Government, drawn up a report of the prophylactic measures he considers necessary. This report has been favorably received, and the Government intend to test, as far as possible, the efficacy of these simple measures of personal hygiene, especially in garrisons, prisons, insane asylums, and other cases where the effects can be carefully studied and recorded by statistics.

At the request of the Bavarian Government, Prof. Bollinger of Munich has reported to the Bavarian Sanitary Council as to the advisability of adopting sanitary measures founded upon the results of Cornet's investigations. Prof. Bollinger, while not disputing the importance of the results, considers that the view taken of the hereditary and more especially the acquired disposition to tuberculosis is too one-sided. He recommends the carrying out of an investigation designed to settle the question as to whether the disposition of the patient or the mere presence of the contagion is the point of greater importance in keeping up tuberculosis. The fact that the enormous mortality from tuberculosis prevailing in German prisons, averaging 18 to 60 per cent., and ranging in some cases as high as 95 per cent. of the total annual mortality, he considers due to the bad hygienic arrangement of these institutions, producing such a condition of mind and body in the prisoners as tends to develop latent tuberculosis, or to render them susceptible to infection in forms which they could withstand in good health. On his recommendation the Bavarian Government are going to try the experiment of repeatedly cleansing and disinfecting the prisons, removing every case of tuberculosis, proved or suspected, at once. If, under these circumstances, the hygienic condition in the prison remains otherwise unimproved, the mortality from tuberculosis should greatly decrease or disappear, he would consider the predominating influence of actual contagion over predisposition to be established.

Dr. Bollinger's experiments, published within the last two years by himself and his pupils (*Muenchener Med. Wochenschrift*, No. 29, 1888, and Nos. 34, 40 and 43, 1889), have shown that the milk of tuberculous cows is capable of producing tuberculosis by intra-peritoneal injection in 50 per cent. of the cases. The dilution of this milk with 40 parts of milk of healthy animals rendered it harmless. Samples of milk purchased on the market were not found to produce infection. The mixed milk of dairies is therefore less likely to infect children than the milk of single animals. Inoculations made with the juice of raw meat in animals with moderate degrees of tuberculosis gave negative results. Inoculations from the juice obtained from the psoas muscles in cases of advanced phthisis in human subjects proved successful in 15 out of 18 experiments made in 9 cases.

The discrepancy between the results in these last two series of cases is probably due to the fact that the tuberculosis was less advanced in the cases of the cattle. It is also probable that the power of the tissues to destroy the tuberculous virus becomes greatly diminished during the last stages of exhausting diseases. A comparison with the flesh of patients dying from some extraneous cause in comparatively early stages of phthisis would be interesting.

Reviews and Notices of Books.

Hunterian Lectures on the Morbid Anatomy, Pathology, and Treatment of Hernia. By CHARLES B. LOCKWOOD, F.R.C.S. Thirty-six illustrations. London: H. K. Lewis.

In these lectures Mr. Lockwood gives the result of investigations made to ascertain the part the peritoneum and suspensory apparatus bears in the pathology of hernia. It is well known that there are two schools of pathologists in regard to hernia, one school believing that the fault lies in the abdominal walls and the other that it is in the attaching membranes of the intestines, the abdominal walls playing a secondary part. That the hernia is a disease, not an accident—a pathological condition, not a merely mechanical lesion; that, in fact, the fault is in the peritoneum. Mr. Lockwood has shown that although it is hard to estimate the share which the length of the mesentery has in the causation of hernia, it may, at any rate, be conceded that those in whom the mesentery is long are more predisposed to hernia than those in whom it is short. Even this latter statement, however, is not always correct, as cases are related of acquired herniæ with short mesenteries. Again, others with very long mesenteries never have hernia.

Prolapse of the mesentery, according to Mr. Lockwood, is a predisposing cause of hernia, not an effect. It would be idle, in the small space that could be afforded us here, to discuss this subject, but we can only say that the careful and painstaking manner in which these lectures have been prepared is deserving of the greatest praise. We recommend every surgeon interested in hernia to carefully peruse this work; he will not only be entertained, but much instructed. Appended is a table giving details of the measurement of 100 subjects without hernial sacs or herniæ. In this table the height and length of the mesenteries are given, and also the amount of downward excision of the intestines. We should have liked to have seen a summing up of results at the end, as it is difficult, without reading carefully the whole work, to find out what exactly were the results obtained by the author. An index would much aid the enquirer in search of information on particular points.

The National Medical Dictionary. Including English, French, German, Italian and Latin Technical Terms used in Medicine and the Collateral Sciences, and a Series of Tables of Useful Data. By JOHN S. BILLINGS, A.M., M.D., LL.D., Edin. and Harv., D.C.L., Oxon. With the collaboration of W. O. Atwater, M.D., Frank Baker, M.D., S. M. Burnett, M.D., W. T. Councilman, M.D., James M. Flint, M.D., J. A. Kidder, M.D., William Lee, M.D., R. Lorini, M.D., Washington Matthews, M.D., C. S. Minot, M.D., and H. C. Yarrow, M.D. In two volumes. Vol. I., A to J. Vol. II., K to Z. Philadelphia : Lea Brothers & Co. 1890.

This truly great work gives a short and clear definition of every medical term in current use in English, French, German and Italian medical literature, together with the Latin medical terminology of all these languages. To give a general idea of the importance and magnitude of this work, it is only necessary to mention that the total number of words and phrases defined is upwards of 84,000, of which 25,496 are Latin, 9,158 French, 16,708 German, and 6,514 Italian. This does not include French, German and Italian synonyms given only in connection with English or Latin primers. In addition to the definition of the medical terms, we have a series of tables, including a table of doses, of poisons and their antidotes, of the inch and metre system of numbering spectacles, of thermometric scales, size of the fœtus at different stages, size and weight of the different organs, and tables showing the metritine value of food and materials.

No medical man interested in the progress of his profession can afford to be without this valuable aid. The distinguished editor in chief deserves well of his professional brethren for having in his multiplicity of duties taken the time and trouble in the preparation of a work which has no equal in the English any other language.

The publishers have produced a work after their best style, and we hope their enterprise will be as successful as it deserves to be.

Society Proceedings.

MEDICO-CHIRURGICAL SOCIETY OF MONTREAL.

Stated Meeting, Nov. 29th, 1889.

G. E. ARMSTRONG, M.D., PRESIDENT, IN THE CHAIR.

Missed Abortion.—DR. G. T. ROSS read a paper on this subject, a full report of which appeared in the January number of this JOURNAL.

Discussion.—DR. TRENHOLME said that missed abortion was very liable to occur in patients of a weak constitution, and this also explains the retention of the fœtus in utero, there being absence of vitality in the membranes, and the uterus requires living structures in contact with it in order to bring about contraction.

DR. ALLOWAY said that unquestionably syphilis and childbearing act as chief factors in the production of missed abortion. He would like to ask Dr. Ross how he explained the rise in temperature twelve days after clearing out the uterus ?

DR. F. W. CAMPBELL remarked that he had frequently had cases where the fœtus was decomposed without the health of the patient suffering in the least. That missed abortion does take place in other than debilitated or syphilitic subjects.

DR. McCONNELL cited a case in which this had occurred, the patient being very robust and had not suffered from syphilis.

DR. ROSS, in reply, said that the rise in temperature was attributable to mismanagement on the part of the nurse. In these cases, if ergot be used, then the os must be widely dilated, otherwise pain and distress are brought about without any beneficial after result. He thought with Duncan that mitral disease had a marked influence upon the life of the fœtus.

DR. JOHNSTON showed for Dr. Springle in this connection an ovum with fœtus and membranes entire. There was cystic and fatty degeneration of the chorion and a marked cicatricial contraction of the umbilical cord. The history gave date of abortion at fourteen weeks, but the fœtus showed a development apparently of only eight weeks, which had evidently been dead some little time. He thought, in most cases of abortion, the expulsion of the ovum did not take place till some time after the death of the fœtus. The cessation of symptoms of pregnancy probably were connected rather with changes in the membranes than in the fœtus itself.

Stated Meeting, December 12th, 1889.

G. E. ARMSTRONG, M.D., PRESIDENT, IN THE CHAIR.

Cystic Myoma of the Uterus.—DR. WM. GARDNER exhibited a specimen of a cystic myoma of the uterus and related the case. The patient was unmarried, aged 41, and began twenty-two years ago to suffer from menorrhagia. This continued to be profuse till about five years ago, when it diminished, and for a few months before operation (on 16th November last) it had almost ceased. The tumor was first noticed ten years ago. Its growth, at first slowly, became much more rapid in the last year. Pain was considerable. The abdomen measured 41 inches and was distended by a large partly fluctuating and partly solid tumor. The patient was extremely anæmic and pallid, with lemon-colored skin. There were no adhesions. Sixteen pounds weight of a yellow transparent fluid were let out by the trocar from a cavity with anterior wall a quarter of an inch thick. This coagulated in a few minutes after exposure to the air. The broad ligaments were tied off to permit the wire of the clamp to be applied low enough over the cervix. Bantock's Welta metal clamp, wire and transfixing pins were used, and the stump of the cervix uteri brought out at the lower angle of the wound. The solid part of the tumor was a multiple myoma. The cavity of the uterus was enlarged. The large cavity whence the fluid was evacuated presented bands crossing from one side to the other. The whole weighed 38 lbs. During the first week there was some high temperature; otherwise recovery had been uneventful, and now (16th Dec.) the patient sits up and is well.

Discussion.—DR. ALLOWAY said the specimen was interesting on account of its extreme rarity. These so-called cysts did not contain a true cyst-wall, but are simply lymphoid spaces. Skeene had applied Kœberle's sœrre nœud without pins ; the pedicle slipped and disappeared without any bad after result, thus demonstrating how the pins can slip and not be followed by any hemorrhage.

DR. SMITH said a case similar to that of Skeene had occurred in his own practice and with a like happy result.

DR. JOHNSTON asked Dr. Gardner how he concluded as to the nature of the tumor ? Multilocular cysts of the uterus are almost unknown. Corneil had seen a sebaceous cyst of the uterus which he considered unique.

DR. GARDNER, in reply, said he had not formed any exact idea as to its being a true cyst; he had not looked upon this as a true cyst, but as dilated lymph spaces. In the after treatment of these cases he cut the constricting wire as early as two days, thus preventing sloughing downwards, and the danger of dropping in of the stump is thus avoided. The dressings were simple, namely, absorbent cotton, the object being to mummify the stump.

Stated Meeting, December 27th, 1889.

G. E. ARMSTRONG, M.D., PRESIDENT, IN THE CHAIR.

Dr. C. O. Brown was elected a member.

Hemorrhage into the Ovaries.—DR. ARMSTRONG exhibited the ovaries of a patient of whom he gave the following history : She had menstruated regularly up to the time of her marriage on May 16th last. On June 14th she was seized with sudden severe abdominal pain and faintness. Menstruation appeared later and continued regularly since that time, but all the time she suffered severe pain on walking, appetite failed, and latterly she had to take to her bed for the greater part of the day. On examination, a partly fluctuating, partly solid mass about the size of an orange was found behind the uterus. Both ovaries were removed through the abdominal incision ; one contained a large hemorrhage into the substance, while a second hemorrhage was found outside, surrounded by a dense capsule ; the other ovary was cystic. No definite traces of chorionic villi were found.

Case of Polyuria with Nervous Symptoms.—DR. STEWART exhibited a man, aged 40, who for the last five years has been troubled with polyuria. For a period of three months during the present year the average quantity of urine passed was upwards of 100 ounces in the twenty-four hours. The patient also presents the following nervous symptoms : There is (1) paresis of the respiratory branches of the left facial nerve ; (2) atrophy of the left half (anterior part) of the tongue ; and (3) paresis of the left half of the palate. No affection of taste or common sensation in the affected parts.

DR. WM. GARDNER asked if there was any known cause for polyuria otherwise than diabetes, and mentioned a case in whom, two weeks after the removal of an ovarian tumor, polyuria to the extent of 150 ounces a day was developed ; no sugar ; appetite was enormous and thirst very great. These symptoms gradually subsided.

DR. HINGSTON found polyuria not infrequent after the removal of ovarian tumors, and regarded it with satisfaction.

DR. STEWART replied that in such cases it was probably due more to mechanical causes than to nervous influences.

Removal of Calculi.—DR. HINGSTON exhibited three calculi from a man 68 years of age. He had suffered from all the symptoms of stone in the bladder and an enlarged prostate, but even after repeated examinations no click was detected. Lithotomy was performed, and even on introducing the finger no stone was felt. Curved forceps were introduced, and by them three smooth, round calculi were removed. Another singular feature of the case was that after the operation not a single drop of urine came from the wound and he could retain his water for many hours. A catheter was used every six hours. The patient made a complete recovery.

A Case of Appendicitis.—DRS. MACDONNELL and SHEPHERD related the case. (*See page* 561.)

Correspondence.

To the Editors of THE MONTREAL MEDICAL JOURNAL.

SIRS,—The spirit of opposition to Provincial Boards, spoken of by Dr. Osler in his letter in your December issue, is not dead; on the contrary it is particularly lively, and though my good friend regrets to see it, yet it is none the less present, and that, too, amongst men whose age is on the near side of the forties. Eighteen months ago, at the annual introductory lecture at McGill College, heretical opinions about Boards, somewhat similar to mine, were expressed, so that in my misguided course I have at least one companion.

Dr. Osler has misunderstood me, probably, because my meaning was not made sufficiently clear. I would not do away with state supervision, but I would do away with the necessity of obtaining a separate license to practice for each province. Canada is one country, and a legally qualified Canadian graduate should be allowed to practice in any part of it. Imagine the city of London, whose population is about equal to that of the Dominion of Canada, divided into a number of parishes, each with an examining board, so that a man who was qualified for one part would have to be examined before he could practice in another, and imagine how unjust it would be were the practitioners of one parish enabled by the legislature to club together and make laws to keep qualified men from practising in their district. And, after all, this is what is going on in Canada.

I would like to ask Dr. Osler (1) whether the Boards are elevating the standard of medicine in demanding so many didactic lectures ; (2) whether he defends the action of licensing boards in exacting from candidates a large money tax, such as the $100 fee in British Columbia, and whether this tax is not exacted more with the object of protecting the profession from competition than of protecting the public from uneducated practitioners ; (3) whether he is not aware that quacks and charlatans still flourish, and that bands of them, protected by a licentiate of one of the boards, visit all the cities and towns of the Dominion ; (4) whether he is not aware that the reforms mentioned in his letter, the compulsory four years, the additional summer session, the grading of courses, did not all originate with the schools and not with the boards.

If Dr. Osler will be good enough to answer these questions he will confer a favor upon a grateful old pupil, and, moreover, he will thus aid in directing public opinion to the educational reforms so urgently needed in our profession.

Yours very truly,

R. L. MacDonnell.

December 26th, 1889.

———————

THE JOHNS HOPKINS HOSPITAL,
BALTIMORE, Jan. 2nd, 1890.

To the Editors of THE MONTREAL MEDICAL JOURNAL.

SIRS,—I entirely sympathize with Dr. MacDonnell in his desire for a Dominion Medical Board, but he has only to read the reports of the Canadian Medical Association on this question to see that it is an impossibility in the present constitution of the country. However much we may regret it, each Province must continue to regulate its own affairs in medicine. When the curricula and the examinations are uniform in all, reciprocity between the Provinces may be feasible, and to this we may hopefully look forward.

As to the questions which Dr. MacDonnell asks, let me reply to them in order.

1. I do not think the Boards are elevating the standard of medicine in demanding so many lectures, but it must not be forgotten that the schools have, until recently, been wedded to the old plan. I do not know a Canadian Faculty in which five years ago it would have been possible to carry out a scheme of graded education. In how many is it possible to-day? Now that a four years curriculum is the rule and the option of a year with the physician is no longer enforced, the Boards and Colleges could easily unite in a scheme of instruction on advanced modern lines. The teaching in each year should be separate, courses of lectures should not be repeated, and laboratory and tutorial work should take the place of much of the didactic teaching.

To carry out this plan effectively, the fees would have to be increased in order to pay for additional instructors.

2. Yes, I think the Boards have a perfect right to protect the public by exacting a money tax.

3. Surely Dr. MacDonnell is aware that prior to the establishment of the Boards the country swarmed with irregulars of all sorts. The Thompsonians and Eclectics were in every town. Where are they now in Canada? Beyond question, the sole reason why the cities and towns are not filled with herbalists, quacks and professional sharks of all kinds, is the wholesome restraints of the Boards. To hold them responsible for the loose practices of their licentiates seems rather hard. The universities themselves are not without black sheep. " Good wombs have borne bad sons."

I willingly allow that the schools have often taken the initiative in reforms, and it should be the duty of school-men, who are members of the Board, to have these good changes adopted. Of this I am quite sure, that the various Medical Boards would accept with pleasure, and adopt without hesitation, a uniform plan such as could be arranged in a conference of representatives of the leading schools.

In conclusion, I would repeat that the Boards have done splendid service for the profession and for the public in the Canadian Provinces. They form permanent organizations which are not likely to be disturbed, and it is of the utmost importance that the Colleges work harmoniously with them.

Yours very truly,

WM. OSLER.

REPORT OF CASE OF PARTRIDGE POISONING.

To the Editors of THE MONTREAL MEDICAL JOURNAL.

SIRS,—On the evening of January 1st, of this year, while spending my vacation at Bedford, N.S., I was called in haste to see Mr. M., of that place, who, the messenger said, had been poisoned by eating partridge for his supper.

I went at once to the hotel and found Mr. M., the proprietor, a strong man, about 35 years of age, semi-comatose, cold and pulseless at wrist, heart beating about 30 per minute and very weak, pupils reacted feebly to light, patient muttering incoherently. Mrs. M. informed me that her husband had eaten the back of a partridge for his supper, and in about two hours was seized with severe pains in epigastric region, accompanied by diarrhœa and dizziness. Mustard and water was administered, and vomiting was induced ; how much he vomited I could not ascertain.

I at once gave apomorphia 1-10th of a grain hypodermically, and ordered hot bottles, brandy, and a mustard plaster. Gave large doses of brandy by mouth, which were followed by 60 minims hypodermically, whenever vomiting began—*i.e.*, in about five minutes. It was very difficult to get patient to take the brandy by the mouth, as his mental condition was so bad ; this fact and the state of the heart induced me to give more brandy hypodermically. I injected in all 180 minims of brandy in this manner. The mustard I placed over the left chest. The first time I got the pulse at the wrist it was beating 36 to the minute, thready and easily compressed. In about one hour after I saw Mr. M. ; he was much improved ; pulse 48, still thready, however ; and said he felt better. I gave more brandy by mouth and told patient to try and sleep, which, on account of the quantity of brandy he had taken (nearly a whole bottle), he did not find difficult. I left at the end of another hour, patient sleeping, pulse 60, quite strong and full. The only complaint on following day was soreness in left arm, owing to hypodermic needle.

Being " only a student," I will not comment on this case as to causes of poisoning, etc., etc., but will say that, in my opinion, had I not had a hypodermic syringe patient would have had a very *narrow* escape, if he would have escaped at all.

F. G. CORBIN, *4th Year, McGill.*

Selections.

TETANY.*

BY JAMES STEWART, M.D.,
Professor of Pharmacology and Therapeutics, McGill University.

Very few observations have been published in America on the extremely interesting disease commonly known as *tetany*. Drs. Henry Hun of Albany, Carpenter of Pottsville, Lyman of Chicago and J. Lewis Smith of New York have each reported one or more cases. It has been my fortune to have observed a large number of cases in Vienna during the winter of 1883 and 1884, and to have had under observation during the past three years a case which presents many points of exceptional interest. I will first give a brief description of the clinical course of this case.

The patient is a male, aged 39. His complaints when he first came under observation were *diarrhœa* and " spasms of the face, arms and legs." He has been troubled with diarrhœa for ten years, and with spasms of an intermittent character for the past eight years. During the late American civil war he served as a private soldier in a number of the Virginia campaigns. During this period he had several attacks of malarial fever, and for a period of eighteen months he suffered from a mild form of chronic diarrhœa. He never had either syphilis or rheumatism, and never drank to excess. The family history is unimportant.

The patient is tall, emaciated and anæmic, with an anxious, careworn expression. For the past eight years he has been troubled with the attacks of tetany. Usually the first subjective symptom of their appearance is double vision. Then the thumbs become strongly adducted and opposed, while the fingers are adducted and semiflexed. These contractions gradually increase in severity day by day up to about the tenth day, when they somewhat suddenly begin to decline, and the parts become normal twenty-four hours after.

When the attacks are what he calls severe, the adductors of the upper arm become involved, bringing the arms crossed in front of the chest, with the forearms semiflexed. For some hours

* Read before the Association of American Physicians, Washington, Sept. 18, 1889.

before and during the whole period of tetany he has a disagreeable feeling of numbness in his fingers. The dorsum of the hands swell and they are extremely painful. The pain is especially severe when an attempt is made to straighten the contracted muscles. The muscles of the face are also frequently the seat of contractions, the upper lip being usually drawn to the left and upward, and the lower to the right and downward. The facial muscles are also the seat of fibrillary twitchings during the period of tetany. The muscular contractions only occasionally affect the muscles of the lower extremities. When affected, the feet and toes are in a state of plantar flexion, the feet being turned inward and the thighs adducted.

The galvanic irritability of the nerves is found to be greatly exaggerated during the period of tetany. The following may be taken as an average result:

	NORMAL PERIOD.	TETANY PERIOD.
Facial, . .	3.00 m.a.	0.25 m.a.
Radial, . .	5.00 "	1.00 "
Median, . .	4.25 "	0.50 "
Ulnar, . .	3.50 "	0.50 "

During the period of tetany usually galvanization of either facial produced lively contractions on closing the kathode with a measurement of not more than 0.25 of m.a., while after the attack passed away it was necessary to employ 3 m.a. to induce a similar contraction. An anode opening tetanus is readily induced by a strength usually not exceeding 3 m.a. A strength of current necessary to induce a contraction during the quiescent period was sufficient in the tetany period to cause a distinct tetanic contraction. There were never noticed any signs of the reaction of degeneration, the KSZ. being always found more marked than the AOZ.

The difference between the reaction to faradization of the muscles during the normal and tetany periods is not very marked. In fact, the interossei require a much stronger current to induce their contraction during their tetany state than after it has passed away. This is no doubt owing to the œdematous tissues increasing the resistance. The mechanical irritability of the muscles

ι a state of tetany is greatly exaggerated. The same
ue of the nerves innervating the affected muscles. Pres-
ι the vessels does not appear to increase the intensity of
the muscular contractions. The muscles, although flabby, are
in a fai ly nourished condition.

Duri g the period of tetany the knee-jerk is greatly exaggerated, I it after it has passed it is always difficult, and at times
impossible, to induce contraction of either quadriceps, when the
patellar tendons are percussed. The same holds true of the
biceps and trice] re is nothing definite to be made
out in regard to irficial reflexes.

Vasomotor ph ιn quently noticed. Mention has
already been made lling of the back of the hands.
Herpetic eruptions on gers are occasionally seen also.
The tongue is constantly for· in a raw-looking state.

During the intervals of m from the attacks, he suffers
from diarrhœa, which mode when the tetany makes its appearance. The stools are copi us, semi-fluid, frothy, and look
like pea-soup. The abdomen is usually distended. During the
attacks the urine has a high specific gravity from an excess of
urea. It contains also a great excess of indican. It is free,
however, from both albumin and sugar. Jaundice frequently is
present ; there is no other evidence, however, of disease of the
liver. The spleen is normal in size. An examination of the
blood reveals nothing abnormal. No evidence of any thoracic
disease.

About one year after this patient came under observation the
following additional symptoms were noticed :

A complaint, not only during the attacks, but also in the intervals, of general numbness. There is noticed a difficulty in speech.
He is able to articulate well, but on attempting to answer a question, it takes him some time to do so, and when he begins to
speak, especially if any thinking is necessary, the speech is slow.
The œdema, which was formerly confined to the back of the
hands, is now more or less general, but is especially marked in
the face. There is no pitting of the tissues, however. There
is no trace of the thyroid gland. The anæmia has also increased
in intensity.

These symptoms resemble closely those of myxœdema. Against that assumption we have the fact that there has been no progress whatever during the past two years, and this is hardly compatible with what is known to be the clinical course of myxœdema. At one time it appeared as if we were going to have a myxœdema engrafted on a tetany. The case is undoubtedly one of tetany, but whether we have, in addition, myxœdema or not, time alone will tell.

Steinheim, in 1830, was the first to give a true clinical description of tetany. Corvisart, in 1852, was the first to propose the name by wnich it is now universally known. It is, however, moinly to the observations of Trousseau, Erb, N. Weiss, and others that we have been made acquainted with many of the more important features of this remarkable disease.

There are three distinct forms of this disease—forms which differ, in the causes that give them origin, in their course, and in their prognosis, but little in the clinical pictures which they present. By far the most common variety of this disease is what is known as rheumatic or epidemic tetany. On the continent of Europe, especially in Paris and Vienna, distinct epidemics occur. In Vienna hardly a winter passes without such an occurrence. In the winters of 1883 and 1884 a very severe epidemic occurred in the latter city.

The course of the disease when it occurs as an epidemic, is acute—usually not lasting over two or three weeks—fatal cases being very exceptional. Extensive epidemics occurred in Paris in the years 1855 and 1876. In England and America no epidemics of this disease have been described.

A second variety of tetany, which is more chronic, is due to either chronic diarrhœa, prolonged lactation, or other debilitating influences. Except in being more chronic, this form differs but little from the epidemic variety. Recovery nearly always occurs. A third form of tetany follows the removal of enlarged thyroid glands. A very considerable number of cases of tetany following this operation are now on record. Up to May, 1883, Billroth performed 78 operations for the removal of enlarged thyroids, and in 13 tetany followed in the course of a few days ; 6 of these

13 cases proved fatal. Two of the fatal cases ran a coure upward of one year, while the remaining 4 terminated within t weeks.

There is a very marked difference between the course of teta following extirpation of the thyroid and that due to debilitati and epidemic influences. The former is a much severer ty being frequently fatal, while the latter is seldom or never fat A fourth variety of tetany is also distinguished by its fatal t dency. I refer to that which occurs in cases of dilatation of t stomach. Kussmaul, Gerhardt, Dujardin-Beaumetz, Müll and others have reported such cases. Müller has collected eig cases of tetany occurring during the course of dilatation of t stomach, with a mortality of 66 per cent. Judging from the statistics, tetany due to this cause is even more fatal than th arising from removal of the thyroid gland. I have purpose excluded the consideration of what is commonly called infant tetany, as it appears to me that true tetany is an exceptiona rare disease in infany. If we are to include, as many observe do, all cases of carpo-pedal contractions under the name of tetan the disease is much more frequent among children than adul Clinically there is a marked difference, however, between t carpo-pedal contractions so frequently seen in conjunction wi laryngismus and tetany.

1. The tetany of adult life is essentially an intermittent diseas while in the so-called tetany of infant life the contractions a permanent until recovery takes place. They may be more inten at one time than another, but they never completely disappea

2. The carpo-pedal contractions of infancy appear in a vei considerable number of cases to be due to cerebral causes, ; eclampsia is a very frequent complication. There is no dou that true cases of tetany do occur in childhood ; what I wish lay stress on is that they are very rare. and that it is an err to say that every case in which we have carpo-pedal contractio is a case of tetany.

Experimental Tetany in Animals.

When the thyroid gland is removed from cats and dogs,

series of symptoms set in in a few days, to which the name of experimental tetany has been applied. The first symptom usually noticed is a peculiar appearance of the eyes, due to a pushing forward of the membrana nictitans on the inner and under surface of the bulb, from tetanic contraction of the internal eye muscles. Simultaneous with this contraction of the eye muscles, there appear fibrillary tremors of the muscles of the extremities and face, and occasionally of the tongue. In some cases these tremors are so marked that it is impossible for the animal to stand erect, at other times they are so weak that it is with difficulty that they can be perceived. In addition to the fibrillary tremors, there is tetanic contraction of the muscles of the extremities. The muscular phenomena described alternate with periods when the animal remains quiet. The respirations are frequent and superficial; the temperature is not increased.

In most animals, after the eighth day, a suppurative catarrh of the conjunctiva sets in, which finally leads to implication of the cornea and its perforation. The death of the animal soon follows, either suddenly from tetanic contraction of the glottis or diaphragm, or more slowly from exhaustion.

In a very large number of thyroid removals in dogs, Fuhr was unable to find any constant changes in the internal organs. Neither the brain nor spinal cord presented any marked changes. The tissues in the neighborhood of the thyroid gland were carefully examined and were found normal.

Exceptionally, a dog may live after complete removal of the thyroid gland. Rabbits, on the other hand, usually recover from the operation, although liable to be affected by the muscular contractions. Man appears to stand midway between these two classes of animals, so far as his power of withstanding the removal of the thyroid is concerned.

The symptoms detailed as following the removal of the thyroid in the lower animals bear a striking resemblance to tetany as it appears in man; that they are essentially the same disease is extremely probable. A valuable proof of their identity has been pointed out by Schwartz. In all his cases—six in number—he found that both the galvanic and faradic reactions were greatly

The reaction of the peroneal nerve to galvanism was ... we often found muscular contraction caused by ... a current not measurable by our ordinary ... AOTe and KaTe were readily brought out by ... current.

... many different forms of trauma that affect the muscles ... tany is the only one in which there is a marked increase ... electric irritability of the nerves, with the positive symptom ... static cholera. Its presence, then, is of great diagnostic ... ance, and leaves little room for doubt that the muscular ... systems which follow the removal of the thyroid in animals ... the same nature as those which follow a similar operation ... man, and also similar to the same disease that occurs epidem... ... and from the other causes already mentioned.

Morbid Anatomy of Tetany.—In the few cases where a ... logical examination of the nervous structures has been ... made after death ... ... during ... ...

The slight changes ... We as having been ... him in the ... cells ... later ... negative a few ... ... described ... ... peritis and ... ... ons of the ... ... died at the age ... ... tetany. Similar ... ... interpreted at this age, and therefore cannot be taken as in any way distinctive of tetany. Seeligmüller and Boyer have each had ... several cases opportunity of making a thorough examination after death of the central and peripheral nervous system, and with negative results in every case.

We may therefore conclude that, as far as we know at present there are no anatomical lesions in cases of tetany. The same is true of the tetany induced in animals by removal of the thy roid gland. Judging from the clinical course of the disease, these negative results are what we would naturally expect.

Before discussing the probable nature of the disease, it will ... lace to glance at the present expressed opinions as to the cause of the experimental tetany of animals after removal of the thyroid glauds. With but very few exceptions, every recent experimenter in this field has arrived at the conclusion that the tetany is directly brought about by the removal of the gland itself, and that it has nothing whatever to do with injury of the nerves in the neighborhood. The very recent experiments of Fuhr, Weil and Schultze establish this, I think, beyond doubt. An interesting experiment performed by Fuhr shows that simple irritation itself does not bring about any of the symptoms of tetany. He injected a hypodermatic syringeful of a 10 per cent. solution of nitrate of silver between the gland and its capsule ; severe and extensive inflammation of the gland and neighboring structures followed, but at no time were there present any fibrillary tremors, muscular contractions, or other symptoms indicative of tetany.

It is a well-established fact that the removal of one gland does not bring about tetany, but if, after the wound is completely healed, the remaining gland is removed, the symptoms of tetany quickly develop, and we then have the usual lethal course as seen when the two glands are removed at the same time. Weil has also shown that if a portion of each gland is removed the result is negative, while the usual symptoms quickly make their appearance when the glands are completely removed.

I think there can be no other conclusion after the consideration of the above facts, than that the cause of tetany in animals is due directly to the removal of the thyroid glands. And no other conclusion is tenable in regard to the tetany which follows extirpation of the thyroid in man.

As the removal of the thyroid glands, both in man and animals, brings about a certain train of nervous symptoms, it follows that these glands have some important relations to the nutrition of the nervous system : whether this function consists in the removal from the blood of matters which would be injurious to the nervous system if allowed to circulate, it is difficult to determine. Experiments performed by Ewald of Strasbourg lend great probability to this view. He injected a number of dogs with the freshly expressed juice from the thyroid glands of healthy dogs, and invariably found that the animals became soporose and cataleptic.

To explain how causes seemingly so diverse in their operation, as rheumatic influences, diarrhœa, pregnancy, lactation, and removal of the thyroid glands, can induce similar symptoms is very difficult. The active cause in the case reported is no doubt in some way due to the diarrhœa; but is the disease induced through impoverishment of the nerve centres, or through the peripheral irritation, or from the absorption of putrid products?

It appears reasonable to conclude that in all cases of tetany we have to do essentially with an unstable condition of the nervous system, a condition which readily reacts to slight peripheral influences. In the great majority of cases the disease is connected with some directly debilitating cause.

No doubt peripheral irritation is an active factor in a considerable proportion of cases. Müller reports two cases of tetany occurring in simple dilatation of the stomach, and where, after death, this organ was found to be twisted on its axis.

I am unable to advance any facts as lending probability to the view that tetany is brought about by the absorption of the products of putrid decomposition.

LITERATURE.

Meinert (Dresden) : Tetanie in der Schwangerschaft. *Archi f. Gynäkologie*, Band xxx., S. 444.

Fr. Müller : Tetanie bei Dilatatio Ventriculi und Achsendrehung des Magens. *Charité Annalen*, 1888, Band xiii., S. 273.

A. Baginsky : Ueber Tetanie der Säuglinge. *Berl. klin. Wochenschrift*, 1886, S. 177.

Ferdinand Fuhr : Die Extirpation der Schilddruse. *Archiv f. Exper. Path. und Pharmak.*, Band xxi., S. 387.

Schultze : Ueber die Folgen der Wegnahme der Schilddruse beim Hunde. *Neurolog. Centralblatt*, No. 8, 1889.

N. Weiss : Ueber Tetanie. *Volkmann's Sammlung*, No. 189.

J. Lewis Smith : Tetany. *Archives of Pediatrics*, June, July and August, 1889.

Henry Hun ; Tetany, etc. *Medical News* (Philadelphia), 1888.

Drobnik : Experimentelle Untersuchungen uber die Folgen der Exstirpation der Schilddruse. *Archiv f. Exper. Path. und Pharm.*, Band xxv., S. 136.

C. Weil; Untersuchungen uber die Schilddruse. *Medicinische Wander-Vorträge,* Heft 10.

Gowers; Diseases of the Nervous System.

H. M. Lyman; Tetany. *Transactions of the Association of American Physicians,* vol. 1.

J. R. Ewald: Versuche uber die Function der Thyreoida des Hundes. *Berl. klin. Woch,* 1887.

Horsley: The Lancet, 1884, vol. ii.

—*American Journal of the Medical Sciences.*

The Disposal of the Sputa in Phthisis.—

(*Ed. Boston Med. and Surg. Journal,* Oct. 31.)—There is now general agreement as to the danger of communication of phthisis by the inhalation of the dried products of expectoration. Experiments on animals compelled to inhale sputa-dust have demonstrated this; such experiments were formerly made by Tappanier, and have recently been made by Cornet. This experimenter also claims to have determined a curious fact by collecting the dust and debris from wards in which phthisical patients were confined, and inoculating those products in animals. Of 21 phthisical wards, 15, or two thirds, contained the tuberculous virus. The patients were in the habit of spitting upon their handkerchiefs, as well as into spittoons. But in a third of the wards no infectious material was found in the air or on the walls; and this immunity was attributed, not only to the presence of spittoons, but also to the precautions enforced to prevent expectoration upon the handkerchiefs or cloths, and the pains taken to promote general asepsis and cleanliness.

Often repeated analyses have proved that the sputa of phthisical persons in very many instances contain Koch's bacillus, and are therefore likely to convey contagion to the predisposed. The chain of evidence seems to be sufficiently complete.

It would seem, then, that the requirement insisted upon by the French Commission—that the constant use of spittoons should be obligatory on the phthisical, and that they should not be allowed to expectorate on the floor, on carpets or mats, or even, except under peculiar circumstances, on cloths or handkerchiefs—should be enforced, both in hospital and private practice. In advanced cases of phthisis it may not be possible for patients to use spittoons, and they may be obliged to expectorate on pieces of cloth or toilet paper ; these should be immediately burned.

It is advised that phthisical patients in their daily walks ought to be enjoined not to spit on the ground, on the sidewalk, etc.; this requirement will be difficult of execution unless such patients be provided with a portable spittoon which they are willing to use in public. Spittoons may be placed in all public rooms, in corridors, closets, about places of promenade, and kept partly filled with water, never with sawdust, ashes, or any other dry material.

Spittoons should not be emptied into privies or water-closets, or upon the soil, but into the fire : or they may be dealt with as Hassal advises in the *Lancet :* " A covered vessel of suitable size, and provided with a rod, should be partially filled with a strong bichloride of mercury solution, and into this the contents of the spittoons should be daily emptied, until it becomes necessary to dispose of the accumulated and now harmless sputa, which may then safely be done by means of the closet or soil. The use of the stirrer is necessary, in order to break up the sputa and allow of the effective action of the germicide."

The sanitarily-ideal apartments furnished to consumptive patients are to have no curtains, carpets or hangings ; and where mats are required, they should be of some non-absorbent material, as rubber cloth. Such patients should be required to sleep alone, and their clothing and bedding should be kept entirely apart from that of other lodgers. Frequent boiling and cleansing of bed linen and underclothing should be enjoined. When a phthisical patient has vacated a room, or has died, the same cleansing and disinfectant measures should be carried out as after a case of any ordinary infectious disease, as scarlet fever or diphtheria.

All these precautionary measures are simple corollaries from facts which have been obtained the past few years as to the parasitic nature of tuberculosis and the contagiousness of phthisical sputa. Their enforcement ought to diminish the extension of tuberculosis but would scarcely increase the content and comfort of the great army of the phthisical.—*Epitome*, Dec. 1889.

Puerperal Fever, a Possible Source of Contagion.

—Mr. R. D. Pedley, F.R.C.S. (Edin.), and L.D.S., Dental Surgeon to the Evelina Hospital for Sick Children, Southwark, contributes to the *Lancet* of Dec. 21st, 1889, a paper which is well worthy the attention of those who are engaged in obstetric practice. He writes:—"Is it possible for a medical practitioner or a nurse whose mouth is in an unhealthy condition to be the means of developing in a patient puerperal fever or any of the local manifestations of septic poisoning, such as pelvic cellulitis or pelvic peritonitis? This question has many times presented itself since reading as a student a case mentioned by Dr. Playfair in Vol. II of *The Science and Practice of Midwifery*, of a medical man who, suffering from chronic ozæna, had to relinquish practice on account of the numerous deaths from puerperal fever among his patients. I have not been able to answer the above question in the affirmative, but I consider there is sufficient evidence to justify a few remarks, thereby placing the matter before those who have better opportunities of forming a correct judgment. Some light may be thrown on this ' possible source of contagion ' by making mention of a case recently reported in the daily press of an inquest held on the body of a woman who had died from puerperal fever. The mother of the patient—an uncertified midwife—had been the means of spreading this terrible disease. Dr. Talbot, in evidence, stated that ' he had attended her for a piece of dead bone in the mouth, and if she had been fingering it, that might account for the outbreak.' This, of course, is an extreme case. Probably the woman was suffering from syphilitic necrosis, and that her mouth was in a very bad condition, also that her acquaintance with antiseptics was practically *nil*. Most mouths are rendered foul by carious teeth, and there can be very little doubt that medical men and nurses are as liable to suffer from carious teeth as their patients, and find, as a rule, far less opportunity of seeking attention.

"The condition I refer to is generally brought about as follows: A tooth is attacked by caries. If neglected this makes its way into the tooth until the pulp chamber is reached, and the nerve

40

is exposed. After a variable amount of pain the nerve dies, and becomes putrid right up to the apex of the fang. A small amount of septic matter escapes through the apical foramen, and sets up an acute alveolar abscess. At this stage, if the tooth is extracted, the trouble is ended ; but if the pus is let out beneath the lip, or makes its way through the thin alveolar plate, the swelling disappears after a day or two and a sinus remains, from which matter is constantly discharged in small quantities. In dental language it becomes a chronic alveolar abscess. The tooth is practically a piece of dead bone ; with this difference, that through its centre is a narrow channel in which rests the remains of a putrid nerve. It is quite common to find several teeth in a similar condition, sometimes cut down level with the gum, having received no further treatment than careful concealment by artificial teeth. Beyond the fact that an occasional swelling takes place in the alveolar plate, and a very disagreeable taste is present, the owner may go on for years with very little discomfort. Is it unreasonable to suppose that a very intelligent nurse (having several teeth such as we have described) may seek to relieve the pain of an aching stump by pressure of the finger ; and, not being aware of any danger, convey septic matter to the body of the patient in the ordinary discharge of her duties ?

“ In May and September of 1886 two cases came under my notice, of which brief notes were taken at the time :—*Case 1*— Miss ——, a nurse, said she should have been before but had been attending a case of puerperal fever. Her mouth was in an unwholesome condition. Front teeth good. Not a single molar sound ; all the back teeth carious. Had two alveolar abscesses in connection with upper bicuspid teeth on the right side, and one in connection with a lower molar tooth on the left side. *Case 2*—Dr. ——, suffering from an acute alveolar abscess over left lateral insisor tooth in the upper jaw. Face considerably swollen. Tooth had been sore for some time ; he could scarcely bite anything with comfort. Teeth generally in bad condition. Several stumps in the lower jaw on the right side and in the upper jaw on the left side. Had suffered for years ; of late the stumps had given considerable trouble. Several sinuses from which pus oozed. Would have sought better advice before, but just after tooth became troublesome had a puerperal fever case to attend to, and had been much worried. No reason to be assigned for puerperal fever; surroundings good and healthy. Good drainage.

" That pus from an alveolar abscess is necessarily septic we cannot be sure; but there are three facts worthy of notice. 1, Pus from an alveolar abscess is often of foul odor. 2, As a consequence of alveolar acscess, necrosis of a portion of the jaw-bone is not at all uncommon. 3, There are cases recorded of patients who have died from pyæmia and septicæmia as the result of alveolar abscess, *vide* Tomes' *Dental Surgery*, Salter's *Dental Pathology and Surgery*.

" It may be urged that the medical practitioner is constantly brought in contact with septic matter, and that the adoption of the necessary antiseptic precautions would exclude all possibility of such direct communications as I have suggested. This is quite likely; also that, if a source of danger is pointed out, the medical man may be trusted to do his best to avoid it. We cannot be so sure of the nurse, who necessarily is brought far more often in contact with the patient, and who, after the first few hours, has the well-being of the patient in her own hands. No medical man can be held responsible should the nurse fail to carry out his instructions; but he can, in most cases, ascertain beforehand that the nurse is not the subject of a malady, be it local or constitutional, which is likely to be a source of danger to his patient. In conclusion I would offer this brief suggestion. It is desirable that midwives and nurses should be subjected to medical inspection before attending obstetric cases."—*Hospital Gazette.*

On the Non-Retention of Urine in Young Girls and in Women.

—May I be permitted to make a few remarks on a paper by Dr. H. Marion Sims on the above subject published in your last September number, read by him at the March meeting of the Obstetrical

Society of New York, in which he recommends mechanical distention of the bladder in cases of incontinence of urine other
than those produced by cystitis or growths in the bladder? In
the paper mentioned, he remarks that at the time he treated the
case related he was certain that he had struck an original idea.
" In looking up the literature of the subject," he says, " I find
very little mentioned in regard to such cases, and only one case
could I find reported where incontinence was cured by forcible
dilatation.   This case was in a girl, after puberty, whom Braxton
Hicks had cured by forcible dilatation with warm water, but in
what quantities I could not find out."   Afterwards Dr. Sims
says : " I only give the above references just to show that there
is no mention made of contraction and hypertrophy and its treatment by forcible dilatation, except in the one case given by
Braxton Hicks."

I do not know from what imperfect source Dr. Marion Sims
derived his report of the case he alludes to, but had he written
to me I should have been happy to answer him and to point out
that if he referred to the second volume of the *Lancet*, 1868,
page 7, he would find that I had done much more.   Under the
head of " Two Cases of Incontinence of Urine from Earliest
Childhood cured by Mechanical Dilatation," the report begins :
" A cause of incontinence of urine is indicated in the following
cases which is not generally recognized.   The treatment which
Dr. Hicks applied was very successful, and we have no doubt
that the record of it will be of great service to practitioners who
have patients suffering from this very troublesome condition."
Then follows the first case and treatment, assisted by injections
of morphia and other remedies: and then : " Dr. Hicks remarked that the constant evacuation of urine permitted by some
mothers to their children allowed the bladder to become so constantly empty that after a time the muscular power of the
sphincter was not sufficient to counteract the contractility of the
organ.   In recent cases, no doubt, this could be voluntarily
overcome by adults ; but in old-standing cases, although we
might do much by lessening the sensibility of the bladder, *yet
we might proceed at once to overcome its resistance by mechani-*

cal force, so that further treatment would not be required."
This is well instanced by Case II, after which follows also :
" Both these girls had been unfit for service from their complaint. Dr. Hicks suggested the applicability of this treatment
to both sexes in cases with similar history. He thought it was
possible that in some cases there were congenitally small blad-
ders, and these possibly might be more difficult to manage."
Then follows a case of contraction following cystitis, in which
relief to a certain extent was obtained by dilatation, in addition
to other local means, but not so satisfactorily as in the above
cases.

It is a source of satisfaction to me to find that Dr. Sims confirms my ideas and treatment by his own independent observations, and I feel sure he will, on the perusal of these remarks,
award me the claim I am making of priority, as it is twenty
years since my cases were published. And I think I may make
another claim of priority respecting the washing-out of the
bladder by various medications, for I believe that prior to my
lectures on " Some Diseases of the Urethra and Bladder" (in
the year previous to the report of the above-mentioned cases),
Lancet, vol. ii, 1867, the washing-out and locally treating
diseases of the bladder was not done ; now it is the rule of
practice, though, of course, with additions to the medicaments
employed, such as boric and salicylic acid, etc.

I have also since tried distention in other cases of contraction,
caused in older patients temporarily by other circumstances than
cystitis and tumors, with great benefit ; and have also pointed
out, some years back, that in distention and washing-out of the
bladder it is not necessary that the bladder should be entered,
if we use an open-ended canula, passed up to but not through
the sphincter, using a little more pressure on the piston. But
I have also shown that generally sufficient pressure for most
cases can be obtained by a rubber tube and funnel attached to
the canula, the water pressure being regulated by the elevation
of the funnel.—*Dr. J. Braxton Hicks in Journal of Obstetrics,*
January, 1890.

THE

Montreal Medical Journal.

| VOL. XVIII. | FEBRUARY, 1890. | No. 8. |

THE PROVINCIAL MEDICAL BOARDS.

The letters of Drs. Osler and MacDonnell, which we publish in this number, will, we hope, direct the attention of the profession in general, and the members of the Provincial Medical Boards in particular, to the weak points in our system of medical education. Dr. Osler, from his extensive experience in teaching and with teachers, is particularly well qualified to point out to us our failings. When he says that "the courses of lectures should not be repeated, and laboratory and tutorial work should take the place of much of the didactic teaching," he has uttered a truth which every teacher in our Canadian medical schools must feel the force of.

We hope the time is not far distant when these desirable reforms will become accomplished facts.

It is useless to expect a Central Examining Board for the entire Dominion, not because there is differences in the requirements of the different Provincial Boards, but owing to the innate incompatibility of the elements that go to make this " Canada of ours." If the different Provincial Boards expressed a wish to hear from the teachers and students propositions for the more effective study of our common profession, they would, we have no doubt, be quickly furnished with schemes which, if carried out, would place the Canadian medical student in a position where at least he would not be at a disadvantage as compared with his brethren elsewhere.

SOME PHASES OF THE INFLUENZA EPIDEMIC.

One of the most striking features of the great epidemic is its universality. It attacks all ages. It spares neither sex. It is as common in the country as in the city. The inmates of the shanty and the magnate's palace are equally its victims. When the approximate mortality returns from its direct and indirect effects come to be written up, it will no doubt be found that they are greater than from any epidemic of recent times.

REGULATIONS AND PROGRAMME OF THE TENTH INTERNATIONAL MEDICAL CONGRESS.

1. The Tenth International Medical Congress will be opened in Berlin on Monday, August 4th, 1890, and will be closed on Saturday, August 9th.

2. The Congress shall consist of legally qualified medical men who have inscribed themselves as members and have paid for their card of membership. Other men of science who interest themselves in the work of the Congress may be admitted as extraordinary members.

Those who take part in the Congress shall pay a subscription of 20 marks (£1 stg. or $5) on being enrolled as members. For this sum they shall receive a copy of the *Transactions* as soon as they appear. The enrolment shall take place at the beginning of the Congress. Gentlemen may, however, be enrolled as members by sending the amount of the subscription to the treasurer* with their name, professional status and residence appended.

3. The object of the Congress is an exclusively scientific one.

4. The work of the Congress will be discharged by eighteen different sections. The members shall declare upon enrolment to which section or sections they intend more particularly to attach themselves.

5. The Committee of Organization shall, at the opening sitting of the Congress, suggest the election of a definite committee or bureau, which shall consist of a president, three vice-presidents,

---

* Treasurer's address—DR. M. BARTELS, Berlin SW., Leipzigerstrasse 75. Please to enclose a visiting-card.

and of a number (as yet undetermined) of honorary presidents and secretaries.

At the first meeting of each section a president and certain number of hon. presidents shall be elected; these latter shall conduct the business of the sections in turn with the presidents.

On account of the different languages employed, a suitable number of secretaries shall be chosen from among the foreign members. The duties of the foreign secretaries shall be confined to the sittings of the Congress.

After the termination of the Congress the editing of the *Transactions* shall be carried out by a committee specially appointed for this purpose.

6. The Congress will assemble daily, either for a general meeting or for the labors of the different sections.

The general meetings will be held between 11 and 2 o'clock. Three such meetings will take place.

The time for the sittings of the various sections will be fixed by the special committee of each section, it being understood, however, that no such sittings are to take place during the hours allotted to the general meetings.

Joint sittings of two or more sections may be held, provided that the bureau of the Congress can offer suitable rooms for such sittings.

7. The general meetings shall be devoted to—(a) Transactions connected with the work and general management of the Congress; (b) Speeches and communications of general interest.

8. Addresses in the general sittings, as well as in any extraordinary meetings which may be determined upon, can only be given by those who have been specially requested by the Committee of Organization.

Proposals relative to the future management of the Congress must be announced to the Committee of Organization before July 1st, 1890. The Committee shall decide whether these proposals are suitable to be introduced for discussion.

9. In the sittings of the sections, questions and problems will be discussed which have been agreed upon by the special Committees of Organization. The communications of those appointed

by the committee to report on a subject shall form the basis of discussion. As far as time allows, other communications or proposals proceeding from members and sanctioned by the Committee of Organization may also be introduced for discussion. The bureau of each section decides as to the acceptance of such offered communications, and as to the order in which they shall come before the meeting, always provided that this point has not been already determined in the sitting itself by a decree of the section.

Scientific questions shall not be put to the vote.

10. Introductory addresses in the sections must as a rule not exceed *twenty minutes in length*. In the discussions, no more than *ten minutes* are allowed to each speaker.

11. All addresses and papers in the general and sectional meetings must be handed over to the secretaries, in writing, before the end of the sitting. The Editorial Committee shall decide whether, and to what extent, these written contributions shall be included in the printed *Transactions* of the Congress. The members who have taken part in the discussions will be requested to hand over to the secretaries, before the end of the day, in writing, the substance of their remarks.

12. The official languages of all the sittings shall be German, English and French. The regulations, the programme, and the agenda for the day will be printed in all three languages.

It will, however, be allowable to make use of other languages than the above for brief remarks, always provided that one of the members present is ready to translate the gist of such remarks into one of the official languages.

13. The acting president shall conduct the business of each meeting according to the parliamentary rules generally accepted in deliberative assemblies.

14. Medical students, and other persons, ladies and gentlemen, who are not physicians, but who take a special interest in the work of a particular sitting, may be invited by the president or be allowed to attend the sitting by special permission.

15. Communications or enquiries regarding the business of separate sections must be addressed to the managing members

thereof. All other communications and enquiries must be
directed to the general secretary, DR. LASSAR, Berlin NW., 19
Karlstrasse.

SPECIAL SECTIONS—COMMITTEES OF ORGANIZATION.

(The names which appear in small capitals are those of the managing members.)

1.—ANATOMY.

Flemming, Kiel.
Hasse, Breslau.
HERTWIG, Berlin W., Maassenstr. 34.
His, Leipzig.
v. Kölliker, Würzburg.

Kupffer, München.
Merkel, Göttingen.
Schwalbe, Strassburg.
Wiedersheim, Freiburg.

2.—PHYSIOLOGY AND PHYSIOLOGICAL CHEMISTRY.

Bernstein, Halle.
Biedermann, Jena.
DU BOIS-REYMOND, Berlin W., Neue
    Wilhelmstr. 15.
Heidenhain, Breslau.

Hensen, Kiel.
Hüfner, Tübingen.
Hoppe-Seyler, Strassburg.
H. Munk, Berlin.
Voit, München.

3.—GENERAL PATHOLOGY & PATHOLOGICAL ANATOMY.

Arnold, Heidelberg.
Bollinger, München.
Grawitz, Greifswald.
Heller, Kiel.
Ponfick, Breslau.

v. Recklinghausen, Strassburg.
VIRCHOW, Berlin W., Schelling-
    Strasse 10.
Weigert, Frankfurt a. M.
Zenker, Erlangen,

4.—PHARMACOLOGY.

Binz, Bonn.
Böhm, Leipzig.
Filehne, Breslau.
Jaffé, Königsberg.
Hugo Schulz, Greifswald.

LIEBREICH, Berlin NW., Doro-
    theen-Strasse 34 a.
Marmé, Göttingen.
Penzoldt, Erlangen.
Schmiedeberg, Strassburg.

5.—INTERNAL MEDICINE.

Biermer, Breslau.
Gerhardt, Berlin.
Leube, Würzburg.
LEYDEN, Berlin W., Thiergarten-
    Strasse 14.

Lichtheim, Königsberg.
Liebermeister, Tübingen.
Mosler, Greifswald.
Naunyn, Strassburg.
v, Ziemssen, München.

6.—DISEASES OF CHILDREN.

Baginsky, Berlin.
HENOCH, Berlin W., Bellevuestr. 8.
Heubner, Leipzig.
Kohts, Strassburg.
Krabler, Greifswald.

Ranke, München.
Rehn, Frankfurt a. M.
Soltmann, Breslau.
Steffen, Stettin.

7.—SURGERY.

Bardeleben, Berlin.
v. Bergmann, Berlin NW., Alexander Ufer 1.
Czerny, Heidelberg.
König, Göttingen.

v. Lotzbeck, München.
Schede, Hamburg.
C. Thiersch, Leipzig.
Trendelenburg, Bonn.
Wagner, Königshütte.

8.—OBSTETRICS AND GYNÆCOLOGY.

Fritsch, Breslau.
Gusserow, Berlin.
Hegar, Freiburg.
Hofmeyer, Würzburg.
Kaltenbach, Halle.

Löhlein, Giessen.
Martin, Berlin NW., Moltke-Strasse 2.
Olshausen, Berlin.
Winckel, München.

9.—NEUROLOGY AND PSYCHIATRY.

Binswanger, Jena.
Emminghaus, Freiburg.
Erb, Heidelberg.
Flechsig, Leipzig.
Fürstner, Heidelberg.

Grashey, München.
Hitzig, Halle.
Jolly, Strassburg.
Laehr, Berlin-Zehlendorf.

10.—OPHTHALMOLOGY.

O. Becker, Heidelberg.
Eversbusch, Erlangen.
v. Hippel, Giessen,
Hirschberg, Berlin.
Leber, Göttingen.

Michel, Würzburg.
Schmidt-Rimpler, Marburg.
Schweigger, Berlin NW., Roonstr. 6.
v. Zehender, Rostock.

11.—OTOLOGY.

Bezold, München.
Bürkner, Göttingen.
Kirchner, Würzburg.
Kuhn, Strassburg.
Kessel, Jena.

Lucae, Berlin W., Lützow-platz 9.
Magnus, Königsberg.
Moos, Heidelberg.
Trautmann, Berlin.

12.—LARYNGOLOGY AND RHINOLOGY.

Beschorner, Dresden.
B. Frankel, Berlin NW., Neustädtische Kirchstr. 12.
Gottstein, Breslau.
A. Hartmann, Berlin.

Jurasz, Heidelberg.
H. Krause, Berlin.
Michael, Hamburg.
Schech, München.
M. Schmidt, Frankfurt a. M.

13.—DERMATOLOGY AND SYPHILIGRAPHY.

Caspary, Königsberg.
Doutrelepont, Bonn.
Köbner, Berlin.
Lassar, Berlin NW., Carlstr. 19.
Lesser, Leipzig.

G. Lewin, Berlin.
Neisser, Breslau.
Unna, Hamburg.
Wolff, Strassburg.

14.—DISEASES OF THE TEETH.

ᵥ rlin NW., Alexander-
  ⸲ 6.
  mburg.
ᵤ ᴌ₀₁pzig.
⸗.ιcke, Kiel.

Holländer, Halle.
Miller, Berlin.
Partsch, Breslau.
Sauer, Berlin.
Weil, München.

15.—HYGIENE.

Flügge, Breslau.
Gaffky, Giessen.
Graf, Elberfeld.
F. Hofmann, Leip⁻ᵗ⁻
R. Koch, Berlin.

Lehmann, Würzburg,
Pistor, Berlin W., v. d. Heydt-
  strasse 13.
Wolffhügel, Göttingen.
Uffelmann, Rostock.

16.—MEDICAL [T]Y AND CLIMATOLOGY.

(HIS.⸗.. . STATISTICS.)

Abel, Stettin.
Brock, Berlin.
Dettweiler, Falkenstein.
Falkenstein, Lichterfelde.
Finkelnburg, Bonn.

Guttstadt, Berlin.
A. Hirsch, Berlin W., Pots-
  damer-Strasse 113.
Lent, Köln.
Wernich, Cöslin.

17.—STATE MEDICINE.

Falk, Berlin.
Günther, Dresden.
v. Hölder, Stuttgart.
Knauff, Heidelberg.
Schönfeld, Berlin.

Liman, Berlin SW., König-
  grätzerlStrasse 46 a.
Schwarz, Köln.
Skrzecska, Berlin.
Ungar, Bonn.

18.—MILITARY HYGIENE.

v. Coler, Berlin.
v. Fichte, Stuttgart.
Grasnick, Berlin.
Grossheim, Berlin.
Melhausen, Berlin.

Krocker, Berlin W., Madge-
  burger Platz 3.
Mohr, München.
Roth, Dresden.
Wenzel, Berlin.

Obituary.

—The death of Prof. Westphal, of Berlin, removes one of the ablest clinical teachers and investigators of diseases of the nervous system of the present century.

—Dr. L. H. Sayre, a son of Dr. Lewis A. Sayre, the well-known New York surgeon, was found dead in his father's reception-room on the 3rd of January. A necropsy revealed organic disease of the heart.

—We regret to have to record the death of Dr. McKercher, of Point Edward. Dr. McKercher, who graduated at McGill last year, when he obtained the final prize, had in the short space of a few months established himself in an extensive and lucrative practice.

—Through the death of Dr. H. M. McKay, of Woodstock, Western Ontario loses one of its most respected and prominent medical practitioners. Dr. McKay was an ex-president of the Ontario Medical Association, and, at the time of his death, a member of the Provincial Board of Health.

—Through the death of Sir William Gull, Bart., England has lost one of her leading physicians. He never entirely recovered from the effects of a cerebral hemorrhage which occurred about two years ago. For many years he was a physician to Guy's Hospital, where he was highly esteemed as a clinical teacher and investigator.

Medical Items.

—Dr. Frank Ferguson, Pathologist to the New York]
pital, has been elected Professor of Pathology in the New Y
Post-Graduate Medical School and Hospital.

—The physicians of the State of Mississippi are, it is ε
endeavoring to pass a bill through the legislature exempt
them from personal taxes.

—The epidemic of influenza has had a marked effect on
consumption of beer in Germany. In Munich the daily ι
sumption is 30,000 gallons less.

—One of the attending physicians on the late King of]
tugal has sent in a bill for $14,000 for ten visits. Ano
has asked $30,000 as a solace for having visited his]
eighteen times.

—After many years of weary waiting, the promoters of
B.A. Bill have succeeded in getting this measure finally pas
That such a measure should find any opposition is, to int
gent people, surprising.

—Professor Rosenthal, Lecturer on Diseases of the Nerv
System in the University of Vienna, is dead. He is the au
of a valuable work on " Diseases of the Nervous System,'
English translation of which appeared a few years ago.

—The following resolution was passed unanimously at
last meeting of the Ottawa Medico-Chirurgical Society,
on Friday, Jan. 24th :—

Moved by Dr. Small, seconded by Dr. S. Wright, "*
whereas Dr. Roome, M.P., at the last session of the Domii
Parliament, moved ' that in the opinion of this House the t
has come when the Federal Government should establis
Central Department of Health, with a responsible head
deputy head, for the purpose of perfecting the collection
vital statistics, educating the public in health matters, and :
venting the spread of disease'; and whereas he is prepared

intends to again bring the motion before the House early during the present session, be it therefore resolved that the Ottawa Medico-Chirurgical Society, in meeting assembled, hereby cordially endorses Dr. Roome's action, and trusts that he may succeed in inducing the House and the Government to take such early action as will secure for the country the much needed legislation as above named."

——Dr. C. A. Stephens, of Norway Lake, Maine, desiring to verify his own researches as to the causes of failing nutrition in aging organisms, offers three cash prizes of $175, $125 and $100 for the best three comparative demonstrations, by means of microscopical slides of the blood capillaries in young and in aged tissues, canine or human. By young tissues (canine) are meant tissues from animals between the ages of 1 and 3 years. By aged tissues (canine) are meant tissues from animals not less than 12 years of age. By young tissues (human) are meant tissues from subjects between the ages of 10 and 20 years. By aged tissues (human) are meant tissues from subjects not less than 65 years of age. While a preference will be given to demonstrations from human tissues, it will be possible for work in canine tissues to take the first and, indeed, all of the prizes. But of two slides equally well done in all respects, one canine the other human, the latter will be given the preference. Canine tissues should be from large animals. Twelve slides from young and twelve from aged tissues must be submitted by each competitor, together with a full description of the subjects, methods pursued, and every detail and circumstance which is likely to throw light upon or account for any peculiarity. The slides are for comparison as to the condition of capillary circulation, the young with the old, and should be in numbered pairs, or groups from the same kind of tissue. The term tissue is used in a general sense—e.g., pulmonary tissue, hepatic tissue, renal tissue, osseous tissue, muscular tissue, nerve tissue, alimentary tissue, etc. No particular schedule of methods for injection or staining will be insisted upon, and no more definite directions or explanations will be given. The slides, carefully packed and boxed,

THE

Montreal Medical Journal.

| Vol. XVIII. | MARCH, 1890. | No. 9. |

Original Communications.

ON ABDOMINAL SECTION IN TUBERCLE OF THE PERITONEUM AND UTERINE APPENDAGES.*

By WM. GARDNER, M.D.,
Professor of Gynæcology, McGill University.

It is foreign to my purpose, as, indeed, it would be outside my sphere of professional work and experience, to discuss generally the subject of peritoneal tuberculosis. I wish merely to present the report of five cases in which a variety of physical signs existed, but in all of which tuberculosis was present, and in each of which I did abdominal section. It must further be added that in none of these cases was the whole condition diagnosed by the ordinary medical attendant or by myself, except in Case 2, in which Dr. Armstrong suspected tubercular peritonitis. Ever since ovariotomy began the ascent to its present magnificent position as one of the great triumphs of surgery, the abdomen has occasionally been opened to take out an ovarian tumor when none has been found, but only an encysted collection of fluid, with more or less matting together of viscera and general studding of the peritoneum with tubercle. Such was my first case, reported to this Society and published in some detail in the CANADA MEDICAL AND SURGICAL JOURNAL for June 1885. I here give an abridged report, as it is the only one of the five in which fluid effusion in the belly-cavity existed.

S. B , aged 23, single, domestic servant, once pregnant, confined at the seventh month one year and a half ago, was sent

---

* Read before the Medico-Chirurgical Society of Montreal, Feb. 7th, 1890.

41

to me by Dr. George Ross of this city for examination. The
large belly had excited suspicion of pregnancy. Nothing definite
as to duration of the enlargement. Her mistress thought about
three or four months. It had rapidly increased. The symptoms
were pain in the belly, absence of menses for four months,
general weakness and wasting, poor appetite, and red tongue.

Examination.—Great enlargement of the belly; recent pink
and old silvery striæ; well marked fluctuation and dull percussion
over the whole anterior and antero-lateral abdomen. In the
flanks and epigastrium, bowel note—the physical signs of ordinary ovarian cyst. The uterus projected forwards, lay just behind the pubes, and measured two inches. Fever of septic type,
profuse sweating, and attacks of vomiting; a red blush and
œdema of the centre of the front of the belly-wall soon appeared.
The diagnosis was suppurating ovarian cyst, concurred in by
Drs. Fenwick, Ross, Roddick, Shepherd and J. C. Cameron.
Operation revealed encysted amber-colored fluid containing
flakes, and in the last portions an obvious admixture of pus. No
cyst-wall could be separated or identified. Drainage and irrigation. Immediate improvement maintained for ten days, then
return of fever and all the bad symptoms. Fœtor of discharge
from the tube. Sudden appearance of cough, with expectoration
rapidly becoming purulent and then bloody. Death six weeks
after operation. Autopsy by Dr. R. J. B. Howard revealed the
following conditions:—

" On opening abdomen a large globular mass presents, of the
size of a man's head, occupying false pelvis; this and the parietes are everywhere covered by a gray rough membrane about
one-eighth of an inch thick. The transverse colon is firmly
adherent to the upper surface, and is also bound tightly down
to the liver. A collection of pus is found below and by the side
of the spleen, and another, smaller, under left lobe of liver in
middle line. The anterior peritoneal cavity is thus converted
into a suppurating cyst, extending from liver down into true
pelvis, nearly filled by the mass, which is found to consist of all
the intestines, except the transverse colon, closely matted together by recent slight adhesions, which are studded with miliary

tubercles. The cyst wall is apparently much older than the inter-intestinal adhesions, and looks like an unhealthy granulating membrane. The walls and viscera of true pelvis are covered by the same membrane. The great omentum has quite disappeared ; but no doubt had been spread out over the intestines, and formed part of the membraue covering them. All the abdominal viscera adherent to one another and to parietes. Liver fatty ; contains a few gray granulations. Kidneys contain a few gray granulations. Lungs universally adherent ; abundantly studded with gray granulations. Tonsils and pharynx—surface gray and sloughy-looking. No loss of substance ; same appearance involves œsophagus opposite cricoid cartilage and about four inches lower down."

Case 2.—E. S., aged 30, unmarried, seamstress, was admitted to the Montreal General Hospital under the care of Dr. Richard MacDonnell. She had been ill for some time with symptoms of acute peritonitis under the care of Dr. Geo. Armstrong. The onset was very sudden, and occurred about the time of a menstrual period, the symptoms being severe abdominal pain, vomiting and marked distension. At the end of three weeks, being still very ill, the patient came to hospital by the doctor's advice. After a time the more acute symptoms had somewhat subsided, but she continued to suffer much from abdominal pain, requiring morphia in full doses, from constipation, and daily vomiting of quantities of greenish fluid. I was then asked by Dr. MacDonnell to see her. The lower part of the abdomen was distended by a nodular, uneven, elastic, insensitive gurgling mass ; not absolutely dull on percussion. By the vagina the uterus was somewhat fixed, and to the left and in front of it a firm mass could be felt. She was much emaciated. On the 14th of May, 1886, nine weeks from the onset of the symptoms, the abdomen was opened by median incision. Numerous parietal adhesions. After these were partially separated, a coil of intestine was found adherent over the surface of the firm mass. This proved to be the small intestines densely adherent to each other and to the parietes and whole pelvis. In many parts, but not universally, the peritoneum was studded with miliary tubercle.

Several coils of intestines were separated.   A drainage tube wa:
inserted and the abdomen closed by silkworm gut sutures. The
patient was greatly relieved of pain, the bowels acted naturall·
and appetite returned for a time.   On the 29th of May a fœti-
purulent discharge came from the drainage tube opening.   0
the 1st June this was bright yellow, and evidently fœcal.   Thi
became more profuse, and continued till the end.   She died ei
hausted about the end of June.

The relief of the pain and vomiting after the operation wa
most marked.   My only regret in this case was that abdomine
section was not done earlier.   In the light of experience c
similar cases on record the results might have been better.

Case 3—Is one of a different character.   Mrs. K. was sen
to me by Dr. Weagant of Dickinson's Landing, and entered m
private hospital on the 31st December, 1888.   Her age, 29
married five years : menses began at 13½, always free ; two mi
carriages during first eighteen months of married life.   A ful
term child in November 1885.   Ever since then pelvic symptom
Ten months after the birth an attack of pelvic inflammatior
Since then repeated attacks of the same nature.

On admission the patient was very fat, but anæmic ; constai
pelvic pain ; unable to walk or do anything without increase ·
pain ; menstruation quite profuse and prolonged.   Uterus pa
tially fixed, very tender.   Through the posterior cul-de-sac, fixe
tender masses to be felt.   On the 2nd January, '89, the abdom·
was opened through at least one inch of fat on the parietes, ai
the uterine appendages removed.   Both ovaries and tubes we
densely adherent.   The tubes were distended like sausage
occluded and filled with pus, their walls ulcerated on the interi
and much thickened.   The left ovary was expanded by a cy
to the size of a hen's egg.   Careful examination by Dr. Finl:
showed that the peritoneal surface of the tubes was thick
studded with miliary tubercles.   None were detected on t
intestines or parietal peritoneum, but as they were not suspecte
they were not sought.   The recovery was tedious, from the d
velopment of pelvic exudation, with pain and fever.   The ex
dation was slowly absorbed, and the patient left for home to

weeks from the date of operation. In a letter received yesterday from this patient, she tells me that until a recent attack of influenza her health had very much improved.

Case 4.—Miss L., aged 22, referred to my care by Dr. Ewing of Hawkesbury last May (1889). She gave a history of a tedious and severe attack of inflammation referred to abdomen and pelvis three years previous. Ever since she has been in poor health ; an invalid most of the time.

On admission to hospital she was weak, had a rapid pulse, cold extremities, anorexia, dyspepsia, insomnia. The abdomen was hard, tender, somewhat distended, but without evidence of tumor or of liquid effusion. She complained of almost constant pain referred to the abdomen and pelvis. Uterus fixed ; behind and to its sides fixed tender masses in the region of the uterine appendages. Her temperature on the evening of her admission was 102°. She was kept in bed under observation for a month, and treated generally by nutritive and general tonics, as well as by local measures, chiefly iodine to the roof of the vagina, but without avail. She continued to suffer and seemed to lose ground. No fever. On the 15th June, '89, the abdomen was opened. The parietal peritoneum was adherent to the omentum underneath, so that there was some difficulty in recognizing the line of adhesion and getting in to the cavity of the abdomen. When this was discovered, the omentum and intestines were found to be matted together. Everything within reach was studded thickly with tubercle. Nothing further was done. The belly was closed without drainage. The recovery from the operation was tedious, but free from important events of any kind. At the end of between three and four weeks she was taken home to die, as I then believed. I heard nothing more from her till October, when in a letter Dr. Ewing wrote me with a case of ovarian tumor he then sent me he said " our patient, Miss L., is very much better. She eats, digests, and sleeps well, and is able to walk and drive a great deal.

Case 5 (still under observation) is that of a lady from Moosomin, referred by Dr. Rutledge of that town. She is 26 years old, married four years. Has been pregnant three times, twice to full term, and had an early miscarriage on the 18th August last. She has always been somewhat delicate. No tubercular family history is to be had. She is of very fair complexion, transparent skin ; very slight causes bring a deep blush to the cheeks. Menstruation has never at any time in her life been regular, the intervals much prolonged. Ever since the birth of her first child she has had pelvic symptoms. The present illness began at the time of the miscarriage, which was followed by symptoms of inflammation in the pelvis and fever. She has been an invalid ever since, suffering from pelvic and abdominal pain ; menses at long intervals, but prolonged and profuse.

Present symptoms.—Pain in groins, especially left, extending to left loin and corresponding thigh, and occasionally across the abdomen. Is menstruating (the flow continued for nearly a fortnight). The morning action of the bowels preceded by pain in lower part of back. Tendency to slight evening rise of temperature and to perspiration after meals, rarely at night. Appetite and digestion good, although patient is thin. The abdomen is not distended, but slightly hard, scarcely tender. By the vagina, the uterus bulky, retroverted and fixed ; the cervix deeply lacerated, much thickened and everted. To its left and behind, closely adherent, lay a mass, rounded and very tender, but somewhat movable.

The diagnosis was inflammatory, probably suppurative, disease of the appendages. She was kept in bed for six weeks and subjected to suitable local treatment, with some temporary improvement in symptoms. The pelvic mass on the left side seemed, however, to become larger and more tender. I therefore decided to open the abdomen. This was done on the 2nd Jan'y, 1890. Immediately on getting through the abdominal wall, which was not adherent to the contents of the belly, the condition was apparent. Everything that could be seen through the 1½-inch incision, and everything that could be felt, was thickly studded with miliary tubercle. No fluid effusion existed. The omentum lay adherent over the intestines, and was adherent to the brim of the pelvis. Beneath it everything was matted together. Nothing was further disturbed. The incision was immediately closed.   For the first few days she was a good deal distressed by belching and occasional vomiting, with some pain and fever. These symptoms subsided by the end of the second week ; since then recovery has been rapid.   Now she is up a good part of each day, eats well, sleeps well, and is practically free from pain. The temperature shows at times a tendency to slight rise.   On the 25th February the patient left my hospital for a trip to the South.   She was then entirely free from symptoms.   Menstruation had not returned.

These five cases constitute the whole of my experience of operation in tuberculosis of the peritoneum and uterine appendages. It will be seen that they present considerable variety, so far as physical conditions are concerned.   *Case No.* 1, with large fluid effusion, simulated ovarian tumor.   In *Case* 2, while there was marked abdominal enlargement, there was no fluid effusion ; the apparent tumor was composed of an aggregation of adherent intestines and omentum with disseminated tubercle.   *Case* 3 presented no evidences of adherent intestines or omentum.   The adhesions existed only about the ovaries and distended Fallopian tubes.   The evidences of tubercle existed only on the Fallopian tubes, or rather were discovered on these organs only after the abdomen was closed.   I feel justified, however, in concluding that if tubercle existed on the general peritoneum, it was so to a very slight extent indeed.   *Cases* 4 and 5 are of the same character, and presented very similar histories and physical signs, namely, of inflammatory disease of the uterine appendages, with, however, much more than the usual amount of impaired nutrition.

I wish to draw especial attention to these last three.   All, especially *Case* 5, following abortion, present histories which show that the first clear evidences of disease were those of pelvic inflammation.   In each the physical signs of diseased appendages were unmistakably well marked.   In *Case* 3 the parts removed were typical examples of pyosalpinx.   It is to be presumed that in *Cases* 4 and 5, if the operation had been completed to their extirpation, equally well-marked conditions would have been disclosed.

Certain prominent German physicians attribute great importance to the pre-existence of a cheesy mass or degeneration somewhere in the body as the real parent of tubercles wherever they appear. The interest and importance of histories, such as those of the last three cases I have related, is, in this connection, surely most obvious. Presuming the theory to be well founded, the primary disease of the appendages was in these cases the parent of the tuberculosis of the peritoneum. In *Case* 3 the tuberculous pus-distended Fallopian tubes may with some, and I think, good reason be regarded as the commencement of a process that would ultimately have extended to the general peritoneum. The whole subject is still obscure. Concurrent observation by the physician, the pathologist, and, I add with some confidence, the gynæcologist will do much to elucidate the question. Meanwhile it may fairly be claimed that the evidence we already possess in support of the theory justifies us in claiming an additional argument for the early removal of the parent condition before opportunity for bringing forth its evil progeny.

I here anticipate a question with reference to *Cases* 4 and 5. Why not complete the operation as intended, and proceed to remove the diseased structures? I reply that in a considerable number of similarly incomplete, merely exploratory operations, the results have been good, some of the patients surviving with fairly good or very good health indefinitely. The extension of abdominal surgery to the removal of diseased uterine appendages is not yet, however, so old an operation as to justify us in speaking now with too great a degree of confidence. Further, completion of the operation in the presence of universal adhesions and general fusion of structures must have been a formidable procedure. The hemorrhage would have been such that the drainage-tube must have been a necessity under most unfavorable conditions from the presence of general tuberculosis of the structures involved. Prolonged suppuration from the track of the tube must almost of necessity have resulted.

Greig Smith has well remarked that the surgical treatment of tubercular peritonitis has been stumbled on by accident rather than carried out by design. The earlier cases were undertaken on a mistaken diagnosis of ovarian tumor or similar condition.

Many of these cases were found to recover, so that in recent years operation is often deliberately undertaken in cases suspected to be tubercular peritonitis.

Kuemmell of Hamburg has collected thirty such cases, beginning with one by Spencer Wells so long ago as 1862. Of these, only two died directly from the operation, while three died from general tuberculosis in from five to twelve months after operation. Altogether of Kuemmell's collection of cases, there were twenty-five cures of from nine months to twenty-five years duration. No doubt, however, many fatal cases are unreported.

Abdominal section for cases similar to *Cases* 3, 4 and 5 of my collection are much more recent, because of the comparatively recent extension of abdominal surgery to the extirpation of diseased uterine appendages. But the result has been, to say the least, equally encouraging as in the cases of encysted collections of fluid simulating ovarian tumor. Mr. Greig Smith has recently suggested a modification of the treatment hitherto adopted in abdominal section for suppurative peritonitis. It consists in keeping the intestines floating in warm aseptic or antiseptic fluid for several days. The solution he prefers is an ounce of boroglyceride to a pint of hot water. This is run in through the drainage-tube several times a day, and kept there by corking the tube. So far he claims encouraging results.

I may here anticipate an objection of some weight that the diagnosis of my cases is not complete, as the bacillus of tubercle was not sought for. I regret this, and in future cases hope to remove this objection. At the same time the naked eye evidences taken with the symptoms were such as to leave little, if any, room for doubt as to the condition I claim to have been present. On this point, as on all others, I invite discussion, and a presentation of evidence of the existence of conditions which to the naked eye simulate genuine tubercle.

I venture to submit the following conclusions :—

1. The hitherto accepted universally fatal prognosis of tubercular peritonitis must, as a result of what we have learnt by abdominal section, be revised. It is certain that recovery has taken place in many cases after abdominal section and probably in others not so treated.

2. My cases 4, 5 and 6 afford some evidence in favor of theory that a cheesy deposit, the result of suppuration, is parent of tubercle wherever found.

3. In these cases the origin was in the suppurative disease the appendages.

4. The early removal of such focus is urgent in certain subjects strongly predisposed to tubercle when other indications may not be strong enough to justify it.

5. Abdominal section in these, as in less serious conditions, has with proper precautions been as an operation recovered from in such a large proportion of cases as to amply justify its performance to clear up a doubtful case.

6. A mass of evidence has accumulated in favor of the beneficial effects of abdominal section in tubercular peritonitis such as it is difficult to resist.

THE LOCAL ASPECTS OF THE PRESENT PNEUMONIA EPIDEMIC.

By J. L. Irwin, M.D., C.M., Chicago.

It is curious to note that, whilst reporters seem to have been scattered broadcast amongst the physicians of the city, by editors, and have created much nervousness and apprehension by their vivid depictions of the spread of the current disease, none of them seem to have sought information as to its domestic treatment whenever they found their medical quarry at his house, possibly nursing himself through an attack. Indeed, few medical men seem to have utterly escaped the grasp of *la grippe;* and those who have done so and have been interviewed, appear to have confined themselves to generalities rather than imparting to interrogators the gist of any special treatment. It is true that to do so has been denounced as unprofessional; but medical ethics vary very much with locality. *Why* it should be wrong for a physician in Chicago to give his views as to the medical treatment of a disease in the daily newspapers, and right for another to brag in a *medical summary* for December that " he does not dread diphtheria more than a bad cold," further setting forth his treatment of it with chlorate of potash and tincture of veratrum, sublimed (?) sulphur and kerosene oil, is difficult to understand; or why papayotin, on the dictum of Jacobi and Dr. Baudry, should have suddenly sprung into fashion for dissolving the diphtheric membrane.

Another curious thing is the disinclination of the health commissioner to ever speak of the connection of influenza and pneumonia with cholera; whereas the fact that it has either preceded or followed that scourge of nations in nearly every instance is established by the report of the Registrar-General of England of January 30th, 1848. It broke out in Paris in 1847 (where 5,000 people died of la grippe) and spread to Madrid, England and Scotland. Fog and rain hung over London. The temperature ran from two to seven above normal, and in six weeks 11,339 people died in that city alone of influenza. It preceded "the black death" in the fourteenth century and the great plague in 1665; also the epidemic of cholera and typhoid fever in 1728-62-67-75-82-88, and 1803 31-42-43-46-47. No part of the world was exempt from it. It travelled from Russia to Ireland, thence to New York, and then swept the States from the lakes to the Gulf. In all cases, it seems to have been preceded by atmospheric vicissitudes, whether in the cold regions of Northern China or Siberian Steppes, or the heats of Peru, Central America and the Antilles. The Cape of Good Hope and Sydney were ravaged, and it did not even spare the English and Dutch ships upon the high seas. In France it was called " coqueluche" (a monk's cowl), from the fact that patients' heads were tied up in caps to exclude air. " Sheep-cough," " the frolicsome," were other names, and the " influence," from its supposed origination in the atmosphere. In Vienna it was believed to be due to an insect swallowed with water.

The original Parisian " grippe" developed symptoms of coryza, cough, sniffing, dyspnœa, aggravated by each paroxysm, fatigue of the limbs and general prostration. Even to the present day has come down the custom instituted on its appearance at Rome by Pope Pelagius II., in A.D. 590, when " the air being impregnated with fœtid vapor, it was customary to ejaculate ' Dominus Tecum ' if a friend sneezed."

The symptoms of modern influenza are well known—malaise, fever, irregular pulse, catarrh of the respiratory and gastro-intestinal tracts, prostration, intense headache, pains in the limbs and distressed expression of the countenance. These, however, usually yield to rest and warmth, stimulating expectorants, tonics, and steam inhalations. The great danger of influenza seems to lie rather in its sequels than in the disease itself. It was formerly believed that influenza predisposed to galloping consumption. We know that it does to bronchitis and pneumonia, and our late daily Chicago reports show the deaths from the latter to be in the ratio of seven from pneumonia to one from influenza. But whether the latter is the genuine Muscovite article is still a matter of controversy.

It is incidentally noteworthy that a disease closely resembling influenza has proven very fatal to cats in this city of late, just as in former years it has attacked cattle, horses, sheep and poultry.

In the *Lancet* of Dec. 28th, 1889, Dr. Bernard O'Connor recommends that the patient be laid on his back and Weaver's powdered periodate crystals dropped in the nostrils and sniffed up. "This," he says, "is the most powerful antiseptic ever used; but it can be swallowed without risk." That paper also casually reports that dengue fever had appeared in a crushing-mill at Edinburgh, where oil-cakes is made from cotton-seed brought from Alexandria, Egypt. Whether this and the Russian influenza are one and the same disease is being warmly discussed by *Le Progrès Médical*, *La Gazette Médicale*, and other Parisian journals.

A curious book, now being revived in London, is Dr. Theophilus Thompson, F.R.S., on the " Annals of Influenza." In it (writing in 1851) he prophetically asserts that epidemics are produced by vegetable germs borne upon the wind, and calls especial attention to the disturbed condition of animal and vegetable life recorded during influenza years. Peculiar seasons recur in cycles : these are associated with recurring developments in the lower forms of life and consequent disordered condition of the health of man. " Is it unreasonable," he asks, " to imagine that some fluctuations in the health of man may have reference to the stage in the condition of some of the despised and even invisible classes of the lower creation ?'' Whether or no, those who help to put together the puzzle of life, and show the exact relations existing between the germs of disease and the environments which determine their growth and distinction, will be the world's benefactors. It is noteworthy that heavy fogs are usually present in influenza epidemics.

Amongst the London physicians who have written this month, Dr. W. Gordon Hogg pins his faith to antipyrine and aconite to relieve muscular pains, with iron and bromide of quinine. He finds spray and inhalations unsuccessful, and that patients " prefer to cough" rather than take opiates. He keeps the head and back of the neck wrapped up in a warm shawl fastened under the chin.

Dr. Horace Dobell says, in the *British Medical Journal*, that he trusts to an inhalation of creosote ʒi, olei caryph. ʒi, olei eucalypt. glob. ʒi, tr. camph. co. ʒii ; a teaspoonful in boiling water to be inhaled for fifteen minutes and repeated every two hours, during which interval gargle with hot water. After the first inhalation a febrifuge of sp. camph., sp. æth. nit., tr. quin. amm. ; with gr. v of antifebrin every hour till the temperature falls to 100°F.

The *Boston Medical and Surgical Journal* points out the importance of observation bearing upon the contagiousness of influenza, and upon relapse, recurrence, remission and second attacks, and advances the theory that the poison is a microphyte multiplying in the air and travelling against the course of the winds. It also notes (Jan. 2nd, 1890) that a case occurred in the middle of December on a steamer in the midst of the Pacific Ocean, and that the disease had developed in Boston before it was reported in London. It also seems that the American squadron picked it up in crossing the Atlantic, and that the *Chicago* alone had 180 cases of the disease on board on January 17th, 1890. The *Record's* account of the treatment at the New York Dispensary shows that it consists of calomel, followed by ꞓ. Dover powder and 10 gr. quinine, morphine, belladonna, camphor and quinine being given if the catarrhal symptoms become marked, expectorants where bronchitis is prominent, and antipyrine and whiskey for frontal headache.

It now becomes necessary to consider for a while the nature of that catarrhal pneumonia apt to occur after an attack of infectious diseases, combined with bronchial catarrh. Anything which develops the latter favors the genesis of the former ; but the extremes of life—childhood and old age—are the most susceptible. After the symptoms of the disease are fairly defined, the bronchial cough ceases to occur in long paroxysms, the patient becomes restless and capricious, the breathing becomes superficial, and the patient becomes drowsy and apathetic. Jürgensen, of Tubingen, finds the disease in the middle-aged chiefly in connection with diphtheria, but less liable to develop rapidly than the pneumonia set up by inhaling irritating gases, in which case dissection shows that the lung has simply collapsed. The disease has no regular type of fever. In the event of recovery, the lungs, heart and intestines appear to become peculiarly vulnerable to other diseases ; the mortality has varied from 48 to 66 per cent. of those seized. Virchow first wrote on pneumonia from embolism : that is, the migration of solid bodies into the pulmonary artery, such as blood-clots which have originated in the general circulation and found their way to the right side of the heart, closing the artery and arresting the circulation leading to the lung. Then supervenes difficulty of breathing, as the interchange of gases stops within the disturbed lung, occasional fever, and chills. The local symptoms are : the expectoration of blood and tenacious mucus, cough and pain in the side, and physical signs of consolidation. The prognosis generally depends more upon the primary disease than the accident of embolism ; but is generally unfavorable, except the healing force of nature join to aid the physician. It is curious that external violence does not appear to excite pneumonia, but grains of wheat or beards of barley frequently set it up in farm hands by finding their way into the bronchi, when gangrene of the lung is apt to supervene, or the breathing into the air-vesicles of the secretions of the bronchial tubes in diphtheria and bronchitis.

Pneumonia is a not uncommon complication in cases of acute rheumatism, albuminuria, and phthisis.

Monsieur H. Huchard, writing to the *Revue de Chim. et de Therap.*, speaks of nervous prostration as being the chief clinical characteristic of severe cases of influenza, requiring for its treatment quinine, alcohol, and, in bad cases, even injections of caffein and ether. Quinine, he says, is indicated on account of the markedly remittent type of fever, and to moderate the evening exacerbation it suffices to give a full dose (5 to 15 grains) of the sulphate or hydrobromate in the morning. Smaller doses more frequently taken are useful for their tonic rather than their antiseptic effect. In the neuralgic or rheumatoid form of influenza antipyrine (15 grains) combined with bicarbonate of soda (7½ grains) is recommended by Mons. Huchard to be taken every four hours; or, instead of antipyrine, phenacetine or salol 7 grains. Influenza often assumes a broncho-pulmonary form, and in certain cases is very grave. In the epidemic of la grippe in 1886, recorded by M. Mentrier, the pneumonia forms were very asthenic. In such cases tonics, milk, alcohol, and, in fact, general restorative measures are indicated rather than local appliances to the chest. If the dyspnœa becomes severe and the condition termed " pulmonary paralysis" ensues, then strychnia is of value; or in case of impending asphyxia, venesection; but when asthenia itself threatens life, there should be no hesitation in resorting to hypodermic injections of ether and especially of caffein. For the gastro-intestinal form, mild aperients, ipecacuanha and the use of salicylates of bismuth or of magnesia, naphthol or iodoform to promote intestinal antisepsis are indicated.

In this country, exalgine, antipyrine, phenacetine, antifebrine and other comparatively new remedies have been tried with more or less success, but the fact remains that prescribing for pneumonia is no more an exact science than any other branch of medicine. We can only hope that change of weather will mitigate the severity of the outbreak of influenza, and that a few days of equable atmosphere and febrifuge treatment will pull a patient through the malady without leaving him prostrated or subject to the more serious trouble of lung, chest and throat complaints. Meanwhile let every American practitioner do his best and record his experiences promptly for the public weal, as his fellows at Vienna, Paris and London have already sought to do. Every case will vary somewhat in its symptomatology, and according to its characteristics the remedies exhibited must be varied alike in nature and quantity, and close watch kept to prevent any epidemic analagous to those which history tells us have already appeared in the train of similar troubles.

A CASE OF ATAXIA IN A CHILD TWELVE YEARS OF AGE.

By A. D. BLACKADER, B.A., M.D.,

Instructor in Diseases of Children, McGill University ; Assistant Physician, Montreal General Hospital.

William Jacotel, aged 12 years, is the second of a family of ten children, of whom seven are now dead. Four of these died during an epidemic of diphtheria in 1885 : the eldest, a lad of 10 years ; the fourth, a lad of 5 years ; the fifth, a lad of nearly 4 years ; and the sixth, of a little more than 2 years. All of these were said to have been in good health, strong and active, before attacked by diphtheria. The seventh, a child of 3 years, died six months ago from scarlet fever. The third, an infant of nine months, is said to have succumbed to an attack of erysipelas in 1879. And this summer, the youngest, an infant two months old, was carried off by diarrhœa. The three survivors are William, of whom we are now speaking, a girl of nearly 4 years, and an infant 16 months old. Both the younger children are at present in good health, with no impairment of the knee-jerk, and no apparent loss of power in the lower limbs.

Both father and mother are said to be in fair health at present. On neither side is there any history obtainable of any relative who suffered from an impairment of gait due to nervous disease. They all appear to have reached a good old age. There is no history either of any special neurosis, syphilis, or tuberculosis. The father and mother are not blood relatives. The father occasionally indulges in alcohol to excess.

William is said to have been quiet as a baby ; was nursed till the tenth month, but was late over teething. There is no history of any convulsions, but as an infant of two years he had a fall, cutting the front of his forehead. This has left a distinct scar involving the bone, still quite discernible on the top of the forehead, a little to the right of the median line. Since the age of five years he has suffered severely from headaches resembling those of migraine. They are described as lasting three or four hours, and as being generally on the same side of the head as the scar ; they were usually associated with vomiting, and passed off during a night's sleep. They recurred somewhat regularly three or four times a month, but were induced by any excitement. Although still recurring occasionally, they are much less severe than formerly. The first distinct symptom of the present illness was noticed six years ago as an unsteadiness in his gait, producing occasional falls, and the lad was in consequence pronounced, by a physician who saw him, to be suffering from St. Vitus's dance. This weakness and staggering gait have gradually become worse, and for this he was brought to the out-patient department of the Montreal General Hospital last June. The strictest inquiry does not elicit any history of true lightning pains. Two or three years ago his mother first noticed some alteration in his speech, and this also has gradually become more marked.

At present he is a fairly-nourished lad, four feet five inches tall, weighs eighty-five pounds, with distinct talipes equinus in both feet and slight curvature in the spine. There is a well-marked ataxic gait. In walking, the body sways from side to side, the legs are widely separated, and the feet are thrown forward. On standing the feet are kept much apart. If placed together there is much swaying of the body, which is only slightly increased by closing the eyes. A very fair attempt is made at walking backward. There is also distinct ataxia in the upper extremities, though much less marked than in the lower. If asked to touch his nose or tip of the ear with his finger quickly, he is generally an inch or two at fault ; but he makes a fair attempt at picking up a pin, even with his eyes closed. There is complete absence of patellar reflex, but the cutaneous reflexes

Retrospect Department.

QUARTERLY RETROSPECT OF SURGERY.

BY FRANCIS J. SHEPHERD, M.D., C.M., M.R.C.S., ETC.

Surgeon to the Montreal General Hospital; Professor of Anatomy and Lecturer on
Operative Surgery, McGill University.

Operative Treatment of Enlarged Prostate.—The treatment of enlargement of the prostate is a problem which constantly presents itself to every surgeon, and so far its solution is not the most satisfactory. In a certain proportion of cases the judicious use of the catheter yields fairly good results, but in many of these cases a day comes when even the friendly catheter cannot be depended upon, and something else has to be tried. Cystitis or other accident may intervene, and to obtain relief operative measures are undertaken. The simplest operation is perineal section, and marked relief is often afforded, but very frequently this relief is only temporary. When the cause of the obstruction to the outflow of urine is hypertrophy of the prostate, no procedure which does not aim at removing this cause will prove of any permanent benefit. At the meeting of the British Medical Association held at Leeds in August last, Mr. McGill opened a discussion on " The Retention of Urine from Prostatic Enlarge- ment " (*British Medical Journal*, Oct. 19, 1889). His paper was based on twenty-four operations of prostatectomy through a suprapubic incision, performed by various surgeons at the Leeds Infirmary. He submitted and discussed the following proposi- tions :—

(1) The prostatic enlargements which give rise to urinary symptoms are intravesical and not rectal.   /

(2) The retention is caused by a valve-like action of the intra- vesical prostate, the urethral orifice being closed more or less completely by the contraction of the bladder and its contents.

(3) That in many cases self-catheterism is the only treatment required.

(4) When the catheter treatment fails, or is unavailable, more radical measures are necessary. He states his belief that a large proportion of cases treated by catheter sooner or later

Cerebellar disease would appear to be excluded by the history of the case, the absence of occipital pain, the absence of optic neuritis, the absence of the patellar reflex, and the presence of the ataxia in the upper extremities. The age of the lad (six years) when symptoms of ataxia were first noticed, the impairment of speech, the absence of lightning pains, of any alteration in the pupillary reflexes, would oppose its being classed as a case of true tabes.

The possibility of insular sclerosis, occurring with somewhat similar symptoms, must not be forgotten; but in my patient this appears to be excluded by the history of the case, by the absence of any paresis or spastic rigidity, and by the absence of any eye symptoms. It differs from most of the recorded cases of Friedreich's disease, in the absence of any other known case occurring in the family, in the history of previous migraine, and in the presence of symptoms indicating some paresis of the bladder.

Retrospect Department.

QUARTERLY RETROSPECT OF SURGERY.

By Francis J. Shepherd, M.D., C.M., M.R.C.S., Eng.

Surgeon to the Montreal General Hospital; Professor of Anatomy and Lecturer on
Operative Surgery, McGill University.

Operative Treatment of Enlarged Prostate.—The treatment
of enlargement of the prostate is a problem which constantly
presents itself to every surgeon, and so far its solution is not the
most satisfactory.   In a certain proportion of cases the judicious
use of the catheter yields fairly good results, but in many   of
these cases a day comes when even the friendly catheter cannot
be depended upon, and something else has to be tried.   Cystitis
or other accident may intervene, and to obtain relief operative
measures are undertaken.   The simplest operation is perineal
section, and marked relief is often afforded, but very frequently
this relief is only temporary.   When the cause of the obstruction
to the outflow of urine is hypertrophy of the prostate, no procedure which does not aim at removing this cause will prove of
any permanent benefit.   At the meeting of the British Medical
Association held at Leeds in August last, Mr. McGill opened a
discussion on " The Retention of Urine from Prostatic Enlargement " (*British Medical Journal*, Oct. 19, 1889).   His paper
was based on twenty-four operations of prostatectomy through a
suprapubic incision, performed by various surgeons at the Leeds
Infirmary.   He submitted and discussed the following propositions :—

(1) The prostatic enlargements which give rise to urinary
symptoms are intravesical and not rectal.

(2) The retention is caused by a valve-like action of the intravesical prostate, the urethral orifice being closed more or less
completely by the contraction of the bladder and its contents.

(3) That in many cases self-catheterism is the only treatment
required.

(4) When the catheter treatment fails, or is unavailable, more
radical measures are necessary.   He states his belief that a
large proportion of cases treated by catheter sooner or later

break down, the urine becomes ammoniacal, the desire to mic-turate continues, and the catheter only relieves for a few minutes at a time. The greatest care does not always prevent this result, nor does the greatest carelessness always induce it. In other cases the patient cannot be taught to pass the catheter himself, and the constant attendance of a surgeon is impracticable. Now the radical measures recommended by McGill are as follows:

(5) Drain the bladder thoroughly for a time and permanently remove the cause of obstruction; the intravesical prostatic growth must be removed.

(6) These two indications are best fulfilled by a supra-pubic rather than by a urethral or perineal operation. Out of 24 cases operated on in the Leeds Infirmary, 8 remain permanently well. There were 4 deaths—1 due to shock, 2 due to shock and hemorrhage, and 1 to retro-pubic suppuration. All the cases were men between 60 and 70; almost all were in a bad state of health, and could not have lived long unless relieved. In seven cases the operation was undertaken for the removal of stone, and prostatectomy was incidental, excluding these and the four cases of death, also one lost sight of and two still under observation, leaves ten still to be accounted for. Eight of these remain permanently well, one only having to use the catheter occasionally; in one case the operation was not satisfactorily completed and no relief was obtained; in the tenth case relief was for a time obtained, but he relapsed and died ten months after operation.

In the discussion which followed, Mr. Bruce Clarke advocated first making a perineal incision and examining the bladder, and seeing what needed to be done, and afterwards to perform supra-pubic cystotomy.

Dr. Kummell of Hamburg has also written on this subject. He reports six cases operated on; the operations were done on severe cases, in which the various ordinary means had been used a long time. He had recourse to suprapubic cystotomy. He extir-pated not only the median lobe, but all portions of the prostate projecting into the bladder. He operates by opening the bladder by a suprapubic incision; uses sponges and iodoform gauze for plugging. The projecting parts of the prostate he seizes with a forceps, burns off what impedes the passage with the galvano-cautery loop or Paquelin's cautery. If necessary the neck of the bladder is dilated and as large a catheter as possible introduced; in a few days it is possible to introduce the thickest catheters. By this time suture of the bladder can be undertaken. The patient should be got about as soon as possible to avoid the dreaded hypostatic pneumonia. He uses continuous catgut suture and removes catheter in eighteen days. One out of the six cases died of broncho-pneumonia the eighteenth day after operation. In his cases Kummell does not claim that the results were so perfect that the after use of the catheter was not needed, but the patient's condition was so serious that in many cases the operation was a life-saving one. He recommends the procedure in those cases where there is nothing to lose, but everything to gain.—(*Eighteenth German Surgical Congres. Centralblatt f. Chir.*, No. 29, 1889, and *Annals of Surgery*, Dec. 1889.)

SURGERY OF THE KIDNEY.

Removal of Kidney.—Schede of Hamburg, at a meeting held in July, 1888, read a paper on twenty cases of extirpation of the kidney. Eleven cases were cured, two improved, and seven died within the first few days after operation, some being operated on under the most unfavorable circumstances. Schede's mortality is only 35 per cent. This is an improvement on that given by Gross in 1885 of 44.6 per cent. Schede uses the lumbar incision, and thinks that the future mortality in this operation will be much lessened.—(*Deutsch. Medicin. Woch.*, No. 52, 1888.)

Nephrectomy in a case of Horse-shoe Kidney where one-half was affected with Hydronephrosis.—In the *Annales des Maladies des Organes Génito-Urinaires* for June last, M. Vignard gives a translation of Prof. Socin's (Basle) paper on the above. A woman, 47 years of age, was admitted into the hospital with symptoms of intermittent hydronephrosis of the right side, severe colic, and vomiting. The diagnosis was not easily made out, for Professor Socin was not clear whether the tumor might not be connected with the mesentery or the pancreas. However, the tumor was aspirated and about 500 cubic centimetres of urinous fluid removed. A urinary fistula remained, which transmitted purulent urine, while the bladder contained healthy urine. A further operation was undertaken in May 1888, at the patient's request. The abdominal incision was made to the outer side of the rectus muscle and the vascular pedicle of the right kidney ligatured, and it only remained to free the lower end of the kidney when it was discovered that it was prolonged by a sort of bridge four centimetres wide across the vena cava and aorta to the opposite kidney, forming thus a horse-shoe kidney. The isthmus was found to be only slightly connected with the front of the vessels, and he therefore divided it by means of a thermo-cautery. Five ligatures proved to be enough to arrest all hemorrhage from the divided surface, the capsule was sewed as a flap over the cauterized surface, and the operation was completed by a lumbo-abdominal drain. The progress was excellent. The urine was albuminous and bloody for a few days only. The patient went out well twenty-five days after the operation. She was seen four months later in good health, with good color, and able to work.

Braun of Heidelberg has reported a somewhat similar case, and the fact that a horse-shoe kidney existed was only made out during the operation for pyonephrosis. The adhesions between the vena cava and the isthmus were so close that hemorrhage occurred, and the patient died at the finish of the operation. Braun, therefore, came to the conclusion that the existence of a horse-shoe kidney was an absolute contra-indication to operation. Socin's case, however, shows this conclusion to be incorrect. The diagnosis is impossible before operation, and the surgeon must treat the case as occasion demands.—(*London Medical Recorder*, Aug. 1889.)

Horse-shoe kidney is comparatively rare. According to Prof. Roth of Basle it occurred five times in 1630 autopsies (1 in 826). I have seen three in my experience, which is not inconsiderable. Normally they have no attachment to the vena cava and aorta, and in Braun's case the adhesions must have

been due to the inflammatory action produced by the pyonephrosis. No doubt in these cases the operation is almost nec es-
sarily a fatal one, but in cases such as Socin's there is no good
reason why success should not follow operation. In some cases
the isthmus is much longer and thicker than others. Prof.
Gruber describes two cases in which the isthmus was membrano-
only. Anomalies of kidneys should be familiar to surgeons. A
not uncommon one is the displacement of one or both organs.
I saw a case last year where the left kidney was situated between
the two common iliac arteries. The hilus was anterior and the
kidney was disc-shaped. It must be also borne in mind that the
kidney may be single. I have seen only one example of this
anomaly.

Renal Surgery at the British Medical Association.—At the
last meeting of the British Medical Association a most interesting discussion took place on renal surgery (*Brit. Medical Jour.*,
Nov. 16th, 1889). It was opened by Mr. Henry Morris, who
drew attention to the following points: (1) The various ways in
which renal calculi are imbedded in the kidney require special
precautions whilst operating. (Mr. Morris is of opinion that
nothing short of a digital exploration of the pelvis and calyces
of the kidney will suffice to discover stone in some cases.)

(2) Tubercle of the kidney, as well as suppurating foci due
to other causes, may give rise to the same tactile sensations as
small calculi.

(3) Tubercular disease of the prostate is a source of fallacy
in diagnosing renal calculi. It is well known that pain may be
transferred to the renal region from disease of the lower urinary
tract; and if there be, in addition, a small amount of pus and
blood in the urine, and no cystitis, the diagnosis is much complicated.

(4) Nephrectomy is of very doubtful value in advanced tubercular renal disease.

(5) Lumbar nephrectomy is the proper treatment for advanced
hydronephrosis, and for large collections of fluid behind the peritoneum, the result of lacerated kidney.

(6) Nephrorrhaphy for movable kidney is of great service.

(7) The changes which the perinephric tissue undergoes, under long continued irritation, sometimes render the search for the kidney very tedious, and, maybe, ineffectual.

Mr. Bennett May had operated on 15 patients for stone or suspected stone—12 males and 3 females. In 13 cases he found a stone and in 2 he did not. In fully half the cases the stone was fixed in the parenchyma of the kidney. These stones, mostly of slow growth, are circular or pyramidal in shape, not branched, and occur in young males. The kidney remains perfectly healthy even in a late stage of the disease. The prominent symptom in these cases is pain, and the main diagnostic test is pain on deep local pressure beneath the last rib. Pus is commonly absent, and traces of blood may be found with the microscope after exercise, The stones are difficult to find, but when removed, give most perfect results. Should the surgeon fail to find the stone by acupuncture, then the kidney should be cut into and explored with the finger and sound. Stones in the pelvis of the kidney commonly grow much more quickly and to a larger size. Pus appears early and is a prominent symptom, and the kidney soon undergoes structural changes, ending in pyonephrosis. These stones are usually easy to find, and the recovery is apt to be imperfect.

Mr. David Newman of Glasgow contrasted the results of nephro-lithotomies with or without suppuration of the kidney. Of the former, of 60 cases, 34 recovered and 26 died (43.3 per cent.) ; of the latter, where there was no suppuration, of 42 cases not one died. This indicates the importance of early diagnosis. In cases of hemorrhage, catheterization of the ureters and estimation of quantity of albumen and hæmoglobin in the urine may aid one in determining the seat of the hemorrhage and ascertaining whether the disease is confined to one kidney. Mr. Newman said that in renal surgery, the condition with which he was most familiar was movable kidney. Out of 27 cases he had met with in private and hospital practice only seven needed operative interference. In the great majority of cases the application of a well-fitting elastic bandage with an air pad was sufficient. When performing nephrorrhaphy, Mr. Newman, in addi-

tion to stitching the kidney to the abdominal parietes, splits th
fibrous capsule and separates it from the surface of the kidney
as it is of little use to stitch the adipose capsule, because it is s
loose.

Mr. Lawson Tait said his first contribution to renal surger
was made in July 1884, though his first operation on the kidne
was performed in April 1874. He gave a list of seventy-fou
operations performed by himself on the kidney with six deaths
The cases were as follows:

Simple exploratory incisions, 4.

Nephrotomy, 44 cases with one death.

Nephrectomy, 22 cases with four deaths.

Incomplete operation, 1 case with one death.

Nephrorrhaphy, 3 cases with no deaths.

Among the nephrotomies 14 were for stone, and of these one
died. He strongly advocated preliminary nephrotomy in doubtful cases; it will save many organs from removal, and make a
subsequent nephrectomy far less risky. Mr. Tait strongly condemns the operation of nephrorrhaphy and will have nothing
more to do with it. One of the three patients operated on has
subsequently died under circumstances for which he thinks the
operation might be blamed. He does not think it matters much
how the kidney is reached. Mr. Tait has several times opened
the abdomen expecting to find ovarian tumors, and has found
soft cancers of the kidney. The conclusions he draws from his
experience are that all tumors of the kidney, all suppurating
kidneys, and all kidneys with persistent, incurable, and unbearable pain in them, should be exposed by incision, laid open and
thoroughly explored by the finger-tip. Stones may then be removed, abscesses drained, and hydatid or cystic growths removed
with trifling risk. He also said that mere exploration in some
cases of tumors leads in a mysterious way to a cure.

Mr. Bruce Clark related an interesting case where, failing to
find stone by needle puncture, he closed the wound. The patient,
not being relieved, returned again. The kidney was again explored, this time by the finger, but no stone found, so the kidney
was excised, and on examining it a small, sharp stone, the size

of a pea, was found hidden away in one of the recesses of the
organ. He advocated the removal of large diseased kidneys by
the anterior incision.

Mr. Kendall Franks of Dublin called attention to a class of
cases which were not uncommon, viz., those in which the diagnosis of renal calculus was almost certain, and in which the
symptoms clearly indicated the affected side, and yet in which,
when the kidney was exposed, the most careful digital manipulation and the most systematic exploration with a long needle
failed to detect the presence of a stone. In such cases formerly
the wound was closed, or, as Mr. Morris had done, the organ
was excised. Mr. Franks advocated incising the kidney *in situ*
and searching for the stone systematically with the finger. Mr.
Franks laid stress upon the importance of leaving the wound in
the kidney to granulate without using any means to close it. He
advocated excision in cases of tubercular disease of the kidney.

Nephro-Lithotomy.—Mr. H. A. Jacobson, in some clinical
remarks delivered at Guy's Hospital (*British Medical Journal*,
Jan. 18, 1890) on the *Symptoms and Conditions which justify
Nephro-Lithotomy*, makes remarks on the following symptoms :
(1) Continued hæmaturia or passage of blood and pus ; (2) pain
or tenderness in the loin and elsewhere ; (3) points connected
with previous history, *e.g.*, habitat, habits, lithiasis, oxaluria,
passage of previous stones, renal colic ; (4) frequency of micturition ; (5) absence of any condition in the rest of the urino-
genital tract to explain the symptoms ; (6) failure of previous
treatment. The chief conditions simulating renal calculus are :
(1) Lithiasis and to a less degree oxaluria ; (2) tubercular
kidney ; (3) pyelitis, not tubercular ; (4) movable and (5) aching kidney, especially if associated with (6) neuralgic conditions ;
(7) disease in organs contiguous to the kidney ; (8) disease of
lumbar spine ; (9) interstitial shrinking nephritis ; (10) malignant disease of the kidney, especially of the pelvis, and malignant disease around the 12th dorsal nerve (a case is reported).
The chief practical points in the performance of nephro-lithotomy
he considers to be as follows :

(1) To count the ribs ; the last rib may be rudimentary and
the 11th mistaken for it.

(2) To make a sufficiently free incision.

(3) To pack away with sponges the colon, which is often troublesomely distended in these cases with flatus.

(4) If a stone cannot be felt in pelvis or after palpation anteriorly or posteriorly, the kidney should be drawn out as far as possible and carefully examined.

(5) In puncturing the kidney, the calyces should be opened systematically.

(6) When palpation and acupuncture fail to find the stone, then the kidney should be opened and carefully sounded.

(7) Hemorrhage from kidney is easily arrested by careful, firm pressure,

(8) Sources of difficulty in finding a stone are (a) mobile kidney, (b) stone in anterior part, and (c) stone in a sacculated kidney.

(9) In large suppurating kidney first incise freely and drain kidney before performing nephrectomy.

I cannot agree with Mr. Jacobson as to the method of exploring the kidney, and my experience has been that in those cases where the stone is small and hidden away in one of the calyces, there is often little chance of its being found either by palpation, needling, or the introduction of a sound. A free incision into the kidney and exploration with the finger is the only certain method of finding these calculi. I have several times cut down on the kidney for suspected calculus, palpated, needled and used the sound, yet failed to find the stone ; but in the last case I made a free incision into the posterior border of the kidney, introduced my finger, and soon came across a small stone encapsuled at upper end of organ. I have never had any difficulty in arresting hemorrhage, and have never found it necessary to plug the wound with gauze ; pressure with sponge or finger easily arrests any hemorrhage, even when it is very free. I have no doubt at all that many of the so-called cases of nephralgia which have been operated on have been cases of stone undiscovered, because not thoroughly searched for with the finger through a sufficiently large incision.

Dr. E. L. Keyes of New York recently read a most interesting

Paper on *Nephro-Lithotomy* before the Medical Society of the State of New York (*N. Y. Medical Record*, Feb. 8th, 1890). His experience extends to six cases of actual or suspected stone. In one case the kidney was filled by a large-branched calculus weighing two ounces, which was extracted in pieces with great difficulty ; there was much hemorrhage, which was arrested by hot water. Dr. Keyes' conclusions are as follows :

(1) The posterior exploratory incision upon a kidney suspected to contain stone is devoid of any serious danger when performed with proper care, and should be resorted to more often than it is.

(2) The best incision is the transverse, below the 12th rib, with as much of a liberating incision downwards along the edge of the quadratus as may be required to gain ample room.

(3) The kidney may be freely cut into and rudely lacerated with the finger, when the stone calls for it, without producing any hemorrhage which hot irrigations will not control.

(4) It is better, in the case of a large branching calculus, to break it up and extract it in fragments rather than attempt to remove it entire.

(5) So little danger attaches to the posterior incision that it seems wiser always to make it the first step, reserving peritoneal exploration for a later resource in cases where the posterior operation miscarries.

Calculus Removed from the Ureter.—A paper was read at a recent meeting of the Clinical Society of London by Mr. Twynam of Sydney, New South Wales (*Lancet*, Feb. 1, 1890), describing how, in a child aged 8 years, a calculus was successfully removed from the ureter. The patient entered hospital suffering from pain in the abdomen and hæmaturia. Pain was felt over the pubes and at tip of penis after micturition. No stone in bladder. Distinct tenderness in left loin. High temperature. On Feb. 6th an exploratory incision was made in the left linea semilunaris and the left kidney and ureter examined, but no stone found. A calculus was found, however, in the right ureter two inches from the bladder, and when pressed upon could be felt through the rectum. The stone was removed by linear incision in a subsequent operation, because patient had a tempera-

ture of 106° and convulsions. Incision was made as if to tie
the common iliac artery. Some difficulty was experienced in
isolating the ureter, but it was ultimately accomplished and the
stone removed with forceps through a linear incision. It weighed
six grs. and was the size of a No. 12 catheter. The wound in
the ureter was closed with fine silk, a drainage tube was introduced into the wound cavity, and the wound dressed with sali-
cylated wool. Urine ceased to flow from wound on the fifth day,
after which it rapidly healed, and the boy made a perfect recovery. The striking points in this case were (1) the difficulty
of diagnosis owing to the fact that a stone in the bottom of the
right ureter caused pain in the region of the left kidney, (2) the
novel method of removing a stone situated so low down in the
ureter.

In his Harveian lectures on the *Surgery of the Kidney*, Mr.
J. Knowsley Thornton (*Lancet*, Dec. 7th, 1889), in speaking of
puncture and lumbar nephrotomy, briefly summarizes as follows :
He would restrict puncture (1) to decide in doubtful cases between solid and fluid tumors of the kidney ; (2) to relieve painful distension when nephrotomy for some special reason is not at
once advisable or possible ; (3) to remove urine, serum or pus
from a very large tumor to reduce its bulk in the performance
of nephrectomy ; (4) as a tentative attempt at cure in some
cases of simple cyst or hydronephrosis ; (5) to localize the position of renal or circumrenal abscess when the physical signs are
not clear enough for free incision ; and (6) to gain time and
relieve harmful tension in some cases of calculous suppression.
He would restrict the use of nephrotomy to (1) calculous suppression in which the incision seems preferable to mere puncture,
with the chance of being able also to remove the stone ; (2) for
the cure by subsequent drainage of simple cysts, abscesses and
hydatids ; (3) for the cure by subsequent drainage of traumatic
pyonephrosis or pyelitis, and in the early stages of tubercular
suppuration ; (4) for the possible cure of more advanced calculous
or tuberculous suppurations when the patient will not submit to
nephrectomy ; and (5) for the performance of nephro-lithotomy
in some cases. Mr. Thornton strongly objects to lumbar nephrec-

tomy for tumors of the kidney, one of the objections being the possibility of not being able to find the kidney, an accident that has happened to experienced London surgeons in a large number of cases; another, that a single kidney may be removed. He being an abdominal surgeon, is altogether in favor of the abdominal method by the lateral incision of Langenbuch along the outer border of the rectus muscle. If it be necessary to drain, a Keith's glass tube is used, and should be cleaned each day under the spray. He says that, as a precise and scientific operation, there is no comparison between the abdominal operation and its lumbar rival. After the operation he allows no opium or stimulants, but if it is absolutely necessary to give a sedative, he gives potassium bromide and chloral injections per rectum. Mr. Thornton has only had a mortality of 20 per cent in his cases of nephrectomy.

Wounds of the Kidney.—M. Taffier of Paris, in an article on *Wounds of the Kidney* (*Archiv Gén. de Med.*, March 1889), says that in cases of wounds of the convex edge of the kidney there occurs a copious hemorrhage from a network of veins in the cortical substance of the organ, this being easily arrested, however, by slight compression. Wounds of kidney are not followed by urinary infiltration; they have a remarkable tendency to heal rapidly and without suppuration,—in 69 cases only seven suppurated. Hemorrhage, in case of injury of the hilus, is, next to shock, the most important symptom, and this may be so profuse as to be followed by death from this cause alone. In bullet wounds, secondary hemorrhage is frequently observed. Hæmaturia in wounds of the kidney is characteristic, though not always present (18 in 31). Anuria is the exception.

Under the head of complications may be mentioned prolapse of the kidney. This may occur without any injury of the kidney having taken place. Suppurative processes are relatively infrequent. Fistulæ are very rare even after suppuration. Among 78 wounds of the kidney recorded in the surgical history of the war of the Rebellion, in only one case did a permanent fistula remain.

The prognosis in cases of wounds of the kidney must be cautiously given. Of course, if other internal organs are inju~ed the case becomes much more serious. When a case prese~ts itself it should be carefully cleansed antiseptically and precipit~te nephrectomy should be avoided.

Treatment of some forms of Chronic Suppurating Kidne~s by Perineal Puncture and Drainage.—In an article on t~he above subject, Mr. Reginald Harrison comes to the followir~g conclusions (*Lancet*, Dec. 7th, 1889):

(1) That in a large number of cases of simple suppuratin~g pyelitis caused by obstruction below, the pus gradually and co~n-pletely disappears as the resistance to the urine is removed. This is exemplified in the ordinary treatment of urethral strictur~e by dilatation or otherwise.

(2) That some advanced forms of chronic double suppurativ~e pyelitis from obstruction below, where the suppuration continue~s to be excessive after the obstruction has been removed or re~lieved, are best treated by an opening in the perineum wher~e the drainage is free and dependent and irrigation can be con~veniently employed.

(3) Perineal puncture (elsewhere described by Mr. Harrison) best meets the requirements of these cases, and may be said to be free from risk. Mr. Harrison says that perineal puncture entails no prolonged confinement in bed. He has had patients going about ten days after operation. Mr. Harrison has devised a very simple contrivance consisting of a soft rubber drainage-tube for retention in the bladder by a T-bandage, to which is attached a continuation-tube fitted with a stop-cock, the end being retained in a belt around the patient's waist.

(4) In cases of suppurating kidneys, where not too advanced, by making a dependent perineal opening, whatever remains of sound suppurating kidneys may be saved and life prolonged, whilst the comfort of the patient is materially added to.

Ligature of the Common Iliac Artery for Hip-joint Amputations.—Dr. Poffert of Giessen reports a case (*Deutsch. Med. Woch.*, No. 29, 1889) in which Prof. Bose had resorted to preliminary ligature of the common iliac artery as the first step in a hip-joint amputation. The patient, a strong, healthy man, aged 40, had noticed for six months that his thigh had begun to swell above the knee, and that the past few weeks the swelling had increased rapidly and caused pain. Examination showed a tumor extending from the condyles to the groin, its upper limit being felt anteriorly under Poupart's ligament, and posteriorly a little below the gluteal fold. The limb was cylindrical in shape, enlarged ; skin over tumor tense and shiny. Veins much dilated. No fracture of femur. Amputation was performed Dec. 11th, 1884. He first proceeded to tie the common iliac artery in the usual manner. The artery and vein were easily exposed, and seen to be surrounded by fat and enlarged glands. The vein and artery were ligated and the glands removed. The wound was closed, a drainage-tube being inserted at the lower angle. The amputation was now performed by anterior flap, consisting of only skin and fascia ; the posterior flap consisted of skin and muscular tissue, which here was healthy. Very little hemorrhage took place. The large wound was drained and closed with silk sutures. The pulse after the operation was excellent, and the patient made a rapid and perfect recovery. Tumor, a spindle-celled sarcoma, starting from bone. Four years after operation patient was perfectly healthy and free from return of disease.—(*Quoted in Annals of Surgery*, Dec. 1889.)

The Use and Abuse of Drainage Tubes.—Mr. Rickman Godlee, in an interesting article on the above subject (*Practitioner*, Feb. 1890), comes to the following conclusions :—

The advantages of doing without them are—(1) The healing is more rapid. (2) The scar is more uniformly linear. (3) The chance of failing with the antiseptic element is much diminished.

Disadvantages are—(1) The temperature does not seem to keep so absolutely normal as we see it in perfectly drained wounds. (2) There is risk of blood or serum collecting under the flaps ; and while in many cases this may be absorbed, in others it will require removal, and then the cure is probably longer than it would have been if drainage had been employed at first.

Dr. Hans Schmid of Berlin, in an article on the *Changes in*

43

Value and in the Manner of Draining Wounds (*Berl Klinik*, Hft. 11, May 1889), says that rubber tubes are frequently compressed by the dressings and bandages, and that their benefit is a delusion. Infection of wounds after operation is represented by two types—either a diphtheritic slough appears on both walls of the wound after union of the skin over the wound, or else a phlegmanous inflammation of the tissues obtains. In neither of these two cases are drainage tubes of any avail. Drainage tubes are frequently stopped at both ends by clots and granulations. They always act as foreign bodies, and may prove disastrous to an aseptic course by containing air. Finally, the presence of drainage tubes calls for an unnecessary change of dressing. Dr. Schmid has treated between 600 and 900 major surgical operative cases without drainage tubes, and in all cases he was contented with the results, and no case gave cause for serious apprehension, but once in a while retention of bloody serum occurred, which occasionally (if not speedily let out) would turn purulent.—(*Quoted in Annals of Surgery,* Nov. 1889.)

Long-standing Dislocation of the Shoulder treated by Operation.—Sir Joseph Lister (*Lancet*, Jan. 1890) reports two cases of the above successfully treated by operation. The first case was that of a man, aged 47, who came to King's College Hospital eight weeks after having dislocated both shoulders. On admission, both limbs presented the usual characters of subcoracoid dislocation. He operated by first making an incision from the coracoid process downwards and somewhat outwards between the deltoid and great pectoral, the tendon of the subscapularis was divided at its insertion, and then with a periosteum detacher proceeded to separate the soft parts from the head of the bone and the inner part of its neck ; pulleys were applied, and after protruding the head of the bone, dividing some tense bands, and separating the external rotators, the bone was returned with difficulty to the glenoid cavity. A week later the other shoulder was operated on in the same way, except that the head of the bone was at once protruded and the attachment of all the rotators divided. In this instance the head, after two attempts, was drawn into place by pulleys. The wounds did perfectly well, and there was no suppuration ; passive motion was employed and kept up; serous oozing for nearly two months ; he was discharged from hospital two months after operation, and returned in about two months for inspection. The arms could be moved to a right angle and rotation was much improved, and patient could do his work as an agricultural laborer.

The second case was that of a young man, aged 23, who was admitted into hospital in July, 1887, seven months after having dislocated both shoulders in an epileptic fit. On both sides the dislocation was subcoracoid. The shoulder was operated on in the same way as the first, but the result was not brilliant, so six months afterwards the other shoulder was operated on in a different way. He decided that he would merely cut down on the head of the bone and remove it piecemeal by means of chisel and hammer without disturbing the attachments of the external rotators. For a study of the skeleton with the humerus in the subcoracoid position had convinced Sir Joseph that the removal of the articular surface without interfering with the tuberosities would allow the bone to drop back in relation with the glenoid cavity. This was done January 1888, and the immediate result was good. The bone went readily into place, recovery of movement was much more rapid than on the other side, and he had almost perfect use of the arm.

Sir Joseph Lister would advise that when the surgeon feels in doubt as to whether it is prudent to make attempts at reduction, or when such attempts do not succeed, he should, in the first place, cut down upon the bone by the usual incision, and then detach with a periosteum elevator the soft parts from the inner side of the upper end of the humerus. This will ensure the avoidance of injury to the axillary vessels. Should these means fail, then detaching the heads of the rotator muscles and removal of the head of the bone will ensure a useful limb.

Note on a possible means of Arresting the Progress of Myxœdema, Cachexia Strumipriva, and allied Diseases.—Mr. Victor Horsley (*British Medical Journal*, Feb. 8th, 1890) suggests that after the removal of the thyroid to prevent cachexia strumipriva a portion of the thyroid gland from one of the lower animals should be transplanted into the peritoneal cavity or into the subcutaneous tissues. The successful growth of the grafted gland would probably bring about arrest of the diseased process by reason of restoration of lost function. Performed under strict aseptic conditions the operation would be without risk or inconvenience. He suggests that the thyroid gland of an anthropoid ape would be best, but this not being obtainable, he advises that of the sheep as most resembling in its anatomical characteristics that of man. One lobe or half of one lobe would be sufficient. Mr. Horsley's suggestion is based on the observations of Prof. Schiff and Dr. Von Eiselberg.

Suture of Nerves.—E. Etzold records (*Deutsch. Zeitschrift f. Chir.*, Bd. xxix, Hft. 5 and 6, 1889) a number of cases occurring at the Dorpat Clinic, in which various nerves, chiefly the ulnar, radial, median and musculo-cutaneous, were sutured at different intervals after their division with great success. After considering the whole subject, he comes to the following conclusions :

(1) Nerves do not unite by either primary adhesion or second intention. The axis cylinders are the extension of the cells of the ganglia, and their re-formation by means of an exudation of cellular elements of mesodermal origin is, for anatomical reasons, not to be expected.

(2) Divided nerves are regenerated by means of a proliferation from the proximal stump. This was established by experiments on animals, and has been confirmed by clinical observation, which shows beyond all doubt that the proximal end of a divided nerve is regenerated earlier and more completely than the distal end.

(3) The return of sensation is of no value in the diagnosis of nerve regeneration. The symptoms indicating its occurrence are—(*a*) active muscular contraction ; (*b*) disappearance of atrophy, especially of muscular atrophies ; (*c*) slow appearance of this improvement ; (*d*) the return of faradic excitability in muscles previously paralyzed. The galvanic current is not of much importance in the diagnosis of nerve regeneration.

(4) Spontaneous union of divided nerves in the extremities is extremely rare. In high injuries of nerves, the prognosis is unfavorable in spite of nerve sutures.

(5) Regeneration of nerves is prevented by the extensive formation of cicatricial tissue.

(6) Nerve suturing is not only a justifiable operation, but in every traumatic case of nerve section it is the duty of the surgeon to adopt it.

(7) The essentials of success are—absolute antisepsis, complete hæmostasis, avoidance of irritation. If after nerve injuries a congested condition of the limb results, it should be elevated and massage employed as soon as the wound is healed. Direct galvanization of the nerve scar should be employed, as well as massage, soon after cicatrization in order to diminish the scar.

(8) It is not proven that electric treatment of the organs supplied by the cut nerves either limits the atrophy or favors nerve regeneration. Massage and passive gymnastics constitute the rational treatment for peripheral paralysis.

(9) The most extensive use of the extremity that is found possible after nerve section appears to have a favorable influence upon the healing.—(*Quoted in American Journal of the Medical Sciences for March*, 1890.)

New Method of Operating for the Relief of Deformity from Prominent Ears.—The deformity caused by prominent ears is very unsightly, especially in females. This deformity, from causes with which I am unacquainted, is peculiarly common in the neighboring United States, so it is quite fitting that an American should devise an operation for its relief.

Dr. Keen of Philadelphia (*Annals of Surgery*, Jan. 1890) describes a case operated on. The patient was aged 19, and the following operation devised for his relief. An oval portion of skin was removed from the posterior surface of the auricle, the cartilage being laid bare by dissection. In the long axis of the oval excision of skin a long, narrow piece of cartilage was removed, V-shaped on cross-section. Great care was taken not to cut through the skin on the anterior surface of the ear. On the left side three catgut sutures were introduced into the car-

tilage itself, in addition to those in the skin. The result was
equally satisfactory on both sides. The two operations were
done at the same time ; they were attended by free bleeding,
which was easily controlled. The result obtained was remarkably good.

Cancer of the Tongue.—Dr. Krause of Halle says that during the period extending from 1875 to 1888 ninety-one cases of
carcinoma of the tongue were operated on at Prof. Volkmann's
klinik. Of these, two died immediately after operation, these
being cases of complete extirpation, of which there were thirty-
five in all. The average duration of life following the operation
in these last-named cases waas twelve months ; but one was absolutely free from recurrence six years after. Of the fifty-six
cases of partial extirpations, seven were found to be free from
recurrence after the same lapse of time. The most rapid recurrence in this class took place in eight months. The microscopic diagnosis was established in all cases.

Prof. Volkmann, after trial of the submental method of operating, abandoned it. He likewise rejects preliminary ligature
of the linguals, as well as preliminary tracheotomy. In the relatively easy cases the tongue is brought well forward and hemorrhage is arrested in the wound ; in more difficult cases Langenbeck's method of temporary section of the lower jaw, with division
of the palato-glossal arch, is adopted ; a drainage-tube is placed
in the recess of the tonsil. Cases involving the epiglottis are
rejected. (*Deutsch. Med. Woch.*, No. 22, 1889 ; quoted in
Annals of Surgery, Feb. 1890.)

New Method of Operating for Thoracic Empyema.—Dr. M.
Ssubbotin says that in long-standing cases of empyema, in which
plastic measures for recurring obliteration of the pleural cavity
by collapse of the chest walls are indicated, he successfully performed the following operation. A portion of the 7th rib is
resected in the usual manner, and the pleural cavity opened and
thoroughly irrigated. This opening is packed in order to prevent
septic infection. A longitudinal incision is now made upon the
external edge of the pectoralis major muscle of about five centimetres in length, by means of which the 6th, 5th and 4th ribs

are bared without removing the periosteum ; from each of these ribs a small wedge is resected, so that the rib becomes movable at this point. A similar longitudinal incision is made in the posterior axillary line, and at this point the above-mentioned ribs are treated in a similar manner. The vertical incisions have no connection with the pleural cavity, and are sutured at once without damage. The portion of the chest wall lying between the longitudinal incisions now sinks in, and, as the healing process advances, becomes fixed in this depressed position, serving the double purpose of protecting the chest cavity and preventing in some measure the scoliosis which occurs so commonly after operations for empyema.—(*Vratch*, 1888, No. 45 ; quoted in *Annals of Surgery*, Feb. 1890.)

Hospital Reports.

MONTREAL GENERAL HOSPITAL.

CONDENSED REPORTS OF CASES IN DR. MacDONNELL'S WARDS.

Exophthalmic Goitre.—Two cases have been before the class. A girl, aged 21, for several years had suffered from palpitations on exertion, and six months ago the thyroid began to enlarge. The area of cardiac dulness was moderately increased. The pulse was rapid (120) ; the cardiac action hurried and violent. There was a systolic murmur, loudest at the 2nd right costal cartilage. The exophthalmos was not so well marked as the two other cardinal symptoms of the disease, but the eyes, though not actually prominent, had a staring appearance, which attracted attention. The remarkable feature in the case was the well-defined brown pigmentation on the upper and lower eyelids. This had made its appearance during the last six months, and seemed to have no tendency to spread. The natural complexion of the patient is fair, and the pigmented skin has the color of a huge freckle. Vitiligo, as I must call these patches, has been noted in cases of Graves' disease, and cases of universal bronzing of the skin have been recorded. The other eye symptoms (Graefe's and Stellwag's) were absent. There was a great deal of nervous excitement, and an inability to remain long in a state of quiet, the move-

ments being almost choreic. There were no tremors. Decided
improvement in all the symptoms followed a period of rest in
bed without any medication. Subsequently the tincture of
belladonna was given in increasing doses until the throat
became dry and the pupils large.

The second case was that of a stout, married woman, aged
35, in whom the exophthalmos was remarkable. The cause of
the disease was probably fright. Ten months ago labor came
on suddenly when she was quite alone in the house, and it was
two or three hours after delivery before assistance arrived.
Almost immediately afterwards the prominence of the eyeball
was noticed and the sight became defective. She presented
herself at the ophthalmic department, where the true nature
of the disease was discovered. The pulse is not very rapid
(100); the heart's action is not hurried. The thyroid is
slightly enlarged, but there is no thrill; the exophthalmos is
very prominent. When the pupil is directed towards the
ground the upper lid remains perfectly fixed in its position,
and it is in a constant state of retraction, so that the cornea is
not covered.

*Lead Poisoning ; Chronic Interstitial Nephritis ; Hemiplegia :
Death.—(Dec. 28th.)*—In the Hospital Reports of the October
number of this JOURNAL, page 291, the reader will find the
history of W. S., aged 58, who, since 1875, has suffered from
symptoms of lead poisoning. On the 11th May of the present
year it was recognized that he was the subject of chronic
Bright's disease of the small kidney variety. He left the
hospital on 31st August. On the 24th of December he was
readmitted, this time profoundly unconscious. It appears that
about a week before admission he had become suddenly unconscious, and had remained so until admission. He died after
being two days in hospital. His condition was as follows:
There was speechlessness without, apparently, unconsciousness, for although he gave no sign of comprehending the
questions put to him, yet his eyes followed one about as if he
partly understood his whereabouts. It would appear as if the
whole body were powerless, but when the neck is irritated the
right hand is raised, but the left arm is never moved. When
the sole of the foot is pinched, the right leg is quickly drawn
away, but this is not observed with the left leg. Knee reflex

is absent in both legs. No evidence of paralysis of the facial nerve. Urine and fæces pass involuntarily. The former contains a very large proportion of albumen. The heart's action regular and the sounds natural. The evidences of hemiplegia were slight, and as he had had transient hemiplegia of the other side on the 18th May last, it was thought that possibly the condition might depend upon uræmia, though the extreme probability of hemorrhages into the brain was fully taken into account. The case is one of exceeding interest, as showing a succession of changes, all resulting the one from the other,—first the lead, then the granular kidneys, the arterial disease, the high tension pulse, and the final catastrophe—the rupture first into one corpus striatum and eight months later into the other. The post-mortem appearances explained all the symptoms which were present. Both might with advantage be represented in tabular form.

SYMPTOMS.	POST-MORTEM APPEARANCES.
Left hemiplegia, with loss of consciousness.	Recent hemorrhage into the right external capsule.
On 18th May, 1889, transient right hemiplegia.	Spot of softening in left internal capsule and corpus striatum.
General mental enfeeblement.	Minute recent hemorrhagic softening in the white substance of the left hemisphere. The smaller arteries of the brain under the microscope show extensive fatty degeneration in the intima and media, with numerous aneurysmal dilatations.
Urine pale amber. sp. gr. 1017; small amount of albumen; quantity usually not much above normal. Hyaline casts.	Kidneys cirrhotic, greatly contracted; weight—left, 80 grammes; right, 70 grammes. Normal weight, 130 grammes.
Normal amount of urea.	
Apex beat displaced downwards and outwards. Increased area of cardiac dulness. High tension pulse.	Hypertrophy and dilatation of the left ventricle.
Ophthalmoscope shows albuminuric retinitis.	Retinitis on right side.
Physical signs of lungs negative when formerly in hospital.	Atrophic emphysema and healed tubercular nodule in left apex. Acute broncho-pneumonia (a late change).

Erythema Nodosum; Phlebitis of the axillary and fem[oral] veins, and subsequently of the external jugular; epig[as-] tric pain and ascites; phlebitis in both legs; evidence[?] of consolidation at the base of right lung; diarrhœa; [?] cutaneous nodules; aspiration of 110 ounces of seru[m]; varicosity of the thoracic veins; rapid dilatation of ri[ght] heart; death; autopsy.

Annie D., aged 43, was admitted into the surgical wards ea[r]ly in September last with erythema nodosum and stiffness of t[he] muscles, especially of the neck. She was transferred to t[he] medical wards almost immediately, and the following state [on] admission was noted. Slight swelling and tenderness of the le[ft] side of the neck and pain on movement. Physical signs of che[st] negative. Urine normal. No digestive disturbance. On th[e] fourth day after admission there was pain and swelling in le[ft] axilla, which was thought to be due to enlarged lymphatic gland[s]. On the twelfth day there was severe epigastric pain, which wa[s] relieved by vomiting and passed gradually away. In the sam[e] evening there was pain and tenderness in left groin. Four day[s] later there was evident phlebitis of the left internal jugular vein, which became distinctly cord-like and very tender. It wa[s] treated in the usual way, the pain and swelling gradually disap- peared, and the patient feeling stronger, left the hospital on the 19th October.

On the 18th November she was re-admitted, this time com- plaining of severe epigastric pain, abdominal distension, and a painful swelling of the left leg. After leaving hospital she had been very well for a fortnight, when she began to menstruate and then to suffer from intense pain at the epigastrium. Tem- perature 100¼°; pulse 96. Nausea and vomiting after food. Evidence of fluid in the peritoneum. Dulness on percussion, bronchial breathing, and crepitant râle at the right pulmonary base. Both legs are enlarged about the calves and very tender to the touch, especially the right. No affection of the joints. Sharp diarrhœal attacks from time to time. The thoracic veins of the left side were noticed to be varicosed. The patches on the legs for which she originally entered hospital never entirely disappeared, but remained as reddish indurations, and now they are inflamed and angry-looking. They are situated about the calves of the legs.

A week later similar physical signs, though not marked to the same extent, were found in the left base.

Nov. 27*th.*—One hundred and ten ounces of a clear fluid were removed to-day by the aspirator ; it contained no pus. The discomfort due to the abdominal distension was removed, but the symptoms were unchanged. The temperature is now generally about 100–101° at night and 99° in the morning. Considerable epigastric pain. As a result of a vaginal examination by Dr. Gardner it was found that the womb was fixed in the pelvis, probably by old inflammatory adhesions.

Dec. 10*th.*—The varicosity of the thoracic veins is becoming very marked.

Dec. 11*th.*—Death occurred to-day, the following symptoms preceding the event. In the early morning she complained of very severe pain in the abdomen, and she became much more feeble. The pulse became rapid (144) and very weak. The thoracic veins became as large as lead pencils, and the general surface of the upper part of the body on the left side was generally cyanotic. The heart's action became visibly turbulent, the cardiac area of dulness became increased, and the sounds became confused, so it was impossible to distinguish one from another.

At the autopsy thromboses were found in the right femoral and the popliteal, as well as in many of the smaller veins of the right leg. There was recent embolism of all the main branches of the right pulmonary artery. Old infarctions in both lungs, over one of which an adhesive pleurisy has occurred. The base of the right lung is collapsed. Pale, colorless clots dilate the right heart to an enormous size. There is chronic interstitial inflammation of the pancreas, with the formation of some large cysts near the splenic end. Several small localized subcutaneous indurations containing pus are found in both legs and in the right arm. Fluid in abdomen and evidences of recent peritonitis.

The diagnosis of this case was very obscure. That some one

cause was producing the stagnation of blood in so many different parts of the body was evident enough. There was no symptom present which could not be explained by the occurrence within the body of what we saw going on outside it. But to find a cause for this general tendency to thrombosis was a different matter. At one time it seemed as if the presence of tubercular peritonitis would account for the abdominal symptoms, but it would not explain the occurrences elsewhere. We must fall back on rheumatism to account for the thrombosis as well as for the erythematous nodules and the peritonitis.

Tubercular Meningitis in an Adult.

J. W., aged 23, had been in hospital two years ago with a tumor of the testis, which, on removal, was found to be tuberculous, and not very long after that he had an attack of pleurisy of the left side, from which he apparently recovered, but soon an abscess formed in the centre of the sternum, from which there came a discharge which continued up to the last. On admission (Jan. 27th, 1890) the chief symptoms were intense headache, which was constantly present, though it was said to be worse at night, and with this headache delirium and noisiness. There was a continued high temperature and a rapid pulse. The expression was remarkably dull and stupid, and the gait staggering. He says that he has felt numbness in his right arm for the last two months. No history of tubercle in his family. The patellar reflex is lost in both legs. Cutaneous irritability is increased. Vision is very dim. Ophthalmoscopic examination reveals slight hyperæmia of the optic nerve and a tortuous condition of the retinal veins. The organs of hearing are unaffected. Physical signs of chest negative. The tongue is clean and flabby. He is not at present suffering from vomiting, but it has been present before admission. Coma put an end to the headache and delirium on the eleventh day after his admission to hospital.

At the autopsy gray granulations were found on the convexity, in the fissure of Sylvius, while large patches of lymph were seen at the base. In the left cerebellar hemisphere a large tubercular tumor was found. A few tubercles were found in the apices of the lungs.

Alleged " Fits" followed by profound Coma in a Young Girl after Mental Emotion ; Death ; General Thrombosis of the vessels of the Brain.

On 3rd February a servant maid, aged 25, was admitted under the following circumstances. She was said to have been in good health until the present attack. Though she had always been nervous and excitable, yet she had never been known to have had fits of any kind or to be at all subject to hysterical attacks. No family history of nervous disease. Five days before admission she complained of dizziness and of dimness of vision, but she continued at her housework for two days, and on the 1st February was said to have fallen in a fit in her kitchen, but re-covered very soon, and was put to bed. On the following day she was said to have had fits every half hour. There was gasp-ing, sighing and rolling of the eyes, but no spasm of the arms or legs. These events were said to have followed some quarrel which she had with her mistress.

On admission she was almost completely insensible ; eyes half closed ; mouth slightly open ; pupils react to light. Pulse rapid and feeble. Tongue heavily coated and abdomen scaphoid. In-continence of urine. Urine normal. The insensibility at the time of admission was not complete, for by an effort she could be roused to give her name and to say " yes" or " no," and she was able to take food offered to her, but immediately afterwards she lapsed into her previous state of insensibility. Reflexes nor-mal. Sensation lost. On the day after admission the coma deepened.

Feb. 5th.—Breathing became rapid and swallowing was accom-plished with difficulty.

Feb. 6th.—Condition much worse. Breathes more rapidly. Mouth continually open ; tongue dry ; mucous rattle in the trachea. Died on the following day.

The diagnosis of this case was a matter of considerable doubt and uncertainty. At the outset there were many symptoms pointing to hysteria. A young, healthy girl, never previously ill, quarrels with her mistress, is put thereby into a state of great mental excitement, is said to suffer from a succession of mild

" fits," during which she does not bite her tongue or pass water involuntarily, and is finally brought to hospital in a semi-unconscious state. But subsequent observations soon dispelled that idea, for the patient presented no appearance of hysteria, but, on the contrary, there was profound stupor and no trace of clonic spasm. The incontinence of urine, which was present from first to last, added to the unlikelihood of hysteria. Though I could make no positive diagnosis, yet the possibility of the symptoms depending upon tubercular meningitis was before me, bearing in mind the case recorded by Gowers, where a young girl under circumstances somewhat similar developed symptoms which were at first regarded as hysterical, but which afterwards became serious, and after being a few days semi-comatose and passing water involuntarily, died on the eighth day after the onset. The post-mortem in this case revealed general tuberculosis of the lungs, peritoneum and intestines, some small masses of yellow tubercle in the cerebral hemisphere, and meningitis of the base, the lymph being specially abundant about the pons and medulla, with opaque tubercular granulations.*

Having just read this case, I thought it possible that a similar condition might be found to exist in my patient. Dr. Johnston kindly furnished me with the following abstract of the post-mortem report, which speaks for itself :

" The vessels of the pia mater are very full, especially in the frontal region, where slight diffusion of blood has taken place into the tissues (post-mortem staining ?). Throughout the whole extent of the corpus callosum, fornix and internal capsule, the white substance is studded with innumerable punctiform capillary hemorrhages. A few similar hemorrhages are also found in the external and inferior part of both crura cerebri. The peripheral region of both optic thalami and the cortex at the spot of diffusion in the first frontal convolution are the only places where the condition extends to the gray matter. The hemorrhages throughout are perfectly symmetrically arranged. The only other lesion found was a moderate degree of broncho-pneumonia, chiefly in the lower lobes. The lungs and all other organs free from hem-

---

* A Manual of Diseases of the Nervous System. London, 1888. Vol. L, p. 323.

orrhages. Examination of the hemorrhagic spots showed them to be accompanied by, and probably caused by, thrombosis of the smaller vessels. The blood at these spots, as well as from other organs, was examined in the fresh condition and in stained preparations for bacteria with negative results."

SURGICAL CASES UNDER THE CARE OF DR. RODDICK.

(Reported by DR. G. A. BROWN, House Surgeon.)

I. —*Excision of Elbow Joint.*

A. B., aged 36, admitted Nov. 8, 1889, complaining of disease of the left elbow-joint. The disease began about twelve years ago after a fall on some ice, which caused the elbow to become swollen, hot and tender. The elbow remained in this condition for about ten days and then apparently got well. After six years it began to swell again, causing stiffness, pain of a dull, aching character, and fixation of the forearm at right angles to the arm. These symptoms remained about the same until four weeks ago, when swelling and pain increased so much that it had to be lanced, and from the wound there exuded about half a cupful of pus. Two months ago it broke again on the outer side of the joint, leaving a large opening. Patient was never a very healthy boy, for when eight years old he had rheumatic fever, which affected the right hip, causing lameness and dislocation on to the dorsum ilii. At present patient is fairly well nourished, sound in all his organs, eats and sleeps well.

On examination, the joint is swollen, and a little distance above the external condyle there is an ulcerated spot with a fistulous opening in the centre leading down to the joint. There is very little movement, as the forearm is fixed at right angles to the arm.

On Nov. 14, '89, the operation of excision was performed, an incision four inches long being made posteriorly over the back of the joint ; the flaps were reflected and the joint opened. Some difficulty was experienced in finding the ulnar nerve owing to the thickened condition of the soft parts. A large amount of thickened synovial membrane was removed. The cartilages were nearly entirely eroded. The head of the radius especially

showed a considerable share of disease, proving that the inflammation was originally located there. The sinus above referred
to was situated immediately over the radial joint. This was
subsequently scraped and pared and the edges brought together.
All the articular surfaces of the three bones were freely removed.
The edges of the wound were sutured, a bone drain introduced,
the joint dressed antiseptically, and forearm placed at right
angles to arm.

Nov. 26th.—Patient has been in a good condition for the last
ten days. Dressing was removed from arm and wound found
healthy, having united by first intention. The sutures and drain
were removed and passive motion performed, and then dressed
with a light dressing.

Nov. 28th—Patient has passive motion performed every day
and wound dressed with dry dressing.

Nov. 30th.—Movement of elbow joint is improving every day.
Wound entirely healed.

Dec. 2nd.—Left hospital with good result. Motion in elbow
joint has steadily improved as result of passive motion. Patient
can straighten his arm and flex the forearm on the arm, almost
touching his shoulder. Pronation and supination good.

II.— *Urinary Fistula.*

G. A., aged 50, admitted Nov. 26th, 1889, complaining of
urinary fistula. Four years ago patient fell astride of a stump,
causing a good deal of bruising of the perineum, but no open
wound. Two years and a half after the fall noticed difficulty
and frequency in making his water and a white sediment in urine.
These symptoms continued up to July 18, '89, when a small
swelling appeared on the left side of scrotum, and steadily increased until it broke, discharging a small quantity of pus.
Since July he has suffered from difficulty and frequency of micturition, pain at the neck of the bladder just before micturition,
and escape of urine through the fistulous opening made by the
bursting of the abscess. Patient is old in appearance, fairly
well nourished, and all his organs are sound.

On examining the urine it was found to be alkaline, with a

specific gravity of 1021, a trace of albumen, and no sugar. With the microscope a few pus cells were found. On examination of the perineum, a small, red, elevated, warty excrescence is seen on the left side of scrotum, about one inch above anus. The parts around excrescence are red and indurated, and in centre of excrescence there is a fistulous opening, which is connected with urethra, and also runs up along the scrotum towards the pubes.

On Nov. 28th, patient was etherized and a median lithotomy staff introduced. An incision was made in the median line at a point midway between scrotum and anus, cutting down on to the staff. A director was passed into the bladder along the staff as a guide and a rubber drainage-tube introduced, and bladder washed out with boracic acid. The fistulæ were slit up, scraped, and the cavities stuffed with iodoform gauze and dressed with a jute pad, held in position by a T-bandage.

Dec. 5th.—Wound filling up; introduced a smaller tube in perineal opening; all induration has disappeared.

Dec. 8th.—Dressing wound with red wash instead of iodoform gauze.

Dec. 17th.—Tube removed; catheterized every four hours during the day, and catheter tied in during the night.

Dec. 23rd.—Stopped passing catheter; can pass his urine all right through penis, but during the act a small quantity escapes through the perineal opening.

Dec. 30th.—Wound almost covered with skin; perineal opening about size of pin's head; tied in catheter night and day, so as to close perineal opening.

Jan. 6th, '90.—Introduced an armed probe of nitrate of silver into perineal opening to stimulate granulation.

Jan. 8th.—Perineal opening closed; wound is entirely skinned over; passes urine all right, no frequency; urine normal.

Jan. 15th.—Left hospital cured.

Reviews and Notices of Books.

The History and Pathology of Vaccination. Vol. I.,
A Critical Inquiry ; Vol. II., Selected Essays. By EDGAR
M. CROOKSHANKS, M.B., Professor of Comparative Path-
ology and Bacteriology in, and Fellow of, King's College,
London. London : H. K. Lewis, 136 Gower street. 1889.

In the study of a great subject such as vaccination, it is well
that, from time to time, some competent person should assume
the duty of collecting, valuing and placing on record the separated facts which form the sum of our common knowledge. Such
a task has been attempted by the compiler of the volumes before
us.

The discovery of an outbreak of cowpox in 1887 led Mr.
Crookshanks to the investigations, of which the present work is
the outcome.   Up to that time he had accepted and taught the
doctrines commonly held by the profession and described in the
text-books of medicine.   The natural cowpox had not been investigated for some fifty years, and the author found that a much
neglected field for research was open to him.   Satisfied that too
much attention was being given to the *technique* of vaccination
whilst the precise knowledge of the history and pathology of the
disease was a matter entirely overlooked, he determined to make
this the subject of a diligent and far-reaching inquiry.

The library of the Royal College of Surgeons afforded some
valuable MSS., and amongst others the original of *Jenner's
Communication to the Royal Society*.   The very small amount
of evidence on which Jenner substituted *vaccination* for smallpox inoculation induced Professor Crookshanks to look carefully
into the biography of Jenner as given by Baron, and into the
vaccination literature of that period ; and in 1888 he made a
visit to the leading authorities in France with the object of obtaining the history of the Bordeaux lymph and of the outbreaks
of cowpox which had been met with in that country during the
time that the disease had been supposed to be extinct in England.

The greater part of the first volume is historical and bio-
graphical, beginning with an elaborate account of small-pox

inoculation both abroad and at home, and it is not until the sixth chapter that we come to read of the investigations of Jenner and the history of his early efforts. An interesting *fac-simile* of part of the first rejected manuscript sent to the Royal Society is inserted in the volume, and the reader can see from the copious extracts of it which are given that there is good reason to account for its want of success. It appears to have been somewhat hastily written, and the part relating to the protection from smallpox is not brought forward with sufficient prominence. Mr. Crookshanks attacks Jenner, or, rather, it would be better to say, he disparages his efforts. According to the author, Jenner was wrong in supposing cowpox to be cow smallpox; he was not the discoverer of vaccination, for the dairymaids found that out, nor was even the credit of introducing the inoculation of vaccine due to this pretender, for, according to Mr. Crookshanks' statement, this was done by Benjamin Jesty in 1774, and a good deal of space is taken up with an account of this worthy, whose portrait forms the frontispiece of the first volume.

Jesty was a farmer in Dorsetshire who had inoculated with virus direct from the cow his wife and two children in 1774. The sons had the disorder in a favorable way, but the arm of Mrs. Jesty (whose portrait is also given) became much inflamed. Fifteen years afterwards the sons were inoculated for the smallpox; slight inflammation ensued, but no fever or other variolous symptom, while all the others inoculated at the same time went through the usual course of inoculated smallpox. Jesty did nothing to persuade others to adopt the safeguard he had found so effectual until thirty years later, when the news of Jenner's rewards reached him, when he attempted to claim the recognition of Parliament also, but in this he failed.

The author in the next chapter deals with the subject of vaccine lymph, taking strong ground on the question that cowpox is not cow smallpox, and that the inoculations practised by Ceely, Badcock, Chauveau and others from the vesicle of a variolated cow, were in reality smallpox inoculations, and differed in no way from the common pre-vaccination inoculations except in the fact that they did not necessarily carry infection.

The following chapters deal with sheep smallpox and goat smallpox, and then we come to the most important heading, " Cowpox as a Source of Vaccine Lymph." The description given by Jenner in the *Inquiry* was the first published account of cowpox. It was soon after more minutely described by Clayton, a veterinary surgeon in Gloucestershire, and, still later, this account was corroborated by Mr. John Sims and by others. Ceely's experiences are given in detail, accompanied by admirable reproductions of his colored plates, and the subject of casual cowpox in man is fully treated.

For an account of the disputed question of the connection between " grease" in the horse and cowpox in the cow we must refer our readers to the volume before us. The author devotes many pages to its consideration, but the limited space at our disposal permits us merely to notice it.

We regret to find that the results of Professor Crookshanks' investigations, beginning with a depreciatory view of the unselfish labors of Jenner, and ending with a page or two on the great subject of the prevention of smallpox by vaccination, are such as to hamper the efforts of those who are making smallpox take its place as a disease of the past along with the plague, typhus, sweating sickness, and other vanquished enemies of the human race. Had the author spent the winter of 1885-6 with us in Montreal and witnessed the awful mortality amongst the unvaccinated, had he seen how smallpox picked out its victims, whether isolated or not, he would never have been guilty of expressing the opinion that when isolation and vaccination have been carried out in the face of an epidemic, that it is to the isolation that the credit of stopping the disease is due.

It is remarkable, too, that after spending so much time, and taking up so many pages, in producing two enormous volumes full of extracts and manifold varieties of padding, he should have disposed of this question in a few words at the end of his first volume, words which will be read and quoted by mischievous persons who will never have the necessary perseverance and industry to read the hundreds of pages and innumerable quotations which precede the unwarrantable opinions the author has thought proper to enunciate.

Of the second volume we have nothing to say, because it consists merely of a number of essays by various authors. Its publication as a second volume uniform with Professor Crookshanks' work cannot be regarded but as an attempt to swell out to abnormal proportions a work which contains the result of some really careful inquiry, but which, if deprived of all that was not written by the author, would shrink into very insignificant proportions.

Bacteriologische und Pathologisch-Histologische.
Uebungen für Thier arzte. (Practical Course in Pathology and Bacteriology for Veterinarians.) By Th. Kitt, Munich. Vienna: Moritz Perles; pp. 328.

The want of some such book as this has long been felt by those who have had to instruct veterinary students in practical pathology. The veterinary practitioner, far more even than the medical, must eep himself practically posted in pathological methods. In spite of this, there is not at the present time a book in any language where this subject is satisfactorily treated.

Prof. Kitt has written not only a thoroughly good book, but one that is made throughout interesting and pleasant to read, from its easy conversational style. The subject is treated in a manner suited to the wants of practitioners who wish to take a post-graduate course and learn the technique in a limited time. The book has met with a large sale in Germany, and is much used as a text-book for students. For this latter purpose it was not intended, but is at the present time the only one available. The only text-books at present obtainable are altogether out of date, and, having been written at a time when next to nothing was known of disease in animals, they all show the same fondness for theorising and disregard of fact which characterized text-books on human pathology written before Virchow's time.

We learn, therefore, with great pleasure that Professor Kitt is also preparing a text-book on comparative pathology of about the same scope as that of Ziegler. It is sure to be a good one, and we can, while heartily recommending the present book to those interested in the subject, only hope that both it and its

successor will be translated and made available to English read...
The value of the work is increased by a large number of origi...
micro-photographs. The get-up and printing of the book ...
both good.

Cyclopædia of the Diseases of Children, Medica... and Surgical. By American, British, and Canadia... Authors. Edited by JOHN M. KEATING, M.D. Vol. II... New York: J. B. Lippincott Company.

The second volume of this magnificent work fully fulfils all the promises made by the first.

Part I. is devoted to the diseases of the skin, which are treated of in a series of articles written by Hyde, Hardaway, Bulkley, Van Harlingen, and others. That on Eczema, by Van Harlingen, is one of the most important. As regards its etiology, the author takes the middle course, and, while urging a careful examination into every weak point in diet, hygiene, hereditary tendency, and general nutrition, he would at the same time enforce the necessity of extreme attention to local treatment, on which his directions are very full. Dr. J. E. Graham, of Toronto, writes on the Hypertrophies and Atrophies in a short, practical article. The Parasitic Diseases are treated by Stelwagon. His remarks on the treatment of tinea tonsurans are disappointing through their brevity.

Part II., treating of constitutional diseases and diseases of nutrition, begins with an excellent article on Scrofulosis, by Henry Ashby of Manchester. It is well up to date. He thinks it wise, in the present state of our knowledge, to give the term only a clinical, and not any definite pathological meaning. The distinctive characteristics of scrofulous lesions are, he says, only clinical; such as their chronicity, their tendency to spread locally, and their tendency to caseate and to involve the lymphatic tissues. He considers that many of the lesions present are unquestionably tubercular, but others, he thinks, are not. He does not wholly agree with Unna in regarding impetigo as a skin tuberculosis, but thinks that the order of events may usually be stated as follows: (1) an impetigo or ozæna or irritation caused by dentition—non-tubercular ; (2) secondary enlargement of lymph-glands—non-tubercular ; (3) caseation of lymph-glands—tubercular. How the bacilli find entrance can often only be conjectured, but they seem to be able to start a tubercular process only in those parts which are in an inflamed or unhealthy condition, and therefore find in the congested or chronically inflamed glands a suitable nidus. Cod liver oil and the iodine preparations, with very careful local measures, is the only treatment recommended. Tuberculosis is very thoroughly treated by Dr. Jacobi, and Syphilis by Dr. Abner Post. Dr. Barlow, of London, contributes very interesting and exhaustive articles, with good illustrations, on Rachitis and Scurvy. Then follows a paper on the Urinary Diatheses, by J. Milner Fothergill. From an appended foot-note we learn that this was the last work of this writer. It is a most interesting article, and should be very generally read. How far this uric acid formation in children is to be regarded as an etiological factor in the production of scrofula, defective or imperfect organisms, the neurotic temperament, biliousness, and chronic Bright's disease, must for the present be only a matter of conjecture, until more complete investigations give us a surer foundation. There are many, probably, who will hesitate to go as far as the author, but the paper is teeming with suggestive thought and will well repay the perusal of every practitioner. An article on Cretinism, by Bury, and one on Diabetes Mellitus, by George B. Fowler, complete Part II.

Part III. is devoted to diseases of the respiratory tract, and begins with a series of articles on Diseases of the Nose, including Nasal Obstruction, by J. N. Mackenzie ; Reflex Cough, by A. W. McCoy ; Epistaxis, by E. C. Morgan ; Foreign Bodies and Tumors in the Nose, by D. Bryson Delavan ; Acute Coryza, by Carl Seiler ; Rhinitis Hypertrophica and Atrophica, by W. C. Jarvis ; and Croupous Rhinitis and Purulent Rhinitis, by F. H. Bosworth. Diseases and Injuries of the Pharynx are described somewhat briefly by E. Fletcher Ingals, and Beverley Robinson contributes an article on Diseases of the Tonsils. Amongst the articles devoted to the larynx there is an excellent one on Intubation, by William Northrup, who also writes on

Spasmodic and Pseudo-Membranous Laryngitis. Tracheotomy is very fully described by H. R. Wharton. In the section on diseases of the lungs the articles are full and exhaustive. The principal ones are written by Minot, Morrill, Shattuck and Whittier, of Boston, and Jacobi of New York.

In *Part IV.*, the articles on the diseases of the circulatory system have been contributed principally by English writers. Mrs. Dr. Osler contributes a short but excellent *résumé* of the Congenital Affections of the Heart. Dr. Cheadle contributes an article on Acute Endocarditis; and Dr. Sansom one on Chronic Endocarditis, both of which are of great value. Dr. Mitchell Bruce writes on Enlargement of the Heart.

In *Part V.*, a series of articles on diseases of the mouth, jaws and tongue, complete the volume.

As a whole, this volume fully sustains the high standard of excellence reached by the first, while its illustrations are more numerous and, we think, of greater worth.

A. D. B.

Society Proceedings.

MEDICO-CHIRURGICAL SOCIETY OF MONTREAL.

Stated Meeting, 24th January, 1890.

G. E. Armstrong, M.D., President, in the Chair.

Myoma of the Uterus.—Dr. W. Gardner exhibited a specimen of myoma of uterus of the submucous variety, there being little uterine tissue existing between the uterine cavity and the tumor itself. The patient was 45 years of age, and had suffered for the last ten years from menorrhagia, headache, confusion of thought, pelvic pain, and general invalidism. Apostoli's method of treatment had carefully been carried out, but without much benefit, so the tumor with the ovaries (these being situated so low at the base of the tumor and cystic) were removed by the extra-peritoneal operation, patient making a good recovery.

Soft Myoma with Cystic spaces.—Dr. Gardner exhibited this specimen, and said that the patient from whom this tumor had been removed suffered only on account of its size : the diagnosis was doubtful, because of its being soft and fluctuating, and it was a question of fibroid or myoma of the uterus. The extra-peritoneal method of operation was performed, followed by good recovery of patient. This patient had, however, during the course of her illness a slight phlebitis of the left leg. He would venture no explanation pathologically of the specimen, but re-garded it as fibro-cystic from its macroscopical appearance.

Fibro-cystic Tumor of Uterus.—DR. SMITH said that the patient whom this tumor had been removed from had been treated by him with apparently good deal of benefit by means of Apos-toli's method for three months, and within two months after treatment size of patient had diminished three inches. Just before starting for home menses appeared and lasted seventeen days, followed by severe pains in left iliac region. Operation for removal of the tumor was successfully performed, the extra-peritoneal method being adopted.

Nine Cases of Hysterectomy for Fibroid of the Uterus, with a new method of treating the stump.—DR. TRENHOLME read a short paper on this subject.

Discussion.—DR. W. GARDNER said that the extra-peritoneal method was early used in Schrœder's clinic and with 32 per cent. deaths. He himself always uses the Kœberle method ; theoreti-cally the intra-peritoneal method was better. The situation of the wire in Kœberle's method was the same as Dr. Trenholme's. Dr. Gardner found hempen ligature strong enough ; the pins he found prevented the mass from moving, and leaving them in until they sloughed through prevented unfavorable vomiting or straining of any kind. He leaves the pins in from ten to fifteen days, and cuts the wire after from forty-eight hours to six days. Dr. Gardner has had ten cases with nine recoveries.

DR. SMITH was struck with the ease by which the uterus could be ligated by the method proposed by Dr. Trenholme.

DR. TRENHOLME, in reply, said he had found that there was little pain attending the use of this ligature. He thought that the hempen ligature would give a broader surface for adhesion than a wire one would. Lays no stress on stretching of the wound, as the snare is sufficient to hold the stump.

Dr. Foley made a few remarks regarding the relationship between dermatology and gynæcology, and said that certain vascular conditions, neuroses, eczema or acne were all associated with menstrual disorders. Even some cases of severe eczema had yielded to treatment after the repair of a lacerated cervix.

Dr. Jack thought that the conditions of the skin were due to a vulnerability of the elements of the skin and not to disorders of the functions of the uterus.

Stated Meeting, 7th February, 1890.

G. E. Armstrong, M.D., President, in the Chair.

Aneurism of Arch of Aorta.—This was exhibited by Dr. Johnston for Dr. MacDonnell. The only attachment of the aneurism was to the left side of the trachea, just above the bifurcation. The trachea was moderately compressed; no erosion present. The left pneumogastric showed marked atrophy. At the spot where it passed over the aneurism it was flattened and widened for an area of half an inch. The left recurrent laryngeal was atrophied. The orifice of the right subclavian was narrowed as to barely admit a No. 5 catheter. Patient was a navvy, and was seized about October last with cough and dyspnœa. There was found to be dulness below clavicles, contraction of left pupil, tugging at the trachea, hoarseness and brassy cough. Dyspnœa increased to such a degree that venesection was performed and followed by a partial relief. The dyspnœa increased three days later, patient succumbing to it.

Dr. MacDonnell showed a photograph of a patient who had suffered from aneurism of the descending aorta, attended with unilateral sweating. Unfortunately no post-mortem was allowed.

Dr. Johnston said he had examined the body externally after death, and found that the tumor was very tense and fluctuating, giving the impression of a closed cyst. This seemed to prove that the pulsating swelling in the back was not a part of the original aneurism, but a pulsating hæmatoma caused by the sac having perforated posteriorly into the tissues of the back.

Chronic Pyelitis.—The bladder showed a chronic cystitis.

In the prostate was a cavity with firm granulating walls containing a small calcified nodule. One kidney was converted into a thin-walled sac full of thick inspissated pus; the other showed commencing suppurative pyelitis. The history of this case was : Patient entered the General Hospital suffering with a distended bladder; urine could only be passed in drops, but after introducing a filiform bougie the urine passed a little more freely. A stricture in the penile portion of the urethra was detected, and this was cut through by the urethrotome. Soon afterwards pus appeared in the urine; the amount of urine passed per diem gradually decreased, and finally patient died.

Laceration of Urethra.—DR. JOHNSTON showed a specimen of extensive laceration of the urethra, produced by passing a catheter for retention of urine for a comparatively slight stricture. The patient had a chill, followed by a temperature of 107°F., and died within five hours, having passed his urine freely after the operation. There was no urinary infiltration, hemorrhage or sloughing in the neighborhood of the laceration, which was situated beyond the bulbous urethra.

Necrosis of Femur.—DR. HINGSTON exhibited the lower half of a femur from a case in which he had performed amputation on account of extensive necrosis of the lower end of the femur. The specimen showed a small opening at the posterior part of the bone, and when a longitudinal section had been made, this opening was found to communicate with the medullary cavity, the walls of which had undergone most extensive caries.

Appendicitis.—DR. SHEPHERD exhibited an appendix which he had removed from a child who had only been ill two days with slight right iliac pain and tenderness. The bowels were moved by purgatives, but without relief. Operation for removal of appendix performed next day; severe vomiting came on, accompanied by protrusion of three feet of intestine; peritonitis developed, followed by a fatal result.

DR. BLACKADER, who was in attendance on the child, said the family history was of peculiar interest. He had attended the mother for an attack of ante-partum peritonitis; two children had died from appendicitis, and another child had succumbed to an attack of *peritonitis.*

The PRESIDENT here related a case of a man, aged 32 years, who for the last year and a half had had several attacks of appendicitis. Last January he suffered with " la grippe," and subsequently was seized with severe abdominal pains, which salines only partially relieved. Decided to operate, and after opening the abdomen found abscess cavity in right iliac fossa enclosed by knuckle of bowel. The appendix had sloughed off, and found to contain the raspberry seeds. No opening in bowel discovered. Patient made a good recovery.

On Abdominal Section in Tubercle of the Peritoneum and Uterine Appendages.—DR. W. GARDNER read the paper, a report of which is to be found on page 641.

Discussion.—DR. SMITH said that if the disease originated in the tubes the prognosis was bad. He thought that the ingestion of tubercular food was a cause of tubercular peritonitis.

DR. JOHNSTON remarked that he had seen at autopsy tubercular peritonitis in which this was not the actual cause of death, and the person had apparently lived without any evidence of it.

DR. ALLOWAY said he thought Dr. Gardner was to be congratulated upon having been able to collect so many interesting cases of this rare disease. He did not think any surgeon had, up to the present time, published the complete histories of so many cases of tubercular peritonitis. He thought that it was a condition more prevalent than was generally considered, and that our knowledge upon this point was due to the rapid strides abdominal surgery had taken of late years. He also thought that many cases of severe pelvic inflammation and death following comparatively trivial operations upon the uterus without due care to antiseptic precautions were probably due to the lighting up of a latent tuberculosis in subjects predisposed by heredity to that disease. He was therefore exceedingly careful with so-called delicate women when he found it necessary to operate upon the uterus or vagina. Dr. Alloway related the case of a lady operated upon by the late Dr. J. M. Drake (dilating the uterus and applying nitric acid to the endometrium), where death took place on the fourteenth day after the operation from general peritonitis. At the autopsy the whole peritoneum was found studded with miliary tubercle. Whether laparotomy and washing out the cavity with water should have the credit of benefitting these patients, or that time and medical care would do the same for them, it is impossible to say. Certainly the majority of such cases that have been operated upon by accident have been improved, and many have remained free from pain and malnutrition for years afterwards.

DR. BELL did not think that abdominal section was called for in cases where the diagnosis was certain, as he could not see what beneficial result would follow such a procedure ; but would advocate such operation only in cases of doubt.

The PRESIDENT remarked that where the operator can find a local focus, then its removal would probably be followed by benefit, but merely opening and closing the abdomen was going to do little good. Until we know the life history of tubercular peritonitis we can expect to do little for such cases.

Trichorrhexis Nodosa.—DR. FOLEY exhibited a specimen, showing the whitish nodules resembling nits and the split or green stick fracture appearance of the hair.

HAMILTON MEDICAL AND SURGICAL SOCIETY.

Stated Meeting, Feb. 4th, 1890.

J. W. ROSEBRUGH, M.D., PRESIDENT, IN THE CHAIR.

Dislocation of the Foot Backwards.—DR. WM. McCARGOW read the following notes of this case :—

The subject of this accident, a large, stout woman, aged 60, I first saw at Oneida, County of Haldimand, August 1858, along with Dr. Jacob Baxter of Cayuga. She stated that three months ago she received a fall, displacing the ankle-joint ; that she was treated for it by a medical man in her neighborhood, who failed to reduce the luxation, and left her in her present state. She also stated having consulted other medical advice without benefit. Upon examination the foot is found to be displaced backwards, with shortening of the foot and lengthening of the heel, with a depression above the latter. The toes are pointed downwards, and the extremity of the tibia forms a projection in front of the

ankle. I gave her to understand that it might not be too late
to remedy the displacement so that she could walk. At this
time the way she went about the house was only by resting the
injured limb on a chair, and with the aid of the other and carrying the chair, move about in that way. Having willingly agreed
to an operation, a plaster cast of the limb was taken. On the
7th September, assisted by Dr. Baxter and Mr. Farrell (subsequently a graduate of Royal College of Kingston), the patient
having been duly placed under chloroform, an attempt was first
made at reduction by the aid of a Jarvis adjuster. Not succeeding by what was considered by us as a fair trial, I divided the
tendo-Achilles, when reduction with the hands was easily effected.
The fibula, broken in the usual place in like cases, was ununited.
The chief after-treatment of the case consisted in keeping the
end of the tibia in place with due support of the heel and foot,
which was done by a well-fitting anterior tin-splint with foot piece,
such as Dr. Kerr of Galt was in the habit of using in simple
fractures of the leg near the ankle joint. She recovered with a
stiff joint. Passive motion was advised after the removal of the
splint, but insufficiently used by her husband, and the distance
from my house in Caledonia being some sixteen miles, it was
out of my power to attend to it. I saw the patient some years
subsequently at the house of her son in London, Ont., when she
was well and had good use of the foot.

This dislocation is very uncommon, which is my only excuse
for bringing this case before the Society. The tibia rests in these
cases from half an inch to three-quarters of an inch in front of its
proper place.

Selections.

The Prevention of Tuberculosis.—In the course of the debate which has been proceeding for some time past in the Academy of Medicine of Paris, and was concluded last week, there has been a republication of curious edicts and rules intended to prevent the spread of tubercular disease among members of communities. Thus M. Germain Sée drew attention to one of those edicts passed over a hundred years ago, namely, in the year 1782, when the King of Naples proclaimed as law : (1) That every physician in practice should be bound rigorously to furnish indications to the authorities as soon as he had discovered phthisis in any of his patients, and if he neglected this announcement should be amenable to a fine of one hundred ducats, and in case of repetition of the offence be condemned, without appeal, to banishment for ten years. (2) That the sick, after the discovery that they were suffering from phthisis pulmonalis, should be taken immediately to the hospital. (3) That the directors of hospitals should be obliged to keep separate the clothes and the linen belonging to the phthisical, with an inventory of all the clothes that had been worn by every individual certified as being tuberculous, and that after the death of such person the director or manager should prove that all parts of the clothes were still present, any infraction of this part of the decree being punishable by imprisonment or even the galleys. (4) That the authorities should be empowered to renew the sick-chambers in which phthisical persons had been lodged ; that is to say, the flooring of the chamber, the bedclothes and the hangings of the bed, and should remove and burn the windows and the doors and replace them by new ones. (5) That severe penalties should also be inflicted on those who bought or sold effects belonging to the phthisical. (6) That every house in which a phthisical patient died should be put under ban, and its proprietor be reduced to the loss of it.

These proscriptions, M. Germain Sée said, were only a copy of still older regulations which had been brought into force against the plague in former times ; and the same rules were applied in Portugal. In the kingdom of Naples this law was applied in all its rigor until the year 1848, and what was the result? The result generally was an evil incalculable. What was the result to the sufferers from tuberculosis? Nothing. The vigorous application of the law for two or three generations to those who were the victims of phthisis proved that it was with-out the least effect. No Neapolitan or Portuguese physician could verify the slightest diminution of phthisis during all this time.

These, says M. Germain Sée, are the results of ignorance; ignorance of the laws which govern the transmission and spread of the most fatal of human diseases among civilized nations. And now what is the true knowledge which M. Germain Sée would have us accept? He himself is as rigorous as the King of Naples ever was in regard to rule and ordinance, only his rule is infinitely simpler, and is one which every nurse could follow without injury or annoyance to any one—a rule which we hope every English nurse does follow scrupulously. The rule is to do away with the sputum expectorated by the phthisical or to des-troy it; then all is said that can be said if this rule be correct.

As will be inferred, M. Germain Sée is a valiant partisan of the school of contagionists. In his eyes heredity as a factor in phthisis plays a very inferior part; and if his points were alto-gether admitted, the part allotted to it would, at the best, be secondary. Take away, he would say, the cause, the source of contagion, and by the act you take away the heredity, since heredity itself requires a root from whence to spring. But he lays himself open to question by his opponents when, in his zeal, he sums up the difficulties lying in the path of all true inquirers into primary causes by attributing every failure to ignorance of the hypothesis, or, as he designates it, the law of the transmission of the tuberculous bacillus. This is not just. It is but fair to assert that they who do not admit the premises of the contagion-ists are *not* ignorant of those premises. Opponents of the hypo-thesis may know the hypothesis as well as the contagionists themselves, but, knowing it, they may not accept the validity of it with such assurance of its certainty as to become convinced of its truth. They may see, in brief, so much evidence in favor of the older and longer recognized views that they feel bound to hesitate, and when they hear of such facts as are disclosed in the working of the edicts of the King of Naples they naturally may hesitate the more. In the English medical fields of controversy the battle on this subject has scarcely commenced in earnest. A good number of men, led into the contagionist camp rather by the novelty of the work there than by the satisfying character of it, have created an impression, and on the question of diagnosis have created an exceedingly strong impression. But the masses of the profession are still in doubt, and before the parasitic and transmissible nature of phthisis is so far proved that the hereditary nature of the disease may be put aside a generation of controversy of the severest kind must be carried out. And, in a matter so momentous, the labor of a generation is worth all the time and all the trouble, since, whichever side ultimately wins, the world at large will, perforce, be the greatest gainer. We have singled out the remarks of Prof. Sée in order to contrast, for the nonce, the two kinds of teaching on this important matter ; but we propose shortly to review the whole discussion, which, it must be confessed, came to a rather impotent conclusion.—*London Lancet.*

The Relation of Dusty Occupations to Pulmonary Phthisis.—(By DR. W. B. CANFIELD.)

This question is by no means new, but it has always been of great interest to those who have much to do with diseases of the lungs. The pulmonary diseases caused by the inhalation of different kinds of dust have received a variety of names, according to the kind of dust inhaled ; but collectively they are all covered by the name " pneumonoconiosis." The pathology of these conditions was not clearly understood. They were spoken of as " miner's consumption," " grinder's consumption," etc., even when their tuberculous nature could not be proven. Even after Koch's discovery of the tubercle bacillus, and the gradually improved classification of the other classes of lung diseases, there seemed to be some doubt whether these dust diseases were tuberculous or not.   45 best writers agree that the inhalation of non-tubercular dust may produce a non-tubercular disease of the lungs. Naturally different kinds of dust, such as sand, coal, soot, slate, when inhaled in large quantities, or by persons enclosed in a laden, crowded atmosphere (unventilated mines, etc.), readily overcome the action of the ciliated epithelium, and advance to the alveoli of the lungs, whence they find their way by their sharp edges through the wounded endothelium—through the pseudo-stomata in the alveolar wall, or between the through the *kittsubstanz* (Osler). Those that are not picked off, rendered harmless or devoured by the greedy phagocytes, remain in their subepithelial bed, and cause an irritation, extermination of blood, inflammation, and resulting hypertrophy and hyperplasia of the connective tissue of the lungs. There results, then, a fibroid condition of the lungs, a fibroid phthisis, or chronic interstitial pneumonia.

This condition seems to be produced by all kinds of dust in some way when inhaled in condensed quantities. Fagge says this condition is only tubercular when tuberculous matter

Although a fact founded on one case, perhaps imperfectly reported, may be of little value, I have thought it worth while to present the following case :—

J. M., Welshman, aged 56, was admitted to hospital about February 1st, 1888, with the following history, imperfect on account of his want of familiarity with the English language. As a boy he had been well, and had been in health up to two years before, in Wales, where he " took a cold," which, growing worse, entirely unfitted him for his work, which was that of a miner. On inquiring more particularly as to his occupation, he said that he had been employed for about fifteen years in the slate mines of Wales, and his particular work was to split the slate. He said that there was always slate dust flying about in the air; but not in such quantities as in coal mines. Upon questioning him further, he said that the slate miners were frequently affected with a cough and a profuse gray or blackish expectoration, and that they usually died from this cough at about fifty. He said their manner of coughing was very hard, and there was much wheezing and shortness of breath. While talking with him, I noticed that he was a tall man, slightly bent, with anxious countenance, showing that he was suffering from dyspnœa or imperfect oxygenation. In fact, he suffered so violently at first that it was very difficult to examine him, and most of the history was obtained at the end of his treatment. Inspection showed a spare man with large chest cavity, but not barrel-shaped. On percussion, which was carried out with great difficulty, a possibly increased dulness was heard over the right apex in front and at the base behind. The left lung was slightly hyper-resonant from increased work. The vocal fremitus was not markedly different on the two sides. Auscultation gave coarse and fine mucus, and dry, sonorous and sibilant râles with expiration and inspiration over the whole chest, the expiration being much prolonged. Cough and shortness of breath were the troublesome symptoms, as was shown in his anxious expression, and in his entire inability to lie in the horizontal position. His expectoration had been dark and also grayish-black ; but recently it was white, as it was when I saw him. In

order to promote expectoration, I put him on oil of turpentine
in fifteen minim doses in mucilage of acacia, cinnamon water
and water three times a day.

> ℞ Ol. terebinthin., - - ℥iii
> Mucilag. acac., - - q.s.
> Aquæ cinnamon, - - ℥ss
> Aquæ q.s. ad, - - ℥vi
>
> S. Take a tablespoonful, well diluted, three times a day,

But as it produced nausea, I changed to the iodide of potash.
with muriate of ammonia dissolved in brown mixture.

> ℞ Ammon. muriat., - - ℥ii
> Mist. glycyrrhiz. co., - ℥iv
> et adde
> Potass. iodid., - - - ℥iii
>
> S. Dessertspoonful, well diluted, three times daily.

This seemed to remove the mucus, but the dyspnœa still continued, and the râles, though dryer, were just as audible as
before.

Dr. Fraser's article on " Dyspnœa in Bronchitis " having just
appeared (*American Journal of Medical Sciences*, Oct. 1887),
it suggested itself to me to use the nitrite of sodium, which resulted in removing much of the dyspnœa.   During the whole
time the sputum was examined for bits of slate dust or pigment
laden cells ; but they were not found.   His diet was regulated
and his bowels kept open.   The urine was tested before turpentine was given, and albumen was found.   It disappeared later.

A few weeks after he entered the hospital the sputum was
examined for tubercle bacilli, not because I expected to find
them, but because I had made it a habit to examine the sputum
for them in every chronic case. They were found in abundance.
Specimens of sputum were examined with care at short intervals,
and the bacilli were always found, and in large numbers. This
surprised me, as I had not thought it tuberculous, and had given
a favorable prognosis. Now, however, I feared a bad prognosis.
Notwithstanding this, he continued to improve under tonics, and
returned to Wales in the spring. I have heard from him within

the last month, and he says he is entirely well. Whether the bacilli have disappeared or not, it is not possible to say. As I have examined the sputa for bacilli many times, I feel certain I made no mistake here, and yet it seems rather peculiar in this case.

Dr. G. Hunter Mackenzie says that the number of tubercle bacilli found in the sputa of any case does not seem to bear any reference to the severity of the cases, and that a case may go on for years with an enormous number of bacilli found at every examination, and yet be well in every other way.

The points of interest in this case are :—(1) Patient had no previous history of or predisposition to tuberculosis. (2) He contracted a disease with which tuberculosis is supposed to be very rarely present. (3) He had tubercle bacilli in his sputa in abundance. (4) He reports himself as entirely well.— (*Trans. of the Medico-Chirurgical Faculty of Maryland.*)

Conclusions Reached by the Hyderabad Chloroform Commission.

—(1) The recumbent position on the back and absolute freedom of respiration are essential.

(2) If during an operation the recumbent position on the back cannot, from any cause, be maintained during chloroform administration, the utmost attention to the respiration is necessary to prevent asphyxia or an overdose. If there is any doubt whatever about the state of respiration, the patient should be at once restored to the recumbent position on the back.

(3) To insure absolute freedom of respiration, tight clothing of every kind, either on the neck, chest or abdomen, is to be strictly avoided ; and no assistants or bystanders should be allowed to exert pressure on any part of the patient's thorax or abdomen, even though the patient be struggling violently. If the struggling does occur, it is always possible to hold the patient down by pressure on the shoulders, pelvis or legs without doing anything which can by any possibility interfere with the free movements of respiration.

(4) An apparatus is not essential, and ought not to be used, as, being made to fit the face, it must tend to produce a certain

amount of asphyxia.   Moreover, it is apt to take up part of the
attention which is required elsewhere.   In short, no matter how
it is made, it introduces an element of danger into the administration.   A convenient form of inhaler is an open cone or cap
with a little absorbent cotton inside at the apex.

(5) At the commencement of inhalation care should be taken,
by not holding the cap too close over the mouth and nose, to
avoid exciting, struggling, or holding the breath.   If struggling
or holding the breath do occur, great care is necessary to avoid
an overdose during the deep inspirations which follow.   When
quiet breathing is insured as the patient begins to go over, there
is no reason why the inhaler should not be applied close to the
face ; and all that is then necessary is to watch the cornea and
to see that the respiration is not interfered with.

(6) In children, crying insures free admission of chloroform
into the lungs ; but as struggling and holding the breath can
hardly be avoided, and one or two whiffs of chloroform may be
sufficient to produce complete insensibility, children should
always be allowed to inhale a little fresh air during the first deep
inspirations which follow.   In any struggling persons, but especially in children, it is essential to remove the inhaler after the
first or second deep inspiration, as enough chloroform may have
been inhaled to produce deep anæsthesia, and this may only
appear, or may deepen, after the chloroform is stopped.   Struggling is best avoided in adults by making them blow out hard
after each inspiration during the inhalation.

(7) The patient is, as a rule, anæsthetized and ready for the
operation to be commenced when unconscious winking is no
longer produced by touching the surface of the eye with the tip
of the finger,   The anæsthetic should never under any circumstances be pushed till the respiration stops ; but when once the
cornea is insensitive, the patient should be kept gently under by
occasional inhalations, and not be allowed to come out and renew
the stage of struggling and resistance.

(8) As a rule, no operation should be commenced until the
patient is fully under the influence of the anæsthetic, so as to
avoid all chance of death from surgical shock or fright.

(9) The administrator should be guided as to the effect entirely

by the respiration. His only object, while producing anæsthesia, is to see that the respiration is not interfered with.

(10) If possible, the patient's chest and abdomen should be exposed during chloroform inhalation, so that the respiratory movements can be seen by the administrator. If anything interferes with the respiaation in any way, however slightly, even if this occurs at the very commencement of the administration, if the breath is held, or if there is stertor, the inhalation should be stopped until the breathing is natural again. This may sometimes create delay and inconvenience with inexperienced administrators, but experience will make any administrator so familiar with the respiratory functions under chloroform that he will in a short time know almost by intuition whether anything is going wrong, and be able to put it right without delay before any danger arises.

(11) If the breathing becomes embarrassed, the lower jaw should be pulled, or pushed from behind the angles, forward, so that the lower teeth protrude in front of the upper. This raises the epiglottis and frees the larynx. At the same time it is well to assist the respiration artificially until the embarrassment passes off.

(12) If by any accident the respiration stops, artificial respiration should be commenced at once, while an assistant lowers the head and draws forward the tongue with catch-forceps, by Howard's method, assisted by compression and relaxation of the thoracic walls. Artificial respiration should be continued until there is no doubt whatever that natural respiration is completely re-established.

(13) A small dose of morphia may be injected subcutaneously before chloroform inhalation, as it helps to keep the patient in a state of anæsthesia in prolonged operations. There is nothing to show that atropine does any good in connection with the administration of chloroform, and it may do a very great deal of harm.

(14) Alcohol may be given with advantage before operations under chloroform, provided it does not cause excitement, and merely has the effect of giving a patient confidence and steadying the circulation.

The Commission has no doubt whatever that, if the above rules be followed, chloroform may be given in any case requiring an operation with perfect ease and absolute safety so as to do good without the risk of evil.—*Lancet*.

THE

Montreal Medical Journal.

| VOL. XVIII. | MARCH, 1890. | No. 9 |

THE CHLOROFORM QUESTION.

As a result of the report made by the Hyderabad Commission, the question of the merits of chloroform are attracting great attention. This Commission, of which Dr. Lauder Brunton was a member, performed a great number of experiments, principally on dogs, with the view of definitely settling the vexed question of how chloroform kills. Ever since the introduction of this agent there have been two rival theories as to the way this lethal effect is brought about. One of these views, mainly held by Edinburgh surgeons and their disciples, was that chloroform induced death by paralyzing the respiration ; the other view was that death almost invariably occurred from cardiac failure.

The experiments performed by the Hyderabad Commission were of two kinds—one being conducted to elucidate what influence is exerted by various conditions upon the relation between cardiac and respiratory arrest, and to point out how far methods at resuscitation are useful ; the second group of experiments, made with recording apparatus, were performed to ascertain the effect of chloroform on the heart and blood-pressure. In the first series, 430 experiments were performed mainly on dogs, with the uniform result that in every case where chloroform was pushed the respiration stopped before the heart. The chloroform was administered in various ways, alone and with morphine, atropine and strychnine. Animals were experimented on who were healthy and suffering from disease. It was given on a full stomach and on an empty one, but no matter what the condition was, the result was invariably respiratory before cardiac failure.

Upwards of 150 experiments were performed to ascertain the influence of chloroform on the heart and blood-pressure, particular attention being directed to demonstrate the influence of all possible conditions that seemed at all likely to affect the blood-pressure during the period of chloroform narcosis.

The conclusion arrived at by the Commission from these experiments is that when chloroform is given continuously by any means which ensures its free dilution with air it causes a fall in the mean blood-pressure. As this fall continues, the animal first becomes insensible, then the respiration gradually ceases, and, lastly, the heart stops beating. However concentrated the chloroform may be, it never causes sudden death from stoppage of the heart.

The above conclusions are directly opposed to the conclusions arrived at by a committee appointed by the British Medical Association a few years ago, and also to the experiments on animals by many independent investigators.

Drs. H. C. Wood and Hare of Philadelphia have recently (*Medical News*, Feb. 22, 1890) investigated this subject, and they arrive at the conclusion that it is possible for the heart and respiration to be practically simultaneously paralyzed by chloroform, and, further, that cardiac arrest may occur before respiratory arrest. They distinctly reaffirm the soundness of the opinions almost universally held up to the present time, " that chloroform acts as a powerful depressant poison both in respiration and circulation ; that sometimes the influence is most felt at the heart, and death results from cardiac arrest ; that in other cases the drug primarily paralyzes the respiratory centres, whilst in other instances it seems to act with equal force upon both medulla and heart."

The experiments of the Hyderabad Commission were conducted with the greatest care, and the only possible way to reconcile the conflicting statements of such competent observers in India, England and America is that the dogs in India are affected differently from those in England and America. After all, it is a very secondary matter how chloroform kills a dog ; the living question is, *How does it kill man*, and what are the best means for combating this lethal tendency ?

On this great question the Hyderabad Commission say that the effects of chloroform are indentical in the lower animals and in the human subject. This surprising statement is followed by the recommendation that the administrator should be guided as to the effect entirely by the respiration. " His only object, while producing anæsthesia, is to see that the respiration is not interfered with." They are further of the opinion that if the directions given by them in respect to attending to the breathing are closely followed, chloroform may be given in any case requiring an operation with perfect ease and absolute safety so as to do good without the risk of evil. As an editorial in the *Lancet* has it, " The practical outcome of the research would appear to be that deaths from chloroform are not inevitable. They are therefore preventible, and by due care in its administration they may be with certainty avoided."

These very extraordinary statements are made with an assurance which will carry conviction to the minds of many medical men, and the inevitable result will be disastrous. If there is a surely established clinical fact, it is, in our opinion, that chloroform does cause death by directly paralyzing the heart, and the only way to prevent and combat this paralyzing influence is to watch the pulse and resort to those measures which experience has shown to be useful in such conditions. Inversion of the patient and the employment of hot applications to the cardiac region are the most trustworthy.

To advise that the administrator should watch the respirations only is going back to that early period in the history of chloroform anæsthesia when clinical facts derived from its action on man were few.

THE PNEUMONIC COMPLICATIONS OF INFLUENZA.

A very striking feature of the recent epidemic of influenza was the complications of bronchitis and pneumonia. In some parts the frequency of the latter complication was so marked as to lead one distinguished observer (Nothnagel) to suggest that there was a veritable endemic of pneumonia in addition to the influenza epidemic. As pointed out by Kundrat, lobular pneumonia was more frequent than lobar pneumonia. The same observer points out several features in the character of this lobular pneumonia which distinguishes it from the ordinary lobular pneumonia which attends bronchitis and the acute infectious diseases. In the first place, the exudate was richer in fibrine than that seen in ordinary lobular pneumonia. It did not affect only the lower and posterior parts of the lungs as the ordinary lobular pneumonia does, but involved also the anterior and superior of the lung as well. The infiltrated patches were much larger than usual, and their centres were usually found in a state of suppurative destruction, resembling in this respect the pneumonic patches that are found in the lungs of horses who have suffered from influenza. Suppurative pleurisy was a feature of most of these cases also.

INFLUENZA.

Prof. Weichselbaum of Vienna has published a report of the results of bacteriological examinations in cases of influenza. (*Wiener med. Wochenschrift*, No. 6, 1890.) The sputum was examined microscopically and by means of plate cultures in 21 cases, in every case showing the pneumococcus to be present, but with only one-third of its usual virulence. In only two of these cases did pneumonia actually occur. The bodies of ten patients who had shown symptoms of influenza, some with and some without lung complications, showed the pneumococcus in every case. Prof. Weichselbaum does not consider, however, that this parasite is the cause of the disease, but that its rôle is only secondary. It is well known to be frequently found in the upper respiratory tracts of healthy persons. In two cases where the blood was examined microscopically for bacteria the result was negative. In one case where symptoms of acute nephritis appeared the urine contained abundant pneumococci. No pneumonia was present and the patient rapidly recovered.

Prof. Klebs has published a short article (*Centralblatt für Bacteriologie*, Jan. 24, 1890) in which he states that in the earliest stages of a number of cases of influenza, he found a flagellate protozoon present in large numbers in the blood. This

was similar to the hæmatozoon found in malaria, but smaller ;
occurred in and between the red corpuscles ; stained with methy-
lene blue ; was present in great numbers in the blood of two
fatal cases. He found bacteria to be absent from the blood in
these cases. He did not succeed in tracing the life cycle of the
parasite or in cultivating it outside the body. He thinks the
lung respiratory affections occurring in the disease are secondary
and not due to any specific microbe. He thinks that the fact
that cases of influenza after a certain lapse of time get well
spontaneously, and that many of the cases afterwards tend to
relapse, is to be explained as showing definite phases of development of the parasite, as is the case in malaria and relapsing
fever. No facts are adduced, however, to support this statement. He thinks the animalcules are probably to be sought for
in the air.

Professor Rippert of Bonn reports finding the streptococcus
erysipelatous in the sputum of cases of influenza. It was found
in the lungs and trachea of five cases.

CLINICAL PSYCHIATRY.

Active steps are being taken to establish, in London, an hospital for the treatment and teaching of insanity. In connection
with it there will be a staff of thoroughly experienced physicians,
whose duty it will be to promote the scientific study of mental
disease. The movement is one of great importance in the interest of the progress of psychiatry as a study, to which it will
undoubtedly give a wholesome and much needed impetus. It
will also be the means of enabling future practitioners to see and
know something of these important class of diseases before they
graduate.

EDITORIAL NOTES.

—From a very interesting report presented to the British Medical Temperance Association it appears that there is a very marked decrease in the amount of alcohol prescribed in 113 hospitals from which a report was received. Collectively the decrease amounts to nearly 50 per cent. as compared with a period twenty-five years ago. There is no doubt that, as a rule, alcohol is too freely and frequently given to hospital patients.

—There is a very instructive lesson to be gathered from the English mortality returns from tuberculosis during the past forty years. In the ten years from 1851 to 1860 the number of deaths from tuberculosis in persons from 15 to 45 years of age amounted to 3,943 in every million. From 1861 to 1870 it had fallen to 3,711. In the following decade, 1871 to 1880, it was 3,194; and from the years 1881 to 1887 it did not exceed 2,666. The decreased rate is more marked in the female than the male sex. It is safe to prophesy that, as our knowledge of this disease increases, the deaths from it will decrease.

—Dr. Sloan of Blyth is a candidate for the representation of the Malahide and Tecumseh division in the Ontario Medical Council. Dr. Sloan is particularly well qualified for the position. For many years he has occupied in the great Huron tract a leading position as a medical practitioner. His popularity in the profession he owes to his ability and sterling integrity. Since the foundation of the Canadian Medical Association he has been one of its most active members, and he has always taken a lively interest in all matters relating to the advancement of the profession. In choosing him as their representative the members of the division will be conferring an honor on one of the most worthy members of the profession in Canada.

—A. Paltauf, Vienna (*Centralblatt f. Path.*) reports four cases where severe injuries and lacerations were not followed by any hemorrhages, though the patients lived ten to thirty minutes after the injury. In all these cases the injuries were multiple, and in three some profuse hemorrhage had occurred elsewhere in the body. He explains the absence of hemorrhage by assuming that the shock of the injury produced spasm of the arteries at the time, and that when this had passed away the lowering of the general blood pressure (from the combined influence of weakness of the heart and free bleeding from other vessels) made it impossible for the blood to be forced into the tissues. The importance of these observations is obvious with regard to testimony as to whether certain injuries were inflicted intra vitam or not; also as to whether multiple injuries, some of which alone show extravasation, could have all been inflicted simultaneously.

Medical Items.

—Dr. Vipond (McGill, '89) has been admitted a Licentiate of the Royal College of Surgeons, Edinburgh.

—The chair of Physiology in King's College, London, is vacant through the retirement of Prof. G. F. Yeo.

—P. T. Hubert, M.D. (McGill, '89), has been appointed Medical Health Officer for the city of St. Johns, N.F.

—Thos. A. Woodruff, M.D. (McGill, '88) has been admitted a Licentiate of the Royal College of Physicians, London.

—Dr. Duquet, President of the Medical Board of Longue Pointe Asylum, has been made an associate member of the Medico-Psychiological Association of Paris.

—It is said that upwards of four hundred graduates attended the New York Post-Graduate Medical School and Hospital during the year 1889.

—The chair of Physiology in the University of Vienna will be vacant, at the termination of the present academic year, through the retirement of Prof. Ernst von Brücke.

—Dr. Sims Woodhead, who, for the past three years, has been Director of the Laboratory formed by the Royal College of Physicians of Edinburgh, has been appointed to a similar position in the Laboratory of the two Royal Colleges of London. The appointment is, we believe, a wise one, for Dr. Woodhead has proved himself to be a worker and investigator.

BRAITHWAITE'S RETROSPECT.—The 100th volume of Braithwaite's Retrospect, being the volume for the last half of the year 1889, has been issued. This periodical, in its long history, has been an admirable exponent of the current views in practical medicine and surgery. The one hundred volumes represent the medical thought of the last half century, a period so prolific in scientific progress.

——Nominations for the quinquennial election of the Council of the Ontario College of Physicians and Surgeons have been made. There are twelve territorial representatives on the Board. Out of these the following have been elected by acclamation :—Dr. Bray, Chatham ; Dr. Ruttan, Napanee ; Dr. Orr, Maple ; Dr. Day, Trenton ; Dr. Williams, Ingersoll ; Dr. Phillip, Brantford ; Dr. Bergin, M.P., Cornwall. The remaining divisions will be contested as follows :—Malahide and Tecumseh, by Dr. Sloan, Blyth, and Dr. McArthur, London ; Burlington and Home, by Drs. James Russel and T. Miller, Hamilton ; Toronto, Midland and York, by Dr. Arthur Dukes Johnson, Toronto, and Dr. H. Machel, Toronto ; Bathurst and Rideau, Dr. J. C. Cranston, Arnprior, and Dr. A. F. Rogers, Ottawa. Election takes place March 25th.

——The fifth annual meeting of the Association of American Physicians will be held at the Army Medical Museum Building, Washington, D.C., on the 20th, 21st, and 22nd of May, 1890. The following is the preliminary programme :—

Discussions—1. Disturbances of Sleep; referees, S. Weir Mitchell, Philadelphia, and Chas. F. Folsom, Boston. 2. Methods of Diagnosis in Diseases of the Stomach ; referee, Francis P. Kinnicutt, New York.

Papers—1. Inflammations of the Appendix and Cæcum and the Duty of the Physician regarding them, Norman Bridge, Chicago. 2. Anæsthetic and Non-Anæsthetic Hysteria, Charles L. Dana, New York. 3. Seizures characterized by Shock and

Loss of Consciousness, Israel T. Dana, Portland. 4. The Dia-
thetic Causes of Renal Inadequacy, I. N. Danforth, Chicago.
5. Certain Points relating to Tricuspid Endocarditis, with specimens, Wm. F. Gannett, Boston. 6. Antisepsis in Midwifery,
Wm. T. Lusk, New York. 7. Varicose Aneurism of the Arch
of the Aorta, Wm. Pepper and J. P. C. Griffith, Philadelphia.
8. Natural History of Typhoid Fever, J. E. Reeves, Chattanooga.
9. What can and should be done to Limit the Prevalence of
Tuberculosis in Man? Edward O. Shakespeare, Philadelphia.
10. Migraine, Wharton Sinkler, Philadelphia. 11. Etiology of
Pleurisy, especially in its Relation to Tuberculosis, A. A. Smith,
New York. 12. Report of Cases of Angio-Neurotic Œdema,
Samuel B. Ward, Albany. 13. Demonstration of Pathological
Specimens, W. T. Councilman, Baltimore.

INVITATION FOR AN INTERNATIONAL MEDICAL AND SCIENTIFIC
EXHIBITION.—In connection with the tenth International Medical Congress, to be held in Berlin between the 4th and 10th of
August, there is to be an International Medical and Scientific
Exhibition. The exhibits will be of an exclusively scientific
nature, as follows :—New or improved scientific instruments and
apparatuses for biological and strictly medical purposes, inclusive
of apparatuses for photography and spectral analysis as far as
applicable to medicine. New objects and preparations in pharmacological chemistry and pharmacy. New foods. New or
improved instruments subservient to any of the departments of
medicine, including electrotherapy. New plans and models for
hospitals, convalescent homes, and disinfecting and bathing institutions and apparatus. New arrangements for nursing, including transportation, baths, etc. New apparatuses in hygiene.
Applications or inquiries inscribed "Ausstellungs-Angelegen-
heit," and accompanied with a printed card containg the name
and address of the firm thus applying, ought to be directed to
the Secretary-General, Dr. O. Lassar, Carlstrasse, No. 19,
Berlin, N.W., Germany.

THE

ONTREAL MEDICAL JOURNAL.

| XVIII. | APRIL, 1890. | No. 10. |

Original Communications.

REPORT OF TWENTY CASES OF SHORTENING
THE ROUND LIGAMENTS AT THE EXTERNAL
INGUINAL OPENING IN THE TREATMENT OF
RETRODISPLACEMENT OF THE UTERUS.

By T. JOHNSON-ALLOWAY, M.D.,
Instructor in Gynæcology. McGill University.

the subject of treatment of retroposition of the uterus has
always been an unsatisfactory one to gynæcologists. It is needless to say that supports of every conceivable form have been
used, and have occupied the attention of the profession for
ages past, without any substantial benefit to patients. So that,
for this unsatisfactory state of things concerning the subject,
was thought justifiable to remedy the condition in question by
direct surgical means. Dr. Alexander of Liverpool was
amongst the first, some seven or eight years ago, to carry into
practice the shortening of the round ligaments by cutting down
the external inguinal ring, taking up the ligaments, suturing them to the wound, and cutting off the slack. As the wound
healed the ligaments united with the tissues in their shortened condition and retained the uterus in its normal forward inclination.

It is not my intention to enter into the question of priority of
the various claimants to originality in suggesting this operation,
also the methods of performing it, as much has of late years
written upon these points by myself and others; but I wish,
in this short report, to bring to your notice some of the main

46

ı the cases in which the operation has been undertaken ʒsults which have been achieved.

Cᴀ —The first case I operated on was in February 1886. The case has been already reported. The lady in question had been for some time a confirmed invalid. Her ill-health was due to chronic metritis and extreme relaxation of the uterine supports, culminating in descent of the uterus and retroflexion. The operation was performed on the 19th February, 1886. She is now, and has ever since been, in perfect health, and leads a very active life.

Cᴀsᴇ II.—T̓ ̓ a young lady who had suffered from constant pɑ... ̓d headache, with other allied symptoms. After a reparatory treatment, I made an attempt to find tl but failed. I operated on one side only. I may say, in ̤ g, that I again operated upon this young lady last Mon̓ ̤k, and found both ligaments without any trouble whateve̓ ̓esult perfect.

Cᴀsᴇ III.—This case was a ɔw, aged 49, still menstruating. Profuse leucorrhœa, old standing laceration of cervix, with extensive hyperplasia. Retroversion to third degree (3°). There had been a progressive state of exhaustion for a year past. Constant headache and backache. I operated upon this lady on the 15th June. First removed the diseased cervix by Schrœder's method and then shortened the round ligaments. This patient recently called upon me in perfect health, free from pain, and is doing considerable work.

Cᴀsᴇ IV.—Aged 37 ; married sixteen years ; twins twelve years ago ; menstruation regular, but profuse and very painful; leucorrhœal discharge ; pain in back and left iliac region ; vertigo and very bad headaches ; extreme nervous exhaustion and insomnia

Examination.—Descent of vaginal walls ; uterus retroverted, enlarged through chronic metritis, and very low down in pelvis.

I performed Schrœder's amputation of diseased cervix and shortened the ronnd ligaments. This lady called several months after the operation to thank me for the benefit she had received. She was then able to do all the work her requirements call upon her to engage in.

CASE V.—Age 50. Had borne one child twenty-five years ago. Had worked very hard all her life. I found her a confirmed invalid, unable to leave her bed. Complained of severe backache, headache, nervous exhaustion and insomnia. Uterus low down in retroversion, cervix appearing at introitus, great descent of vaginal walls, and incomplete rupture of perineum, with atrophy from pressure. She was removed to a private hospital, where, after a few days preparatory treatment, I repaired the perineum by the flap-splitting method and shortened both round ligaments. This patient is now conducting a retail store and is doing heavy work. Uterus high in pelvis and in anteversion.

CASE VI.—This was the case of a young lady who had suffered from severe backache for some years past. Menstruation very profuse and over-frequent, accompanied with pain. Great prostration, but little or no headache. She can scarcely walk, movement causing her so much pain. Uterus very low down, retroverted, and fundus exceedingly tender. Cervix elongated and congested. Endometritis present.

After a few weeks of preparatory treatment, I shortened the round ligaments September 27th. November, returned to her work as saleswoman. Uterus anteverted, lying close to the pubic symphisis. Absolutely free from tenderness and all symptoms formerly complained of.

CASE VII.—This was a young lady who had suffered from severe backache for some years past, but especially severe during the latter four months; also severe intermenstrual, hypogastric pain and irritability of bladder. Feels an inability to walk much, as, if she should have a sudden jar, it causes her very severe pain. Uterus retroverted and fixed in cavity of sacrum. Exudation mass in Douglas's pouch. Utero-sacral ligaments very tense and tender by rectal examination. This patient was confined to bed for one month on preparatory treatment.

Sept. 26th—I shortened the round ligaments. They were extremely thin on both sides.

Nov. 6th—Called to say she was going home the following

day. All symptoms disappeared, and feels much pleased to be free from pain. The uterus in this case was well forward, but not so much so as in other cases.

CASE VIII.—An unmarried lady of 32 years of age. She has not menstruated for about one year. While lifting a heavy case, about one year ago, was suddenly seized with severe pain in her right side. Three months ago she began to eject all food taken, and this condition has existed to the date of consultation. She says she cannot retain even a teaspoonful of water. She has almost constant headache and insomnia. Removed a soft rubber ring pessary which had set up a distressing vaginitis. The uterus lay in 2° of retroversion.

After some days of preparatory treatment, I shortened the round ligaments. Since the operation, now sixteen days, she has been taking fairly large quantities of food, and has not once vomited. She sleeps well and is very little troubled with headache. Uterus, on examination, is well anteverted, and parts free from tenderness.

CASE IX.—This was a case of a married lady, aged 28 married three years, one child. Menstruation over-frequent and profuse. Complains of a dull, dragging pain in back and hip. Profuse leucorrhœal discharge. The principal subjective symptom (intense headache), however, was continued, which had become almost intolerable during the past two years. There was also a constant feeling of nausea, with disinclination for food. I found, on examination, cervix bilaterally lacerated and segments everted; uterus in retroversion, with contraction of utero-sacral ligaments; endometritis, with glairy discharge. I had this patient in bed on preparatory treatment for four or five weeks.

Dec. 20*th.*—I performed trachelorrhaphy and shortened the round ligaments. Found them very large and strong. The patient made a good recovery, and has not had a headache or feeling of nausea since, neither has she had a return of her former back and other aches.

I have now given a short history of a few of my private cases, and it was my intention to place before you the history of at least twenty of those I have operated on ; but, on second thought, it occurred to me that it would be hardly fair to inflict upon you so many cases of so similar a nature. I will therefore be content with publishing the remainder when sufficient time has elapsed since operating to determine definite results. I would, however, here say that I have already, in my hospital reports, published the minute histories of six cases operated upon last summer at the Montreal General Hospital. In two of these cases I completed a cervix, a perineum, and the round ligament operation at the same sitting. One of these patients had complete prolapse of the displaceable portion of the pelvic contents (uterus outside vulva). The other case was one of incomplete prolapse. In the other four hospital cases the operation was also more or less combined with either perineorrhaphy or trachelorrhaphy. I may say that these cases have turned out satisfactorily in so far as relief given and the deformity being rectified. I have ensured the attendance of these patients during the period between the operation and the present time at the gynæcological clinic, and they have expressed their gratitude for the relief afforded them by the operation. In one of these cases the wounds suppurated, but still the uterus was found sharply anteverted, although the sutures had to be removed on the seventh day. Of all my cases, hospital and private, I have had two cases in which the wounds suppurated, but the accident did not prolong convalescence or interfere with the good result of the operation. One of my patients thought she felt a " weakness " in one of the wounds, and as a prophylactic measure I fitted a truss. She is now sometime without it, and no protrusion has taken place.

The other case, the one of complete prolapse, did not return to the clinic as desired. She could not be found. But a few days ago (six months after the operation) she was sent to me through the kindness of Dr. England, whom she had consulted about a lump in her groin. I found, on causing her to force down strongly when in the erect posture, that some protrusion did take place on the right side, and undoubtedly would have in time become a full-sized hernia if it had not been attended to.

I cannot account for this condition in her case, as the wou...nd
was very small and the disturbance of the parts little. She ...eft
hospital rather soon, fully two weeks before I generally g...ive
them permission, and I think privation, hard work, and a p... en-
dulous condition of the abdomen tended largely to cause a sli...ght
separation of the pillars of the external opening. We must n...not
forget here also the great beneficial change which had be...een
brought about as a result of the operation. The woman now ...is
carrying her pelvic floor high up in the pelvis and her uterus ...as
high up as the finger can reach, instead of it being totally ou...ut-
side the vulva—between her thighs. From this it can be easi...ily
seen how the intra-abdominal weight became directed again...nst
the pillars of the inguinal canal, instead of being carried dow...wn
past them through the pelvic outlet as a true pelvic hernia—th...the
condition in which I originally found the case. So that it solve...es
itself into the question, Where would this poor woman prefer t...to
have her hernia ? I may say here in passing that the hospita...al
case-book states this patient had been operated on three time...es
in London, Eng., and twice in a special hospital in Canada, fo...or
the relief of her complete prolapse (perineorrhaphy) without an...y
benefit whatever. These facts speak sufficiently in themselve...es
for the great advantage of Alexander's operation over all other
methods of treatment for this distressing deformity. I have
fitted a simple hernia truss, which has relieved her of the tenderness in the wound caused by the constant spreading of the
pillars of the ring, and the patient is now free from suffering
and able to undertake her regular work.

In regard to suppuration in these cases, I think causes tending in this direction should be avoided, although Polk of New
York states that he regards it as of advantage. Dr. Polk uses
the open wound method of dressing—i.e., packing the wound
with iodoform gauze. I do not think, however, that suppuration involves any danger to the patient so long as we ensure
good drainage. I do not think there is any doubt about the
direct cause being the introduction of septic matter. In both
of my own cases I traced it to this cause, although not directly
connected with myself or instruments. In future I shall do the

operation under irrigation of plain boiled water, and not allow nurses through the medium of sponges (however clean) to cause me to run any chance of infection from without. It is now well acknowledged that spongy connective tissue is extremely liable to break down under the influence of septic infection. It has not the same degree of vitality as muscle or the peritoneum. The latter, in fact, is a veritable digester of filth, and is difficult to influence in this way. On this account I now never make a vaginal examination on the day of the operation, and am more scrupulously careful in every way than in the case of any other operation. I think that the prolonged use of pressure forceps to keep the wound open while the ligament is being searched for has a tendency to cause severe injury to the connective tissue. I have therefore devised a very convenient wound speculum which answers as a reflector as well. This instrument is inserted directly the inguinal opening is reached ; it is self-retaining, and acts also as a good reflector.

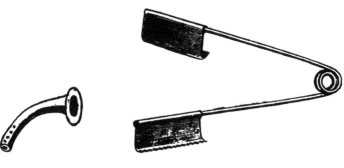

DRAINAGE TUBE.
(*Full size.*)

WOUND SPECULUM.

In regard to protection of the wounds, I think it will be well to cause the patient to wear a double truss for a few months, especially if a hospital patient with a pendulous condition of the abdomen. I am having such an one made with a large soft pad, which will be worn with more comfort than the ordinary double hernia truss.

ñdering the operative methods for retroversion, Dr. H.
says :—

" ander's operation for shortening the round ligaments
is now been performed several hundred times, and is established
s a safe and effective procedure. The position of the uterus
obtained s one of moderate or normal anteversion. Relief of
symptoms is not always immediate, since the traction of the
shortened round ligaments upon the tender or contracted tissues
about the broad ligaments, or contrariwise, the dragging of the
rigid resisting u upon the newly healed round
ligaments, may forts for some weeks or months.
Adjustment of ace after a time, however, and
all symptoms due lacement, together with many
others, eventually : unmeaning argument has been
trumpeted throughout ñc world about the inadequacy
of the round ligamer ; the uterus against abdominal
pressure, and about . er structures beside the round
ligaments play in causing re rsion. It is not pretended that
the round ligaments support the womb in its natural position—
they merely draw the fundus in position so that its weight and
abdominal pressure will act to antevert the uterus. The effect
of their action upon the uterus may be likened to the effect of
the action of the rudder upon the boat—directing merely, not
antagonizing the displacing or propelling powers. This brings
us to the methods by which the fundus has been fixed in front
of the axis of the superior strait. Kœberle was the first to
stitch the uterus to the abdominal wall by suturing the stump,
after abdominal oöphorectomy, in the wound. Olshausen recommended suturing the broad ligaments to the abdominal walls by
a laparotomy performed expressly for this purpose. Since then
Kelly and Sænger have prominently associated their names with
this operation. By it the uterus dislocated toward the front of
the pelvis and swings on a somewhat rigid fundal attachment
near the reflection of the peritoneum over the bladder. The
position of the uterus is not at all comparable to that after
Alexander's operation, since there is a dislocation forward and
a fixation of the fundus. The Germans calls it ventro-fixatio-

uteri, or ventral fixation of the uterus, while Kelly has named it hysterrorhaphy. Laparo-hysterrorhaphy, or anterior fixation of the uterus, as it might more properly be called, must be reserved for those in which Alexander's operation may not be available or practicable, or for those in which it may become necessary to perform laparotomy for breaking up of adhesions or other purposes."

In conclusion, I would say that, carefully judging from experience, I think there is a good future for this operation in affording relief to that most distressing of conditions—retroversion with descent. In recent discussions at American societies it is fast gaining in favor. Its difficulty of successful performance is its greatest drawback, and it requires a great deal of experience and careful manipulation to overcome this difficulty. When, however, the pelvic floor is in the slightest degree functionally impaired and the uterus enlarged, the three operations I have spoken of should be done at the same sitting—and should be properly done. To simply suspend a heavy, bulky uterus by the aid of the round ligaments over a prolapsed pelvic floor is unreasonable, and the bad result obtainable will only tend to bring the round ligament operation into discredit, and very unjustly so.

The following are a few letters I have received from some of the above patients or their husbands, which I thought might be interesting to read :

" *Dear Sir,*—Words cannot express my thanks and gratitude to you for the successful result of this case.
  " Yours faithfully,   A. G."

" *Dear Sir,*—I am happy to tell you that since the operation performed by you I am feeling very much stronger and improved in health in every way. It is now seven months since the operation, and I may say that I have felt well and am able to do my work. Thanking you very much for your kindness during my illness,
  " Believe me, dear sir, yours truly,   M. M."

" *Dear Sir,*—Allow me to tell you how well I am now feeling, the result of an operation performed by you.   Previous to the operation I suffered for years with backache, excruciating headaches, loss of appetite, insomnia, a depressed feeling and lowness of spirits, besides other troubles which you are well aware of. Now I am happy to tell you that I feel like a new woman. No more aches or pain, have fair appetite, rest and sleep well.

"I remain, yours most thankfully,   R. L. McL."

"*Dear Dr. Alloway*,—Allow me to express my gratitude for the happy results of the operation performed by you some time ago. I may say that the result was far beyond my anticipations.
                    Yours truly,   M. H."

CASE OF MUMMIFIED FŒTUS.

CONTRIBUTED BY M. W. LANG, M.D., LAKE PORT, MICHIGAN.

Early on the morning of 30th January, 1890, I was called to attend a primipara, æt. 24, presenting symptoms of threatened abortion. She had last menstruated about the beginning of August, and reckoned herself in the sixth month of pregnancy. About 1 A.M. on 30th January she was awakened with a sharp hemorrhage, followed in an hour by expulsive pains. About 4 A.M. I saw her and found the abdomen of normal size and appearance —fœtal movements distinct—fœtal heart-sounds 160 per minute, head midway between the umbilicus and the middle of Poupart's ligament. On vaginal examination a slight flow was found still persisting, the parts were moist and soft, the os slightly dilated. Rest and full doses of opium were prescribed; in consequence the pains soon subsided and the flow ceased for a few hours. At noon she had a severe rigor, followed shortly by strong expulsive pains. When I saw her again at 4 P.M. it was quite evident that abortion could not be prevented, so I stopped the opium, dilated the os with the finger, and ruptured the membranes; in an hour a living child was born, but died in a few minutes. The placenta and membranes were delivered *entire* by expression. The uterus, however, remaining abnormally large, I made a vaginal examination and found another fœtal head protruding through the os; I hooked my finger over the neck and brought away the fœtus, cord, placenta and membranes all together. The fœtus was 4½ inches long, flattened antero-posteriorly, well preserved, and of a leathery consistence. The cord was 12 inches long, almost straight (only two twists in its entire length), tough, leathery, and requiring considerable force to break or tear it. The placenta was brownish, tough, leathery, and odorless; the membranes were shrunken to mere threads, no liquor amnii being present. On the maternal surface of the placenta there was no appearance of recent detachment from the uterine wall, nor was there any sign of lateral attachment to the other placenta. It seemed as though the fœtus and placenta had remained unattached in the uterine cavity for some time.

There was no specific history; the patient was somewhat anæmic, but otherwise in good health. Most likely this was a case of the survival of the fittest, the stronger and more favorably situated twin crowded out the weaker and pushed it to the wall. The interesting point in the case is the spontaneous separation of the placenta from the uterine wall, and the retention of fœtus and placenta *free* in the uterine cavity while another fœtus was developing there. When was the placenta separated? How long afterward did labor set in? Was abortion brought on by the irritation of the dead fœtus and placenta *in utero?* Unfortunately I was not permitted to take away the specimen for examination, and these interesting questions cannot be definitely answered.

CASE OF SUPERNUMERARY BREASTS.

By J. Herbert Darey, M.A., M.D.,
of Granger, Minnesota.

I was summoned on December 2nd, 1889, to attend Mrs. D., who was at the time in labor with her sixth child. She had had four living children and one born dead at full term. Nothing of any importance occurred with regard to any of her previous labors. I found, on examination, the os moderately dilated and the membranes unruptured. After waiting some time till the os was fully dilated, I ruptured the membranes and she was shortly delivered of a healthy male child. She informed me of a peculiarity in her organization which had caused her a great deal of trouble during each pregnancy and for some time after delivery, viz., the existence of an extra breast in each axilla, which secreted milk very freely and were very hard to dry up. For the latter portion of each period of pregnancy these extra breasts would increase in size, the same as the normal ones, and cause her great distress and discomfort by pressing on the brachial plexus and the axillary vein, causing the arms to swell up. The only way she could get any rest at all at nights was to lie flat on her back, with the arms stretched away out from the sides. If she attempted to lie on either side the gland crowded on the plexus of nerves would cause her such excruciating pain that she could not stand it. During lactation the extra breasts would secrete very freely and wet her night-clothing completely in the course of the night, thus rendering her very uncomfortable.

On examination I found two normal mammæ in the natural situation, and, in addition, in each axilla a mamma as large as a medium-sized lemon, with a distinct areola, but no nipple at all. The ducts opened in the areola, of course, or no milk could flow out. The hair in the axilla grew over these extra glands. The glands were freely moveable under the skin, and had the ordinary consistence of the normal breast. There was no connection whatever between the normal breasts and the supernumerary ones. I advised her to get a breast pump for the two extra breasts, as she said she had never used one; but she informed me of a method she had tried in her last three pregnancies to dry the milk up and so be done with it. As it is very simple, and I had never heard of it before, I will mention it, as it might prove useful in cases where it is advisable to diminish or dry up the secretion of milk. It is simply to make a hot saturated solution of common table salt and apply it constantly on cloths as a fomentation. I saw her again a week after her delivery, and she said that the extra breasts had secreted freely for two or three days, but that under the influence of the salt solution they had almost ceased to flow. She had plenty of milk for the child in the normal mammæ. I thought the anomaly an interesting one, and worth putting on record, as I have never seen any account of a precisely similar case.

EXALGINE AS AN ANALGESIC.*

By James Stewart, M.D.,

Professor of Pharmacology and Therapeutics, McGill University.

The following paper is based on observations made with exalgine for the relief of pain from various causes. In all it was given in 95 cases, with the result of a marked relief in fully 74 cases, or upwards of 77 per cent. In the remaining 21 cases, the effect was slight or negative. The group of cases where relief was most marked were those of facial neuralgia. In all there were 23 cases of facial neuralgia, and in only three was there a negative effect or slight relief. In other forms of neuralgia it was given four times, with a good result in three of the four cases. It was administered in 31 cases of simple headache. In 20 cases relief was obtained, while in 11 the effect was practically negative. In one case of the lightning pains of tabes, marked relief followed its use. In four cases of acute pleurisy relief was marked. A similar result followed in four cases of acute rheumatism. In two cases of severe gastric pain the relief obtained was marked. In 10 cases of abdominal pain from various causes, only six received a beneficial effect. The remaining 16 cases comprised pains of a general and anomalous

* Read before the Medico-Chirurgical Society of Montreal.

The writer is indebted for the majority of the reports on which these observations are founded to Drs. Campbell, England and Brown, Medical Residents at the Montreal General Hospital.

character, due to traumatism, etc. Relief followed in 14 of these cases, while in only two was the result negative.

It will be noticed, from these observations, that the action of exalgine was most marked in cases of *pure* facial neuralgia, while it was least successful in headache. The cases of the latter where the drug was employed comprised headache from various causes. It is generally a difficult and frequently an almost impossible problem to ascertain with any degree of exactitude the cause of headache. This is the only excuse I have to offer for the vagueness of the term headache as here employed.

Now what conclusions are fairly derivable from the experience here related ? Exalgine has marked analgesic powers. To estimate the real worth of a drug, it is necessary, however, to take into account not only the good it does but also the evil ; and, unfortunately, nearly all of our agents of this class possess some very undesirable qualities.

The untoward effects, up to the present, observed in the agents derived from the aromatic series are nausea and vomiting, cardiac depression, dyspnœa and lividity from destruction of the red blood corpuscles, and rashes on the skin. In the 95 cases where exalgine was given, slight nausea was complained of in one case and nausea and vomiting in four. In only two cases, however, was the vomiting apparently directly traceable to the drug. A complaint of numbness in the left arm was made by one patient, but it is doubtful whether the exalgine had anything to do with it. Another patient complained of bad dreams. A feeling of coldness in the feet and legs was another complaint, but the patient was, as a rule, unreliable in her statements, and little weight has been placed on this complaint. The only untoward effect of any moment in the entire 95 cases, or, if we count several doses at intervals in some cases, we have upwards of 150 administrations, were two cases of vomiting, and in both it was but transitory.

No depressing action on the heart was observed in any case, and this is an important point. Neither was there noticed any dyspnœa or other sign of a destructive influence on the red blood cells. Sweating appeared in some cases, but was never profuse enough to exhaust the patient.

It follows, as far as these observations lead us, that exalgine is freer from any deleterious effect than any other analgesic of its class or power.

Exalgine is a compound anilide, being the methyl acetanilide, and is prepared by acting upon sodium acetanilide with iodide of methyl. It appears in needle crystals, hardly soluble in water, but readily soluble in water containing a little alcohol. The dose varies from one grain up to six grains. Fraser of Edinburgh says that he has found marked analgesic effects from quantities as small as half a grain. In a few cases I have tried these small doses, but not with any satisfactory result. Not infrequently it has been found necessary to have to administer a second dose of five grains in the cases reported. The greatest quantity given in twelve hours was 30 grains.

Two doses of five grains at intervals of two or three hours I should consider to be a maximnm quantity.

Its action begins usually in about half an hour and reaches its maximum in about an hour or an hour and a half.

As compared with antipyrine, antifebrine and phenacetine, exalgine is, I think, fully as reliable. It is not more so than any one of these agents, but it is comparatively free from the untoward effects not uncommonly following the action of these agents, the special advantage of exalgine being its good effects in small doses. It is especially interesting, as opening the way to the discovery of other agents belonging to this class which which will exceed it in activity for good and harmlessness.

A very important point which is still unsettled is the mode of action of the aromatic group as analgesics. How do they relieve pain ? We know that opium and agents belonging to its class act by numbing the susceptibility of the sensory centres. The aromatic group, however, do not act in this way.

All the agents of this series, it is found, have a peculiar action on the spinal cord, and from this action there is more than a probability that through it we can explain the analgesic effects of these agents. This effect on the cord was ascertained first in regard to antipyrine. It has been found that this agent, in medium doses, depresses the reflex functions of the cord ; larger doses, on the other hand, cause convulsions, followed by paralysis. The primary diminution of spinal excitability is followed, when large doses are given, by an increased excitability, and this in turn by absolute loss of reflex function. Now there is a very intimate connection between agents which tetanize and those which relieve pain. Both of these properties are commonly found together in the one agent. This point has been prominently brought forward by Lauder Brunton.

The primary depression is supposed to be due to a stimulation of the inhibitory muscular nerves or tracts, the muscles responding but slightly owing to the greatly increased inhibitory influence. As a result of excessive stimulation, we have exhaustion of the inhibitory mechanism and, in consequence, convulsions and rigidity; the final paralysis being explained by the exhaustion of the motor nerves.

Physiology has not, as yet, unravelled the mysteries of the nature of pain. It is surprising how little is said on the essential nature of pain in physiological works. No doubt the seat of pain is in the brain, and we know that there are influences capable of inhibiting pain—that there are higher centres which inhibit the sensory centres. Intense concentration of the mind destroys pain, or as the poet says, " The labor we delight in physics pain."

A constant feature, and one common to all forms of hypnotism, is insensibility to pain from pricking, pinching, burning, etc. while the sensibility to touch may be present or actually increased. Now, although we are unable to explain the phenomenon of hypnotism, it is clear that it is essentially owing to an inhibitory influence, and the most plausible explanation that I know of to account for the analgesic action of the group of aromatics is that given by McAllister. He thinks " that this class of drugs acts, not by numbing the sensory nerves, but by stimulating the inhibitory centres."

This hypothesis may appear to many as too highly imaginative. For true progress it is very necessary to have hypotheses. It requires no effort of the imagination to conceive the time when we can explain the true nature of pain, and then the day will not be far distant when the modern chemist can put into our hands agents more powerful for its relief than any we at present possess. It is even not unphilosophical to assume that we may yet be put into possession of agents which will relieve not only bodily but *mental* pain.

Retrospect Department.

QUARTERLY RETROSPECT OF OBSTETRICS.

PREPARED BY J. CHALMERS CAMERON, M.D.,

Professor of Obstetrics, McGill University ; Physician-Accoucheur to the Montreal Maternity, &c.

Mummified Fœtus Retained in Utero.—Slow death of the fœtus, with mummification and retention in utero for weeks or months, occurs in multiple more frequently than in single pregnancies. Usually the placentæ are attached by their borders and anastomose freely, or else one placenta serves for both children. When one fœtus is much stronger than the other, or is more favorably situated, it is apt to take the lion's share of the nutriment and push the weaker to the wall. This latter slowly perishes and is compressed more or less by the other's growth, and sometimes even flattened out like a sheet of parchment, when it is known as *fœtus papyraceus.* Dr. Lang reports a case in the current number of this JOURNAL, which it is interesting to compare with one reported by Dr. E. W. Mulligan in the *Buffalo Med. Soc. Journal* (quoted in the *Brit. Med. Journal*). On 21st Nov., 1888, Dr. Mulligan was called to a patient six months pregnant, with symptoms of threatened labor, the pains recurring every half hour. The abdomen was so large that he thought the patient's calculations must be astray, and that she was at or near full term. He left directions with the nurse to send for him when labor pains became more active. Soon after he left the house the waters broke and nearly a pailful came away. The pains ceased and the patient continued in good health and attended to her domestic duties till the end of February, 1889, when labor set in. The abdomen was then much smaller than in November. A ten-pound child was delivered, followed immediately by a dead mummified fœtus, whose cord had a velamentous attachment to the border of the placenta. Here there were

47

two amniotic sacs with but one placenta ; the rupture of the one
sac and death of the first fœtus did not bring on labor prematurely or affect the growth of the other fœtus. In Dr. Lang's
case there were two sacs and two placentæ, apparently unattached and not communicating with each other ; the one fœtus
perished and mummified, its placenta separated from the uterine
wall, both fœtus and placenta apparently lying free in the uterine
cavity for some time. It is very unfortunate that Dr. Lang was
unable to secure the specimen for examination.

A Remarkable Case of Fœtal Retention from Fibroid Disease.
—Prof. Alphonse Hergott of Nancy presented the report of a
remarkable case to the Academy of Médicine in December last.
(*Annales de Gynécologie.*) The patient, æt. 24, II-para, was
admitted to the hospital 26th March, 1889. She menstruated
regularly from her fifteenth year, was married at seventeen,
and bore a child two years later. She enjoyed excellent health
till the middle of August, 1888, when her menses ceased ; then
for three months she suffered from difficult and painful micturition, at times necessitating the use of a catheter. The abdomen
enlarged irregularly, fœtal movements were first felt on the right
side at the sixth month, symptoms of peritonitis appeared in the
seventh month, whereupon the fœtal movements became gradually feebler, and finally ceased about the middle of the eighth
month. The abdominal distention then declined somewhat, but
her general condition became so bad that she sought admission
to hospital. On examination, the abdomen was found to be irregularly enlarged. Palpation was painful. The right corner of
the uterus in which the fœtus had developed occupied the right
flank and extended almost to the border of the false ribs, while
a large, firm, fibroid tumor extended from the superior strait in
the middle line up to the umbilicus. It was impossible to induce
labor on account of the situation of the cervix, so there was
nothing to do but to wait for the onset of labor and build up the
patient's strength meanwhile. On April 6th the liquor amnii
began to drain away, a few days later there was a reddish discharge with shreds of membrane, which continued till April 24th;
meanwhile the abdomen was getting smaller and the breasts

larger and more turgid. The diagnosis was fœtal retention from fibroid disease of the uterus. The patient's condition grew rapidly worse, signs of fœtal decomposition and septic absorption appeared, and it became imperative to remove the putrid contents of the uterus by abdominal section. On May 22nd an incision was made to the right of the linea alba obliquely downwards over the site where ballottement had been made out, the uterus was freely incised, a quantity of dark fœtid, purulent fluid came away, and a macerated fœtus extracted. It was about seventeen inches long and weighed a little over five pounds. The placenta was attached to the left side and was firmly adherent throughout. As uterine contraction was feeble, and the patient very weak, it was deemed unsafe to peel off the placenta or attempt the amputation of the uterus; so the edges of the uterine wound were sewn to those of the abdominal wound and the placenta left to separate spontaneously. To guard against septic absorption, the uterine cavity was thoroughly irrigated with the naphthol β solution so highly recommended by Pinard and Bouchard, and tamponed with iodoform gauze. A large thread was attached to the cord and three soft rubber drainage tubes carried down beside the placenta. The sutures were then placed and the dressings applied. Every day gentle traction was made upon the cord and the uterine cavity irrigated with the naphthol solution. On the thirteenth day after the operation the placenta began to come away in fragments, and by the twenty-fourth day it had all been fished out. From that time improvement went on rapidly; on July 18th cicatrization was complete, and on August 1st she left the hospital. The rapid growth of the fibroid in this case is remarkable; so small as to give rise to no symptoms before gestation began, it grew so rapidly that it filled the pelvis, displaced the uterus, and formed the bulk of the uterine tumor. Prof. Hergott wishes to draw the attention of obstetricians to the fact that in certain exceptional cases when the surgeon is obliged to do a Cæsarian section, he may, after suturing the uterus to the abdominal wall, leave the placenta adherent to the uterine wall, thereby avoiding the hemorrhage which is so formidable after its immediate artificial separation and extraction. Naphthol β, a non-poisonous antiseptic, diminishes considerably the danger of septic absorption, and enables him to await the spontaneous separation of the placenta without fear of hemorrhage.

The Influence of La Grippe upon Diseases of the Female Genitals.—Biermer states that the grippe is apt to cause uterine hemorrhage, and in cases of amenorrhœa sometimes re-establishes menstruation. Jacquemier and Kiwisch say that in their experience the disease does not exert an injurious effect upon the course of pregnancy. Dr. Sigmund Gottschalk of Berlin (*Centralblatt f. Gyn.*, 1890, No. 3) gives his experience and confirms the views of Biermer. He found the uterine hemorrhage to be a true metrorrhagia, not merely a menorrhagia. Blood appeared either on the first or second day of the attack, was profuse and accompanied by sacral pain and dysuria. This latter symptom was referable to inflammation of the urethra and vulva. The bleeding lasted from five to eight days; partial relief was obtained by the use of Hydrastis Canadensis and hot vaginal irrigation. In all his cases the uterus was markedly enlarged, its cavity lengthened 1—1½ cm., its walls softened as in pregnancy, its mucus membrane thickened and softened. The uterus was tender to touch and the passage of a sound painful. There seemed to be no special engorgement or sensitiveness of the appendages: he considers the hemorrhage attributable rather to inflammation of the uterine mucous membrane than to any reflex effect from the appendages. It has been asserted that pregnant women are less liable to be attacked with influenza; this was not Gottschalk's experience. Abortion occurred in two cases, pains setting in about the second day of the attack. In both the uterus was very sensitive to touch. In neither was the rise of temperature high enough to account for abortion. He thinks that the influenza acts by inflammation of the uterine mucous membrane in the pregnant as well as the non-pregnant, a condition which may readily lead to abortion in the first half of gestation especially. Gottschalk's observations coincide very closely with my own, made during the recent epidemic in Montreal. In three cases abortion occurred within five days from the onset of influenza, and the loss of blood was unusually great. In another, ten days confined and not yet allowed up, the influenza was ushered in with severe hemorrhage and marked uterine tenderness. In another who was confined while sickening with influenza, there was marked uterine inertia during labor and atomy afterwards. Considerable blood was lost during the third stage, the lóchia continued profuse and bloody for a long time, and the convalescence was slow and tedious. Symptoms of cardiac weakness were marked in most of my cases, in two severe enough to cause great anxiety. Ergot seemed to be of little use ; quinine, digitalis and stimulants were of most service.

Case of Air Embolism after the Iodoform Gauze Tamponade in Placenta Prœvia.—(*Centralblatt f. Gyn.*, No. 1, 1890.)— Vàvra of Prague reports the case. Patient, æt. 38, II-para, was delivered spontaneously. The placenta, attached low down and to the side, came away in half an hour. Atonic hemorrhage followed, which was not controlled by massage, ergotin, hot and cold douching. After several strips of iodoform gauze had been introduced the patient became suddenly cyanosed, and died. At the post-mortem, air was found in the veins of the broad ligaments, both internal spermatic veins, the inferior vena cava, the right heart and pulmonary artery. Moderate anæmia and œdema of the lungs were also found. Vàvra calls attention to the necessity of care in tamponing, because in this case the air was pressed into the uterine veins while the strips of gauze were being placed *in situ.*

The Antiseptic Value of Acetic Acid in Obstetrics.—(*Centralblatt f. Gyn.*, No. 6, 1890.)—Dr. Schæffer read a paper before the Berlin Obstetrical and Gynæcological Society criticising the views of Battlehner and Engelmann upon this subject. In Veit's laboratory he carried out a series of experiments upon the relative germicidal power of acetic acid and carbolic acid upon anthrax spores and the staphylococcus aureus. A 5 per cent. solution is as strong as can safely be used ; the following are the results :

{ A 5 p.c. sol. of carbolic acid destroyed anthrax spores in 36 hours.
{ A 5 p.c. sol. of acetic acid   "   "   " in 15 days.
{ A 5 p.c. sol. of carbolic acid destroyed staph. aureus in 1 minute.
{ A 5 p.c. sol. of acetic acid   "   "   " in 7 hours.

In the treatment of puerperal septicæmia, the carbolic acid solution is consequently 420 times as powerful a germicide as the acetic acid solution. Battlehner advocated acetic acid, because it is always readily obtainable in the form of vinegar; Schæffer considers the intrauterine injection of vinegar objectionable on account of fermentative and other germs it is liable to contain.

A Case of Ectopic Gestation without characteristic symptoms. —(*Medical News.*)—Dr. J. M. Baldy records a very interesting case where he diagnosed pyosalpinx and operated, but found an unruptured tubal pregnancy. The patient, æt. 24, had two children, no miscarriage. The last pregnancy was six or seven years ago. After this labor she was confined to bed for eight weeks, and has never since been free from pelvic and abdominal pain, and has been once confined to bed for a week with abdominal pain. Her menstruation has been regular but profuse. On November 15 she applied to Dr. Baldy, stating that her regular period had come on five weeks previously, and that she had been losing more or less ever since. She had chilly feelings, a high temperature, and rapid pulse. On examination, the uterus was found of normal size and in good position. On each side were irregular cystic masses, the largest being on the right. Manipulation was painful. The diagnosis was double chronic pyosalpinx with acute pelvic peritonitis. Six days later abdominal section was performed and a tubal pregnancy six or seven weeks old was removed from the right side, and an ovarian cyst the size of a hen's egg from the left side. Subsequent questioning elicited no other signs of gestation, ectopic or otherwise. During the past year no menstrual period had been delayed, scanty or missed. None of the ordinary signs of pregnancy were present, such as she had previously noticed. There were no mammary changes, no decidual discharge, no stomach symptoms, no enlargement of the uterus, no discoloration of the genitals. Sterility for six or seven years, bleeding for five weeks and pain were the only symptoms usually present in ectopic gestation, symptoms altogether too indefinite to make diagnosis possible. This case is of interest in view of the dogmatic statements that are made from time to time as to the early diagnosis of ectopic gestation. Dr. Baldy calls particular attention to the following points :—

1. That this was an unruptured or primary tubal pregnancy.

2. That there was no missed or scanty menstrual period.

3. That there was no decidual discharge.

4. That there were no breast or stomach symptoms or other signs of pregnancy.

5. That the woman did not think she was pregnant.

6. That the uterus was of normal size.

7. That the character of the pain was not markedly distinctive.

8. That there was a tubal pregnancy on one side and an ovarian cyst on the other.

The Influence of Menstruation upon Lactation.—(*Medical News.*)—It is and always has been a popular belief that in nursing women menstruation impairs the quantity and quality of the milk. Some trace rickets to the continuance of lactation after menstruation has been re-established, while one observer claims that bacteria appear in the milk during menstruation. Schlichter has recently published some important observations on this subject in the *Wiener Klinische Wochenschrift.* In the foundling hospital for five months and a half, careful note was taken of the general health, evacuations and weight of fifty-two children nursed by women whose menses had returned, thirty-three milk analyses being made. It was found that children nursed by menstruating women sometimes increase wonderfully in weight, the average increase being greater during and just after the appearance of the menses than before, and the condition of the child during the menstruation period being excellent. Only one child became dyspeptic at this time, and even then did not cease gaining in weight. The milk analyses showed less difference between the milk of the menstruating and non-menstruating than between specimens of the same woman's milk collected at morning, noon and night. The conclusions drawn are as follows :—

1. Menstruation returning during lactation (that is, after the sixth week from delivery) is not necessarily injurious to mother or child.

2. Metrorrhagia before the sixth week may retard the development of the child.

3. Diseases in the nursing child, as dyspepsia, colic, enteric catarrh, occurring during menstruation in the nurse, should be regarded as coincidences, and, therefore,

4. Should not, à priori, be treated by a change of nurses or artificial feeding, but should be managed in the usual way by medication and regulating the length of the nursings and the intervals between them.

The writer of the *Medical News* editorial concludes that these views of Schlichter's are in accord with his clinical experience, and that menstruation not excessive in amount or duration, nor accompanied by other pathological conditions, does not of itself interfere with lactation.

Changes in the Tubes and Ovaries in Pregnancy and the Puerperal state.—(*Zeitschrift f. Geb. und Gyn.*, Bd. XVIII., Hft. 1.)—*Dr. Thomson* of Dorpat, from a series of investigations upon rabbits, comes to the following conclusions:—

1. The tubes in pregnancy and the puerperium undergo very appreciable changes. In pregnancy the connective tissue is richer in blood and more succulent, and seems somewhat thickened. The tubal musculature hypertrophies, but in a less degree than the uterine. In the puerperium the muscle cells involute in the same way as the uterine.

2. The ovaries manifest no appreciable change in their structure during pregnancy or the puerperium.

Abdominal Section for Congenital Umbilical Hernia.—In the January number of the *American Journal of Obstetrics*, Dr. McDonald reports a case which resisted reduction by taxis, but was cured by section. At birth it was noticed that the cord was the seat of an umbilical hernia ; a temporary ligature was applied about eight inches from the abdomen and repeated attempts made to return the bowel. The child was normal except the hernial protrusion at the umbilicus the size of an orange. The sac-wall was thin and translucent, permitting a view of the already congested bowel beneath. Taxis having failed, immediate operation was decided upon. The child, wrapped in warm flannel, was placed in a good light and put under chloroform. The abdomen and cord having been made aseptic, the sac was divided between two artery forceps to the left of the umbilical vessels. The external layer (amnion) was freely incised, and Wharton's jelly having been carefully cleared away, the inner coat (peritoneum) was freely incised between artery forceps, care being taken to avoid adherent intestine. The sac contained portions of the ileum, ascending colon and cæcum. All non-adherent portions were at once returned and a hot sponge applied to close the ring; adherent intestine was relieved by resecting the inner wall of the sac and adherent omentum ligated and removed. The intestines were then returned, hemorrhage controlled, the entire sac down to the integument excised, and the wound closed by through-and-through silk sutures, introduced well back from the edges of the wound. The patient made a good recovery. The author gives a table of all the cases of abdominal section for umbilical hernia he has been able to find, nineteen in all—with seventeen recoveries and two deaths. He has also collected from various sources twelve cases treated by the expectant method (compress and bandage)—with three recoveries and nine deaths.

The operation should be done as soon as possible after birth, as the delay of a few hours may be followed by commencing gangrene of the cord and peritonitis. The indications for operation are—

1. The character of the sac must be such that delay will lead to its sloughing.

2. The hernia must be irreducible.

3. If reducible, it must be incapable of retention by suitable mechanical appliances.

Pregnancy in the rudimentary horn of a bicornate uterus mistaken for Tubal Gestation; Laparotomy; Recovery.—Dr. Mundé (*Amer. Jour. Obstet.*, Jan. 1890) reports the case of a woman who had a tumor to the right of the uterus which he supposed to be an ectopic gestation. He opened the abdomen, and discovering his mistake, aspirated the liquor amnii, whereupon the uterus regained its normal outline. The uterus was returned to the abdominal cavity and the abdominal wound closed. The patient aborted that night, as expected, and made an uninterrupted recovery.

The subsequent behavior of cases of Ectopic Gestation treated by Electricity.—In May, 1888, Dr. Brothers of New York reported a case of ectopic gestation successfully treated with electricity, and gave a resumé of forty-three cases collected from various medical journals (*American Journal of Obstetrics*) In the February (1890) number of the same journal he reports ten more cases, and gives the results of his enquiries respecting the subsequent behaviour of cases so treated. It is well-known that in the majority of reported cases the use of electricity has been followed immediately by an abatement in symptoms due to growth, and a marked diminution in the size of the tumor. In order to determine more accurately the subsequent course of such cases, he opened a correspondence with those operators who had used this method or knew of cases where it had been used. An answer was requested to the following two questions: I. What secondary dangers has your patient undergone as a result of the treatment? 2. What is the present degree of health of your patient, or when last seen? From replies to these questions he is able to state positively that 25 patients (reported cured) have been heard from, after the lapse of one to eight years, and that at last accounts all were well. Many still carried traces of the old trouble, but not such as to cause any inconvenience. From a careful study of the facts he has collected, Dr. Brothers draws the following conclusions :—

1. The risk of rupturing the sac of an ectopic pregnancy and causing death by internal hemorrhage is slight. In but one case has this possibly occurred, but the reporter himself thought that the damage existed prior to the employment of electricity.

2. Suppuration of the dead fœtal mass has not occurred in any case in which electricity was employed before the third month.

3. Beyond the third or possibly the fourth month, electricity should not be resorted to.

4. Electro-puncture is to be condemned in all cases.

5. In cases of mistaken diagnosis, no harm is done by the electrical treatment.

6. Under galvanism or faradism early ectopic gestation can

be checked in its growth and caused to disappear entirely or become shrivelled up. The remaining masses have thus far caused no subsequent trouble.

Embryotomy vs. Cæsarian Section.—Dr. Barnes replies to Dr. Wathen's criticisms of his views on this subject in the *American Journal of Obstetrics,* March 1890. Dr. Barnes discriminates between cases of labor at term with conjugate diameter under 2 inches, and those with a conjugate of 3 inches and more. In the first class of cases he advocates C. section. If the conjugate is under 2.5 inches and the child is not viable, he thinks abortion should be induced. If the conjugate is 3 inches or more (too narrow to allow a mature fœtus to pass alive) he advises to temporize till the fœtus is viable and then induce labor. He says it is the mother's right to turn the scale in her favor when there is a doubt. He maintains that neither craniotomy nor Cæsarian section can be absolutely accepted or absolutely condemned; each has its own proper field, and in particular cases we are bound to consider which is to be preferred. "It has become the fashion of late to accept without reserve the dogma that fœticide, done for the purpose and with the high probability of saving the mother, is murder. May it not be said with more justice that to encounter the serious risk of matricide with the doubtful hope of saving the fœtus is near akin to murder? There are two sides to the question; they are not incompatible."

RETROSPECT OF PATHOLOGY.

By Wyatt Johnston, M.D.,
Demonstrator of Pathology, McGill University.

Peritonitis.—Dr. H. J. Waterhouse of Edinburgh has published some interesting experiments upon purulent peritonitis. Grawitz had shown, in 1886, that the injection of even large quantities of pyogenic bacteria into the peritoneal cavities of rabbits and dogs was not sufficient to produce suppuration unless they were mixed with some substance difficult of absorption (blood, etc.), or unless the peritoneum was at the same time inflamed by some substance such as turpentine or croton oil. Dr.

... these results on rabbits and
... experiments to bring out certain
... in explaining the conditions under
... laparotomies, intestinal strangulation,
... that very small quantities of decomposing
... injected into the peritoneum were capable
... peritonitis, but when largely diluted
... Injection of a few drops of any fluid
... with simultaneous irritation of the peri-
... caused fatal peritonitis. A laparotomy
... predisposing cause for peritonitis, be-
... injection of staphylococci gave negative
... of the angles of the wound itself
... failed to produce peritonitis. Inocu-
... but not opening, the peritoneum
... in the abdominal wall, but no periton-
... intestine, the peritoneum showed itself
... resulting in one case where resection
... injection of staphylococci. Artificial strangu-
... always spontaneously recovered from
... the constriction had only lasted six
... cavity was infected with staphylo
... peritonitis, even when the constriction
... A similar fatal result was obtained
... into the veins of the ear,
... abscess or osteomyelitis. On the other
... injection of staphylococci into the stom-
... intestine was not followed by peritonitis.
... injection of a very few drops of the
... in every case purulent peri-

... —Prof. E Ponfick of
... the results of a re-
... this subject, to ascertain to
... be dispensed with.
... others were chiefly con-
... with the uniform result of

leath within a few hours. Ponfick found to his astonishment
.hat by ligaturing the long tongue-like processes of the rabbit's
iver near their roots, close to the vena cava, he was able to
xcise, either at a single sitting or by repeated operations, from
ne-fourth to three-fourths or even more of the organ without
eriously affecting the general health of the animal. The rabbit's
iver consisting of five lobes bearing a uniform ratio to the
ntire organ, the removal of one or more of these signified respectively the removal of one-fourth, one-half, three-fourths, four-
ifths, etc. The immediate effects of the removal of one-fourth
were a temporary venous congestion of the spleen, stomach and
mall intestine. When one-half or three-fourths were removed,
his condition was more marked, a few ecchymosed and infarcted
pots being observed. The spleen in these cases was increased
) double its normal size. The large intestine and cæcum were,
owever, quite free from congestion. This portal congestion was
ily transitory, disappearing completely in the course of a few
ays or even hours. These immediate effects were observed in
iese animals dying from various causes soon after the operation.
he majority of the animals survived.

The ultimate effects of the operation.—Since the individual
eight of each of the five lobules bore a constant ratio to the
tal weight of the liver, and the total weight of the liver to the
dy weight, it was interesting to estimate the degree of com-
ensatory hypertrophy in those portions of the liver left intact.
t was found that the animals, after removal of one-fourth, at
rst lost weight but soon regained or even exceeded the weight
revious to the operation. In attempting subsequent further
emoval of another lobe the operation in several cases was
ttended with fatal hemorrhage. The autopsy showed that the
ntact portions of the liver had compensated for the portion lost,
he actual liver weight being greater than that estimated at the
ime of operation. When one-half or three-fourths of the liver
iad been removed, this compensation was even more marked,
ind took place within even the incrediby short spaze of eight to
ifteen days. An attempt to remove subsequently the remaining
ourth of the liver in thirteen cases resulted uniformly in the
leath of the animals from hemorrhage.

successful
B. sebach
made upon
impossible t
and indep
by exclu
growing
bu
the boo
disinf
y 5
us are
ate.
prod
H
note th
produc
ame symp
some unkr
determinin
as a
uction of leu
Bact.
other animals

ventricle. The disease is frequently fatal in from six weeks to as many months. The symptoms appear to depend upon a progressive paresis of the diaphragm, and much benefit is derived from faradization of the course of the phrenic nerve. Dr. Minra considers that this obscure neurosis is produced by eating certain species of tunny fish. (*Fam. Scombridæ.*) It was formerly very prevalent in the Japanese navy, but disappeared entirely about a year ago when fish was abolished from the sailor's diet. It was common amongst the jailors in the prisons, but the prisoners who lived on a vegetable diet were free from it. It was present only during the summer months, when this fish was obtainable, and existed chiefly among those persons who were in the habit of eating it (probably in a condition not perfectly fresh).

Acute cases of poisoning from these fish had been long well known, and went by the name of fish-drunkenness, the symptoms being headache, vertigo, palpitation and dyspnœa.

Malignancy in Tumors.—There seems to be a growing tendency to accept the theory so long upheld by Sir James Paget, that tumors are due to some specific virus whose nature we have yet to learn. The announcement by Scheuerlen some three years ago that a specific bacillus had been discovered in cancer, led to the careful investigation of this point by numerous competent men with negative result. It seems well proved that the virus, if it exist, is not bacterial in nature. At present it seems probable that some tumors, at all events, are due to parasitic protozoa (psorospermia) belonging to the family of Gregorinidæ. The conditions known as epithelioma contagiosum and Paget's disease of the nipple appear due to the coccidium (or spore case) form of these parasites. These are forms of cutaneous epithelioma due to psorospermia. The parasitic nature of the disease was first pointed out in 1889 by Darier, of the Hospital St. Louis in Paris, who calls it follicular psorospermiosis. The small oval parasites were found in large numbers in the sebaceous follicles and in the deeper layers of the rete Malphigii, which showed a marked tendency to proliferation and infiltration of the deeper tissues. In the laster stages ulceration occurred.

L. Wickham of the Hospital St. Louis has since investigated six cases, finding parasites present in every instance. Inoculation experiments were unsuccessful. Cultivations in moist sterilized sand were attended with some degree of success, certain changes in the protoplasm being observed to take place. These changes remained absent when the cultures were mixed with powdered iodoform.—(*Archives de Médecine Experimentelle*, Jan. 1890.)

Bland Sutton (*British Medical Journal*, 1889) has described similar bodies in cases of mucous papillomata of the cervix uteri in monkeys. In these cases, however, the conditions did not appear to be malignant. The parasites were not detected in some cases of uterine cancer in the human subject.

Thoma (*Fortschritte de Médecine*, No. 11, 1889) reports having met with cell-like bodies apparently parasitic in nature lying within the nuclei of cancer cells.

It is possible that these may have escaped detection through the close resemblance they bear to the histological elements; unless some method of cultivation and inoculation is discovered the microscopic appearances alone cannot be considered conclusive.

A contagious form of epithelioma also occurs in fowls, and in this L. Pfeiffer has recognized similar parasitic protozoa.— (*Zeitschrift f. Hygiene*, Bd. IV.)

Hanau of Zurich (*Fortschritte de Médecin*, 1889) reports the successful inoculation of a form of carcinoma affecting the testicles of white mice. He transplanted portions of the tumor into several other mice both subcutaneously and into the peritoneum.

Wehr (*Arch. f. Klin. Chirurg.*, Bd. XXXIX.) was able to successfully transplant minute portions of a medullary cancer from the prepuce of a dog into the subcutaneous cellular tissue of healthy dogs. The grafts attained the size of hazel nuts and then disappeared. In one case, however, secondary carcinoma was found six months later in the lymph, glands and spleen.

Hospital Reports.

MONTREAL GENERAL HOSPITAL.

CONDENSED REPORTS OF CASES IN DR. MACDONNELL'S WARDS.

The Influenza Epidemic in its Relation to the Mortality from Pneumonia.—According to the various records of previous epidemics of influenza there has been, during the period of the visitation, an unusual mortality from lung diseases, and more especially from pneumonia. It was my lot to have had charge of half of the medical patients in the Montreal General Hospital during the period in which Montreal was visited by the influenza, and inasmuch as many lung cases found their way to my beds, it has appeared to me that some account of the cases may not be uninteresting.

Most writers on epidemics give some six to eight weeks as the period during which influenza visits a place. So I shall take the months of January and February as the *grippe* period here, as it was during Christmas week that the first cases made their appearance. The field of observation, I confess, is very small, some thirty beds all told, many of them occupied during all that period by those suffering from chronic diseases, but, perhaps, had our records extended over more patients we might, as has happened during typhoid fever visitations, become so overworked as to render the accurate recording of all the symptoms and physical signs an impossibility.

There were admitted 15 cases of lobar pneumonia ; of these 9 died. Of the whole number but two had a previous history of *la grippe*. In all the other cases in which a connected history could be obtained there was the story of the pain in the side, the chill and sudden illness. These two cases were both fatal. One was a consolidation of the whole of the right lung, occurring in our nurse who, having had the influenza, struggled to attend to the patients under her charge. The second case was in one of our chronic patients who had been under treatment for aortic regurgitation. After having had febrile symptoms for some days, pneumonia developed, and death was speedy.

48

change.   After the crisis, in addition to the sweating, there had been sharp diarrhœa and very copious mucous expectoration, but there had been no perceptible change in the physical signs. To-day, however, it is evident that fluid is rapidly forming. The apex of the heart is displaced to a point half an inch outside the nipple line.   In the right lung, below the nipple line, all round there is silence ; above this level the breathing is bronchial. Two days later the signs of fluid became more manifest ; the right chest was perceptibly larger than the left, and did not undergo any perceptible movement during the act of inspiration. The temperature, which had fallen to normal after the crisis, now began gradually to rise at night.   Aspiration with a hypodermic needle withdrew fluid suspiciously sero-purulent.   The physical signs are now indicating very copious effusion ; 20 ozs. of fluid were withdrawn with an aspirator on the 4th February. This fluid, on microscopical examination, was reported to contain pus.   On 9th February another aspiration was practised and 46 ounces of decidedly purulent fluid were taken away.   The general condition having somewhat improved, the chest was opened by Dr. Bell on the 11th February and a considerable quantity of very thick pus was removed.

March 19th.—Progress of the case satisfactory.[*]

Small as was our experience of the relation of epidemic influences to the frequency of pneumonia, it enables us to say (1) that during the period of the visitation there were an unusually large number of admissions for pneumonia, (2) that of these persons so attacked a large proportion were either drunkards or aged persons, (3) that the prognosis in pneumonia during this period was no worse than any other time.   All the single lung

---

[*] The following references to Metapneumonic Empyema have recently come under my notice :—

In the *Revue des Sciences Médicales,* Jan. 1890, there is an abstract of a case reported by Sevestre, of a boy aged seven, son of a consumptive mother, who in the course of a left apex pneumonia presented the physical signs of effusion into the pleura with displacement of the heart.   Three hundred grammes were withdrawn from the 7th interspace. Ten days afterwards another tapping had to be made in the 2nd interspace to empty a second collection of fluid.   Finally the operation for empyema was performed, and recovery ensued in the space of two months.

The *American Journal of the Medical Sciences* for June, 1888, contains (p. 621) an abstract of an article by Penzoldt (*Munch. med. Wochensch.* 1888, 227) on this subject, in which he relates his experiences of seven cases.

pneumonias not complicated with alcoholism or age recovered. The proportion of deaths to recoveries corresponds very closely to what has been observed elsewhere. Thus, in Vienna Prof. Rettenbacher reports eight deaths in ten cases. Nothnagel reports a high mortality from pneumonia, and states that the peculiarity of the disease is the tendency to spread to both lungs. In the " General History of the Epidemic of Influenza " by Dr. Jacobi, in the *New York Medical Record* for February 22nd, 1890, it is stated that in St. Luke's Hospital there were fifteen cases of lobar pneumonia, seven deaths; both lungs involved in four cases.

Reviews and Notices of Books.

The Principles and Practice of Surgery. By JOHN ASHURST, JR., M.D., Barton Professor of Surgery and Professor of Clinical Surgery in the University of Pennsylvania, Surgeon to the Pennsylvania Hospital, Senior Surgeon to the Children's Hospital, &c. Fifth edition, enlarged and thoroughly revised. With 640 illustrations. Philadelphia: Lea Brothers & Co. 1889.

We had the pleasure and privilege of reviewing the last edition of this excellent work on surgery, and the only regret regarding it we had then to express was the continued antipathy of its able author to the great principle of modern antiseptic surgery. Now, however, we are happy to be in a position to state that Dr. Ashurst has at last become a convert, and is now almost as strong in his advocacy of Lister's methods as before he was opposed to them. This is a great gain, because there are few teachers on this continent who wield a more widespread influence than the author of the work under review.

We have pleasure in making the following quotation from the article on the treatment of wounds : " In previous editions of this work I have expressed a doubt as to the superiority of the *antiseptic method* over other plans of wound-treatment. Having now employed it for over two years in large clinical services at the University, Pennsylvania, and Children's Hospitals, as well as in private practice, I feel compelled to say that I have modified my opinion, and that while I cannot subscribe to the extravagant laudations which this plan of treatment receives at the hands of its most enthusiastic advocates, I believe that, when used with judgment, and, if I may be pardoned the expression, when *diluted with common sense*, it is capable of affording very valuable aid to the surgeon. I have not, indeed, found any diminution in the mortality after operations by its employment, but I find that the average period of convalescence is shortened ; that the violence of the traumatic fever and the frequency of secondary fever are both lessened ; that upon the whole the comfort of the patient is promoted ; and that the labor and anxiety of the surgeon are very materially diminished. For all which I am duly thankful."

While the general arrangement of this edition is very much the same as that of previous volumes, all parts have been carefully revised and much new matter incorporated. The chapters on Diseases of the Eye and of the Ear have been thoroughly revised by Drs. De Schweinitz and Randall, both former pupils of the author. The number of illustrations has, moreover, been considerably increased by original cuts, especially of new and improved forms of instruments and apparatus.

We can, in conclusion, strongly recommend the work, and we predict for it a large sale both among students and practitioners.

Chronic Bronchitis and its Treatment. A Clinical Study. By WM. MURRELL, M.D., F.R.C.P. London : H. K. Lewis. 1889.

This little book consists largely of abstracts of various papers published by the author during the past ten years, but strengthened by much additional experience. Various forms of treatment are discussed by the writer, many of which are either original or have been largely worked out through his industry. The routine treatment with counter irritants, stimulating expectorants, etc., is dismissed in a few words as proving unsatisfactory in many cases. A strong case is presented for the wider introduction of the ipecacuanha spray, and cases are cited in which great relief to the cough and more especially to the dyspœa were obtained. This remedy may now be looked upon as an established method of treatment, and its value has been corroborated by many continental and American observers. Terebene, cubebs and other remedies are spoken of favorably. Although it seems probable that the views expressed are too sanguine, yet any attempt to alleviate the distressing symptoms of this complaint will be welcomed. The author has evidently made a careful and systematic study of a large number of cases, and his work can be confidently recommended as a valuable contribution to the therapeutics of the disease.

A Manual of Obstetrics. By A. F. A. KING, A.M., M.D.
Fourth edition. Philadelphia: Lea Brothers & Co. 1889.

In each successive edition, Dr. King's manual exhibits evidence of growth; it now numbers 431 pages. No doubt in a few years it will have expanded into a full-fledged systematic treatise on the science and art of obstetrics. The sooner the metamorphosis takes place the better will it be for both author and student. In many respects the book is excellent; it is well written, contains much valuable information, and is particularly good in its illustrations. In its present form it may serve a good purpose as a synopsis for review, but it can not be safely permitted to take the place of a good standard text-book. Such manuals, useful perhaps to the diligent, are liable to great abuse by the idle and indifferent, and cannot be recommended for general use.

Lehrbuch der Hebammenkunst. Von DR. BERHARD SIGMUND SCHULTZE (Jena). Neunte Auflage. Mit 96 Holzschnitten. Leipzig: Wilhelm Engelmann. 1889. (Text-book of Midwifery. By Dr. B. S. Schultze of Jena. Ninth edition, with 96 woodcuts.)

Among the poorer classes in Germany, the practice of midwifery is almost exclusively in the hands of women, a physician being summoned only in cases of difficulty or danger. It is necessary, therefore, to prescribe a more extended course of

study for midwives in Germany than is usually considered necessary in this country where common usage is so different. Dr.
Schultze's manual is prepared especially for the use of midwives
and contains a good deal of matter not usually found in English
text-books; it is clear, plain and practical, and the illustrations
are excellent. It is divided into seven parts and an appendix.
The first part is devoted to the anatomy of the female pelvis
and fœtus; the second describes the course and symptoms of
normal pregnancy, the development of the ovum, the position of
the fœtus in utero, the methods of making external and internal
examinations, the diagnosis of pregnancy, and gives directions
for the diet, dress and care of the pregnant woman; the third
and fourth parts treat of normal labor, the puerperal period and
lactation; while the fifth, sixth and seventh are devoted to a
consideration of the abnormalities which may occur during those
periods. The appendix treats briefly of ethical and medico-legal
duties, conduct in emergencies, the use of the douche, catheter,
etc. The chapter on the resuscitation of still-born infants is
particularly good.

**Handbook of the Diagnosis and Treatment of the
Diseases of the Throat, Nose, and Naso-
Pharynx.** By CARL SEILER, M.D. Third edition.
Philadelphia: Lea Brothers & Co. 1889.

The popularity of this book is evidenced by the fact that it
has, in a short space of time, reached its third edition. The
subjects discussed have been thoroughly revised in the former
edition, and brought to the views most generally accepted,
omitting many points upon which so much has been said without
anything definite being arrived at, thus saving the student of
laryngology invaluable time. The chapter on the physiology of
the voice and articulate speech deserve particular commendation,
for this matter, a thorough knowledge of which is absolutely
essential to the correct understanding of certain pathological
conditions and of their successful treatment, is, unfortunately,
almost neglected even by so-called standard works on laryngology. There is one point which does not commend itself, and

that is a classification of subjective symptoms of the larynx and naso-pharynx, for symptoms in this class of diseases are so varied and so ambiguous even in the same disease, that the student is apt to lay too much stress upon subjective symptoms and neglect the more important ones, viz., *objective*.

As a guide to the study of diseases of the throat and naso-pharynx, we cordially recommend it to students and practitioners.

Society Proceedings.

MEDICO-CHIRURGICAL SOCIETY OF MONTREAL.

Stated Meeting, Fvbruary 21st, 1890.

G. E. Armstrong, M.D., President, in the Chair.

Orbital Tumor.—Dr. Buller brought before the Society a young girl, aged 18 years, whom he had operated on for tumor of the right orbit. The eyeball, provious to operation, was displaced outwards, downwards, and half an inch forwards. The growth had been slow and painless, blindness being the first symptom ; the movements of the eye were not restricted : ophthalmoscopically choked disc was seen. The tumor was reached after tenotomy of the right internal rectus, and found, by digital examination, to have extended as far back as the apex of the orbit and to have involved the optic nerve. The tumor was carefully separated from the orbit and that portion of the optic nerve which was imbedded in its centre removed along with it. The internal rectus was then re-attached. Now, three weeks after the operation, the action of the right external rectus was defective ; with this exception, it was extremely satisfactory to have retained the eyeball *in situ*, this being the third case on record where such a result had been obtained.

Sarcoma of the Sole of the Foot.—Dr. James Bell exhibited this specimen, and said that it had been removed from a young girl 18 years of age. The first appearance was a small nodule on the sole of the foot, about the size of a bean, which was noticed three months ago ; this had been incised, with the result that it rapidly increased in size. Symes' amputation was performed, with a happy result.

DR. JOHNSTON, who examined the specimen, said it was a round-celled sarcoma, originating in the structures beneath the cutis, and it had not infiltrated the surrounding tissues.

DR. FOLEY then read a paper entitled " *The Influence of Clothing upon the Skin.*"

DR. F. W. CAMPBELL, in discussing this subject, advocated the disposing of woollen clothes for night use as being decidedly healthier. In acne, he had noticed tight collars acting as an exciting cause.

DR. SHEPHERD thought that no rules could be laid down as a guidance to proper clothes to be worn, and that common sense was the best guide. In children, the speaker had observed urticaria as a result of suddenly changing the clothes.

Pathological Specimens.—DR. ALLOWAY exhibited a uterus he had removed by vaginal hysterectomy from a patient three months ago. The patient was aged 42 ; had had one child twenty years ago. She was a heavily-built, florid woman, in apparent good health. She had suffered some pain of late, and on passing her finger into the vagina found a large tumor obstructing the way. This was the first intimation she had of there being anything abnormal. On examination he found a large fungating epithelioma, about the size of a Florida orange, springing from the cervix uteri. The surrounding parts were uninvolved. During the operation he employed both ligature and clamp. The clamps on the broad ligaments were removed on or about the fiftieth hour. The patient made an uneventful recovery, and the cicatrix at present looks very healthy and smooth.

Dr. Alloway also exhibited an interesting specimen of a blood cyst of the ovary, about the size of a large walnut. The patient, a young lady aged 24, had been a great sufferer all her menstrual life. The hemorrhage into the ovary probably took place within a few weeks. A drainage-tube was used for twenty-four hours, as considerable adhesions had to be separated. The patient made a rapid and uninterrupted recovery, and is now, four months after the operation, free from pain and has gained much in flesh. Menstruation has not returned.

from within. A deep groove was made in the right maxilla parallel to the alveolar process on the right side, at a level slightly above the floor of the nasal fossæ, the bony nasal septum was then divided with bone forceps and the left maxilla was sawn through from the left nasal fossa to the side of the canine tooth, and backwards and inwards through the hard palate. The soft palate was then separated from the hard by the knife, and the piece of bone severed by bone forceps, cutting in the groove first mentioned and connecting its posterior extremity with the opening between the hard and soft palates. The bone was then depressed by bone forceps and completely separated by cutting a few shreds of soft tissue. The parts were well douched with warm water frequently. She was sitting up on the third day, when two of the stitches in the lip were removed and plaster strip substituted. The three other stitches were removed on the 30th, two days later. By the 20th October the mouth was solidly healed and has remained so ever since.

Microscopic slides from the tumor showing epithelial nests were exhibited by Dr. Olmstead.

The patient was shown to the members of the Society. There appeared little or no disfigurement, and everything nicely healed as above described.

Case of Lead Poisoning.—DR. ALGERNON WOOLVERTON then read the notes of a case of lead poisoning :

J. S., aged 26, of strong and muscular development, with good family and personal history, was first seen by me on the evening of 20th December last. He was moaning and tossing himself about, and complained in distressing tones of an agonizing pain in the abdomen, but which was chiefly referred to the upper half. He said the pain was continuous, but had frequent exacerbations, when it was almost unendurable. His face had a drawn, anxious expression ; the skin was cool ; respiration thoracic, and a little increased in frequency ; the pulse I found to be quite slow and soft, about 46 per minute   On inquiry I learned that he worked in a factory where lead was manufactured from the refuse material derived from the distillation of coal oil. He had been working but a few days prior to the

furnace having been shut down on account of a fire
ing taken place in the factory. Prior to the fire he had been
orking at the business for some months, and had never felt any
effects from the work. Preceding the attack he seemed as
well as usual, and showed none of the symptoms of lead poisoning. He worked during the whole night, but had to give up in
the morning on account of severe pain. It is somewhat peculiar
that the symptoms usually preceding lead poisoning were not
present in his case. There was no constipation, loss of appetite,
colicky pains or emaciation ; he attack seems to have developed almost sudden examining the mouth, the
characteristic blue trail p ed along the gums. I found
the bowels had not been open it day. Upon inspecting the
abdomen, there was no retrac f the walls, which is said to
be characteristic of lead pois but rather a slight distension
accompanied with very marked lity of the abdominal muscles,
which I may say continued m rsistently until after all other
symptoms had abated. This tom I think worthy of your
particular attention, being one that impressed me more forcibly
than all others, on account of its persistent and unyielding
rigidity. It was as tense as that characteristic of peritonitis,
but was not accompanied with pain and tenderness on pressure.
Relief of the pain demanded first consideration. I injected half
a grain of morphia hypodermically and left several half grain
powders to be given at intervals of two hours if the pain persisted. I also ordered two ounces of castor oil to be given at
once, to be followed by two ounces of mag. sulph. if the bowels
would not act. I also directed hot fomentations to be applied,
and which were to be frequently changed.

On visiting the patient next morning, I expected that there
would have been some abatement of the pain, but found that
such was not the case, nor had the bowels been opened. He
had taken 2½ grs. of morphia during the night. I then directed
that injections of hot water and soap-suds should be given and
the morphia to be continued. Two or three of these injections
were never returned per anum, having become absorbed, being
retained on account of spasm of the sphincter.

.he temperature still remained normal and the pulse slow
il the evening of the third day, when the pulse rose to 110
the temperature to 100½°F.   There was also at this time
e vomiting ; the bowels remained obstinately constipated,
pite frequent doses of mag. sulph. and copious injections
iwn up through a long tube.   The pain still persisted, although
pupils were contracted to pins points, showing the patient
thoroughly narcotized.   He was in a stupid, dazed state,
would answer on being questioned.   When the temperature
pulse began to rise I became anxious as to the result and
uested a consultation.   Dr. Miller being called in, we decided
give chloroform to relieve the intense sufferings and to (if
iible) overcome the great rigidity of the abdominal walls.
also passed a long tube along the rectum and injected as
:h water as we could, but nothing came away with the injec-
.   Chloroform was given until the conjunctivæ were insen-
i to the touch and the muscles of the extremities became
:id and unresisting, and yet the abdominal muscular spasm
not yield ; chloroform narcosis being kept up until a two
:e vial was exhausted.   When the effect of the chloroform
e off the pain was as bad as ever.   The prognosis at this time
in to look unfavorable.   We decided to substitute hydrate
hloral for the morphia, and obtained much better results.   I
iot think it would have been possible to have relieved the
with morphia unless you had killed the patient, it almost
ned to aggravate the pain and caused a feeling of great
:ression in the head.   Thirty-grain doses of chloral repeated
·y two hours gave some relief and some sleep, and that drug
continued more or less frequently as long as the pain per-
:d.   The next day, after the substitution of the chloral, the
ie again became slow and the temperature normal, but the
els still refused to act, though no purgatives were given at
time on account of the vomiting, for I considered them use-
, if not injurious, as long as the great rigidity and spasm of
bowels continued.   It was not until the sixth day that the
im of the bowels was overcome to such an extent that a
sage from them was secured, from which time improvement

set in. On the tenth day he was able to be up and about, considerably reduced in flesh, but not otherwise much the worse for the attack. At no time was there albumen in the urine.

This is the severest case of lead colic that has ever come under my notice, and was especially interesting to me on account of the persistency of the spasm. Although the mortality is stated to be only from two to three per cent., I at one time feared a fatal termination to this case. The conditions for lead poisoning must have been very favorable in the factory, as all the employees, four or five in number, were attacked, with more or less severity, at the same time. One man had been employed at the business for over twenty years, and had heretofore had no trouble from the lead. The method of procuring the lead is briefly as follows :—

In distilling coal oil, 3 lbs. of litharge (a prob. oxide of lead) is used for each barrel of oil. This is deposited in the black tar-like refuse which is collected after the distillation of the oil. This refuse is burnt in some open place, and a brown, flaky, dry substance remains. This residue is put in a crucible furnace and a very strong heat applied, which causes a large portion of the lead to flow in a molten state from the furnace, while a considerable part is also driven off in a state of fumes, carried into pipes under ground, and in which the lead is deposited as a white oxide. The workmen are constantly inhaling these fumes, and as no great precautions are taken to prevent lead absorption, it is surprising that poisoning does not take place more frequently. The amount of lead taken in these cases must have been excessive, but harmful results are not always proportionate to the quantity of lead taken in. Small amounts, even 0.0015 per cent., if long continued, has been known to cause lead poisoning, and, on the other hand, large doses have been given for weeks with seeming impunity. Lead may be introduced into the system in a variety of ways, and it is often a difficult matter to discover the origin of the poison. Sometimes it is due to the water in lead pipes or cisterns, especially when the water is soft ; sometimes from drinking cider and beer or soda-water kept in lead utensils ; also from eating food kept in badly glazed vessels ;

and sometimes from canned fruit, the acid of the fruit acting upon the solder. It is well known that various trades and occupations are favorable to lead poisoning, such as plumbers, potters, type-workers, enamellers and painters. The colica pictonum must not be confounded, as is often the case, with the colica pictorum (the colic of painters). The former is a name given to a form of colic common among the people ot Poitou, which is probably due to impure wine. Lead-poisoning was known to the Greeks and Arabians, who recognized the arthralgia and paralysis which sometimes follow this disease. In modern times Tanquerel des Plauche's (1830) work remains an authority upon this subject. It would seem that lead poisoning was more common sixty years ago than at present, as no less than 1,217 cases came under Tanquerel's observation. In every one of these cases colic was present; arthralgia in 755 cases, paralysis in 107, and encephalopathy in 72—17 of these latter cases were fatal. One attack predisposes to another, and may occur years after the first attack. Tanquerel relates the case of one painter who for nine consecutive years had attacks of lead colic and other symptoms of lead poisoning, although he had ceased to follow his trade. Cats, dogs and horses have been known to have symptoms of lead poisoning produced both experimentally and from living in a lead-infected atmosphere or from drinking lead-contaminated water. Horses working in lead factories have had tracheotomy performed on account of paralysis of the larynx. Tanquerel was the first to point out that the blue line seen along the edge of the gums was due to a deposit of sulphide of lead in the substance of the gums, the decomposition of food affording a supply of sulphuretted hydrogen which combined with the lead, and caused the dark discoloration which extends in some cases to the whole mucous membrane of the mouth. The three most common sequelæ of lead poisoning are the arthralgia, paralysis and encephalopathy. The last is the severest form of lead-poisoning, and is found only among workers in lead. It may come suddenly with violent headache and sometimes amaurosis or severe convulsive attacks. Post-mortem appearances in these cases only give negative results. Lead paralysis may occur as

ie third day after exposure or not till after years have
ʋₗₐpsed. t affects chiefly the upper extremities and the extensor
muscles, especially the extensor communis, then the triceps and
then the deltoid. This is in singular contrast to the nyalgia
which chiefly affects the lower extremities and the flexor muscles.
The paralysis may be confined to a single muscle, as the extensor
of a finger, or involve the whole limb, or by gradual extension
even the whole body. Sensibility is not usually affected, though
there may be some circumscribed areas of anæsthesia. But the
most characteristic chat ⸱ ⸱ place in the nutrition of the
paralyzed muscles. In a ieks the muscles become very
much wasted and atrophied rked contrast to the surrounding muscles, which retain their rmal development. The prognosis is, as a rule, proportion o the extent of the paralysis
and of the atrophy. Post-mo n examinations show but few
pathological changes except in tl affected muscles and peripheral
nerves, and negative results in · e central nervous system, thus
rendering it very difficult to d a satisfactory explanation of
the various symptoms of the disease. Different investigators
have described different pathological changes in the cord and
medulla and brain, which is presumptive evidence that no definite
pathological lesion has yet been discovered which may be stated
to be characteristic of the disease. It was at one time thought
that the lead acted upon the muscular fibres, especially the un-
striped variety, but Heubel shows that this not the case. He
states that lead exists in the blood and all the organs in chemical
combination with albumen. He says that lead cannot be detected
by chemical tests prior to the destruction of the organic substances containing it. The amount of lead found in the system
is comparatively small, not amounting in the average to .02 per
cent., too small a quantity, one would think, to produce such
grave results, and it probably can only be accounted for in some
such manner as chronic alcoholic poisoning, that the circulation
of a foreign poisonous material in the blood causes an abnormal
nutrition of the whole system, but why it should cause colic
(which is supposed to be a neurosis of the intestinal plexus) in
one case, arthralgia in another, and encephalopathy in another,

is not yet understood. I will not dwell upon the general treatment of this disease, for I believe time is the chief element in it, but the general indications are the relief of the pain and the overcoming of the obstinate constipation. And my experience points to chloral as being the drug best adapted to accomplish this purpose.

Selections.

The Isolation of Consumptives. (By Dr. P. H. Kretzschmar, of Brooklyn, N.Y.)—

At the Congress of American Physicians and Surgeons, held in Washington during the month of September, 1888, one of the most prominent members of the profession, from the city of New York, made the statement that the time had come when pulmonary consumption should be classified among the contagious and infectious diseases, and consumptives should be cared for in like manner as small-pox patients are. At that the writer entered his protest against any such proposition ; but so much has been said since regarding the probabilities of transmitting the disease from the patient to the healthy, that a discussion of this very important subject seems to be advantageous.

The fact that the " International Congress for Tuberculosis," which will meet in Paris this year, has among other subjects the question of " Isolation " on its programme, is evidence that a portion of the medical profession *does* seriously consider the advisability of such a proposition. Since Dr. Koch first demonstrated the specific cause of tuberculosis, it has been asserted that consumptives are a source of danger to their surroundings, and it has been claimed that many cases of pulmonary tuberculosis are directly traceable to infection by contact only. As long as one hundred years ago the theory, now preached by many, that consumptives are liable to infect healthy persons by contact *only*, was accepted as a fact, and appropriate laws were issued. In Naples a law existed during the latter part of last century for over fifty years, compelling the attending physicians to report every case of pulmonary consumption—l'ulcera pulmonale—and the fine for the first failure to comply with this law was three hundred ducats, to be followed, in case of repeated neglect to report this class of cases, by expulsion from the country for a period of ten years. All poor consumptives were at once removed to a hospital; the clothes and bedding belonging to consumptive patients had to be destroyed after death; the dwellings of all patients who were fortunate enough to die outside of the hospital had to be entirely renovated and nobody was allowed to occupy them until one year afterward. Similar laws and restrictions were in force in Portugal, without, however, influencing the prevalence of pulmonary consumption in any marked degree. Rigorous laws, strictly enforced for fifty-six years, would certainly have shown *some* fovorable results if isolation and *public supervision* of consumptives were of any practical value whatsoever.

In a paper read before the American Public Health Association during its meeting in October last, the writer used the following language : " If the advocates of isolation would reflect for a moment and consider the hardship and injury which would follow its introduction, affecting, as it would, a large proportion of the human race and seriously interfering with our entire social life, without giving the slightest assurance of better results than those obtained after many years of trial in Naples and Portugal, one would think that they would hesitate to advocate so inhuman a proposition. It will not be denied by them that a very large proportion of consumptives are phthisical subjects long before they themselves are aware of it, and even physicians frequently treat alveolar catarrh as bronchitis until the microscope demonstrates the fact that the patient's expectorations are full of tubercular bacilli. What benefit would be derived by isolating advanced cases of pulmonary consumption, if cases during the early stages are permitted to deposit millions of microbes with their expectorations upon our streets, in our churches, public halls, railroads, and all over their own residences ? And, finally, what advantage would it be to have isolation enforced in the State of New York and not in New Jersey, Pennsylvania, or other neighboring States : or, if adopted by the United States and not in Canada !"

Careful consideration of the subject has strengthened the

writer's former opinion about the infeasibility, cruelty, and absurdity of any attempt to carry into practical effect the teachings of those advocating isolation of consumptives for the purpose of diminishing or destroying the danger of infection, although it is admitted that, *theoretically*, the isolation *of all consumptives* would do much to lessen the quantity of tubercular bacilli floating in the air, and thereby the danger of infection. *Practically*, the same favorable results would be obtained if the lessons taught by Dr. George Cornet's experiments would be made the basis for proper teachings regarding the expectorations not only of people known to be consumptive, but of all persons suffering from prolonged coughing, depending, apparently, upon other deranged conditions of the human system. We know that the source of contagion is contained in the sputa ; we also know that as long as these expectorations remain in a moist state they are not apt to infect anybody, but that the dry sputa, becoming pulverized, allowing the poisonous germs to be carried away into the surrounding atmosphere, are alone responsible for the dissemination of the disease. The short pamphlet issued by the Board of Health of the City of New York regarding this matter gives most excellent instructions, and it seems to the writer to be an act of vital importance for this Society to do *its share* that these instructions, or others of a similar character, be published by every health officer or every county society of this State.

To obtain the views of the most advanced phthiso-therapeutists the writer entered into correspondence with some of them. Dr. Hermann Weber, of London, England, writes under date of January 2nd, 1890 : " In answer to your note I beg to say that it would not only be a great cruelty to isolate consumptive patients, but it would also be an impossibility. . . ." Dr. P. Dettweiler's answer is dated Naples, December 24th, 1889, and reads, . . . " regarding the effect of isolating consumptives, I can only say, most minute cleanliness, the rigorous use of the spittoon, and the general introduction of the ' blue flask ' are the best means to prevent the spreading of the disease ; isolation is unnecessary." Dr. Ernst Meissen, of Falkenstein, Germany, writes December 19th, 1889, about as follows: " The isolation

profession loses by his death one of its brightest stars, and those especially interested in the subject of phthiso-therapy their foremost teacher, writer, and active practical worker. For over thirty-five years Dr. Brehmer conducted his now world-renowned institute for the cure of consumption in Goerbersdorf; beginning with almost no capital and upon the smallest scale, his institution has grown to a most marvellous extent, and more than 14,000 patients have visited it during the last three decades. Of Dr. Brehmer's writings the most important are: "Chronic Pulmonary Consumption and Tuberculosis of the Lungs: Its Cause and Cure," published in 1857; "Etiology of Chronic Pulmonary Consumption," 1885; "The Treatment of Chronic Pulmonary Consumption," 1886, second enlarged edition, 1889; and his latest work, "Communications from Dr. Brehmer's Institution for the Cure of Consumptives, in Goerbersdorf," 1889.

Strongly opposed to *isolation* of consumptives for the purpose of diminishing the spread of the disease, the writer is one of the most enthusiastic advocates of the *separation* of consumptives from the healthy, and their removal to institutions properly conducted and located, and conducted solely for the cure of this class of patients. It is a great pleasure to the writer to see that the profession in France—as shown by the writings of Professor Nicaize and Drs. Daremberg, Pouzet, and Frémy—is adopting the view that consumptives find the greatest probabilities for a cure within sanitoria and not in so-called open "health resorts." The excellent results obtained in the Adirondack Cottage Sanitarium by Dr. E. L. Trudeau, of Saranac Lake, are so encouraging, that it is surprising that other institutions of similar character have not been established, and it is to be hoped that the profession in the United States will soon recognize the importance and the value of special institutions for the cure of consumptives.

I repeat what I stated in a paper read before the American Climatological Association in Boston, during the month of June, 1889, that "if anything is to be done tending to restoration to health for those who are consumptive, whether rich or poor, it can be accomplished with the greatest promise of success in a properly located and rationally conducted sanitarium."—*The Sanitarian*, March, 1890.

A Sanitary Wash-house.

—Albert Shaw has a most suggestive paper in the March *Century* entitled " Glasgow, a Municipal Study," from which we quote :—

" Not the least important feature of the health department's work in Glasgow is the Sanitary Wash-house. A similar establishment should be a part of the municipal economy of every large town. In 1864 the authorities found it necessary to superintend the disinfection of dwellings, and a small temporary wash-house was opened, with a few tubs for the cleansing of apparel, etc., removed from infected houses. For a time after the acquisition of Belvidere a part of the laundry of the hospital was used for the purpose of a general sanitary wash-house. But larger quarters being needed, a separate establishment was built and opened in 1883, its cost being about $50,000. This place is so admirable in its system and its mechanical appointments that I am again tempted to digress with a technical description. The place is in constant communication with sanitary head-quarters, and its collecting waggons are on the road early every morning. The larger part of the articles removed for disinfection and cleansing must be returned on the same day, to meet the necessities of poor families. I visited the house on a day when 1,800 pieces, from twenty-five different families, had come in. In 1887, 6,700 washings, aggregating 380,000 pieces, were done. The quantity, of course, varies from year to year with the amount of infectious disease in the city. The establishment has a crematory, to which all household articles whatsoever that are to be burned after a case of infectious disease must be brought by the vans of the sanitary department. The carpet-cleaning machinery and the arrangements for disinfection by steam, by chemicals, and by boiling I cannot here describe.

" The department's disinfecting and whitewashing staff is operated from the wash-house as headquarters. A patient being removed to the hospital, the authorities at once take possession of the house for cleansing and disinfection. It is a point of interest also that the city has provided a comfortable 'house of reception' of some ten rooms, with two or three permanent servants, where families may be entertained for a day or more as the city's guests if it is desirable to remove them from their homes during the progress of the disinfecting and clothes-washing operations. The house is kept in constant use, and it is found a very convenient thing for the department to have at its disposal.

" As net results of the sanitary work of the Glasgow authorities may be mentioned the most entire extinction of some of the worst forms of contagious disease and a mastery of the situation, which leaves comparatively little fear of widespread epidemics in the future, in spite of the fact that Glasgow is a great seaport, has an unfavorable climate, and has an extraordinarily dense and badly housed working population. The steady decline of the total death-rate, and its remarkably rapid decline as regards those diseases at which sanitary science more especially aims its weapons, are achievements which are a proper source of gratification to the town council and the officers of the health department."—(*Medical and Surgical Reporter.*)

A Test for Albumin in Urine.—In the *Johns Hopkins Bulletin*, Feb. 1890, D. Meredith Reese calls attention to an editorial note in the *British Medical Journal*, Nov. 16, 1889, in which a new test for albumin in urine was given. Trichloracetic acid $CCl_3 COOH$, a substitution product of acetic acid, formed from acetic acid by the replacement of three of its hydrogen atoms by three chlorine atoms occurs as a crystalline salt, and is colorless and readily soluble in water. Boymond claims to have been the first to make mention of the reagent, and since this it has been adopted by Raabe. Boymond begins his article by saying that Marsalt and Languipin have described albuminous urine in which a precipitate by heat was gotten, but in which urine the precipitate was re-dissolved by acetic acid. Patein, in a note quite recently made, attributes this fact to the presence of a special albumin differing from serum albumin and globulin. Boymond has observed this phenomena repeatedly, and considers that the condition is much less rare than supposed, and that the peculiarity has much import; for in a rapid examination of urine where heat and acetic acid are used alone, we might perhaps conclude that albumin was absent, when the urine might contain considerable proportion of this special variety of albumin. He has been accustomed for some time to employ trichloracetic acid instead of acetic acid. Other agents which precipitate albumin also precipitate this variety, but trichloracetic acid presents some advantages, and particularly that of not changing the albumin. The reagent precipitates albumin in cold solution, and is considered to rank among the most delicate tests. Raabe, in the article referred to above, considers it sensitive, superior to HNO_3 and to metaphosphoric acid, advocated by Hindenlang. Raabe gives the relative amounts of albumin recognized by metaphosphoric acid, nitric acid, and trichloracetic acid as in the proportion 1 : 3.7 : 6.2. He also states that .0295 grm. of albumin can be recognized in 250 cc. of urine.

It may be employed as a solid or a liquid. When used as a solid a crystal of the salt is dropped into the urine in a test-tube, and touching the bottom is dissolved, producing a diffuse turbidity or turbid zone definitely marked out. When used in liquid form, the solution may be saturated or of medium strength. The saturated solution is used after the method employed with HNO_3 in Heller's test, by floating the urine on the acid. A characteristic ring will be formed, as one finds with the HNO_3 test, but without the production of the colored zone between the urine and acid caused by the oxidation of the pigments. When urine is rich in urates of soda error will be avoided, an error common to all reagents, by diluting the urine with the addition of distilled water. Boymond closes his paper by saying that he confirms the observations of Marsalt and Languipin, and that he wishes to draw attention again to trichloracetic acid as a useful test in not only this particular variety of albumin, but in the ordinary forms.

In the last few months this reagent has been tried in the clinical laboratory of the Johns Hopkins Hospital. The article was obtained from Merck and found to be, as Boymond describes, a crystalline salt, colorless and deliquescent. In all the tests a saturated solution was used, making a liquid of the consistency of HNO_3. This was kept well stoppered to keep it of uniform strength in the experiments. It was employed as above described by pouring the acid beneath the urine by means of a pipette.

In all, eighty-seven different urines have been tested, the urine filtered, and that from women drawn by catheter. At first only those urines showing albumin by control tests, such as heat, HNO_3 and picric acid, were used, and in all cases trichloracetic acid gave a distinct, clearly defined zone, produced immediately, with no discoloration whatever between the urine and acid. Generally the zone was produced more quickly than with nitric acid, and was of a greater thickness and intensity. On standing for some time a slight pinkish discoloration may in some cases be obtained below the urine in the acid when trichloracetic acid is used.

In forty-three cases where the control tests gave albumin a precipitate was obtained by trichloracetic acid, not dissolved, but made more distinct by heat. In twenty-five cases no reaction whatever was obtained by any test. In fourteen cases where there was no reaction by control tests, the trichloracetic acid gave a precipitate. In eleven of these cases granular, epithelial and hyaline casts were found, and in three of these eleven cases the post-mortem showed distinct changes in the kidneys. In three cases where heat and acetic acid and nitric acid gave no precipitate of albumin, a precipitate was obtained by picric and trichloracetic acids. In all three of these cases casts were found. In two cases where the precipitate on heat was dissolved again by acetic acid, trichloracetic acid gave a good precipitate. In conclusion it may be said that trichloracetic acid has proven a most delicate test for albumin in urine ; that it is prompt in its reaction ; that it gives no discoloration or colored zone ; that it is a test easily applied and one worthy of more extended use.—
(*Medical and Surgical Reporter.*)

The Cold Bath Treatment of Typhoid Fever. A REVIEW OF RECENT DISCUSSIONS.—(By DR. SIMON BARUCH, New York.)

—The experienced hydrotherapeu-
tist never uses ice-water for a prolonged application. Water
below 50° is sometimes used in the douche for ten to twenty
seconds. But the aim of all hydrotherapeutic measures is to
refresh, to stimulate the nerve-centres, never to induce a sedative effect. This must be clearly understood as the first principle of scientific hydrotherapy, and it is even well understood
by the empirical hydropath to-day.

It has been objected to Brand's rule for bathing, that the intelligent physician should not be hampered by strict rules, that
he should be allowed to use his judgment in each individual
case. Brand's rule, however, is not inflexible, as the following
extract from a letter received on Saturday, February 15th, from
Dr. Brand, illustrates· Referring to a case where bath treatment was detailed in one of our journals, he says: " By following my rule is not to be understood such treatment as was given
by Dr. —— to the child, which was so far reduced in strength
and nerve-power that it should not have been put into a cold
bath, but into a warm one, until it gradually became accustomed
to the cold bath, for twenty-four hours. To me it is surprising
that Dr. —— did not obtain greater disadvantage from the low
temperature used in this case ; it was a special piece of good
luck. I always use warmer baths for twenty-four hours, usually
temperature of the room, if the patient has been ill over four
days ; often, also, from the beginning." From this extract it
will be gathered that Brand does not advise the plunging of
every case into a bath of 6 ⸳°F. without regard to individual
condition. The truth is, that in no method of treatment is good
judgment more necessary than in the management of typhoid
fever by the cold bath.ʻ

But how is this method to be tested, if, as is evident in the
recent discussions, there is no uniform method of treatment ;
when gentlemen class cold sponging, the wet pack, the ice-
sprinkled sheet, the graduated bath of all temperatures, from
70° to 90°F., as the cold bath treatment ? It is remarkable

that American physicians, who are usually so practical and ready to utilize the most successful methods, have so long stood aloof from this well-proven treatment.

The statistics furnished by Juergensen and Vogl are the best possible guide for this or any country, because they are obtained from hospital practice, civil and military, and they represent the comparative merits of various methods. Vogl is the chef of the Garrison Hospital at Munich. He offers us the records of 8,325 cases of typhoid fever treated there during forty-seven years. (Military records in Germany are proverbially accurate.) Vogl mentions each year the type of the disease, derived from symptoms and autopsies, the treatment pursued, and the results. The mortality ranges from 40.3 per cent. (1843) to 23 per cent. (1877 and 1878). Since 1875, when the cold bath treatment was systematically begun, the mortality per cent. has never exceeded 4.7 per cent., and the average was 2.7 per cent.; neither one of which figures had ever been reached before (the lowest was 9.9 per cent. in 1865, under quinine and camphor treatment; the next, in 1869, 11.5 per cent.).

In the Poliklinik at Tübingen Juergensen had observed even better results. During nine years 217 cases were treated by strict bathing, according to Brand. Only one of these died.

I desire to emphasize the fact that it is not at all difficult to place typhoid cases under the cold bath treatment before the diagnosis is clearly made. Every suspicious case of fever should be placed in the bath, if the temperature reaches 103°F. This is the course pursued at Munich and Stralsund. That no harm can result from it may be easily demonstrated. I pursue it constantly in private and hospital practice. If this rule is adhered to in all suspicious cases, many would come under treatment before the fifth day, and almost surely be saved. If the case be one of simple fever of an ephemeral type, no harm will ensue, especially if the graduated bath be used, until the diagnosis is clear.

Bahrdt says that the mortality of typhoid fever in the Jacobs Hospital at Leipsic was reduced by the bath treatment from 18.2 per cent. to 9 per cent. Riegel reports a reduction in

Bamberger's clinic from 20 per cent. to 4.4 per cent. by bath
Schulz, in Bremen, reduced the mortality to 2.7 per cent.
strict bathing.

Guttstadt, who is the censor of the Statistical Bureau i
Berlin, said, in a lecture before the Verein für innere Medizin
in Berlin, in 1887, that " an important factor in the diminution
of mortality is the more successful treatment now used, especially
Brand's method."

The most important question in this review of the recent discussions is : What constitutes the *cold bath treatment* ?

The statistics referred to, showing a reduction of mortality to
less than three per cent., and in 1200 cases treated before the
fifth day to less than one per cent., were not obtained from cold
sponging, wet packs, cold coils, cold affusions, graduated baths,
or any other agreeable substitute. They were the result of
methodical bathing according to Brand's original method. As
there seems to be much vagueness of conception on this point,
I deem it important to furnish an outline of the method, as I
have learned it from the study of Brand, Vogl, Tripier, and
Bouveret, and correspondence with Brand himself.

1. The first principle is to bathe early ; even before diagnosis
is clear. No harm is done at least by a graduated bath, viz.,
reduced from 90° to 68°F. for a quarter or half an hour. This
is the only modification of the method which is advisable. It
accustoms the patient to the treatment and gains time. It should
be resorted to as soon as the temperature in the rectum reaches
103°F. I am in the habit of bathing the patient's face and
chest with ice-water before placing him into any bath.

2. As soon as the case becomes defined or even suspicious,
the strict bath (65°F.) should be used. The tub must stand at
the patient's bedside, filled two-thirds with water at 65°. The
patient receives a stimulant, and has his face and chest washed
with ice-water. He is undressed and gently lifted into the water.
A gasp or shudder follows, perhaps an ejaculation of distress ;
but gentle reassurance by word and deed, a calm demeanour
devoid of haste, and avoidance of force, will do much to quiet
the patient. With one hand under his head, if necessary, the

other is used to gently practice friction over the submerged parts. Another nurse pursues the same course, if possible This important feature of the Brand method is, I have observed, frequently neglected, and to its neglect may be charged the occurrence of collapse, cyanosis, and chill. Gentle friction with the outstretched hand produces a rosy hue of the skin ; the superficial vessels are dilated. By thus exposing a large supply of blood, the cooling is more rapid. The bath should be continued in this manner for fifteen minutes, no matter how urgently the patient desires to be removed. A pinched countenance, chattering of teeth, unless excessive, or a small pulse, must not be taken as indications for removal. If the face becomes cyanotic, or respiratiod embarrassed, the bath must cease. Every five minutes during the bath, water at about 60°F. should be gently poured from a pitcher over the head of the patient, after a folded handkerchief has been tied like a bandage with the knot over the nucha. This prevents the water from running over the face, and spreads it over the head.

Before the patient is removed from the bath, a linen sheet should be spread over a blanket to receive him. If his temperature has been high, this sheet alone is wrapped around him, while his lower extremities are also covered with the blanket. If his temperature has not been over 103.5°, the whole body may be wrapped in the blanket over the sheet and hot bottles placed to the feet. He is then left to dry for ten or fifteen minutes ; something hot is now given him ; his night-gown is replaced and his temperature is taken. A piece of old linen sheeting (cotton should never be used for any purpose in this treatment) is now folded into a compress of four folds, gently wrung out of water at 60°F., and placed upon the entire anterior portion of the body, from the neck to the pubis. It is renewed every half-hour if patient is not sleeping. This process is repeated every three hours, so long as the temperature reaches 103°, night and day, unless the patient is asleep naturally.

Stupor, coma or delirium are always indications for the bath, even if the temperature is below 103°. In these cases, placing the patient semi-recumbent into a half-bath at 95° and pouring

effeet arising from the infective process in typhoid fever, before it accumulates and overwhelms the system, we accomplish the same result that we reach in opium poisoning by early faradization and other measures, viz., we endow the system with nerve-stimulus or force to tide over the danger of toxæmia, until the offending elements are eliminated   Our antitoxic measures will prove efficient in proportion to the earliness, persistency, and good judgment with which we apply them, in the one case, just as they will in the other.   For the object is almost analogous in both cases, although the conditions are not.

Regarded in this light, and not in the light of a heat-reducing measure, this mode of bathing (not sponging, wet-packing, or ice-coil) must save many lives that are now daily sacrificed.

The main object of the treatment by cold baths is not to reduce temperature, but to furnish a restorative and stimulant to the nervous system.   Brand, indeed, now claims that his method is antipyretic.   It was Liebermeister who was the leading spirit in proclaiming that the benefit derived from cold baths was due to their antipyretic effect, and, after giving a bath, he often administered forty or fifty grains of quinine, for the purpose of keeping the temperature down after it had been reduced by the bath.   But the result of this treatment was a mortality of 18 per cent.

My object, then, is to show that the cold bath is not meant for the purpose of antipyresis.   Antipyrine, as I have found to my cost, will bring down the temperature much more efficiently than the cold bath.   As to my analogy between typhoid toxæmia and opium poison, I grant that the comparison might be defective in some particulars; but, at the same time, the main points will hold good.   In both cases we have a profound poisoning of the system, though in one case the poison acts rapidly and in the other slowly.   In both, the poison will become eliminated in the course of time, if we can but support the patient and prolong life until nature can accomplish this; and in both, therefore, the indication is simply to fortify the flagging powers until this can accomplished.   I do not claim that we can *cure* typhoid; but it is a self-limited disease, and what we have to do is to maintain

life until it has run its course.   In regard to statistics, it is true
that twenty or thirty, or even a hundred cases, are of no practical value ; but if we have vast numbers of cases, the correctness of whose data is vouched for by men of the highest scientific attainments and reputation, I believe that such statistics are
to be trusted.

The omission of medicine in the strict bath treatment is perhaps, as Dr. Delafield has suggested, of great value.   It seems
probable that often the medicinal treatment employed has actually damaged our patients, and in what is known as the combined
treatment, in which drugs of various kinds are employed in
addition to cold baths, the mortality, as has been shown in the
paper, is very large.—*College and Clinical Record,* April, 1890.

Chronic Morphinism.—A valuable communication
on the subject of morphinism was recently made by Dr. Arthur
Wynne Foot to the Royal Academy of Medicine in Ireland.
To us the most important parts of the paper are those relating
to prognosis and treatment.   As regards prognosis in morphinism,
Dr. Foot does not consider it so favorable as was at one time
believed.   In the opinion of some authorities the morphine habit
belongs to the category of diseases which are almost incurable.
The weaning from it is a laborious task for the patient as well as
the physician, and yet thereon rests the only hope of recovery.
It is considered by those who have had the longest experience
of such cases to be easier to cure a morphine eater of his craving
than a morphine injector.   The probability of a cure may be
estimated by attending to the following points : (1) The duration
of the habit.   Cases of short existence are more successfully
treated than those in which the habit of long standing has exercised a deleterious influence on mind and body.   (2) The persistence or not of the condition which gave rise to the exhibition
of the drug.   If this condition be irremovable, a cure is scarcely
to be expected.   (3) The physical and nervous constitution of
the patient.   Bad effects follow the withdrawal of morphine in
cases of weakly individuals, or in those of specially nervous temperament.   The magnitude of the dose does not much affect the

prognosis, except in so far as the larger doses indicate chronicity of the habit. It is a hopeful consideration that in most cases to break the habit means to get well, because, unlike alcoholism, the morphine habit does not entail structural lesions of any vital organ. Relapses, however, are very frequent, being more common in men than in women. So great is the tendency to relapse that Jaeckel does not consider a cure to be accomplished by the mere suppression of the morphine hunger, but considers the continuance of control over the patient in a proper institution of the greatest importance. Dr. Wynne Foot's practical remarks on the treatment of morphinism may be summarized as follows: The process of cure or of " demorphinization" requires a degree of moral and physical courage seldom at the disposal of a morphine *habitué*. His abject mental state calls for firmness, gentleness and tact on the part of the physician and the attendants. Neither the intensity of his craving nor the reality of his sufferings should be underrated or disputed. Four methods of treatment have been tried—(1) the deceptive plan ; (2) the substitution plan ; (3) the tapering-off plan ; (4) the abrupt withdrawal plan. The deceptive and the substitution plans are not worthy of serious consideration in the management of confirmed morphinism, the latter simply handing the sufferer over from one enemy to another. Not only is the substitution of cocaine for morphine dangerous, but there is a risk of developing a cocaine habit which is worse than morphinism. As to the tapering-off plan and the abrupt withdrawal plan, there seems to be no unanimity of opinion as to which mode of treatment should be employed. The first-named plan consists in the gradual reduction of the dose until none of the drug is required. Dr. B. W. Richardson considers it better to reduce the dose at each administration than merely to lessen the number of injections in the twenty-four hours. The abrupt discontinuance of the drug is attended in all cases by indescribable sufferings, and in many by serious dangers. When morphine is suddenly cut off in those accustomed to its use, a remarkable group of severe and alarming symptoms ensue, called the *Abstinenz-systome* or reactionary effects. These comprise acute diarrhœa, insomnia, great excitement, amounting

Q. " Definition of Organic Chemistry ?" *A.* " Of flesh, stomach, bowels, liver, or any organic matter."

" The Sterno-Cleido-Mastoid muscle takes its origin from the mastoid portion of the temporal bone, runs down the neck, and is inserted into the upper and back portion of the scapula."

" The coverings of the femoral artery is the same as of hernia, it lies between the femoral vein and sciatic nerve."

" The pulmonary artery is a branch from the great arto, fully supplying the lungs with arterial blood."

" The coverings of the femoral artery are three in number, and in Scarpia's triangle, include the vein and nerve."

" The kidney is a muscular formation, in shape oblong, color quite dark, weight about one pound to one and a half, but may vary considerable."

" Parts severed in amputation at upper third of thigh—just avoiding the insertion of the glutei musels, passing through the Taylor's musel, periostum and femer."

" Coverings of oblique inguinal hernia—skin superficial facia, transversalis mussle peritoneum and omentum."

" The sympethetic system is composed of all the filament of nerves that start from the spinal cord, and are distributed to all parts of the system, especially the brain. The cervical portion ramifies the encephalon in general. The dorsal portion ramifies the anus."

" Extra uterine pregnancy may be a fungoid groth or tumor fibroid in its character or any extra groth in the uttrous would be called extra-uterine pregnancy."

" A breech presentation may be known by the sense of touch, the buttox being different in formation from the cranium. The anus is different from the mouth, absence of tongue and nose, get your finger in the inguinal reagion soon as possible and assist your patient by ferm but gentle tention."

" Trismus neynatorum—a peculiar trouble of the eye, generally congenital, falling of the lids giving a unnatural look to the ordinary face of a child."

Q. " Tests for Arsenic." *A.* " Separate the juices or secre-

at times to mania dan.
the physician, hallu
habit is denied or
the occurrence of t
supervene during th
is needed in the
because incautious
according to some
the loss of the f

To Show
ing Board
the answers giv
Examiners du
with the *Nort*
that " it is a
ciate the imp
ining Board
ignorance
literatim
who, with
as prac
the pr
they d
ing fr
"
husk
I w
a b

de
re

THE

Montreal Medical Journal.

| VOL. XVIII. | APRIL, 1890. | No. 10. |

DESTRUCTION OF BACTERIA WITHIN THE BODY.

A number of researches have been made upon this subject during the past few years. When Metschnikoff published his observations upon the immunity of the frog towards anthrax, and founded the doctrine of " phagocytosis," he certainly introduced a very plausible explanation of a previously unexplained fact. From a theoretical side, the doctrine that the leucocytes eat up the bacteria leaves nothing to be desired, but, unfortunately, it does not seem to be in accordance with the facts. Careful observers have failed to recognize these alleged powers of devouring bacteria not only in the white-blood corpuscles, but in the other cells of the body. Baumgarten* has published a larger number of observations upon the destruction of bacteria within the body, and finds that in animals which possess immunity from anthrax, the bacilli are not taken up by the leucocytes. Osler (lecture before Alumni Association of New York Academy of Medicine) failed to observe anything like phagocytosis in malarial blood. On the other hand, the fluids of the body appear to possess a marked power of destroying bacteria. Nuttall (*Zeitschrift f. Hygiene*, 1888) and Buchner (*Central. f. Bacteriologie*, 1889) have shown that, while blood serum which has been sterilized by heat forms an excellent culture medium for bacteria, serum which has been received into sterilized vessels, but not heated, is capable of destroying anthrax and typhoid bacilli. T. M. Prudden of New York has recently confirmed these results, and has tested ascitic and pleuritic exudations to

* Beiträge, Path. Anat., Vol. VII.

see if they possess this power.   He found them capable of destroying anthrax and typhoid bacilli, but not the pyogenic bacteria—a point of interest with reference to the tendency of these exudations to become purulent.

THE MEDICAL COURSE.

The Commission appointed to enquire into the methods of teaching in the Scotch Universities will soon assemble to hear the views of all interested in this important subject.   As yet nothing has been made public as to proposed changes in the methods of conducting the medical course, with the exception of a pamphlet by Dr. James Finlayson, Physician and Lecturer to the Western Infirmary of Glasgow.   Dr. Finlayson's chief recommendation is for the supersession of courses of systematic lectures by courses of practical instruction.   He would make attendance at systematic lectures voluntary, and attendance on practical courses compulsory.   He says that " the day is probably not far distant when systematic lecturing, in many subjects, will be almost abandoned, except in so far as is required for practical instruction."

MUNIFICENT DONATIONS.

Through the princely liberality of Mr. W. C. McDonald, of Montreal, McGill University is to receive donations of upwards of $400,000.   Of this sum, $150,000 is to be devoted to the Faculty of Law and the remainder to the Science Faculty.   This is the largest single gift ever received by McGill.

FIRST SURGEONS OF MONTREAL.

The following interesting notes were given to us by Mr. W. McLennan :—

Etienne Bouchard, born at Paris, parish of St. Paul, master surgeon, signed his engagement with the Company of Montreal, 10th May, 1653, received 147 livres on account of his wages ; born 1622, married Marguerite Boissel at Quebec, 6th Oct. 1657, died at Montreal 20th July, 1676.   Lived in Notre Dame street, near the site of the present City Hall.   Had 9 children.   (Tanguay

Dic. Gen.) By a contract dated 30th March, 1655, he agreed with 26 heads of families to treat the husband, wife and children "born and to be born" for 100 sous each, with the right to either party to withdraw at will. (Faillon II., 198.) Before this he was paid by the Company. By deed before Basset, notary, No. 277, Bouchard engages Nicolas Colson for one year as "serviteur chirurgien," for which he agrees to pay "sept vingt dix *livres tournois*"—*i.e.*, seven times twenty + ten, 150 livres, equal, with the difference of purchasing power in money, to about as many dollars to-day, and board and lodge him.

Louis Chartier came out in 1653, the same year as Bouchard, as surgeon. When he came out he received 120 livres on account of wages. Born 1633. Drowned while bathing 20th July, 1660. Unmarried. He seems to have lived with LeBer and LeMoyne, as it was in their common house that Basset, notary, made his inventory on the 22nd July, 1660. Among the articles enumerated are :

6 shirts of white linen, valued at..............	26 livres.
4 " de traites neuves (for trading)........	12 "
5 pair drawers, bleached linen..............	10 "
2 old shirts.................................	3 "
3 " pair drawers	4 "
10 pair ruffles for sleeves	10 "
8 pair socks, white	8 "
8 " stockings........................	
3 cravats, cotton	6 "
4 others	3 " 10
27 handkerchiefs	100 "
12 falls of cambrick (*i.e.*, bands)..............	12 "
3 " of lace	10 "
1 " (must have been very fine)........	100 "

SUITS.

A pourpoint with breeches of grey serge, façon de Raz (I find in Cotgrave Ras de Milain—the finest kind of bare serge or a silk serge), garni de rubans couleur de feu et vin, very much used, &c., &c., &c.	
1 pair of double or lined chamois gloves......	30 "
A cloak of Bergame grey, lined with Ras de Chalons	30 "
A sword with silver hilt and baldrick.........	18 "
Another without sheath	6 "
A gun, the barrel 4 ft. in length (probably for ducks).................................	80 "
A musquetoon, mounted	16 "
A pistol and belt	18 "
2 powder horns.........................	50
A beaver muff	10 "
A case with silver spoon and fork............	18 "

TENTH INTERNATIONAL MEDICAL CONGRESS.

To be held in Berlin, August 4th to 9th.

The Committee of Organization of the Tenth International Medical Congress—R. Virchow, President ; E. von Bergmann, E. Leyden, W. Waldeyer, Vice-Presidents ; O. Lassar, Secretary-General—have appointed the undersigned members of an American Committee for the purpose of enlisting the sympathy and co-operation of the American profession.

We are assured that the medical men of our country will receive a hearty welcome in Berlin. The Congress promises to prove of inestimable value in its educational results, and in securing the ties of international professional brotherhood. It is most important that the American profession should participate both in its labors and its fruits.

Delegates of American Medical Societies and Institutions, and individual members of the profession, will be admitted on equal terms. The undersigned therefore beg to express their hope that a large number of the distinguished men of our country will appreciate both the honor conferred by this cordial invitation and the opportunity afforded us to fitly represent American medicine.

The Congress will be held at Berlin, from the 4th to the 9th of August.

The arrangements in regard to a few general meetings and the main scientific work, which is delegated to the sections, are the same as in former sessions. A medico-scientific exhibition, the programme of which has been published a few weeks ago, is to form an ingredient part. It is to the latter that the Berlin Committee is very anxious that both the scientific and the secular press should be requested to give the greatest possible publicity.

The office of the Secretary-General is Karlstrasse 19, N.W., Berlin, Germany.

S. C. Busey, Washington, D.C.	Wm. T. Lusk, New York.
Wm. H. Draper, New York.	Wm. Osler, Baltimore, Md.
R. H. Fitz, Boston, Mass.	Wm. Pepper, Philadelphia, Pa.
H. Hun, Albany, N.Y.	J. P. Porcher, Charleston, S.C.
A. Jacobi, New York.	J. Stewart, Montreal, Can.

110 West 34th Street,
New York, April 7th, 1890.

Mr. Editor,—In a letter dated Berlin, Karlstrasse, 19, March 22nd, Dr. Lassar, the Secretary-General of the Tenth International Congress, directs me to inform the medical profession of America that a programme of the Congress and other communications will be distributed two months before the meeting amongst those who will have registered previously and received their tickets of membership.

The latter can be obtained by sending application and five dollars to Dr. Bartels, Leipzigerstrasse, 75, Berlin, S.W. By so doing the members will save much crowding and time during the first days of the Congress.

For the American Committee of the Tenth International Medical Congress,   A. JACOBI, M.D.

The following additional programmes of the work of Sections have been published :—

SECTION OF DERMATOLOGY AND SYPHILOGRAPHY.

(1) Pathogenesis of Pigmentations and Discolorations of the Skin ; (2) Diagnosis, Prognosis, and Treatment of Chronic Gonorrhœa in the Male and in the Female ; (3) Treatment of Syphilis—(A) Results (*a*) of excision, (*b*) of general preventive treatment ; (B) Beginning, Duration (chronic, intermittent, or temporary ?) and best method of Treating Constitutional Syphilis ; (4) Treatment of Inflammatory Diseases of the Skin ; (5) The Special Indications of the Different Modes of Applying Mercury in the Treatment of Syphilis ; (6) On What Etiological Factors does the Outbreak of Tertiary Forms of Syphilis Depend ? (7) The *Rôle* of Diathesis, Nervous Causes of Disease, and Pathogenic Parasites in the group of diseases designated as Eczema ; (8) The Nature of Medicinal Eruptions ; (9) Lupus Erythematodes, its Nature and Treatment. Communications should be addressed to Dr. Lassar, 19, Karlstrasse, Berlin, N.W.

SECTION OF OTOLOGY.

A discussion on the relations of Micro-organisms to Diseases

of the Middle Ear and their Complications, will be introduced
by Drs. Moos and Zaufal; one on Cholesteatoma of the Ear, by
Drs. Duhn and Bezold; one on the following question: Can
opening the mastoid process from the external meatus be con-
sidered as equal to the more usual method? by Dr. Hessler.
4. One on the After-treatment of the Trephined Mastoid, by
Dr. Kretschmann; one on the Indications of Excision of the
Malleus and Incus, by Dr. Stacke; one on the Pathological
Anatomy of the Labyrinth, by Dr. Steinbrügge; one on the
Condition of the Organ of Hearing in Diseases of the Central
Nervous System, especially in Tabes Dorsalis, by Dr. Morpurgo;
one on Otitis Interna as a Sequel of Hereditary Syphilis, by
Dr. Wagenhauser; one on Statistics of the most important Ear
Diseases, by Drs. Bürkner and Jacobson; one on Testing the
Hearing and Notation of the Auditory Capacity, by Drs. Mag-
nus and Schwabach; one on the Diagnosis, Prognosis and Treat-
ment of Progressive Deafness in Chronic Non-suppurative Otitis
Media, by Drs. McBride and Gradenigo. Communications
should be addressed to Prof. Lucæ, 9, Lötzowplatz, Berlin, W.

SECTION OF FORENSIC MEDICINE.

1. Are gonococci so thoroughly established that the finding
of them in the vaginal secretion of a child can with certainty be
referred to gonorrhœa in a supposed ravisher? 2. On impotence
in the male, and the criteria in which it can be established in
court. 3. Can Air drawn into the Lungs by Respiration disappear from them in Dead Bodies, so that the Lungs of New-
born Children may present the Signs found in those who have
never breathed? 4. Can the Changes produced in the Anus
by Passive Pederasty disappear after discontinuance of the
Pederastic Acts, and in how long a time after? The discussion
on this subject will be introduced by Professor Liman. 5. Can
the Lungs of a Newborn Child that has never breathed present,
owing to Schultze's Vibrations, the signs of having done so?
6. When Sepsis is found in a person who has secretly miscarried,
can a strong suspicion or certainty be expressed that the Abortion was deliberately induced, or does Sepsis also occur after

Spontaneous Abortion ? 7. Is there an independent "Moral Insanity," or is that Complex of Symptoms one of the Manifestations of other forms of Mental Disease ? 8. Is Mummification of a Corpse confirmatory evidence of Arsenic Poisoning, or is it quite without significance in that respect ? 9. The significance of Proofs of Life. 10. On the Influence of the Recent Development of the Doctrine of Infection on Medico-legal Examinations in cases of Death occurring after Bodily Injuries ?' 11. The Significance of Ptomaines in Forensic Medicine. 12. What position must the Medical Jurist take up as regards the question of Auto-infection in Puerperæ ? 13. Observations of Medical Jurists on the recognition of the Simulation of Neuroses, especially of Traumatic Origin. 14. Medico-legal Observations on the Occurrence and Significance of Rigor Mortis. Communications should be addressed to Professor Liman, 46A, Königgrätzerstrasse, Berlin, S.W.

SECTION OF MEDICAL GEOGRAPHY AND CLIMATOLOGY (HISTORY AND STATISTICS).

1. Influence of Tropical Climates on Immigrants from Higher Latitudes, the resistance of Immigrants to Diseases prevalent in the Tropics, and the Possibility of the Acclimatisation of Europeans and North Americans in the Tropics. 2. Influence of Climatic, Telluric, and Social Conditions on the Occurrence and Course of Pulmonary Tuberculosis, with special reference to the Disease in the Torrid Zone. 3. Endemic and Epidemic Spread of Yellow Fever, and the Influence of Climate, Soil, and Trade thereon. 4. Beri-beri from the standpoint of Etiology and Treatment. 5. Leprosy, with special reference to its Transmission by Heredity and Contagion. 6. Malarial Diseases, with special reference to the Geographical Distribution of the Various Forms thereof : Are all forms due to one and the same or to different poisons ? Communications should be addressed to Professor A. Hirsch, 113, Potsdamerstrasse, Berlin, W.

SECTION OF DISEASES OF THE TEETH.

1. Bromide of Ethyl as an Anæsthetic in Dental Practice.

2. Causation, Course, and Treatment of Pyorrhœa Alveolaris.
3. The Part Played by Micro-organisms in Caries of the Teeth.
4. Crown and Bridge Work.   5. The Bonwill Method of Articulation in Artificial Dentures.   Communications should be addressed to Professor Busch, 8, Alexanderufer, Berlin, N.W.

Medical Items.

—We regret to announce the death of Dr. Trélat, the famous
French surgeon.

—The Influenza has about completed its circuit of the globe.
It is reported that it is now very prevalent in Persia.

—The Jefferson Medical College, Philadelphia, had 220
graduates at its recent convocation.

—The *Transactions* of the recent Intercolonial Medical Congress of Australasia, held in Melbourne, has been issued.

—Sir Andrew Clark has been re-elected for the third time
President of the Royal College of Physicians of London.

—Prof. Bramann, late assistant to Prof. Bergmann, has been
appointed to the chair of Surgery in the University of Halle.

—Professor Grashey of Munich has been appointed to fill the
chair rendered vacant by the death of Prof. Westphal of Berlin.

—The next annual meeting of the American Medical Association will be held in Nashville, Tenn., on the 30th of May
next.

—An effort is being made to establish a medical school at
Cardiff in connection with the University of South Wales and
Monmouthshire.

—The University of Basle has thrown open its doors to women.
Zurich and Berne for some time have admitted the fair ones to its
different faculties.

—An excellent portrait of the late R. Palmer Howard, M.D.,
has been placed in the library of the Medical Faculty of McGill
University.

—Prof. Henoch, the Director of the University Clinic for Diseases of Children in the University of Berlin, will celebrate his seventieth birthday on the 16th of July next.

—The death of Dr. Aquilla Smith, of Dublin, at the advanced age of 84 years, is announced. Dr. Smith was for many years the representative of the College of Physicians on the General Medical Council.

—A proposal recently brought forward to establish regular chairs for the teaching of Medical Jurisprudence in the German Universities has been negatived on the ground that the subject is not of sufficient importance.

—The Pennsylvania State Board of Health is anxious to obtain information from practitioners throughout the entire country as to any evidence they may have as to the alleged value of smoking in the prevention of tuberculosis.

—We have received the first number of a new centralblatt, called the *Osterr-Ungar. Centralblatt für die Med. Wissenschaften.* It is published by Moritz Perles of Vienna. The editors are Paschkis and Zerner of the same city.

—Dr. Caroline White, in a recent issue of the *Forum*, has an article denouncing the practice of vivisection. The article is hardly worthy of serious consideration, the author being deeply ignorant of what has been done in scientific medicine during the past two decades.

—The following additions have been made to the Faculty of the New York Post-Graduate Medical School and Hospital:— Charles B. Kelsey, M.D., Professor of Rectal Diseases ; Charles H. Knight, M.D., Professor of Laryngology and Rhinology ; Reynold W. Wilcox, M.D., Professor of Clinical Medicine ; Dr. S. Lustgarten, formerly Privat Docent in Vienna University, Instructor in Syphilis and Dermatology.

—The first election of the Council of the newly-formed College of Physicians and Surgeons for the North-West Territories took place at Regina on February 11th. The five practitioners required by the Act who received the highest number of votes were the following in order: Dr. O. C. Edwards, Qu'Appelle Station; Dr. Jas. Lafferty, Calgary; Dr. R. B. Cotton, Regina; Dr. R. G. Brett, Banff; Dr. H. C. Wilson, Edmonton. The first meeting of the Council was held at Regina on March the 10th, when officers for the ensuing year were elected as follows: Dr. O. C. Edward, President; Dr. J. Lafferty, Vice-President; Dr. Cotton, Registrar and Treasurer.

VIRCHOW AND THE SHOEMAKER.—So the great Professor Virchow, as a politician, has had to bow to an obscure Polish shoemaker. This seems to strike a certain section of the press with awe, but in reality there is no cause either for surprise or mortification. Admirably as the illustrious scientist might represent a university town, we can perfectly understand that his lofty ideals (if he has any) do not correspond to the objects which Berlin electors have just now in view. Fancy Sir Joseph Lister or Sir Andrew Clark putting up for Mile End! Whatever their views as stated at the hustings might be, it is morally certain that their opinions upon matters in general would clash with those of their constituents, and since the object of an election is to obtain a representative—that is, a mouthpiece—the elector of the particular district, if afflicted with advanced views, would do wisely to choose some one whose life and education were most calculated to bring him into touch with them and their aspirations.—*Hospital Gazette.*

SIMPLICITY THE SEAL OF TRUTH.—Dr. Robert Koch, in minds of many the foremost scientist and physician of living Germans, is in manner of life the personification of simplicity. His demeanour is said to be so plain and free from self-assertion that, by comparison with him, certain others of his *confrères* the Berlin profession appear haughty and unapproachable. As an illustration of Dr. Koch's habits, it is said that when he travels he is quite as apt to be found taking a third-class railway ticket as any other, while the majority of his students would consider their dignity compromised by anything less than a second-class passage. In other matters as well are indicated attributes of mind and character which place him in the right line of descent the great Boerhaave, whose favorite motto was " *Simplex lum veri.*" And this is the legend that is graven on his ıment in the St. Peter's church at Leyden by her grateful ɔns—a fact which has put in the mouths of thousands the ırable sentiment, " simplicity is the seal of truth," hundreds hom have probably dwelt but lightly on their debt to the t professional talents of him whose life was squared to that

Simplicity is the trait of the master, while the lack of it ıs entirely natural to the novice. As it is the single flower produces the seed, while the double one beside it perishes its beauty, so there is that singleness of purpose and simty of method that bear the fruit of life-saving discoveries, as the genius of Boerhaave gave to his generation, and as Koch's labors promise to yield in surpassing measure.— ·. *Amer. Med. Association.*

OMŒOPATHY.—The New York *Graphic* having recently ı out of its artistic way to inform its readers that " quite half of the medical practice of the world is governed by the ɔsophic discoveries of Hahnemann," the *N. Y. Medical ɔrd* sets forth the facts as follows :—" In the United States e were, in 1885, twelve homœopathic and eighty-eight ılar medical colleges, with 1,088 and 9,441 students res- ively. At the most liberal estimate the homœopathic prac- ɔrs of this country form one-eighth of the total number. re is no homœopathic medical college in the country which be said to be even fairly well equipped and endowed, as pared, for example, with the leading regular medical colleges lew York, Boston and Philadelphia. The only school which ly flourishes is in Chicago. The statement that ' homœopathy recognized branch in most of the great medical schools of ope' is absolutely untrue. Homœopathy has no place what- · in any of the universities of Germany or France, nor has school of its own anywhere in Germany. There is a small .œopathic hospital of one hundred beds in London, with a ll medical school attached. There are said to be only about homœopathic physicians in Great Britain and Ireland. The ıber on the Continent is proportionably even less." Accord-

ing to the most recent official statistics in Austria, there are
only 118 homœopathists out of the whole number of medical
men (7,183), and only 44 of these profess to practise homœopathy exclusively.   There are none at all in the Italian districts,
and only 19 in Vienna.   The number also is said to be steadily
decreasing.—(*Dublin Jr. of Med. Sc.*)

—Dr. Willard's Rest Cure establishment at Burlington, Vt.,
offers all the comforts of a first-class hotel, at rates no higher
than are charged at many boarding-houses, including the professional services of the doctor himself, who is a regular graduate
and an expert in mental diseases, as well as a lecturer at the
medical college. The Rest Cure is a handsome building, delightfully situated in the fashionable part of the city, away from the
noise and turmoil of business, and just the place for a man who
needs the restful seclusion which this retreat affords.   The
advertisement will be found on another page.

—Dr. F. F. Henwood, of Thompson, Pa., writes : " In a case
of acute neuralgic headache I used Peacock's bromides with
complete success, and find it to be the best nerve sedative prepared."

LILLY'S IMPROVED GLYCERIN SUPPOSITORIES.—These invaluable peristaltic persuaders are prepared in a most excellent and
improved manner by Messrs. Eli Lilly & Co., of Indianapolis.
Their suppositories contain 95 per cent. of glycerin, and a beauty
of their construction is the peculiar water-proof covering of each
suppository, which is readily and easily removed.   By simply
pressing upon or slightly squeezing the suppository between the
fingers it slips out with astonishing ease, leaving the covering
between the fingers. A great improvement, as any one will
readily recognize who has ever made the effort to divest one of
the ordinary suppositories from its lead foil and tissue paper
envelope.—*Southern Practitioner*, Oct. 1889.

THE

MONTREAL MEDICAL JOURNAL.

| VOL. XVIII. | MAY, 1890. | No. 11. |

Original Communications.

VALEDICTORY ADDRESS

DELIVERED TO THE GRADUATES IN MEDICINE AT THE ANNUAL
MEETING OF CONVOCATION OF McGILL UNIVERSITY,
APRIL 1ST, 1890.

BY J. CHALMERS CAMERON, M.D.,

Professor of Obstetrics, McGill University; Physician-Accoucheur to the Montreal
Maternity, &c.

Gentlemen, Graduates in Medicine :

It is the time-honored custom in the University for the
Faculty to select one of their number to address a few words,
in their behalf, to the graduating class—words of congratula-
tion, encouragement, advice and cheer.

First, then, we congratulate you most heartily upon the
successful completion of your Collegiate Course. Four long
years of patient, steady work culminate to-day in your Doctor's
degree. The parchment you have just received testifies that
you have attained to the standard laid down by the University, have fulfilled all her requirements, and are fit and proper
persons to practise Medicine ; while you on your part have
solemnly sworn to practise your profession *carefully, honestly*
and *uprightly.* The diploma you now hold is one of which you
may well be proud, for in whatsoever part of the civilised
world your lot may be cast, you will find that the reputation
of your Alma Mater has preceded you, and will bespeak for
you the confidence of the public and the respect of your confrères. You will never have cause to be ashamed of your
Alma Mater ; look well to it that you never, by word or deed,
give her cause to be ashamed of you.

51

To-day is with you a red-letter day, marking a great epoch in your lives. Four long years you have been toiling up the hill, with eyes fixed upon graduation day as the great final goal of your efforts. Other realities of life have been obscured or overshadowed by the intense reality of *this.* Your degree has been your *summum bonum,* and every nerve has been strained to win it. To day the degree is yours; you have climbed the hill, reached the goal, but as you look around, lo! the realities, responsibilities and possibilities of life open out before you. Your perspective is wholly changed, your life-climb has but begun. You were students before, if you would succeed you must be students still. You worked hard before, you must work harder still. Toil, the birthright of mankind, must still be yours, if you are not to be laggards in the race. Under the careful guidance and supervision of your teachers, you have learned first to creep, then to stand, and at last to walk. The way has been marked out for you, its roughness smoothed, your faltering steps steadied. Now you are cut loose from leading strings, you must choose your own road and make your own pace; how far you will manage to push along will depend very much upon the energy, perseverance and singleness of purpose you henceforth display.

In welcoming you to our ranks, we would remind you that our profession is one of intrinsic nobility and dignity. In it science and charity, knowledge and sympathy, skill and pity go hand in hand, ministering to the sorrows and sufferings of human kind. Its annals teem with deeds of heroism, self-sacrifice and devotion. When pestilence stalks the earth, when panic and fear seize upon the people, the physician will be found at the post of danger "firm, fearless and faithful." When human pity may wipe away a tear, human skill ease a pain, or human sympathy comfort and console, there, too, will he be found. Of all the brave and gallant deeds by land or sea, none are more truly great and noble than those of men who amidst the horrors of pestilence, in the privacy of daily life, without the stimulus of excitement, publicity or hope of reward, have toiled without repose to assuage the misery of the sick and dying, and at last without a murmur have laid down their lives for their fellow-men.

Such is our profession. Would you prove yourselves worthy

of it ? Would you emulate the brave deeds and noble spirit of your predecessors ? Then you must begin well, and as you begin so must you continue to the very end.

Duties to yourselves.—Your owe certain duties to yourselves. First and foremost, your character must ever be above reproach. Honor, uprightness and integrity must be the very *Warp* of your lives. Then to the best of your ability you must keep well abreast of the times, and strive always to be accomplished, educated physicians. Though now, no doubt, you *" know everything about medicine that is worth knowing,"* you can not maintain that happy state of affairs without constant diligent study. He who is content with what he knows soon drops out of the ranks and is left behind ; in the medical profession, there is no such thing as standing still ; you must either push on or fall back. An eminent professor was once asked by a young graduate what he should do to secure success in his profession. " Three things," replied the Professor, " 1st, observe; 2nd, observe; 3rd, observe." Careful observation is the surest road to success ; it is the magic key which unlocks the mysteries of Nature and reveals her secrets to the studious enquirer. Train eye, ear and touch ; investigate every case thoroughly and systematically ; observe everything, considering nothing too trivial or minute. Study the laws of cause and effect and apply them in your daily practice ; consider each case as a problem you are called upon to solve. Study out carefully and estimate at its proper value the *personal* factor ; aim to treat your patient, not his disease, and you will find the practice of medicine an absorbing, fascinating study—a never-failing source of pleasure and gratification, the best antidote to jealousy, irritation and querulous discontent. I pray you, do not allow yourselves to degenerate into the routine practitioner—a sort of peripatetic prescribing machine. Such a man cares very little for principles or deductions therefrom. The prescription is his great stand-by; and with a pocketful of them he is armed for any emergency. He poses as a *practical* man ; no theory or nonsense about him. At Medical Societies and Conventions he comes out in full force. Notebook in hand, he goes about buttonholing prominent men for their favorite prescriptions ; if he succeeds in capturing any, he goes home happy and

proceeds to use them upon all and sundry for the balance of
his professional life, or until he can replace them by some
newly-captured favorites.

While you study the cases which come under your care and
train your faculties of observation and reflection, do not fail
to acquaint yourselves with the results and opinions of others.
Attend Medical Societies and Conventions, for there you come
in contact with fellow-workers of riper experience, and mutual
benefit is derived from criticising and being criticised. *Read
diligently.* Read the current journals; they give you the
latest news from the front; the pioneers of thought, the original workers and investigators are there, like pickets and
skirmishers, spying out the land, sometimes advancing,
sometimes retreating, sometimes gaining new positions, sometimes abandoning old ones no longer tenable. At all events
it is news from the front, of absorbing interest, though subject
to much alteration and correction, and not always trustworthy.
In the text-books you find the solid ground that has been won.
And so you perceive the professional army marching along;
pickets, pioneers and skirmishers away at the front, busily
exploring, prospecting, making roads and bridges; the rank
and file with baggage and equipments moving more slowly,
trying and proving the ground, testing the strength of roads
and bridges. On they march with face ever to the front,
fighting disease and death. Alas for the stragglers who face
to the rear, who sleep by the way.

Duties to patients.—In the practice of your profession you
have certain well-defined duties to your patients. There is in
fact an implied contract between you. They on their part
place confidence in you and trust you. In your hands are placed
sometimes health and happiness, honor and reputation, the
issues of life and death. You on your part, in accepting such
grave responsibilities, are bound to possess and maintain a
competent knowledge of your profession, to devote due care
and attention to your patients, and exercise your best skill.
In your professional relations, you will be admitted into the
privacy of the family circle; in sickness the society mask is
off and you will see poor humanity in all its weakness. You
will know the shadows that darken many a home, the hidden
sorrows that embitter many a life; weighty secrets, important

confidences may be committed to your care; and thus not only the lives, but often the prospects and fortunes of individuals, the peace, honor and happiness of families, and even the welfare of the community may rest in your hands. Upon your prudence and caution great interests may hang, beware how you betray them.

Remember, too, that the personal factor enters very largely into the problem of success. By your patients you are valued, not only for your medical skill, but also for the refreshing or soothing influence of your own personality. To the pain-wracked sufferer your daily visit may be the one bright oasis in the dreary monotony of life; a gentle manner, a gentle voice and sympathy are potent factors in the cure. While you strive to be skilful in your profession, do not forget that when human skill is of no more avail, sympathy and kindness may temper a blow you can not ward off, or lighten a sorrow you can not avert. Be honorable, honest, upright; a sympathetic listener, a wise counsellor — but a *gossip*, a *talebearer*—never. Strive to be a ray of sunshine in every home; let the sick brighten at your entrance; let the little ones long for your visits; then, when your life work is drawing to a close, when you are old and grey, men and women grown, whom you have watched and tended from infancy, will love and revere you and cherish your memory in the tenderest esteem.

Duties to Confreres.—When you begin the practice of your profession you will be at once thrown into contact and competition with other medical men. Remember you are fellow-workers; let no unseemly rivalry or jealousy mar your friendly relations. Pay no attention to those who laugh at the strictness of our professional etiquette. Follow strictly our *Code of Ethics*, for it is nothing more or less than a practical application to medical matters of the Golden Rule in its negative form, "*Do not unto others that which you would not have them do unto you.*" Be modest in your demeanor, especially to older men. Perhaps they may not be as well up as yourselves in the latest teachings of the Schools, but from long personal observation and experience they have gathered rich stores of knowledge which no mere book lore can give, and which you must work many years to acquire. Do not forg that there is often room for honest difference of opinion. We sometimes hear it said that doctors differ. Of course they differ. And so do all men who are not mere machines, men who reflect, weigh evidence, balance probabilities, and use their own judgment and common sense. The clergy differ— witness the multiplicity of sects and parties, the wide divergence of opinion and belief in the religious world. Lawyers and judges differ—witness the elaborate machinery of our courts, with appeal, review and final appeal, one court modifying or reversing the finding of another. Philosophers, men of science, politicians, political economists, thoughtful men everywhere differ—and so do doctors. In the practice of your profession, not only is there room for honest difference of *opinion ;* there is room also for honest difference in *treatment.* You wish to go from McGill College to the Post Office; you have your choice of many different ways, each of which will eventually bring you to your destination—some longer, some shorter, some pleasanter than others ; if time is no object you may go around by Cote St. Antoine, and yet finally reach the Post Office. Your choice of road is really very much a matter of taste and urgency. So you will find in practice, the same end may be accomplished in many different ways ; the ultimate choice of method being largely a question of taste and tact on the part of the practitioner. How very foolish and unjust, therefore, to criticise the methods of a confrère and act as if your own way was the right way, the *only* right way. The wise man is always glad to learn from his neighbours, observing wherein their methods are better than his, and modifying his own accordingly.

Duties to Science.—Besides our more immediate duties to our patients, there are other indirect obligations none the less binding. We cannot directly repay our parents for their love and care to us during our infancy and childhood. We repay them indirectly by bestowing like care upon our children. So in medicine, from the past we inherit the accumulated knowledge and experience of the ages ; it is incumbent upon us not only to transmit this goodly inheritance unimpaired but also to contribute all we can to increase the store. Science entrusts us with various talents ; in return she demands from us a profitable service. The best men in the profession everywhere consider it one of the first duties to record for the benefit of the profession their cases, methods and results. In this way only can science be advanced. Deeds of darkness love darkness, but science and truth love the light. Secrecy begets carelesness and ignorance, and is the favorite refuge of the charlatan. But some of you may say, that is all very well for the city men with their great hospital and other advantages, it is easy enough for them to do original work and advance the cause of Science; but what can be expected from a poor country practitioner, isolated from converse with his confrères, with limited experience, few books, scanty means and opportunities all too few. No man's lot is so humble that he cannot cherish the scientific spirit. Your books may be few, but the great book of Nature lies ever open. Read thoroughly the few lines or chapters spread before you, and by mere concentration of attention you may discover therein a hidden meaning undetected by those who perforce must skim from page to page. The country practitioner has one great advantage over his city confrère ; *he has time to think.* The rush and whirl of city life are fatal to steady, fruitful thought, and we find that many of the brightest discoveries of scientific medicine are the contribution of quiet, thoughtful men with limited opportunities, but imbued with the scientific spirit. You are begining your career in a time of unusual scientific activity. Chemistry, experimental physiology, pathology, and pharmacology are rapidly changing the aspect of practical medicine. Sanitary science and preventive medicine offer specially rich fields for original research. The problems are legion and demand for their solution carefulness of observation, accuracy of thought and soundness of judgment. Every one of you can do something; will you try? You will not be losers thereby, for if the true scientific fire burns in your hearts and illumines your daily work, you will find work no longer wearisome, poverty no longer despicable, disease and death no longer loathsome or terrible. Above all, have faith in yourselves; have faith in your art. Let a firm abiding faith be the mainspring of your practice. No human theory is perfect. Science and art are progressing, improving. Be ready to abandon the *old* when proved *false*, to accept the *new* when proved *true*. But do not throw away the faith you have until you are sure of another

to take its place. An imperfect, defective faith is far better
than no faith at all. It is after all very easy to pose as a
sceptic or iconoclast, to sneer and rail at prevailing belief and
practice, to profess disbelief in the efficacy of drugs, and the
possibilities of nature, science and art. But such a mental
attitude betokens weakness, not strength,—conceit, not knowledge. I beseech you, do not join the ranks of the medical
nihilists; the man without faith in *science,* in his *art,* in *himself,*
is like a ship without ballast or rudder, tossed about hither
and thither with every wind of doctrine.

Duties to the University.—Now, finally, you have some duties
to the university. Hitherto you have been students of medicine, and your chief allegiance has been to your own professors. To-day your Alma Mater enrolls you among her sons
and sends you forth into the world bearing her name. In all
her departments she has claims upon your life-long interest
and sympathy. While her reputation is in a manner your
reputation and her success your success, do not forget that in
like manner your reputation is her reputation and your success
her success. Strive to be worthy of her. Guard well the
charge this day entrusted to your care. According to ancient
Jewish legend, the patriarch Abraham ever wore upon his
breast a jewel whose light raised those who were bowed
down, and healed those who were sick. And when he died
the jewel was set in the heavens, where it still shines among
the stars. May the badge conferred on you to day be as mighty
for good as the patriarch's jewel of old; and if you guard it
untarnished to the very end, your names will shine forever
among those starry hosts to whom the eyes of humanity ever
turn with admiration, gratitude and love. Go forth, graduating
class of '90, bearing aloft as your banner the motto " *Excelsior,*"
ever onward and upward, and may success attend your efforts.
In the name of your professors, in the name of the University,
Godspeed and fare you well.

IAL HYSTERECTOMY FOR UTERINE CANCER.

By T. K. HOLMES, M.D., CHATHAM, ONT.

insatisfactory results that have followed the various plans
ng uterine cancer have led surgeons to resort to opera-
ore and more radical until complete removal of the organ
a resorted to. The number of times this has been done
fully warrants the hope that with the improved methods
,ting the mortality may be reduced, many lives saved
ers prolonged, or, if death result from recurrence of the
it may at least be less painful and loathsome.

certain that a careful selection of cases must be made for
ration of hysterectomy if this surgical procedure is not to
disrepute. Conditions applicable to the surgical treat-
cancer elsewhere in the body should guide us in the
nt of cancer uteri. The rule should be to resort to that
n by which the whole of the disease can be removed
least risk to the patient's life. If the disease be in the
the uterus, or if beginning at the os uteri, it invades the
canal far up to the body or even to the internal os, ex-
a of the entire organ is the most reliable means of cure.
tissues than the uterus be involved, hysterectomy could
palliative, and is too serious an operation to be under-
ith no prospect of a radical cure. If the disease be so
to the cervix that the whole cancerous part can be
l by supra-vaginal amputation, this should be the opera-
:cted.

ollowing case was one in which cancerous growth began
.he external os and extended beyond the internal os, so
.rpation of the uterus offered the only means of cure.
opic sections prepared by Dr. Caven and exhibited before
iological Society of Toronto showed the extent of disease
stated above :

C., aged 55, has had several children, and has always
good health until nine months ago, when she began to
norrhagia, which gradually grew worse until she came
ie care of Dr. Jenner of Kingsville, who applied nitric

acid to the diseased part of the cervix. This controlled the hemorrhage, so that for six weeks it has been much less profuse. Dr. Jenner, through whose advise I saw her, had recognized the nature of the disease, and I was told by the patient that Dr. McGrath of Detroit had pronounced it malignant. The macroscopic and microscopic appearance left no doubt as to its malignancy. The operation was performed at Kingsville, on October 7th, 1889, with the assistance of Drs. Jenner and Campard of that place, Dr. Dewar of Essex Centre, and Mr. Pearson, medical student, of Chatham. A saline aperient was given the morning before, and the bladder and rectum were evacuated before anæsthesia. The patient was placed in the lithotomy position, the external genitals were shaved and washed with soap and water and bathed with a bichloride solution 1 to 1000, and the vagina thoroughly douched with the same. A large Sims' speculum was introduced under the pubic arch and the vulva held apart by retractors. Owing to the shortness of the vaginal portion of the cervix and the fragile character of the diseased part it was impossible to draw the uterus down either by a silk cord passed transversely through the cervix or by volcellum forceps, and it became necessary to operate *in situ*. A curved incision was made with scissors through the vagina at its line of junction with the posterior surface of the cervix, and extended each way to the base of the broad ligaments; the connective tissue was separated by the finger until the peritoneum was reached, and this was then opened and the incision extended laterally to the broad ligaments. A similar procedure in front of the cervix was followed, and the uterus was held now only by its ligaments and by a small portion of vaginal tissue at each lateral fornix. The latter was snipped through on each side, care being taken not to divide the tissues high enough to wound the uterine arteries. The second and first fingers of the left hand were next passed up so as to include the broad ligament between them, and the clamp was guided so as to compress as much of it as the jaws would reach, and the part so clamped was then divided between the clamp and the uterus. It was necessary to use a second clamp for the upper part of the ligament and the tube, which were then divided as before. The opposite side was managed in the same way, and the uterus then came away through the wound. As soon as Douglas's sac was opened a portion of omentum prolapsed, but it received no further attention than the avoidance of its being wounded. The vagina was gently cleansed with the bichloride solution, no material of any kind was placed in the vagina, and the only dressing consisted of bichloride gauze placed over the external genitals and renewed as often as it became soiled. The catheter was used for three days, the clamps were removed in thirty-six hours, and the case did well under the care of Dr. Jenner, to whose skill and watchfulness the successful termination of the case is largely due.

In the performance of this operation care is necessary to avoid injury of the rectum, bladder and ureters. Keeping close to the uterus is the safest way. The ureters pass about one-third of an inch from the antero-lateral surface of the cervix, and must be carefully avoided. Where the vaginal portion of the cervix is very short and fragile, as in this case, the operation is more difficult. The use of the clamp simplifies the operation very much. The operation occupied forty-five minutes, but would have been completed in half-an-hour had not some time been lost in efforts to draw down the uterus with a cord passed through the cervix. The patient gained her former weight, and at the present time looks and feels well.

Retrospect Department.

QUARTERLY RETROSPECT OF MEDICINE.

By R. L. MacDonnell, M.D.,

Professor of Clinical Medicine in McGill University; Physician to Montreal General Hospital.

Lithæmic Manifestations in the Upper Air Passages.— In the *American Journal of the Medical Sciences* Dr. A. Whiteh Hinkel calls attention to this subject as one which has hitherto received but slight attention. The author uses the term *lithæmia*, as Murchison used it, to express a condition of suboxidation and overcharging of the blood and excretions with excretory matter in a state of faulty elaboration, due to inherent and hereditary abnormality of function or to prolonged exposure to depressing environment. Lithæmic manifestations in the upper air passages fail to present conditions that invariably announce their origin, and they are not uniform in type, but at the same time certain given appearances or symptoms are more or less connected with lithæmia and suggest treatment for that condition, whatever local measures may be indicated. A patchy congestion of the laryngeal face of the epiglottis, extending along the arytæno-epiglottic folds and over the posterior aspect of the ventricular bands, is occasionally seen in cases of irritable sore throat associated with lithæmia. There is a harsh, dry cough, with a sense of extreme irritation about the larynx. This patchy congestion of the mucous membrane has been observed by means of the cystoscope in the bladder of a lithæmic patient. A case cited, which was aggravated by aromatic inhalations, mild astringent sprays, etc., was promptly relieved by alkalies and antizymotics, together with inhalations of diluted lime-water and a carefully arranged diet. This patchy condition may exist in the pharynx, extending in streaks along the postero-lateral walls, with a sense of uneasiness or pain on swallowing   The pain of gouty sore throat appears severe, out of all proportion to the degree of inflammation. Lithic storms have been accompanied by marked naso-pharyngeal catarrh, not present in appreciable degree during the intervals, the symptoms appearing several days before the digestive and other disturbances.*

---

* The New York Medical Journal, Feb. 15th, 1890.

Cheyne-Stokes Breathing in Granular Kidney.— At the meeting of the Clinical Society of London, held on the 28th Feb., 1890, an interesting discussion on this subject took place. Dr. Samuel West read the notes of a case of granular kidney of three months duration, in which the phenomenon was present. The patient, a man of 53 years of age, with a history of gout occasionally, had been suffering from shortness of breath, especially after exertion, for eighteen months. Six months before admission he was suddenly seized with severe dyspnœa at night that he thought he was going to die. After half an hour he rallied, but he had two similar attacks in the course of a month, and then remained well until three weeks ago, when the worst attack of all came on, since which time his breathing remained short. He had a pale, sallow, earthy complexion, with tortuous and thickened arteries, and a pulse of high tension. Pulse 104 ; respiration 48. Heart not manifestly hypertrophied ; no murmur. Urine of low specific gravity (1010), and contained about one-sixteenth of albumen. The retina was natural. The case was diagnosed as one of weak heart resulting from granular kidney. A few days later Cheyne-Stokes breathing developed. There were several minor points of interest connected with the phenomenon itself, for which the reader is referred to *The Lancet* of March 8th, 1890.

Dr. Charlton Bastian said that old writers had remarked on the association of Cheyne-Stokes respiration with fatty degeneration of the heart, but he had seen no such cases ; he had observed it in connection with cerebral lesion. It might be, he supposed, produced by the blood-poisoning associated with renal disease.

Dr. Stephen Mackenzie had observed in a patient of 80, with dilated heart, granular kidneys and a little albuminuria and Cheyne-Stokes breathing, that in the commencement of the series of ascending respiratory acts a distinct movement of the arms towards the head took place. He had seen two patients recently in whom, during the apnæic period, a distinct convulsive seizure took place ; one had between 150 and 200 such fits in twenty-four hours. He asked if any one had seen a case of Cheyne-Stokes breathing apart from injury of the head which had recovered.

which time there were two or thre
lasting from a quarter to half an l
administered. On recovery fron
breathing was resumed. The foll
fell to normal, and the breathing r
The second case occurred in Mr.
months. The illness began with
but after a week Cheyne-Stokes l
tinued for four days. The paus
between the respirations (somet
marked. The temperature befo
noticed was raised, but afterward
vulsive attacks occurred at interva
ing, which commenced a few da
illness, existed for several weeks.
Stokes respiration lasted the fonta
and remained so for two weeks.
symptoms ceased hydrocephalus
bulging of the fontanelles and o
symptoms ceased to increase afte
head is more square than normal
since ceased to grow out of propo
body, and perfect health has beer

Mr. Lawford Knaggs reports a case of recovery after Cheyne-Stokes breathing, but death occurred in three months and a half. Such cases are by no means uncommon. I can recall three instances occurring in the practice of the Montreal General Hospital, where the phenomenon was present for a similar period. It seems that Cheyne-Stokes breathing is more readily produced in children. Some readers may remember a discussion of this very subject at a meeting of the Canadian Medical Association in 1884, where Dr. Osler reported a case of Cheyne-Stokes in a child otherwise quite healthy.

So far as the discussion has gone, no real case of recovery after Cheyne-Stokes breathing has developed is on record, though an anonymous correspondent of the *Lancet* reports the case of his own father, in whom the symptom has been present for many years, having been observed as long ago as 1874. The old gentleman is 93 years of age, and otherwise enjoys good health.

Thirty-two Cases of Basilar Tubercular Meningitis.—Hermann Rieder relates the history of 32 cases of this disease which occurred in Ziemssen's service in the General Hospital of Munich[*] from the years 1880 to 1889. Of the 32 patients, 23 were men, 9 were women, and their ages ranged from 10 to 70 years. The age of the majority was between 21 and 30 years, and two cases occurred between the ages 61 and 70. The result of the autopsies showed : well marked chronic tuberculosis of the lungs in 10 cases, disseminated caseous foci of tubercle in various stages in 12 cases, caseous pneumonia in 1 case, caseous glands in 1 case, solitary cerebellar tumor in 1 case, and fibrous changes of the apex in 1 case without any caseous or tubercular centres. In the remainder of the cases the presence of tuberculosis could not be established, but in fourteen instances general miliary tuberculosis was found.

In the majority of cases the meningitis began without any specially predisposing cause, and in almost every instance with headache, dizziness, constipation, wakefulness, severe attacks of vomiting, and in but two cases with rigors. In one case there occurred, even in the beginning, paralytic manifestations in the

---

[*] Munchn. med. Wchnchr. xxxvi., 49-51, 1889.

right side with perverted sensations and epileptiform attacks in another patient a facial palsy was one of the first symptom[s]

Among the important symptoms were : rigidity of the nec[k] 20 cases ; contraction of the muscles of the back, 20 case[s] unilateral contraction of the cervical muscles, 6 cases ; scapho[id] retraction of the abdominal walls, 5 cases ; general convulsion 5 cases ; spasm of the masseter muscles, 2 cases ; hiccough, cases ; palsy of the facial muscles, 9 cases ; complete rig[ht] hemiplegia, 1 case ; paraplegia of the lower extremities, 3 case[s] retention of urine, 3 cases ; incontinence of urine, 11 case Eye symptoms : Ptosis in 3 ; variations in the size of the pu[pil] in 16 ; general hyperæ[sthe]sia in 19. The pulse was, at t[he] outset, unaffected or slowed but later accelerated ; the temper[a-] ture varied in most cases between 100.4°F. and 102.2°F.; t[he] respirations were in most cases accelerated ; in eight patien[ts] Cheyne-Stokes breathing was observed. Vomiting was comm[on] at the outset, but seldom occurred in the course of the diseas[e.] There was persistent constipation and rapid emaciation.

Fatal Cases of Ear Disease.—In the Gulstonian lecture[s] delivered at the Royal College of Physicians, Dr. G. Newton P[*] dealt with this very important subject, confining his observatio[ns] to the unpublished records of Guy's Hospital, dealing only wi[th] those cases which proved fatal. First, with regard to the ca[ses] of ear disease which have proved fatal from the secondary co[m-] plications they have set up in the cranial cavity—two of [the] commonest complications to which they may give rise are ce[re-] bral abscesses and thrombosis of the sinuses. In twenty ye[ars] there were 57 post-mortem inspections of cases where ear dise[ase] had set up disease in the cranial cavity which ultimately pro[ved] fatal. During this period there were nearly 9,000 inspectio[ns] No case of simple otitis media with or without disease of [the] mastoid cells was fatal during the whole of this period, and [only] twice was the fatal complication outside the cranial cavit[y] being in one a retropharyngeal abscess, and in the other hem[or-] rhage from ulceration into the internal carotid artery. [The] difficulties of diagnosis in ear disease are much increased by

---

* The Lancet, vol. i., 1889, p. 739.

fact that not only may a patient die without any otorrhœa being noticed, but in two instances the membrana tympani was found intact at the inspection.

Of the 57 cases 34 were males and 23 females ; the left ear was rather more frequently affected than the right. Seventeen of the patients were under 10, seventeen were between 10 and 20, fourteen between 20 and 30, and only nine over 30. The acute symptoms in ear disease appear to come on spontaneously ; at others, they have followed exposure to cold, a blow on the ear, mastoid suppuration, the introduction of foreign bodies into the external meatus, or the removal of a polypus. If the pus is pent up under tension, earache and headache will develop ; but only those cases, in this series, proved fatal in which the inflammation had spread outside the petrous bone. The majority of the cases, if freely drained by opening up the mastoid cells, recover, and many of them ultimately discharge their pus externally without surgical aid. Toynbee thought that affections of the external meatus and mastoid cells produced disease in the mastoid cells, lateral sinus and cerebellum, that affections in the tympanic cavity produced disease in the cerebrum, and that affections of the vestibule and cochlea produced disease in the medulla oblongata. As the lecturer shows later on, thrombosis of the lateral sinus often has originated from caries of the posterior wall of the tympanic cavity, and mastoid disease sometimes spreads to the middle fossa of the skull : still, the usual sequence is that indicated by Toynbee. Disease of the internal ear appears usually to set up meningitis in the posterior fossa of the skull. Postmortem evidence shows that the condition of the mastoid cells and of the roof of the tympanum and the situation of the lateral sinus play the most important part in determining the direction in which the disease shall spread, and that therefore too great stress should not be laid on the presence or absence of disease of the mastoid, although it may be somewhat of a guide to the seat of the mischief. The condition of the wall of the middle ear teaches nothing which can be of assistance in diagnosis. The most convenient arrangement of the complica-

52

tions to be discussed will be according to their site: (1) dura
mater, (2) cerebral tissue, (3) sinuses, (4) pia-arachnoid.

Owing to the thinness of the tympanic roof, the dura mater
over the anterior surface of the petrous bone is rather more often
inflamed than that over the posterior wall of the middle ear, but
less often if we include the part bounding the mastoid cells as
well. The otorrhœa in these cases is of old standing; generally
the bone beneath is inflamed, discolored, carious or necrosed
and in some of the cases the bone presented carious apertures
through which the infection had spread directly. Inflammation
or sloughing of the dura mater occurred in ten out of twelve
cases of temporo-sphenoidal abscess, and probably seven of these
could not have recovered unless the dura mater as well as the
abscess could have been allowed to drain. In extra dural abscess
which may produce optic neuritis, the inflammation has probably
spread along the lymphatics around the veins. In three cases
of mastoid disease which recovered after trephining and one
without trephining, there was optic neuritis.

Of 18 cases of cerebral abscess, 9 occurred on each side of
the brain. All the patients were men, and 13 of the case
occurred between the ages of 10 and 29, the only case over 4
being one of pontic abscess. They agree with the general
experience that otorrhœa does not set up cerebral abscess unt
it has lasted months or years, for in only two was its duratio
under a year. Three of the abscesses were in the cerebellum
one in the pons, two in the cerebrum ovale, and the remainin
twelve in the temporo-sphenoidal lobes near the tympanic roo
The dura mater in this latter group was healthy in only two,
eight it was sloughing, in two inflamed, and in one there was
localized extra dural abscess.

When there is healthy brain tissue between the tempor
sphenoidal abscess and the bone it is probable that the infecti
has been spread by the veins which empty into the superi
petrosal sinus from the temporo-sphenoidal lobe on the one han
and the tympanum on the other, by means of a septic phlebit
or more probably by means of the peri-vascular lymphatics; l
if it had been due to a phlebitis, thrombosis of the superi

petrosal sinus would have been occasionally noticed. Only five of the abscesses were less than an inch in diameter, while ten exceeded two inches.

Thrombosis of the lateral sinus occurred twenty-two times. In some there was well-marked phlebitis; in considerably more than half the thrombus was suppurating, and in others where not breaking down it had set up a pulmonary pyæmia, thus demonstrating its septic nature. The disease more often spreads from the posterior wall of the middle ear than from the mastoid cells; this is important, for any treatment to be successful must deal with the condition of the bone and dura mater as well as with the sinus. Whenever the mastoid vein, which perforates an inch and a quarter behind the meatus and on a level with it, is found thrombosed, the sinus should be explored. The clot may be a small one, or it may occupy the whole of the sinus and spread into the internal jugular or general venous system of the skull. Thrombosis is a fatal lesion, but there is some evidence that patients with the typical symptoms appear to recover, at any rate for a time. The otorrhœa is generally, but not always, of long standing; in only five it lasted less than seven weeks. The onset is usually sudden, the chief symptoms being pyrexia, rigors, pain in the occipital region and in the neck, associated with a septicæmic condition. Earache, as distinct from headache, is more common than with meningitis and abscess; vomiting and coma were also met with. In no other complication are erratic pyrexia and rigors so constantly present, and it will be always justifiable to assume that they probably indicate thrombosis in any patient in whom freely opening the deeper mastoid cells and draining the ear have not been followed by their subsidence. Well marked optic neuritis may be present, and is more suggestive of sinus thrombosis than of other lesions. The appearance of acute local pulmonary mischief or of distant suppuration is almost conclusive of thrombosis; and, as death in three-quarters of the cases ensues from pulmonary pyæmia after a course of but three weeks, treatment, to be of any value, must be directed to the prevention of the pyæmia.

QUARTERLY RETROSPECT OF GYNÆCOLOGY

By T. Johnson-Alloway, M.D.,

Instructor in Gynæcology, McGill University; Assistant Surgeon to the Montreal
General Hospital; Gynæcologist to the Montreal Dispensary.

The Surgical Treatment of Puerperal Peritonitis.—Matthew
D. Mann says that there is no reason why pus within the abdomen should not be let out as well as pus within the pleural sac,
or within any other serous cavity. Under such circumstances
the cavity is simply converted into a large abscess, and as such
should be drained. Nor does it make any difference what the
origin of this pus may be. It is all the same whether it comes
from the bursting of an abscess of one ovary or from the gonorrhœal salpingitis, or from a suppurative process originating within
the uterus after confinement and extending through the tubes to
the peritoneal cavity. The pus, if present, must be evacuated
before recovery can take place. Several things stand in the
way of the general adoption of the operation. One is the traditional fear of the peritoneum—a fear which still lingers in the
minds of the general profession, but which has long since van-
ished from the thoughts of the laparotomist. If there is already
inflammation with pus formation, what worse can happen? What
harm can the opening of the cavity do? Such incision, if made
with due care, is in itself absolutely without danger, as has been
proven over again. So, if no good is done, or might happen in
the case of mistaken diagnosis, no harm will result.—(*Trans.
New York Medical Society.*)

Non-Retention of Urine in Young Girls and Women —No
disease is more annoying or more depressing to a patient than a
disease of the bladder which calls for an almost constant evacuation of that organ. Frequent micturition is usually due to
cystitis, or urethritis, or to the presence of a tumor or foreign
body in the bladder, but at times it is due to indifferent causes.
After a time in certain cases the walls of the bladder contract,
owing to hypertrophy of the muscular layer, and the capacity of
the bladder is reduced to one or two ounces. Such patients are
obliged to urinate every few minutes during the day, and at night
when asleep the urine dribbles almost continually. Dr. H. Marion

Sims advocates the systematic use of injections of warm water to dilate the bladder and increase its capacity, for the alleviation and cure of this distressing condition; and reports a number of cures effected by the method. The apparatus used by Dr. Sims is a silver catheter attached by means of a rubber tube to a Davidson's syringe. He injects water, comfortably warm, into the bladder by means of this apparatus until the bladder is distended. This is indicated by the sensations of the patient. The process is quite painful, and, sometimes, to the patient, "unbearable," and requires patience on the part of the physician and bravery on the part of the patient to bring about good results. The injections are practised daily for one, three or more months, until the bladder will hold a pint of water, and then not so frequently. Improvement in the patient's condition and ability to retain urine usually keeps pace with the dilatation. The water injected should not be allowed to remain, but should be drawn off at the conclusion of each treatment. This method of treatment appears logical, and the results in the hands of Dr. Sims have been quite brilliant, as many of the cases had been the rounds of physicians and had been subjected to many methods of treatment. Apparently the only danger inherent in the method is the risk of rupturing the bladder, which could only occur under exceptional conditions of the walls of that organ, or when undue violence was used in giving the injection. Dr. Sims is to be congratulated for having perfected a successful method of treating a distressing class of cases.—(*Med. and Surg. Reporter.*)

Corporeal Endometritis.—It is considered that the increasing attention that is being given to affections of the interior of the uterus is being productive of great benefit to women suffering from uterine affections. Treatment implied as a necessary step dilatation of the cervix and os internum, and this dilatation is believed to be of itself a great, even in some cases the chief, factor in giving relief. Further, the fact that such dilatation could be done at one sitting, under anæsthetics, and without any previous use of dangerous tents, rendered it possible to examine and relieve many cases which formerly would have continued to suffer for years, imperfectly relieved by other methods. Dr.

Robert Bell considered that endometritis was not a rare disease. With regard to the diagnosis, he considered there was not much difficulty ; in fact, it might almost be diagnosed by the subjective symptoms alone. For example, if a patient complained of a bearing-down sensation, accompanied by pain and a burning sensation in the pelvis, acute suffering over the sacrum, dysmenorrhœa, a copious purulent or muco-purulent discharge, and an irritable condition of the bladder and bowel, and also suffered from lowness of spirits, irritability of temper, disturbed sleep, on a vaginal examination the uterus would be ascertained to be hyperplasic and flabby, while from the os a copious purulent or muco-purulent discharge would be seen to exude. In addition, there might be exaggeration of pain in the pelvis at the menstrual period ; in consequence of this aggravated congestion, there was coagulation of the blood occurring at the moment of its exudation which necessitated the clots being expelled by uterine contractions. The inflammatory conditions might be so acute that coagulation actually took place within the lining membrane itself, and thus there would be, if not absolute absence, yet paucity of discharge, and from the same cause there might be an absence of catarrhal discharge also. He held that salpingitis never occurred without a prior endometritis having existed, and that the inflamed condition of the tubes was due to the inflammation having spread by continuity of tissue. In treatment, the first object must be to dilate the os internum, then to swab out the uterine canal, and apply freely some form of stimulating antiseptic (iodized phenol).—(*Pridgin Teale, M.D.*)

The Surgical Treatment of Local and General Peritonitis.—The author (*Gill Wylie*) reports five successful case of laparotomy for intestinal trouble, in two of which perforation of the intestine and general septic peritonitis were present. He presents the following conclusions, which are based upon his large experience in abdominal surgery :—

When there are symptoms of local peritonitis, intense pain and tenderness, followed by tympanites and vomiting, with chilly sensations and rise of temperature, search should be made for the cause. As a rule, the pain will soon become localised over the region of the Fallopian tubes, the cæcum, or gall-bladder, or some old ventral or inguinal hernia. If signs of a tumor or exudation can be definitely made out, and the general symptoms indicate the formation of pus, then the patient should be ether-ized and the pus reached by incision, the pus evacuated, and the cavity washed out and drained. If it is in, or involves, the tubes and ovaries, the abdomen should be opened, and if the tube or tubes are occluded and pus found, they, with the ovary or ovaries, should be removed. If the abscess is around the appendix ver-miformis or cœcum, an incision should be made near the crest of the ilium and the peritoneum dissected up till a place is reached where the peritoneum is adherent to the tumor, which should then be carefully opened, the pus evacuated, the sac washed out, and a drainage-tube introduced without opening into the free cavity of the peritoneum. If it is about the gall-bladder, if the signs of pus can be made out, an incision over the sac should be made and the pus evacuated.

If the general symptoms are severe and no localized centre of pus made out, then an incision should be made in the median line and the peritoneal cavity explored with the index finger. If then a pus sac is found, if it be so situated that it can be reached by another lateral incision and the pus evacuated with-out allowing the pus to escape into the free peritoneal cavity, it should be made, and the median incision closed. If it cannot be reached by a lateral incision where the wall of the sac is adherent to the abdominal wall, then the pus should be drawn off from the sac by an aspirator or trocar, and the cavity washed out clean with an antiseptic solution before it is freely opened, and a drainage-tube inserted.

If signs of general peritonitis show themselves—that is, by vomiting, obstinate constipation, tympanites, etc.—then a free incision should be at once made in the median line and the start-ing-point of the peritonitis found if possible. If it is over the cæcum an incision should be made over it, and the pus washed out by means of hot water of a temperature of 110° to 115°F., run from a large fountain syringe with a large-sized glass drain-age-tube attached to the rubber. After the free pus about the cæcum is well washed out, several fingers or the whole hand should be put in the abdominal cavity and the intestinal adhesion broken up, and all puddles of pus completely washed out. Then a glass drainage-tube should be introduced into each opening and the wounds closed around them, etc.

In pelvic peritonitis, as a rule, the operation is not necessary to save life ; but it may be, and it is, better to operate during the first attack, if there are symptoms plainly indicating the formation of pus, for the adhesions are much more easily broken up, and more complete removal of the diseased organ can be done than after contraction and dense adhesions have formed, as they do after repeated attacks of inflammation. Besides, dangerous pelvic abscesses are avoided and the bad influences of chronic invalidism are prevented. Of course, I refer to severe cases of local peritonitis, where there are symptoms either subjective or objective, indicating beyond reasonable doubt the presence of pus.

In typhlitis the operation should be done before the fourth day, the earlier the better, so as to prevent the chance of rupture and septic general peritonitis, which is, as a rule, attended by so much shock that no operation can do any good. As a rule, general peritonitis from a rupture of a septic abscess is likely to be attended with more shock and rapid failure and death than peritonitis from direct perforation.

In all cases of general peritonitis an exploratory incision should be made as early as possible, after trying to lessen the tympanites. If an exploratory operation does no good, it is not likely to add much to the danger.

There may be cases of idiopathic peritonitis, but I have never seen one proved by anything to be relied upon. Certainly in septic peritonitis, where shock is not too great, free opening, washing out, and drainage will cure some cases. It helps, if it does not cure, tubercular peritonitis, and exploratory incision has proved to be, in the hands of experts, almost entirely free from danger, and it must become the practice in all cases of septic peritonitis, or intestinal obstruction.   Many cases of local peritonitis due to salpingitis may never necessitate a laparotomy, for they often become encysted, and give comparatively little trouble.   Not infrequently the symptoms are due to a severe metritis, where the peritoneum covering the enlarged and inflamed uterus becomes so sensitive as to give in a marked degree almost all the symptoms of a peritonitis due to salpingitis, and repeated attacks of this kind are often mistaken by good physicians for genuine cases of salpingitis.   But I am referring here to cases where a distinct tumor can be felt in the broad ligaments, accompanied by other symptoms indicating the formation of pus, which, when not operated on, rarely fails to cause a general peritonitis, and kills or makes the patient a confirmed invalid.

In typhlitis the diagnosis is, as a rule, comparatively easily made, and I believe it will soon become the general practice to operate early in all well-marked cases.   What I wish to especially advocate is early operation in cases of general peritonitis, both those starting from a local peritonitis and those due to the escape of septic matter into the peritoneum, and to make it plain that to succeed in such cases it will not do to merely open the belly, allow pus to escape, put in a drainage-tube or gauge, and leave intestinal adhesions causing obstruction to remain to kill even more certainly than septic poison, or fail to empty and wash out puddles of septic fluid encysted among the coils of intestines ; but we must make free incisions large enough to introduce the hand, to break up all adherent intestines, and freely wash the whole cavity of the peritoneum and put in two more drainage-tubes.   Without question, in many cases where the patients are debilitated weeks before the starting of the peritonitis, and in those cases where the septic poison is too virulent to be successfully washed out, our patient will die in spite of an early operation.   But are the chances of this class of cases getting well lessened by the operation ?   I think not.   Death may be hastened, but that is all.   But the majority—the large majority—of cases of general peritonitis taken early are not in this desperate condition, and yet, if not operated on, at least four out of five die.
—(*W. Gill Wylie, M.D.*)—*Medical Record.*

Injuries of the Bladder during Laparotomy.—The author
(Reeves Jackson) has collected 67 cases of injury of the bladder
during the performance of láparotomy among 41 operators, and
thinks that this list is sufficiently large to show that the accident
is by no means infrequent. Considering the conditions under
which bladder injuries may happen during laparotomy, it is not
discreditable to any surgeon to meet with them, for they may
not be due to any carelessness or lack of skill on his part. In
many of the foregoing cases no possible degree of diligence could
have averted the accident. Adhesions of the peritoneal surface
of the elongated bladder to that of the anterior abdominal wall
frequently cannot be known In advance, and their existence is
only demonstrable after the viscus has been opened. The use
of the catheter as a diagnostic means is not always available,
because the compression of the bladder against the pubis may
prevent the introduction of the instrument beyond that point.
Certainly, however, this should always be attempted in any case
of suspected difficulty, and would seem to be even a proper and
unobjectionable routine method. Another useful precaution is
to avoid prolonging the abdominal incision far down toward the
pubic bone until the openlng into the peritoneum has permitted
the relations of the bladder to be ascertained. The mortality
of the cases in which the bladder has been wounded is large,
namely, about 30 per cent. ; but this is due to the complicated
and serious character of the cases in which the accident has
occurred, the consequently increased length of the operation and
the greater danger from shock, rather than to the mere vesical
injury. Inasmuch as the bladder is recognizable with more difficulty when empty than when full, it would be better, in cases
presenting doubtful features, to commence the operation with
the viscus wholly or partly distended. When its position has
become known, after the completion of the abdominal incision,
it may be emptied by an assistant.

Treatment.—When it is known at the time of operation that
the bladder has been cut or torn, the opening should be at once
closed with a continuous suture of catgut or fine silk, applied so
as to invert the edges of the wound and bring together the peri-

toneal surfaces.   A permanent catheter ought to be used during the first two days.   After the expiration of that time its constant use is usually unnecessary ; and if the wound has been small—less than one inch in length—the instrument may be subsequently dispensed with.   If, however, the wound has been large—exceeding two or three inches—the bladder ought to be artificially emptied as often as every three hours during three or four days additional.   The catheter should be used so long as the urine contains blood.

In the cases in which urine appears through the abdominal wound subsequently to the operation, at a time and under circumstances which might make it dangerous or inexpedient to reach the seat of the vesical injury, the catheter ought to be used either continuously or at short intervals, for the purpose of lessening the amount of urine which escapes through the fistula, and thus aid in the closure of the latter.   If, however, the fistulous opening should show no disposition to close after two or three months, the edges ought to be freshened to the depth of half an inch or more and stitched together.

In exceptional instances it may be expedient to affix the edges of the wounded bladder within those of the abdominal incision, in the manner detailed by Thomas and others ; but as this method must interfere to some extent with the subsequent contractility of the bladder, it is not to be commended as a usual practice.   The suturing and "dropping" of the vesical wound is the better method.—(*A. Reeves Jackson, M.D.*)—*Journal American Medical Association*, Feb. 22, 1890.

The Surgical Treatment of Cancer of the Uterus.—The author for convenience divided the uterus into three parts as they are affected by the disease, viz., the vaginal, cervical, and body, and then proceeded to explain his views as to the palliative and radical methods of treatment.   In very bad cases, or any such that were beyond operation, he advised the patient to be kept at perfect rest, and that the vagina should be washed out twice daily with sanitas or some other antiseptic lotion, and then through a speculum carefully wiping out the cavity with plugs of wool, and finally applying tampons of wool soaked in equal parts of pinus Cana-

Jessis and glycerine in ten parts of sanitas oil, ten grains (
chloride of zinc, and one ounce of vaseline. By adopting the
methods, it is claimed that the patients are freed from pain a
... and odors, and that they improve in general health, strengt
... gain weight in cancer of the vaginal and cervical portio
... Jessett discussed the treatment by caustics, the cautery a
... and finally said he objected to all of these, and c
... that the disease could be more easily and certainly
... by dragging the uterus as far down as possible, and tl
... scissors bent on the flat he snips cautiously the muc
... membrane, and by pushing the vaginal portion with the adjac
... upwards and dragging the uterus freely downwards, i
... snipping, he claimed to be able to remove as much
... uterine tissues as he required, even to the fundus of
... as explained by Dr. John Williams. Mr. Jessett qu
... cases in more or less advanced states, in which he had o
... with success in all; nine months after the operation tl
... recurrence. Mr. Jessett finally discussed extirpatio
... uterus for cancer of the body of the uterus, but expre
... that owing to the severity of the operation and
... as to whether the disease had extended to the
... and varies, he did not think the operation wa
... except when the disease was recognized
... state.— Mr. Fred. B. Jessett.)

... mentum.—Several authorities have observed
... operations for the removal of the uterine a
... adhesions are often found to be very exte
... The omentum may adhere to the par
... tissues, the uterus, or the appendages
... the tube and ovary upwards high out (
... one, however, the omentum is drawn
... pulling after it the transverse colo
... of small intestine to which it ad
... to cause much local trouble. (
... that, after very careful removal of in
... the surrounding parts being dis
... the patients often suffer as much pa

discomfort after convalescence as before the operation. On the other hand, in similar cases, where the ovaries and tubes are found too adherent to neighboring structures to allow of removal without great risk, the patient is often permanently cured of the pain and gastric and intestinal trouble for which she sought relief. The " exploratory operation" has proved a cure, not by the faith of the patient who feels sure that an operation will cure her, but by the breaking down of troublesome omental adhesions. In the *Hospitals-Tidende*, 1889, Dr. Howitz describes a case of strongly adherent omentum, with displacement of the stomach and intestines, as described above. The patient had been treated for gastric ulcer, also for " the womb " ; pessaries had been applied, and douching and massage of the hypogastrium practiced in vain. Dr. Howitz carefully liberated the omental adhesions, so that the displaced viscera returned to their normal positions. All the pain and discomfort from which the patient had so long suffered rapidly disappeared.—*Brit. Med. Journal.*

Malignant Disease of the Corporeal Endometrium—In the *New York Medical Record*, April 5th, 1890, Dr. Henry C. Coe writes a very valuable essay on the above subject. Under malignant disease of the corpus he includes, in the order of frequency, carcinoma, sarcoma and adenoma. He cannot speak positively regarding the relative frequency of occurrence of these different varieties, due, he says, to the unfortunate negligence of those who are in a position to form statistics. In regard to frequency of sarcoma of the corpus. statistics are often based upon the microscopic examination of scrapings, or the naked eye examination alone ; this method, of course, should not be in evidence at all. Dr. Coe draws attention to the difficulty of deducing facts of value from hospital statistics because of the biased views and inaccurate statements of the men who make them. Dr. Coe states that in spite of statements of clinical observers to the contrary, sarcoma of the endometrium, especially the diffuse form, is very rare. In speaking of diffuse recurrent adenoma, he states that our statistics are still more imperfect. Cases, however, have been recorded by Winckel, Gusserow, Schrœder, Thomas, Goodell and himself. The author shows that in between nitrates

of total vaginal extirpation. He believes that the curette is a dangerous instrument in these cases; he has made several autopsies in fatal cases and found perforation of the uterus by the curette. He concludes his most instructive paper by a detailed report of four cases.

Dr. Coe also writes a paper upon *Laparotomy for Intestinal Obstruction following Vaginal Hysterectomy* (*Amer. Journal Obstet.*, vol. xxiii. No. 2, 1889). He reports one case rather fully, in which symptoms of obstruction set in on the fourth day after the operation. He delayed re-opening the cavity until about the sixth day. He found a coil of intestine firmly adherent to the wound in Douglas's pouch and obstructed. The patient died next morning from shock following the second operation. He regretted very much he did not operate earlier, but was otherwise influenced by council. He mentions six other cases reported by other surgeons which had been operated upon a second time. All of these cases died as a result of the second operation. This experience is consistent with what is generally known of secondary operation for the relief of obstruction, if not done immediately after onset of symptoms. Dr. Coe says:—
" In reviewing these seven cases (including my own), one is struck with the fact that the pathological conditions and the clinical symptoms were almost identical. In each one there was an adhesion of one or more coils of small intestine to the edge of the vaginal wound, with distention and bending of the gut above the point of adhesion, thus obstructing the lumen. Although there was intense congestion of the serous covering of the intestines, in no instance was general peritonitis found at the operation. In all but one case death seemed to be due primarily to exhaustion or, where laparotomy was performed, to the shock of the operation. The symptoms continued to be indefinite until after the fourth day, and the classical symptoms of intestinal obstruction (especially fæcal vomiting) appeared when it was too late to profit by them. Certain points are to be noted in this connection, as emphasized by Reichel, bearing on the differential diagnosis. Ileus is most likely to be mistaken for general peritonitis, especially if there should be general tender-

ness. But, as I noted in commenting on my case, pain is conspicuous by its absence. There is little, if any, elevation of temperature, the pulse may not be accelerated for several days, and tympanites is not excessive. As in the case reported, it may be unsymmetrical, being more marked on one side; this I regard as an important sign, in fact almost confirmatory when taken in connection with the visible movements of the distended gut. The absence of flatus and faecal movements after the repeated administration of cathartics and high enemata should at once awaken suspicion, especially if four or five days have passed without an evacuation, even though the patient may be entirely free from nausea. It is important to note that the passage of scybalous masses which were contained in the large intestine may mislead the surgeon as well as the nurse, and lull the former into a sense of security. Nothing but the thorough clearing out of the small intestine and the free escape of gas, with lessening of the tympanites, can justify him in feeling certain that his suspicions of obstruction were unfounded. Faecal vomiting is, of course, conclusive evidence, but the histories of these cases, as of those in which the obstruction has followed laparotomy, show that it usually occurs at a stage in the case when the time for successful operative interference has passed."

Total Extirpation of the Uterus.—Dr. Münchmeyer describes in a recent number of the *Archiv für Gynäkologie* an account of 110 cases of total vaginal extirpation of the uterus in the Dresden Women's Hospital. Eighty-eight were cancerous; the mortality in these malignant cases was five per cent., and 65 per cent. of the patients who recovered remained over two years free from recurrence. The appendages were latterly removed entire whenever that step was practicable, as in two cases where they were left behind they became involved in the cicatrix at the top of the vagina and caused so much pain that an operation was needed for their removal. Parametritic induration was frequent, but it gave less trouble than narrowness of the vagina. Dr. Münchmeyer did not particularly dread injury to the bladder, as if immediately sutured a wound in the vesical walls was not serious. Recurrence of cancer did not appear to be more frequent when inflammatory infiltration in the parametrium and utero-sacral ligaments existed at the time of operation. Carcinoma of the cervical canal proved the most serious form ; cancer of the body was less, and cancer of the vaginal part of the cervix least prone to rapid recurrence. Total extirpation was also performed for small fibroids, which crippled the patients, in 17 cases ; the mortality was given as 11 per cent. Five of these operations were performed, all successfully, for total prolapse of the uterus ; eight, also all successful, for disease of the appendages, on the plea that without tubes and ovaries the uterus was useless, and that the operation was less dangerous than an abdominal section. In this country it is doubtful whether many authorities approve of total extirpation of the uterus excepting for malignant disease. The above statistics will be interesting in reference to the recent dis-cussion on Dr. Cullingworth's paper at the Obstetrical Society.

Technique of Vaginal Hysterectomy.—The late Dr. Jas. B. Hunter of New York published shortly before his death a paper upon the above subject in the *Transactions of the New York State Medical Society*. The author emphasized the necessary demonstration of two facts in regard to this operation. First, the immediate mortality from the operation must be small ; second, the results, immediate and remote, must be such as to show that the benefit to the patient is sufficient to compensate for the risks incurred.

The principal dangers following this operation are shock, hemorrhage, peritonitis and septicæmia. The author points out in very emphatic language the great necessity for rapidity of action on the part of the surgeon in this as in all gynæcological operations. Shock has been the cause of death in a large number of patients in which the operation was prolonged to over one hour. Much valuable time in such cases was lost in secur-ing vessels with ligature. He refers to the advantage of Péan's method with hæmostatic forceps, and gives him priority of claim in this matter over Richelôt. He shows how vastly superior the forceps are to any form of ligature in this operation. In eight cases recently he used no ligature of any kind. In several cases the time occupied for the operation was forty-five minutes, and in one case it was thirty-five. The forceps favor drainage when it is most required. There is less danger of injuring the ureters than with the ligatures, as they can be applied more closely to the uterus. More traction on the tissues is required in applying a ligature than in applying the forceps. Dr. Hunter did not try to include all of the broad ligaments in one instrument. He used a Tait forceps having a bite of about one inch and a half. Richelôt's forceps are too long in the blade and needlessly heavy.

ABSTRACT OF TRANSACTIONS OF THE AMERICAN PEDIATRIC SOCIETY.

By A. D. BLACKADER, B.A., M.D.,

Instructor in Diseases of Children, McGill University; Assistant Physician, Montreal General Hospital.

The first meeting of the American Pediatric Society was held in Washington last September. Its transactions are just published. The meeting was opened by an address by Dr. Jacobi of New York. Among the papers read was one on *Two Cases of Double Empyema, by Dr. Francis Huber*. The first, a lad of 13 years, fell into an excavation eighteen feet deep, from which he was taken out unconscious. To restore him to his senses he had been thoroughly drenched with water, and shortly afterwards taken home. In a few hours he was seized with a chill, intense pain in the chest, fever and cough with bloody sputum. There was no vomiting of blood. On the third day he came under observation. There were no evidences of injury to the head, nor were any of his ribs fractured. A diagnosis of double pleuro-pneumonia was made, the percussion note being absolutely flat on the right side. The heart's action was very weak. On the fifth day he was seen by Dr. Jacobi in consultation and the diagnosis confirmed. In view of the extensive pulmonary œdema present anteriorly, it was not thought probable he would live longer than twenty-four hours. Free stimulation was ordered, half an ounce of brandy every half hour, one minim of digitalis with three grains of camphor hourly, and carbonate of ammonium every two hours. Morphia was given hypodermically to relieve pain and restlessness. He made a slow improvement. At the end of a fortnight an exploratory puncture revealed pus in the right pleural cavity, and a pint was drawn off by aspiration. Two days afterwards the left cavity was opened posteriorly and two large drainage tubes inserted. Large quantities of pus escaped. No broken down clots were discovered, nor any evidence of an old hemorrhage into the cavity. Four days later the right side was freely incised, allowing a large amount of pus to escape. Antiseptic gauze dressings were applied in both cases. The patient made a good recovery.

The second case had a somewhat similar history of a fall, followed by pyrexia, with somewhat indefinite symptoms pointing to the lungs. On the eighth day an exploratory puncture revealed the presence of pus in the right pleural cavity, which was opened, a drainage-tube inserted, and antiseptic dressings applied. On the left side there was dulness on percussion, and bronchial breathing with friction sounds at the posterior and lower parts. A week later, evidences of pus being obtained, the left side was treated similarly. The boy made an excellent recovery.

Remarking on the cases, the doctor says the most careful examination gave no evidence of any direct injury to chest wall in either case. Both lived under poor hygienic conditions. In both cases the excessive dyspnœa contra-indicated the use of any anæsthetic. In reviewing the literature of the subject, less than a dozen cases of double empyema were met with.

In the discussion which followed, Dr. Osler said that he considered empyema a surgical affection. Free, full and satisfactory incisions should be made in the case of adults, but in children aspiration should first be tried. Many cases at an early age are cured by one aspiration. The aspiration should not be repeated, but if the pus re-accumulates, incision should be practised.

Dr. O'Dwyer, of New York, read a paper *On the apparent physical paradox involved in the Re-expansion of a Collapsed Lung, while a free opening remains in the Pleural Sac.* He said none of the theories so far advanced offer any satisfactory explanation of the mechanism by which this process is accomplished. If the inspiratory movement be nothing more than the production of a partial vacuum within the chest, with consequent inrush of air, until the pressure is equalized there can be no force developed by this movement to overcome the contractility of the of the lung, because the atmospheric pressure being the same in both situations the power to create a vacuum is destroyed, and the lung will simply remain contracted as long as the external wound remained patulous. But every one who is familiar with the treatment adopted for the cure of empyema knows that the clinical teaching is directly opposed to the teaching of physiology in this instance. He knows not how it is accomplished, but he knows that a lung that has been completely collapsed and compressed becomes so fully reinflated that in after years it is impossible to distinguish any difference between the two sides, and that the principal part of this inflation takes place while free communication exists between the pleural sac and the atmosphere. The theories usually advanced are: 1. The small size of the opening or its valvular form produced by the dressing or otherwise, tends in some measure to exclude the air. 2. The presence of old adhesions, which prevent complete collapse of the lung, or the presence of new ones acting in a similar way. 3. The force brought to bear on the contracted lung by the recoil of air from the sound side on the act of coughing or other forcible expiratory effort. Dr. O'Dwyer thought that, judging from his own experience, the size of the opening or its valvular arrangement has no influence whatever in aiding the expansion of the lung. Old adhesions seldom exist in cases of empyema in young children. Before new adhesions can form, the opposing surfaces of the pleura must not only be brought in contact, but held in that position for some time. The last theory to be considered is the effect of forcible expiration on the collapsed lung while the glottis is either partially or completely closed. Here we have to deal, not with the presence of the atmosphere as in inspiration, but with compressed air, the amount of compression being in proportion to the muscular effort brought to bear, and the obstruction offered to its escape by the degree of closure of the glottis. Cough is probably the most powerful of these efforts, and were this act repeated with sufficient frequency, it might be sufficient to re-expand a contracted lung, and even keep it in contact with the costal pleura sufficiently to allow some adhesions to take place ; but it is not frequent, in fact some children with empyema cough very little, and it can have no influence when both pleural cavities are open at the same time, as in the cases reported by Dr. Huber. Every inspiratory expansion of the chest operates in the opposite direction, drawing away the ribs from the lung and so tending to prevent adhesions.

In a previous paper the author has suggested the possibility of a physico-chemical force generated by the interchange of gases in the pulmonary vesicles, possibly as the result of an attraction between the oxygen and the hæmoglobin. The mechanical theory of the circulation which assumes that the action of the heart is sufficient to propel the blood through the whole circuit from the left back to the right does not explain the important fact that venous blood will not circulate in the systemic capillaries.

Dr. W. P. Northrup, in opening the discussion, referred to the Bradshawe lecture on Pneumothorax by Samuel West, F.R.C.P., Lond., in which the lecturer says : " The fact, therefore, that the pleural cavity may be laid open, and that yet collapse of the lung with consequent pneumothorax may not occur must be accepted, and an explanation sought." Again, " when the lung does not contract after the pleura is opened, it must be kept on the stretch by some force greater than the force of the normal elasticity of the lungs, and . . . . this force is probably to be found in the cohesion between the two serous surfaces." Then follow elaborate experiments with disks of wood, upon which were stretched stomachs and other membranes, the cohesion of which upon one another, according to the lecturer, demonstrated that a lung would not let go its hold upon the parietal pleura except under force directly applied. Dr. Northrup then related experiments conducted on dogs in the Loomis laboratory by himself, with the assistance of Prof. W. Gilman Thompson, to determine whether there was sufficient cohesion between the two pleural surfaces to maintain them in apposition after the costal pleura had been opened without violence. A dog was placed under ether—the tissues carefully dissected away till the parietal pleura was reached; through it the fully expanded lung could be seen gliding back and forth in respiration. A small pinhole opening was then carefully made through it, when there was an instantaneous recession of the lung. On the next expiration a fine thread of air was expelled, and by the second respiration the lung was not to be seen at all and a probe passed two and a half inches straight down before it reached the lung. The experiment was repeated under varying conditions on different dogs, but always with the same result. In one, a glass disk was buttoned quickly through the slit so as to act both as a valve and as a window. Respiration at once improved. With each respiratory movement a few bubbles of air escaped at the margin of the glass, but none entered. Finally the lung appeared fully expanded, and glided rhythmically back and forth upon the glass as upon the pleura-covered wall. The dog, which had by this time recovered somewhat from the ether, got upon the floor, evinced great activity, walked about, and wagged his tail. All the dogs, while recovering from the ether, made repeated attempts at vomiting. In the repeated retchings one dog failed to express the contents of his stomach, but did compress the sound lung and force air from it into the contracted lung till, from being small and cyanotic, the latter became aerated, rose-colored and expanded, but there being nothing to maintain its expansion, it contracted as soon as the effort was over. This muscular action is similar to, and almost identical with, that of coughing, and the incident serves to fortify the position taken by Dr. O'Dwyer that cough exerts the strongest expiratory force.

As the result of his experiments, Dr. Northrup concluded that Mr. West was wrong in his conclusions; that it seemed to him that there was not a complete collapse on the opening of the pleura, but the lung fluctuates in the anterior and upper portions in a state of equilibrium between the elasticity of the lung on the one side and on the other by the pressure of the air within, assisted by a certain amouut of force from the blood, the blood-vessels acting to a certain extent as erectile tissue. The experiments suggested to him the desirability of a valvular canula with which to drain empyemic chests, but he thought that all dressings which catch the tenacious discharge from an empyemic cavity can act more or less as a valve, allowing the exit of pus and air, but on inspiration more or less effectually applying itself to the aperture, sufficiently at least to disturb the equilibrium in favor of diminished external pressure.

Dr. W. H. Welch, of Baltimore, said—I have never noticed any expansion of the lung exposed freely to the atmosphere by an opening in the chest wall. I have made experiments upon animals bearing on this point, and am prepared to assert quite positively that under these conditions no expansion takes place, nor can I conceive it possible that the physical conditions admit of any expansion. I apprehend that the basis for the discussion of the point, as to the possibility of expansion of a lung while there is still an opening in the chest-wall, must be observation of cases where adhesions have formed between the pleural surfaces. Such adhesions must alter the physical conditions, and and it is quite possible to understand how these adhesions could be arranged as to permit of considerable pulmonary expansion even when there is an opening in the thoracic wall.

Dr. Jacobi said—I understand that Dr. Welch says that no expansion of the lung can take place while there is an opening in the chest. We know, however, as the result of clinical observation, that the lung does expand nevertheless. No reasoning can gainsay the fact. Dr. O'Dwyer, in conclusion, said there can be no inspiratory force that will have any effect on the contracted lung under such circumstances. I claim that there is no other way of explaining the inflation of a collapsed lung except by the mechanical effect of forced expiration.

Dr. C. W. Earle, of Chicago, described a case of *General Subcutaneous Emphysema occurring in a Child of 3½ years*. The child had been ailing for nearly three weeks. Its illness had commenced as an ordinary cold, but had developed into a catarrhal pneumonia. Its progress had been apparently satisfactory till the sudden onset of the emphysema. When seen the subcutaneous tissues of the forehead, cheeks, neck and of the entire trunk anteriorly to Poupart's ligaments and posteriorly to the iliac crests were filled with air. The respirations were hurried, the pulse moderately rapid, and the face, in addition to its peculiar appearance, had a worried and anxious look. The swelling had appeared in the neck at first, and rapidly extended to every other part of the body except the scalp and legs. The child was bandaged from its feet to its chin, and a stimulating and supporting treatment administered. At times it seemed to improve, but at last began to show signs of exhaustion, and died on the tenth day after the appearance of the complication.

So severe and such almost complete subcutaneous emphysema occurs comparatively seldom in children, and in most cases has a fatal termination. The possibility of the occurrence of subcutaneous emphysema is sometimes alluded to in text-books, but very few cases are recorded. It is generally due to some interference with or obstruction to respiration, and is occasionally met with as a complication of catarrhal pneumonia, pertussis, croup, and diphtheria. It may arise from perforating laryngeal ulcerations, from rupture of the tracheal rings either by force or the results of disease, and from rupture of the œsophagus. The prognosis is good unless the preceding disease has induced great asthenia. In weak children suffering from a grave malady, a fatal result may be expected. The means at our command are limited. The skin may be punctured where the emphysema is most prominent, the body may be bandaged, and the most sustaining treatment should be employed.

The report of a case of *Membranous Croup in a Girl of* 12 *years*, when tracheotomy was performed, with eventual recovery, was read by Dr. A. Caille. Speaking on this case, Dr. Jacobi said the disease was rare at this age. He agreed with what Dr. Caille had done. He had been converted to a belief in the value of intubation, but where the membrane was below, and where the croup was ascending, tracheotomy should be employed. He recalled twenty or thirty cases of fibrinous bronchitis terminating in diphtheritic tracheitis and laryngitis. In these cases, when this ascending form of croup reaches the larynx, cyanosis sets in very rapidly, and as a rule tracheotomy yields but little relief, if any. Still it ought to be performed, furnishing the only way in which access to the pseudo-membranes can be had.

The *Artificial Feeding of Infants* is discussed in two papers —one by Dr. A. V. Meigs, the other by Dr. J. Lewis Smith. Dr. Meigs again emphasizes the fact that in all his analyses of human milk it never contained more than one per cent. of casein, whereas cow's milk contains three or four. He thinks that much of the difficulties in the artificial feeding of infants are due to this fact, which is so often disregarded. He has somewhat altered the formula which he published some years ago, on account of the difficulty in obtaining good fresh cream. He recommends now fresh milk should be allowed to stand in a tall pitcher or other vessel for three hours in a cool place. From this the upper third or half is then slowly poured off, so as to obtain the upper layer, which contains much of the cream. When the child is to be fed there should be taken of this weak cream three tablespoonfuls, of lime-water two tablespoonfuls, and of sugar-water three tablespoonfuls. The sugar-water is to be made in the proportion of eighteen drachms of milk sugar to the pint of boiled water. Dr. Rotch recommends the sugar in powder to be used, and has constructed a little measure that will just hold the quantity for each half pint of food. He also recommends a smaller proportion of lime-water. Dr. Meigs leaves these suggestions to be acted on or not by the physician as he finds his experience guide him, but finds that his own formula has given him excellent results in one of the large foundling hospitals in Philadelphia. Dr. J. Lewis Smith strongly recommends sterilization of the milk and the use of a cereal in which a considerable portion of the starch had been converted into dextrine. He now uses largely barley or wheat flour which has been subjected to the heat of boiling water for seven days in a double boiler. If there is indigestion or gastro-intestinal catarrh, he peptonizes the milk or makes use of one of the preparations of pepsin at each time of feeding.

Dr. Huber, of New York, read the notes of a case of *Acute Peritonitis following Vulvo-vaginal Catarrh in a Girl of 7 years*, simulating a porforation of the appendix ; laparotomy—death. The patient had been troubled with a vaginal discharge for a short time. She was very anæmic, and though frail, did not complain much. The vulva was inflamed ; there were a few drops of pus about the urethral orifice. The hymen was intact. Close questioning failed to discover any cause for the catarrh. Unfortunately an examination for the characteristic coccus was not made. The patient was treated at the office for a few days. Complaint of soreness was now made about the lower pelvic regions, and she took to bed. On the following day, June 1st, she vomited a little blood, being mixed with contents of stomach. Slight soreness was complained of on palpation over pubes. The pulse was good ; no distinct pain ; a little diarrhœa ; temperature normal. The little one at this point was laughing and in excellent spirits. At the evening visit a state of collapse had set in. The temperature was subnormal, pain in right iliac fossa was marked, and there was distinct muscular rigidity of abdominal walls. She had vomited a number of times. A perforation of the appendix was now suspected. The parents only consented to an operation on the evening of the 3rd. The operation was performed at 1 A.M. June 4th. Chloroform was cautiously given. The abdomen was opened by lateral incision. Considerable sero-purulent fluid was found in abdominal cavity ; the intestines were distended with gas, congested, and here and there coated with lymph. The appendix was found and presented a normal appearance. The right fallopian tube, however, with its fibrillated extremity, was inflamed and thickened, and evidently had formed the channel by which the infecting process had gained access to the peritoneal cavity. The abdomen was washed out, a rectal injection of hot water and brandy administered. Twenty hours later death occurred from heart failure.

Dr. A. F. Currier, in an article on *Vulvo-Vaginitis in Children* (*Med. News*, July 6th, '89), says : In adults this disease not unfrequently extends to the uterus, the fallopian tubes, the ovaries and the peritoneum, and may end fatally. I can find but one recorded case in which such an extension occurred in children ; but it seems to me extremely probable that many of the deformed and undeveloped uteri, with which are associated so much dysmenorrhœa, sterility and domestic unhappiness, are the legitimate consequence of vulvo-vaginitis in early life.

Dr. A. Caille, of New York, read a paper entitled *A Plea for a general adoption of Personal Prophylaxis in Diphtheria.* The author regards the usual measures for the prevention of diphtheria—isolation, disinfection, etc., of each particular case—insufficient. Although of certain value, it is not all that we as physicians should insist upon. Diphtheria is without doubt primarily a local disease, due to the invasion of a micro-organism which provokes tissue necrosis, and to the formation of ptomaine, which enters the circulation and produces constitutional effects. It is agreed by all that a hyperæmic mucous membrane offers favorable conditions for its development, and that different forms of micro-organisms, identical in appearance with those supposed to be pathogenic, are found in the naso-pharynx in individuals in good health, and thrive in naso-pharyngeal mucus. Hence the value of keeping in a healthy condition the mucous membranes usually affected, and in avoiding the accumulation of catarrhal secretions. This may be done by the use of gargles, the nasal insufflation of harmless antiseptic solutions several times a day, the removal or reduction otherwise of enlarged tonsils, and the proper treatment of carious teeth by a competent dentist. Any one who will make it a rule to enquire will find that in most cases of nasal or pharyngeal catarrh, filthy gums and carious teeth had existed for some time previous to the diphtheritic onset. Similar preventive measures should be used in all cases of scarlet fever, measles and pertussis to avoid the development of diphtheritic exudations.

The Necessity of Prolonged Rest after some attacks of Diphtheria was emphasized in a short paper by Dr. C. W. Earle of Chicago.

Aneurism in Early Life was the subject of a paper by Dr. Jacobi, with the history of a case of aneurism of the abdominal aorta occurring in a girl of five, the subject of tuberculosis, with destructive disease in the hip joint. Unfortunately the specimen was lost before an exact examination had been made, but it must with such a history have been tubercular. The literature of aneurism occurring in the young is scanty. This makes the twenty-ninth case of which any report in modern literature can

be found. The causes have been various. In the case reported
by Mr. Hutchison the cause was *an abscess* which had ulcerated
into the aorta. The lining membrane was smooth and perfectly
healthy up to the edges of the orifice of communication (one-
fourth by one-eighth of an inch) with the sac. This was the size
of two chesnuts placed side by side, and hung from the arch of
the aorta into the pericardium. The heart was normal, but in
the lungs were tubercles. The child died of acute pericarditis.
Embolism depending on valvular disease has been the cause in
several. *Endarteritis* was the cause in a boy of two years, who
had an atheromatous arch and a hypertrophied heart. *Co*-
genital incompetency of the walls of bloodvessels has been found
in a few cases. A fifth cause is to be found in morbid *histolog-*
cal alterations of the bloodvessel walls, especially in the pulmonary artery, owing to the formation of " hyaline" substance
principally in the middle coat. Some of the cases reported were
small aneurisms in the pulmonary artery occurring in connection
with excavation of the lung.

Both Dr. Booker of Baltimore and Dr. Jeffries of Boston have
long and excellent papers on their recent investigations *on the*
bacteria found in the fœces of Infants affected with Summer
Diarrhœa. Dr. Jeffries says " Bacteria I believe to be at the
bottom of the disease—that is, rule bacteria out of all foods and
the alimentary canal, and summer diarrhœa would cease to be."
Passing to the mode of introduction of the bacteria, it is probable, judging from cases, that certain forms are able to slip in,
multiply, and produce disease in the healthy infant. Other forms
need assistance ; they are not able to thrive in the normal
healthy infant intestine ; it is here that the predisposing causes
of heat, food, catching cold, and the like come in. They throw
the digestion sufficiently out of order to give the plants a start.
Improper feeding offers fine opportunities, affording good food
for bacteria, scarcely acted upon by the disturbed digestion of
the infant. That these bacteria do not cause more trouble in
adult life is probably due to the greater power of resistance of
adults, the more stable nervous system, and the more active
chemistry of digestion. In regard to prophylaxis, it is clear that

bottle-fed infants should have sterile food. The stomach can then start fair and work unhampered on the, at best, unsatisfactory substitutes for the breast milk. Once given an attack of summer diarrhœa, the desire to kill the bacteria in the digestive tract at once suggests itself. Unfortunately, we have yet to find a germicide which is not an infanticide also. Escherich, who has gone deeply into the subject, suggests starving the bacteria by giving albuminous foods in cases of fermentation, and vegetable in cases of putrefaction. The difficulty is to tell which is going on in the child, or perhaps both may be acting at the same time. Where sterile food is not well borne, therefore it seems desirable to cut off food for a time as much as possible. The writer recommends a sort of series from breast milk to sterilized milk, wine whey, and, lastly, spirits and water ; and places himself among those having more or less faith in the alkaline treatment. In closing, he says : Over and above the bacteria, it must not be forgotten that we have a child with lesions of the digestive tract to consider.

Dr. A. Seibert, of New York, gave a report on *Two years of experience in the Treatment of Gastro-intestinal Disturbances in Infants*, by washing out the stomach and the large bowel with sterilized water, or water rendered slightly antiseptic. Since September 1887 he has records of 1404 cases of infants under three years of age treated in this way. Stomach washing was used in 521 cases. Every infant stood the washing well, and was evidently relieved. In not one case did depression, convulsions or death occur shortly after the procedure, although in several cases it was in a state of severe collapse before the washing. The same thing can be said of the bowel washing. The nausea and vomiting ceased in every instance. In the majority, pain subsided and the temperature was lowered. The youngest patient on which he used the stomach washing was only thirty-six hours old. The results were certainly good, but the author gives no exact percentage, as most of the cases were treated at the Dispensary, and many could not be followed up. Only fifteen deaths out of the whole number are definitely recorded. For stomach washing, a soft rubber velvet, eye catheter, in size cor-

responding to No. 10 steel bougie ; attached to this, by rub
tube, is either a regular irrigator or small glass funnel, a sm
piece of glass tubing being inserted in the tubing to judge
the character of the escaping fluid. In bowel washing, a fount
syringe answers all purposes so long as the child's buttocks a
sufficiently elevated to let the water run up into the transver
and ascending colon.

Reviews and Notices of Books.

The Refraction of the Eye.   A Manual for Students

By GUSTAVUS HARBRIDGE, F.R.C.S., Consulting Ophthal
mic Surgeon to St. Bartholomew's Hospital, Chatham
Surgeon to the Royal Westminster Ophthalmic Hospital
formerly Assistant Surgeon to the Central London Oph
thalmic Hospital, and Clinical Assistant to the Royal Oph
thalmic Hospital, Moorfields. Fourth edition. Two hundred
and forty-nine pages, with ninety-eight illustrations. Philadelphia : Blakiston, Son & Co. 1890.

This fourth edition is considerably enlarged by the addition of
new matter, and some chapters have been partly rewritten,
though the original plan of the work is maintained. The author
has quite discarded the old or inch system in dealing with the
subject of refraction, and it is to be hoped that all writers of
ophthalmic text-books will in this respect follow the same plan,
since the metric system has met with the general favor which
its manifest advantages justly merit.

This work is, perhaps, somewhat too comprehensive for the
ordinary student of medicine during a college course, but for the
student of ophthalmology who can devote sufficient time to the
clinical study of refraction, it is all that could be desired, and
undoubtedly may be ranked as one of the best text-books of the
kind now in print. The first chapter deals with the elementary
principles of optics as far as necessary to elucidate the action of
convex and concave lenses, and is neatly illustrated with numerous
diagrams. Three chapters are devoted to the physiology of
vision and the determination of visual acuteness, both in the

normal state and in the presence of errors of refraction: These comprise also a full discussion of visual tests and the use of glasses in measuring refractive errors. Then follows a description of the use of the ophthalmoscope in estimating refraction. his instrument plays so important a *rôle* in the study of refraction that a discussion of the optical principles involved in its use could not well be omitted from a work of this kind. The chapter on rhinoscopy is particularly well written, and is well worthy of careful study, especially to those who have not given to this recent and important addition to the uses of the ophthalmoscope the attention it deserves. There is, of course, nothing new in the chapters on presbyopia, hyperopia, myopia, and astigmatism, but they are given in a readable and attractive form. If the author has failed to present any portion of his subject in a satisfactory manner, it is in his discussion of muscular defects and their treatment, and it may safely be predicted that should he ever bring out another edition this part of the work will not appear at all in its present shape. The practical value of this work is greatly increased by the detailed description of illustrative cases, so arranged as to afford to the student of refraction a guide in the clinical part of his work, which in reality is by far the most difficult part to master.

The work is one which should be in the library of every advanced student of ophthalmology, and is certain to continue in favor with the profession.

A Guide to the Diseases of Children. By J. F. Goodhart, M.D., F.R.C.P. Re-arranged, revised and edited by Louis Starr, M.D. Second American from the third English edition. Philadelphia : P. Blakiston, Son & Co. Montreal : C. Ashford.

The American editor, while claiming to have altered in the least possible degree the author's forcible descriptions of disease, has certainly by his re-arrangement given us a much more convenient and readable volume than appeared in the first edition. It is an eminently practical work, and very pleasantly written. Dr. Goodhart quotes largely, throughout the work, from the

records of his clinical cases in the Evelina Hospital, and the
American editor, in addition to inserting typical tempera ... are
charts wherever practicable, has given us valuable additio ... al
material. On the matter of infant feeding the directi ... ns
are particularly full. We regret he has not given Dr. Le ... is
Smith's directions for preparing the boiled wheaten and bar ... ey
flour, which give, in our opinion, a much superior article to ... the
plan here recommended. Following this is a series of excelle ... nt
articles on diseases of the digestive system. In all severe   or
persistent cases of diarrhœa, a thorough irrigation of the bo ... el
as far as the cæcal valve is recommended, with either pure wat ... ter
or some weak antiseptic solution. The acute infectious disea ... s
with their various complications are fully described in Part I ... II.
In speaking of the diagnosis between pertussis and enlarg ... ed
bronchial glands, the author recommends strongly Dr. Eusta ... ce
Smith's method of examination, which is as follows : If the chi ... ld
be made to bend back the head so that his face becomes almo ... st
horizontal and the eyes look straight upward, a venous hum var ...
ing in intensity is heard with the stethoscope placed upon th ...
upper bone of the sternum. As the chin is now slowly depresse ...
the hum becomes less audible, and ceases shortly before th ...
head reaches its ordinary position. Part IV., treating of Diseases of the Nervous System, is particularly interesting, from
the number of illustrative clinical cases which are given by Dr.
Goodhart. The whole work has been brought thoroughly abreast
of the recent advances in pediatric science, and can be very
cordially recommended as a text-book to the student and practitioner. The type is large and clear and the binding excellent.

The Diseases of Children, Medical and Surgical. By
HENRY ASHBY, M.D., M.R.C.P., and G. A. WRIGHT, M.B.,
F.R.C.P. Longmans, Green & Co., London and New York.
Montreal : E. Renouf.

The authors tell us in their preface that the book is written
chiefly from a practical point of view, with but little pathological
detail. Their experience has been an unusually large one. It
has been gained during ten years' service at the General Hos-

Hospital for Sick Children, Manchester, an institution at which some 1200 in-patients and some 10,000 out-patients are annually treated. The original feature of the book is that it has been written conjointly by a physician and surgeon, and therefore, perhaps more than any other similar treatise, presents a complete account of disease in children. Both the authors are already well known by their previous contributions, and in the present work have presented us with a most excellent volume, which can be cordially recommended both to the advanced student and to the practitioner. Not only do they draw largely on their own extensive experience, but full justice has been done to all recent writers on the various subjects. The illustrations are all good, most of them original. Numerous temperature charts are introduced wherever they are likely to be of service. The type, though small, is particularly clear.

Transactions of the Second Session of the Intercolonial Medical Congress of Australasia, held in Melbourne, Victoria, January 1889. Melbourne: Stillwell & Co., printers, 195A Collins street. Pp. 1029.

The handsome volume of reports before us reflects the highest credit upon the energy and talent of the medical profession of Australasia. The Intercolonial Medical Congress represents in the main our Canadian Medical Association. It is an assembly of the medical men of all the colonies, and its members number some five hundred. The papers read at this meeting were very numerous, and of a high order of merit, a large proportion representing really good scientific work. We cannot notice separately, in the brief space at our disposal, any of the papers; we can merely mention those of Dr. Bancroft on Filaria and the various papers by J. Davies Thomas and others on Hydatid Disease, which called forth a most instructive discussion. Typhoid Fever, more especially its etiology, was the subject of another special discussion. The surgical section was well represented. Gynæcology, too, held its own, but failed to take up all the time of the meeting as it does in some not distant countries. All the other special branches showed great activity and progress, and

54

tho meeting appears to have been most thoroughly successf
To our Australian brethren we offer our hearty congratulati
on the success of their publication.

A Treatise on Materia Medica, Pharmacology a
Therapeutics. By JOHN V. SHOEMAKER, M.A., M.
Professor of Materia Medica, Pharmacology and The
peutics in the Medico-Chirurgical College of Philadelph
and JOHN AULDE, M.D., Demonstrator of Clinical Medic
and of Physical Diagnosis in the Medico-Chirurgical Coll
of Philadelphia. In two volumes. Vol. I. Philadelp
and London : F. A. Davis, publisher.

This important work adds another to the already long lis
works on Materia Medica and Therapeutics. The first volu
is devoted to Pharmacy, General Pharmacology and Therapeut
and remedial agents not usually classified with drugs.

Following a preliminary chapter on General Pharmacy,
have a description of a classification modified somewhat from
usual physiological classification of drugs. It will be seen f
the following quotation that the authors recommend drugs fr
even in trifling states. Referring to the abortive treatmen
colds, they say " medicinal treatment will include attentio
the condition of the skin, the kidneys, and the bowels, with
use of aconite, gelsemium, veratrum or other suitable rem
to reduce the activity of the circulation and overcome any
dency to fever. As soon as that has been properly effected
patient should be placed under the influence of quinine and
sulphide of calcium, so that within twenty-four hours he wi
fully charged with both remedies." We would be very slo
recommend any one to adopt such heroic treatment.

Under the list of vascular stimulants the authors place chl
form. The pronounced action of chloroform on the heart is q
the contrary.

Under the head of vascular sedatives, acting especially o
heart, we have placed digitalis. This is an unfortunate e
for if there is any well established therapeutical fact, it is
digitalis is the type of cardiac tonics.

The second part of the volume under consideration deals with Electro-therapeutics, Hydro-therapeutics, Massage and other less commonly employed agencies in the treatment of disease.

Society Proceedings.

MEDICO–CHIRURGICAL SOCIETY OF MONTREAL.

Stated Meeting, 7th March, 1890.

G. E. ARMSTRONG, M.D., PRESIDENT, IN THE CHAIR.

DR. MILLS exhibited two specimens illustrating so-called hermaphroditism in the pig. True hermaphroditism, while common in invertebrates (*i.e.*, the tapeworm, earthworm, etc), is unknown among vertebrates. In the true hermaphrodite, both male and female organs exist, and are functionally active. In the specimen shown, in one case the penis was well developed, in the other but indifferently. In other respects both specimens closely resembled each other. The testes were of good size and the urethra embraced by the prostate. What was most remarkable was the large development of the Müllerian ducts, which usually atrophy in the male into an organ greatly resembling the two-horned uterus, the walls of which were as thick as in the gravid condition of the organ. Apparently these served as the vas-a deferentia, while the latter seem to be fused with them. The specimens were obtained at the abattoir by members of Dr. Mills' class in physiology, and the butcher who first noticed them says they are the only specimens of the kind seen there in fifteen years.

Ruptured Tubal Gestation.—DR. WM. GARDNER exhibited the fœtus, placenta and umbilical cord from a case of ruptured ectopic gestation on which he had done abdominal section. The patient, aged 31, had been married fourteen years. One pregnancy to full term twelve years ago, and one early miscarriage shortly after. Since then she had suffered more or less from pelvic symptoms. Emmet's operation for laceration of the cervix had been done eighteen years ago. Menses had been regular till the last period in October, 1889, whether beginning middle or end of the month she could not tell. She had some of the signs of pregnancy and suspected it. Early in January, 1890, she was seized with pelvic pain and collapse, but rallied. Symptoms recurred, and at the request of her medical attendant, Dr. England of Point St. Charles, Dr. Gardner saw her with him. Pain was not severe, but the patient was blanched. The uterus was soft, bulky, fixed and discharging blood in moderate quantity. Behind it lay a small mass. Nothing could now be felt through the abdominal wall. Dr. Gardner again saw her on the 4th February. There had been little change till three days previous, when an increase of pain and faintness had occurred. A tumor-like mass had now appeared in the hypogastrium, and per vaginam the uterus was pressed forward by a firm mass which filled the pelvis. Four days later pain and collapse became alarming, and the abdominal tumor now reached above the umbilicus, distending uniformly the whole of the lower part of the belly. On the 9th February, at 4 A.M., the abdomen was opened. On reaching the peritoneum it bulged through the incision; the omentum being adherent, was cut through. An enormous quantity of clot and fluid blood was removed with fœtus and placenta. The sac on the left side of the uterus was grasped, tied and trimmed off. A second bleeding point in the pelvis needed ligature. The pelvis and abdomen were then thoroughly washed out by Tait's large tube. The value of this instrument in carrying a large volume of water to the deep parts of the cavity and forcing out clots was beautifully shown. A large glass drainage-tube was carried to the bottom of Douglas's pouch and there left. When put to bed the patient was very weak, but steadily rallied. She, however, died on the sixth day apparently from septic peritonitis. The fœtus, cord and placenta were perfectly fresh-looking, their being neither discoloration or any other evidence of death for more than a few hours before operation. The length of the fœtus was seven inches, and the points of ossification and other evidences present indicated a fœtal age of four or five months. The absence of very urgent symptoms till the day before operation, and the rapidly-growing abdominal tumor, were the grounds for waiting in the hope that a viable child might develop in the abdomen. The result well shows the danger to the mother of inaction.

Report on fœtus in Dr. Gardner's case of ruptured tubal gestation :

" Received in good condition, with shreds of placental tissue and some fibrinous blood-clot. No trace of amnion. Umbilical cord inserted 1 cm. above pubes ; seems rather small ; vessels pervious. Fœtus measures 12.5 cm. in length ; surface gela-tinous-looking, no traces of vernix. Skin over back of neck œdematous. Penis and scrotum distinct ; anus pervious. Nails on hands and feet rudimentary, but distinctly visible. No hair. Eyelids not separated. Brain diffluent. Liver large and soft ; gall-bladder small and empty ; small intestines contain bile ; testes lie in iliac fossæ ; kidneys size of beans, lobulation distinct ; lungs pale and firm, undilated, microscopically no pneumonia ; heart pale. Extremities (leg, upper arm and fore arm) measure 2 cm. ; femur 2¼ cm. Centre of ossification distinct in calcaneus on both sides. Microscopically, in subcutaneous tissue nuclei abound ; mucin absent."

Stated Meeting, 21st March, 1890.

G. E. ARMSTRONG, M.D., PRESIDENT, IN THE CHAIR.

DR. JAMES STEWART read an interesting paper on *Exalgine as an Analgesic,* which appeared in the April number of this JOURNAL.

Discussion.—DR. FINLEY—How do the members of the aromatic group compare with croton-chloral or gelsemium in their action ?

DR. BELL—Would it compete with opium in relieving pain due to traumatism, or only suited to pain of a nervous origin ?

DR. ARMSTRONG—I have used exalgine extensively within the last few months, and found it reliable in many cases of simple neuralgia which did not yield to antipyrin ; the dose requires to be increased. I have tried it in a case of cellulitis of the hand and in cases of inflammation about the cæcum, but without effect, and had to fall back upon morphia. It possesses advantages, in small doses, of (1) easy administration, (2) heart not affected, and (3) stomach not deranged. What influence has it upon the temperature ?

DR. GARDNER—What effect has it upon migraine, which is found so frequently to accompany gynæcological cases, and which, in my experience, yields only to morphia ?

DR. STEWART, in reply, said chloral and gelsemium are simply peripheral nerve sedatives, attacking only special nerve areas. It will not, I think, take the place of opium. The drug has, like all members of the same group, an antipyretic action, but in doses larger than four grains.

Epithelioma of the Cervix Uteri.—This specimen was exhibited by Dr. Alloway at a previous meeting.

DR. WM. GARDNER remarked that he had met with two cases of typical sprouting epithelioma of the cervix uteri in which no symptoms at all were present, the existence of such a grave condition being accidentally discovered by the patients themselves. A great deal can be done in relieving these by high amputation of the cervix rather than complete extirpation, where the disease is localized in the cervix. Dr. Skeene's (Brooklyn) statistics of cases operated upon by the galvano-cautery knife look as if we might expect better results than by other methods now existing.

DR. TRENHOLME exhibited two specimens. (1) *Hydrosalpinx,* which he had successfully removed. (2) *Par-ovarian retro-peritoneal cyst*—This tumor proved difficult to remove on account of the peritoneum being pushed away from it. After tapping cyst it was readily shelled out.

DR. GARDNER said he had met with several cases of cyst of the broad ligament which easily shelled out, but had not met with one similar to that now under consideration. He would substantiate the remark that often the pain was severe with objective symptoms being almost *nil* and *vice versâ*. Many cases did not seem to improve at once ; but when nutrition improved then pain became lessened.

Stated Meeting, 4th April, 1890.

Dr. Hingston in the Chair.

Peri-œsophageal Inflammation.—Dr. Johnston exhibited the specimen for Dr. Bell. The patient, a young girl aged 15 years, about a week ago, whilst swallowing a piece of tongue, was suddenly seized with a sensation of choking. Slight relief followed the passing of an œsophageal bougie. This difficulty of swallowing had existed since an attack of scarlet fever, which patient had had when five years old. There was a sensation of something like a lump in the throat. Upon examination, a saccule was seen between the pharynx and larynx. The next day after this obstruction occurred there was a marked cellulitis of the pharynx and neck; temperature 103°F. Forty-eight hours later there was emphysema about chest and neck, and breathing labored. The patient died suddenly 60 hours after first attacked with dysphagia. The mucous membrane of the œsophagus was found perfectly normal, and free from traces of laceration or any foreign body. Posterior to the pharynx was a large saccular space extending from one side to the other, about the size of an egg. This sac was partly filled with fœtid putty-like substance. It communicated with the pharynx low down on the left side. The tissues about the larynx were normal. The cellular tissue between œsophagus and trachea was in a state of acute phlegmon, being infiltrated with fœtid pus. The sheath of the vessels of neck was involved in this infiltration. The right pneumogastric nerve was swollen to the thickness of a slate pencil. There was slight emphysema of cellular tissue at root of neck, for which no cause could be detected. There was caseating tuberculosis of the bronchial and mesenteric glands and spleen, with acute tuberculous peritonitis; thoracic duct free.

Dr. Shepherd asked why the swelling could not have been reached by an incision behind sterno mastoid muscle?

Dr. Bell—On account of the uncertainty as to the nature of the case.

Papilloma of Ovary.—Dr. Gardner exhibited this specimen and related the history of the case. Patient, 27 years old, unmarried, suffered for the last two years from pelvic and abdominal pain, with enlargement.   Examination by palpation and percussion revealed the presence of fluid in abdomen; but, strangely, percussion in the flanks, with patient lying on the back, gave a clear note.   An exploratory abdominal incision was made, giving exit to a large quantity of pale straw-colored fluid. On the ovary was seen a cauliflower excrescence surrounded by a wall.   The parietal and visceral layers of the peritoneum were studded with nodules of a similar nature.   Examination microscopically of the tumor by Dr. Springle showed it to be made up of large round cells imbedded in a scanty stroma.

DR. GEO. ROSS asked Dr. Gardner how he would explain the presence of a clear note in the flanks, patient lying on the back, when there were evidences of fluid in the abdomen.

DR. HINGSTON said that from the appearance of the tumor, and from its having invaded the parietal and visceral peritoneum he would adjudge it to be a round-celled sarcoma. He would like to know how Dr. Gardner came to operate in view of the fact that the symptoms were so indefinite.

DR. GARDNER, in reply, said that the clear note in the flank was explained by the fact that the omentum was adherent to the abdominal wall.   He was in doubt himself as to the exact nature of the case, as the symptoms were so anomalous, and thought that the best way of ascertaining it was to make an exploratory incision.

Embolism of Abdominal Aorta.—Patient, female, aged 4 was admitted into the General Hospital suffering from gastric and nervousness, the effect of a drinking bout.   Shortly afterwards one leg became cold and insensitive, gangrene setting in; then, after a short period of time, the other leg was attacked in a similar manner, patient subsequently dying of heart failure.

DR. JOHNSTON, who exhibited the specimen for Dr. Bell, said there was gangrene of the right foot and lower half of left leg. An embolus had lodged at the bifurcation of the aorta.   In the left auricle, loosely attached, was a rounded thrombus, softened in the centre, and moderate mitral stenosis.

HAMILTON MEDICAL AND SURGICAL SOCIETY.
Stated Meeting, April 1st, 1890.

J. W. ROSEBRUGH, M.D., PRESIDENT, IN THE CHAIR.

Malignant Disease of the Bladder.—DR. COCKBURN reported the case as follows :—

About the latter end of November, 1888, my father came to me complaining of a feeling of discomfort just over the pubes, not severe, which eased at times, but never quite disappeared. During the next four or five weeks it gradually and almost imperceptibly became more palpable, till one day, about Christmas 1888, a small clot of blood was washed out with the urine, which from its shape, must have been lodged in the urethra. I now began to feel some anxiety, for the sequence of symptoms tallied unpleasantly closely with the earliest symptoms of malignant disease of the bladder. On January 7th, 1889, Dr. Leslie saw my father, and took a favorable view as to any vesicle trouble, but (if I remember aright) thought he suffered from lithiasis, an opinion afterwards confirmed by Dr. Osler. After this my father went about as usual; he did not complain much, but when questioned, always said the pain was getting slowly worse, and small casts of blood were passed from time to time. Still feeling very dissatisfied with my father's condition, I mentioned my suspicions to Dr. Bertram of Dundas, the family physician, and suggested he should examine per rectum, which was done. Dr. Bertram discovered nothing abnormal, and at this time took a hopeful view. On March 26th my father had a sort of hysterical attack and took to his bed. Under Dr. Bertram's care he improved for a time, but he now began to pass small particles of tissue. These were carefully examined microscopically on several occasions by Drs. Malloch, Osborne and myself; their appearance was suspicious, but by no means pathognomonic. Some of these shreds of tissue were sent to Dr. Osler of Baltimore, who very kindly examined them and (to the best of my recollection) said such particles were often passed by patients suffering from chro degenerative changes in the kidneys. The pain graduall creased, but no great change occurred till May 26th, wh

considerable discharge of blood occurred at the end of micturitio
On May 30th, Drs. Malloch and Bertram met me in consultatio
over my father's case. A perineal section was suggested pen
ing an examination of the urine. The urine showed a consid
able quantity of albumin and the operation was abandoned. Fr
this date my father commenced taking morphia hypodermical
His general condition became worse, the pain over the pul
became more severe, and the whole hypogastric region beca
intensely tender on pressure. The albuminuria continued to
crease, but although the urine was examined for casts by :
Malloch and myself on several occasions none were found.
August 9th, 1889, Dr. Osler saw my father in consultation v
Dr. Malloch, Dr. Bertram and myself. (Speaking from re
lection) Dr. Osler was unable to detect anything by firm press
over the pubes, and digital examination per rectum gave a ne
tive result. Dr. Malloch examined my father per rectum on
first visit, and both he and Dr. Osler agreed in pronouncing
prostate normal and no pathological condition to be detect
On this occasion my father was sounded by Dr. Malloch wit
negative result. To the best of my recollection, Dr. Osler
lieved it to be a case of gouty kidneys, remarking that
cause of the hæmaturia was obscure. Dr. Osler oppo
any operation. This opinion, expressed by so eminent
authority, gave myself and my family great relief, and I be
to hope I might be wrong in my view of the case. From
time my father went steadily down hill, the pain became m
severe and constant in the region indicated, and blood and
were constantly being passed. The morphia was gradually
creased. As time went on he began to emaciate; blood
constantly passed at the end of micturition, and the suffering
these occasions became intense, especially towards the close
the act. The pain spread down the penis as in cases of a calcu
Uræmic symptoms appeared from time to time, and the u
became loaded with albumin, but in spite of repeated exam
tions no casts appeared. Morphia was given in increasing do
to mitigate the constant suffering. All the symptoms beca

worse and worse. From time to time large quantities of blood were passed, sometimes mixed with pus. Albumin was always present in large quantities, and the pain in micturition became most intense. On January 28th, 1890, I was telephoned for, as there was some obstruction in the bowel. I found a hard mass blocking the rectum, which was with difficulty removed. Three days later a second mass presented, and was removed under chloroform. The chloroform was pushed to complete anæsthesia, and I then proceeded to explore per rectum. I easily mapped out the prostate and satisfied myself that it was normal. In the situation of the bladder I was able to make out a hard, irregular mass, movable, and, to a bimanual examination, apparently about the size of the gravid uterus at the fourth or fifth week. I now felt absolutely certain I had a case of malignant disease of the bladder to deal with. From the feel of it, I judged it to be most probably scirrhus cancer, involving principally the fundus. From this time my father began rapidly to sink. The suffering became so terrible that he was kept more or less constantly under chloroform, as the morphia seemed to lose all power, an injection of 4½ grains producing no appreciable effect. He died Feb. 15th, 1890 ; the duration of the case from the earliest onset of symptoms being therefore about one year and three months. From May 30th, 1889, to February 15th, 1890, he took over 2,000 grains of morphia hypodermically, and that with only partial relief to the suffering.

Remarks.—The specimen showed a growth on the posterior wall, which it infiltrated, measuring about 1¼ inches in width, 1½ inches in depth, and 1 inch in thickness. Over its free surface were numerous elongated papillæ, which formed a fringe-like covering to the growth. The tumor had not a very firm consistence, although it had been in methylated spirits for two weeks.

In the discussion which followed, Drs. Mullin, Malloch and Olmstead dissented from the view of it being scirrhus.

Oöphorectomy for Chronic Ovaritis.—DR. H. S. GRIFFIN reported the following case :

Mrs. H., aged 41, married, nullip. Family history poor,

several members having died of phthisis. Spare and nervous; menstruation regular. December 3rd, 1888, on making an emergent night visit, I found her suffering from intense pain referred to the lower part of the back and extending into the left inguinal region. She gave a history of previous tenderness and uneasiness in the same locality extending over several weeks, but not sufficiently severe to call for treatment. A vaginal examination discovered a small-sized mass posterior to the uterus, movable, but intensely tender ; making steady pressure in Campbell's position I readily succeeded in placing it above the pelvic brim. This relieved the intense pain, but considerable distress and soreness still remained. She was instructed to lie on her face and side as much as possible.

Dec. 4th *to* 14th—A few hours after replacing the ovary it again prolapsed, with return of the severe pain. It was quite impossible for her to retain a pessary, but persisted attempts were made to support the ovary with cotton wool tampons, aided by rest and posture. It would, however, invariably descend within twenty-four hours and have to be replaced with the finger. Nausea and anorexia were prominent symptoms.

Dec. 14th—Menstruation occurred with amelioration of her condition. She was able to be up and attend to her household affairs to some slight extent.

Jan. 2nd *to* 12th—The severe pain returned. All local treatment seemed only to aggravate the trouble and irritate the parts. She had to be constantly visited and the ovary replaced. Until the beginning of March this condition persisted ; then occurred an improvement, and for two weeks she did not require a single visit.

March 22nd—In response to a call, I found her suffering intensely. Examination showed the ovary firmly pressed down and so intensely painful that I had to abandon attempts at reduction. Under sedatives and hot water douches I was able to replace on the 28th. I still hoped that patient treatment would succeed in releasing her, but towards the end of April it was apparent that operative measures were necessary. She had become unable to take sufficient nourishment, and loss of rest with continuance of the pain had greatly reduced her.

April 30*th*—Operated at 11 A.M. Dr. Miller gave chloroform and Dr. Leslie assisted at the operation. A two-inch incision in the usual place enabled me to hook up the left ovary from Douglas' pouch ; the pedicle was tied and dropped, the right ovary examined and found normal, and the wound closed. The operation occupied about twenty minutes. On returning to the patient a few hours after, I found her suffering from the most severe retching I ever saw. It was promptly relieved, however, by a half-grain hypodermic of morphia.

May 14*th*—The patient convalesced rather slowly owing to irritability of the stomach. The temperature, which was 100° on the day of the operation, has never reached that point since, and is now normal.

June 1*st*—Patient able to leave her room, and feeeling quite well.

Since then (nearly a year ago) she has enjoyed perfect health, and has never had a pain since the day of the operation. The ovary removed was but slightly enlarged, and had three small cysts about the size of marrowfat peas.

Selections.

How to become Strong.—Mr. William Blaikie recently delivered a most invaluable lecture upon this subject. It was our pleasure to hear Mr. Blaikie lecture at Germantown. It was not only an invaluable discourse, but a highly interesting one. We were much impressed with the forcible way in which the speaker dwelt upon the importance of physical development and the health, strength and long and happy life it brought. We here publish some extracts from the lecture :—

" As I came along I saw that your town was dotted with three public libraries. Along Chelton avenue I noticed handsome churches. You have here valuable agencies ; one trains the mind and the other trains the moral nature. This is what constitutes our American system of education. What do we do for the body ? Oh, they say, the body will take care of itself. Well, so will the mind. How about the men and women who cannot read and write ; they are no worse off than the man whose body has not been trained. A man whose body is trained has an annuity fund laid in on which he can draw. I see you have a sort of make-believe gymnasium down stairs. There are so-called gymnasiums in this country. The man in charge takes your money, and generally takes plenty of it. You go in to get your money's worth ; you take hold of the big dumb bell, and try everything in the place ; next morning you've got your money's worth, and you go around asking, what ails me ? This is very much as if you should fill a school-room with desks and slates, and blackboards and books, but provide no teacher, and then say to the boys and girls, educate yourselves. There would be lots of education going forward, wouldn't there ? Brains are needed in a gymnasium.

" Oh, but we have lots of athletics. The papers are full of them. But what good does it do you ? The old Greek and Roman athletics could not compare with our records. They sent a famous courier to bring up the hardy Spartan troops, and he made 149 miles in 48 hours. A few years ago, in Madison Square Garden, New York, little Charlie Rowell made 150 miles in 24 hours. Rowell would have warmed the old Spartan's jacket for him in a go-as-you-please race. Vanderbilt's Maud S, out at grass, would not be brought in and put in a race right off. She would be got in condition, and then let that other horse look out. But the portly citizen of Germantown runs along Chelton avenue for a train and topples over, all because of his ignorance of elementary knowledge.

" We develop our muscles in a one-sided, partial way. There's rowing : it exercises us in pushing and pulling. I was referee at the race between Hanlan and Courtney, where the latter's boat was so mysteriously cut. I asked Hanlan to try the simple experiment of resting his hands on two chairs and then letting himself down between them. How often did he do it ? Well, he got down and could not get up. He hadn't trained the right muscles. There is a great man—John L. Sullivan, a man of striking ability, who always makes a marked impression. He trains the other muscles. But put him in a shell against Hanlan and the Canadian would pull clear away from him. Change the scene a little and the symmetry of Hanlan's head would be seriously impaired inside of two minutes. Had they started in a race with Rowell they would both soon have been hopelessly behind.

" Our mechanics train only the muscle each wants in getting bread and butter.

" Among American women walking is a lost art. I don't know how it is here in Germantown, but in New York I have seen them shopping on Fourteenth street ; they go dawdling along at about a two-miles-an-hour gait. Some one has said that a woman in America runs fast enough for a man to catch her. Some of them can't do that. There is 70,000 of them in Massachusetts. Once I went up to Vassar College to see their gymnasium. They had lots of apparatus there that looked like as if it was the kind that Noah used when he was loafing around in the ark. Then the girls showed me how they ran. After a few trials they came in puffing and blowing, and their hearts beating about 140 to the minute. ' What do you think of the running ?' they asked. ' What running ?' said I. Then I showed how the sandal of the runner was made, with no heel, and how he ran on his toes with his head up and his chest out, and they admitted that the y couldn't run."

He told the girls how to develop weak arms, make them strong and so that they would be well rounded and shapely when they wore evening costumes. "One of the hardest problems is how to keep the girls who go into this training from doing too much hard work at the beginning. Ham is a good thing for breakfast, but no one wants to eat a whole ham for breakfast. They must start off easily. A man at Englewood came to me about his daughter. She was low-spirited and weak. 'Well,' I said, ' what does she do ?' and he said, ' she went five miles to school every day and carried a great strap full of books.' ' Does she walk ?' ' No, she rides in a horse-car.' Oh, the lovely horse-car ! Oh, the beautiful horse-car ! Sidewalks deserted to hang by a strap in a crowded horse-car. Give up walking to be hauled home in a lovely horse-car. Get her a pair of Waukenphast shoes, broad enough at least for two of her toes to touch the ground. Ugly, of course they're ugly ; but they are comfortable. Let her go off the car one mile from home the first week. Rain ? Well, let it rain ; I hope it will. Rain doesn't look half so bad when you are in it as when you look at it through the window. Then let her try two miles the second week, and so on up to five. I met the father in two months. He said : ' The aches are all gone, and we are afraid she'll eat the table-cover. Her brother has taught her boxing, and we are all afraid of her around the house. She's actually getting good-looking.' "

He compared Bernhardt's attenuated proportions with Lily Langtry's fine physique. "The Lily had six brothers, all athletes. She joined in their sports, she became a practical yachtswoman, and her average daily walk now is ten miles. This accounts for it all. She says American girls don't take exercise enough. The finest figure in all Europe is the Empress of Austria. At fifty-five she is a great horseback rider. When Dr. McCosh's daughters came to Princeton, one of the young men took them out for a stroll. They walked him to Trenton and back, some twenty miles. That young man could have been called a sub dude when he got back.

"Did you ever hear of neuralgia, nervous prostration, insomnia? Ask any expert in neural disorders what to do. He will not advise drugs and chemicals as an antidote, but exercise. Get your muscles in grand running order and you need have no fear for the nerves. The dyspeptic needs exercise. Some one has said dyspepsia was a disease of the legs. When an old woman heard that John Bright was coming to the United States she wondered whether he was going to bring his disease with him. She needn't have asked; we have it, it is insidiously but surely undermining our bodies.

"John Morrisey was told by his physician that he must die in two weeks of Bright's disease of the kidneys. He considered what he should do. He went into the same course of training that he used when he was preparing for a prize fight. It made him a new pair of kidneys, and he was a vigorous man for twenty years afterward.

"I could name four young fellows at Harvard who wouldn't take exercise; said they didn't need it; in five years they were laid under the sod. You all know Tom Corwin. He's the man who stood up in the United States Senate and said : ' Mr. President, I deny the allegation, and I can thrash the alligator.' One time his son, who was in college, wrote home : ' Dear father, I am studying very hard, so hard that I fear I will die.' Corwin wrote back : ' My dear son, it would give me great pleasure to attend your funeral under the circumstances. Your affectionate father.' I don't know whether this applies in Germantown or not. You see them digging up a street for a sewer. The men in the offices complain of malaria and go home and get nourished and coddled. The Irishmen who do the digging don't complain of malaria. Men who are great accomplishers are men of great bodies as well as great brains."

Then the speaker went on to illustrate by, "Alexander the Great, whose teacher, Aristotle, withdrew him from the Court and trained body as well as mind; Julius Cæsar, who was an athlete; John Wesley, who had a sturdy, well-knit frame; Gladstone, who cuts down an oak four feet in diameter between luncheon and dinner, when he is at his Welsh estate. Washington was a man of grand physique. He was six feet two inches in height and weighed 213 pounds. If he had been in training, John L. Sullivan couldn't have stood five minutes before him. He was a straight-sided man, and was a great wrestler when a young man. Frazer has made the running-board jump record twenty-three feet; Washington did twenty-four feet. They talk about throwing a baseball four hundred feet; Washington threw a silver dollar six hundred feet. A United States senator showed Chief-Justice Coleridge the place where he did it, and when the Englishman asked how it was done, the Yankee replied, ' a dollar went farther in those days.'

" What kind of school-yards have you got? In New York they have them a little bigger than a postage stamp. Every school should have a large yard for the children to run and leap in and exercise."—*Anti-Adulteration Journal; Cincinnati Lancet-Clinic.*

Some Points in the Treatment of Gonorrhœa.

—The early use of astringents in gonorrhœa is advocated by many practitioners. We do not agree with those who advise the use of astringent injections in the early stage of the disease. The effect of astringents is to thicken the mucous membrane upon its surface, and seal up the gonococci in the meshes of the areolar tissue and the deeper portions of the mucous membrane. Aside from this effect, injections in the early stage of the disease are pernicious from their mechanical effect. We believe that they often cause stricture, not because they are used in too powerful solution, but simply because they act mechanically on the inflamed canal. One of the most potent causes of stricture, independent of cases treated by the use of injections, is the passage of urine over certain portions of the canal (normal points of contraction). The entire calibre of the canal is lessened. There is a good deal of friction during the passage of urine, and consequently the epithelium becomes abraded, and a habit of rapid proliferation and removal of epithelium supervenes. It is at these points of extreme friction that granular patches occur, which result in a perpetuation of gleet and a liability to the formation of stricture. Injections very often act in the same way if used frequently.

We do not believe in the practice of passing into the urethra medicated applications in the acute stage of the disease. We have tried soluble bougies, hot water irrigations, and various other things that have been recommended, with but little benefit. We do not believe any antiseptic in combination with an ointment is capable of paralyzing the gonococci, as has been stated. When the surgeon passes an instrument into the canal it carries the discharge into the deeper portions of the urethra, and unless the ointment is sufficiently powerful, he will defeat the very object he aims to secure by his applications.

We have noted objections to the use of irrigation by the recurrent catheter in gonorrhœa. Dr. Palmer, of Louisville, recently wrote an able article on a particular method of treatment of urethritis by irrigation. After reading Dr. Palmer's article on the subject we tried the method, and immediately had a succession of cases of inflammation of the vesical neck and prostate. A number of cases of epididymitis arose, and seemingly were also due to the manipulations of the canal. The poison is carried by the catheter into the deeper portions of the canal, and the inflammation extends to the deep urethra by affecting contiguous structures. By any of these mechanical methods a greater number of cases will be affected by complications and become chronic than under ordinary conservative methods of treatment.

The probabilities are that if we treated cases of gonorrhœa as we treat other diseases of like severity and importance as regards serious complications and results, we would have very few cases of stricture, very few cases of abscess, and very few cases of epididymitis or bladder troubles secondary to gonorrhœa. If every man with a gonorrhœa went to bed and remained there for two or three weeks there would not be one-tenth part of the number of strictures which we have now to treat.

The regulation of the diet is a most important feature of treatment of genito-urinary troubles of an inflammatory character. The patient should be instructed to live on bread and milk. This particular dietetic regimen continued for a few days affords more benefit than almost anything else we could give. Large quantities of milk produce alkalinization of the urine, and produce it more effectually than does the administration of drugs during the acute, or, what Van Buren and Keys have termed, the ascending stage of the disease.

When the disease has come to a stand-still—when the purulent discharge has begun to diminish, antiseptic injections should be given ; the bichloride of mercury is the most reliable remedy we have. It may be used in a solution of half a grain to four ounces of rose-water. There is one very important point with reference to the bichloride of mercury which we will mention. If there is any remedy to which there is a varying susceptibility on the part of the mucous membrane, it is this drug. Some patients using the drug in the strength of one-eighth grain to the ounce may not complain of any immediate effects of the injection, but after its use for a few times will find that urination is painful. Retention from inflammation may occur in a few patients who are using solutions much milder than those which have been found to perfectly agree with others. In using bichloride of mercury, it should be given in a strength of, on an average, half a grain of the drug to four ounces of rose-water and glycerine. In a few days, or perhaps a week, it will be found that the bichloride has lost its beneficial effect. After a few days it will be necessary to substitute astringent injections, and if these are properly and carefully used, it makes no difference what form of astringent is selected. Matico, hydrastis, etc., are as useful as anything. In the way of minereal astringents the sulpho-carbolate of zinc, glycerine and rose-water form a good combination. If the case does not get along well, the explanation is not that the injection is improper, or that some other form of astringent would be better, but usually that the patient is carousing with women, drinking or over-exerting himself. Patients are very apt to tell us that an injection does not work well in spite of their good habits, but as a matter of fact they lie in a great many cases.

As regards balsams, we believe that they have decided virtues in the treatment of gonorrhœa. We use at first sandalwood, subsequently, in the later stages of the disease, copaiba and cubebs in the order named. If they are used in this way they are decidedly efficacious and beneficial.

One point that is worthy of attention is that gonorrhœa is a self-limited disease. The normal duration of gonorrhœa is from three to six or eight weeks. There are exceptionally few cases that recover in three weeks or less. If a case comes to us early for what we suppose to be gonorrhœa, and we cure the disease in a few days, we conclude that the patient did not have a virulent urethritis. When we use the term *gonorrhœa*, we do not speak of it as an entity. By *virulent urethritis* we mean that the poison has arrived at its highest degree of culture and always produces definite results.—*Western Medical Reporter.*

THE

𝕸𝖔𝖓𝖙𝖗𝖊𝖆𝖑 𝕸𝖊𝖉𝖎𝖈𝖆𝖑 𝕵𝖔𝖚𝖗𝖓𝖆𝖑.

| VOL. XVIII. | MAY, 1890. | No. 11. |

THE ABUSE OF COFFEE.

Mendel, of Essen, has recently pointed out that when coffee is taken too freely for long periods it induces a peculiar train of symptoms which are characteristic. It affects not only the nervous system, but also the circulatory and muscular systems. The nervous symptoms include a feeling of general weakness, apathy and mental depression. The motor symptoms noticed were loss of power and tremor in the extremities, while the circulatory disturbance was evidenced by a small, weak and irregular pulse, with palpitation. Nervous dyspepsia and constipation were usually present also.

THE GERMAN CONGRESS FOR INTERNAL MEDICINE.

At the recent Congress held this year in Vienna, several very important discussions took place. The distinguished president, Prof. Nothnagel, opened the proceedings of the Congress by an able address on the past, present and probable future of medicine. Immerman, of Balse, introduced a discussion on the treatment of empyema. He prefers puncture of the thorax with aspiration of the pus contained in the pleural cavity, while Schede recommends the more radical operation of resection of the ribs with the subsequent antiseptic treatment of the wound. It was decided to form a collective investigation committee to report at a subsequent meeting of the Congress.

Prof. Mosler read a paper on the pathology of pemphigus. He looks upon it as being due to nervous influences, repeated examination having failed to discover any micro-organisms. He has found changes in the spinal cord in fatal cases. Kaposi referred to the great mortality in cases of pemphigus, the death-rate in two hundred cases that came under his own observation being 90 per cent.

Probably the most important discussion held was that on the treatment of Albuminuria. The subject was introduced by Prof. Senator, who remarked that the prognosis is not at all as grave as it is commonly held to be. The great importance of dietetic treatment was insisted on. Albuminous food should be sparingly taken, while fats and carbo-hydrates are indicated. Fish and the meat of young animals might be taken, but eggs should be avoided. The milk and koumiss cure were frequently of great service. Several of the speakers looked upon bodily quiet as being of great importance.

INTERNATIONAL MEDICAL CONGRESS.

The preliminary programme for the discussions on subjects connected with internal medicine at the coming International Medical Congress at Berlin has been published. It includes—

(1) The Treatment of Disease of the Heart, by Nothnagel of Vienna.

(2) The Treatment of Diseases of the Kidneys, by Lepine of Lyons and Grainger Stewart of Edinburgh.

(3) The Treatment of Anæmia, by Osler of Baltimore and Laache of Christiana.

(4) The Treatment of Diphtheria in America, by Jacobi of New York.

(5) The Treatment of Pulmonary Consumption, by H. Weber of London and Loomis of New York.

(6) The Treatment of Diabetes, by Pavy of London, Dujardin-Beaumetz of Paris, and Seegen of Vienna.

(7) The Treatment of Gallstones, by Ord of London.

(8) The Nature and Treatment of Uræmia, by Landois of Greifswald.

(9) The Nature and Treatment of Tabes, by Strümpell of Erlangen.

(10) Myxœdema, by Ord of London.

(11) Dengue Fever, by Fleras of Constantinople.

It will be seen the above include subjects of great and pressing importance. There is every reason to hope that much will be added to our knowledge as the result of these discussions.

CANADIAN MEDICAL ASSOCIATION.

The twenty-third annual meeting of the Canadian Medical Association will be held in Toronto on Tuesday, Wednesday and Thursday, the 9th, 10th and 11th of September next.

LEGACY TO THE POST-GRADUATE MEDICAL SCHOOL AND HOSPITAL.—Among the legacies of the late Honorable Daniel B. St. John, of Newburgh, N.Y., was one of ten thousand dollars to the above-named institution.

—The death-rate in the city of New York for the year 1889 was 25.1 per 1,000. The deaths exceeded the births by upwards of 2,000.

—It is sad commentary on the boasted civilization of our mother country to find that nearly two millions of the surplus revenue for the past year was made up from the increased consumption of alcoholic liquors.

Obituary.

—We regret to announce the death of Dr. Allison of Bowmanville, at the advanced age of 85 years. Dr. Allison has been for over half a century a leading and much-respected practitioner in the Bowmanville district. He was for a number of years a member of the Council of the College of Physicians and Surgeons of Ontario, and during 1880-81 he was president of this body.

McGILL UNIVERSITY.

FACULTY OF MEDICINE CONVOCATION.

The annual public meeting of Convocation for the conferring of Degrees in Medicine, and in comparative Medicine and Veterinary Science, was held in the William Molson Hall, on Tuesday, April 1st, at 3 p.m.

Sir Donald A. Smith, the Chancellor, presided, and at his left was the Principal, Sir William Dawson. Around him were the Governors, Mr. John H. R. Molson, Mr. W. C. MacDonald, Mr. Samuel Finley, Alexander Johnson, L.L.D., Dean of the Faculty of Arts; Dr. Craik, Dean of the Medical Faculty; and Dr. Ross, the Vice-Dean; Prof. Bovey, Dean of the Faculty of Applied Science; N. W. Trenholme, Q. C., Dean of the Faculty of Law; Dr. McEachran, Dean of the Faculty of Comparative Medicine; Dr. Stewart, Dr. Shepherd, Dr. Wilkins, Dr. Cameron, Dr. Mills, Dr. Girdwood, Dr. Gardner, Dr. Rodger, Dr. Grant, Dr. Birkett, Dr. Johnston, Dr. Finley, Dr. Ruttan, Dr. Baker, Dr. McEachran, Rev. Principals MacVicar, Shaw and Barbour; Prof. Penhallow, F. W. Kelley, Ph. D., Prof. J. Clarke Murray, John Dougall, M. A., Prof. C. E. Moyse, Rev. Dr. Cornish, Rev. Prof. Scrimgour, Mr. Justice Cross, Rev. Prof. Coussirat, Dr. Godsgen, J. W. Brackenridge, B.C.L.; W. Skaife, B. A. Sc.; P. Toewes, M.A.; E. H. Hamilton, B.A. Sc.; J. A. MacPhail, B.A.; M. W. Hopkins, B.A. Sc.

Rev. Dr. Cornish opened the proceedings with the usual form of prayer, and then Dr. Craik, Dean of the Medical Faculty, presented the report for the past session. The number of students attending were:—From Ontario, 111; Quebec, 71; New Brunswick, 26; Nova Scotia, 20; Prince Edward Island, 11; United States, 7; Manitoba, 7; Newfoundland, 2; British Columbia, 2; West Indies, 2; England, 1. The number this year is greatly in excess of former years, as the following statement shows. Dividing the period into decades, the Dean showed that sixty years ago—in the session of 1829-30—there were but thirty students in attendance;—

	Students.
In 1839-40	20
In 1849-50	44

In 1859-60 108
In 1869-70 141
In 1879-80 186
In 1889-90 261

It will be remembered that in '39 an '40 the rebellion occurred, and for two or three years the classes were closed. Only eight or nine years ago the university had almost reached the limit of its accommodation; the class rooms and laboratories were overcrowded and students unable to obtain admission were forced to go elsewhere. Then it was that the Chancellor came to their aid (cheers), and enabled them to further extend their usefulness. The Campbell Memorial fund had also enabled them to extend their class rooms, laboratories and equipments. They had accordingly endeavored to increase the useful working of the institution. He felt that their efforts had been fully appreciated by the class from which their students are drawn. But while congratulating themselves they must face a feeling of anxiety. They had seen one period of stagnation owing to overcrowding; that must not occur again; they could not afford it. They must keep constantly advancing. Medical teaching is not a remunerative employment; advanced methods have to be employed with the forward move of the times. The Dean felt sure that their wants only require to be made known to friends in Montreal to gain the help necessary to carry on their work as it should be carried on.

Continuing, he said :—The following gentlemen, 56 in number, have fulfilled all the requirements to entitle them to the degree of M.D., C.M., from the University. In addition to the Primary subjects mentioned, they have passed a satisfactory examination, both written and oral, on tho following subjets:—Principles and Practice of Surgery, Theory and Practice of Medicine, Obstetrics and Diseases of Infancy, Gynæcology, Pharmacology and Therapeutics, Medical Jurisprudence, Pathology and Hygiene —and Clinical Examinations in Medicine, Surgery, Ophthalmology, Obstetrics and Gynæcology conducted in the wards of the General Hospital and Maternity :—

G. A. B. Addy, St. John, N.B.; C. A. Ault, Oshkosh, Wis.; C. P. Bisset, River Bourgeois, N.S.; E. J. Bowes, Ottawa, Ont.; E. J.

Broderick, B.A., Fredericton, N.B.; C. H. Burritt, B.A., Mitchell, Ont.; F. M. Campbell, Longueuil, Que.; J. W. Clarke, Tatamagouche, N.S.; J. Clune, Warkworth, O.; A. H. Coleman, Belleville, Ont.; F. G. Corbin, Bedford, N.S.; I. B. Curtis, Hartland, N.B.; T. H. Ellis, Pembroke, Ont.; D. J. Evans, Montreal, Que.; A. S. Gorrell, Brockville, Ont.; T. J. Green, Appleton, Ont.; H. D. Hamilton, B.A., Montreal, Que.; N. M. Harris, Ormstown, Que.; John Hayes, B.A., Richmond, Que.; W. E. Inksetter, Copetown, Ont.; A. F. Irwin, Chatham, Ont.; E. Jenkins, Conquerell, N.S.; C. P. Jento, Mellville, Ont; D. N. Fordyce, Ont.; H. D. Kemp, Montreal, Que.; A. C. Leslie, Grand Forks, Dak.; A. A. Lewin. St. John, N.B.; G. L. Liddell, Cornwall, Ont.; O. Morris, Pembroke, Ont.; E. A. Mulligan, Aylmer. Que.; M. W. Murray, Beachwood, Ont.; M. S. Macdonald, Scotchtown, Q.; F. Brown, Winnipeg, Man.; H. H. McKay, Pictou, N. S.; R. E. McKechnie, Winnipeg, Man.; G. L. McKee, Coaticook, Que.; A. C. McLellan, Indian River, P.E.I.; H. D. McManus, B.A., Fredericton, B.; G. A. McMillan, St. St. Agnès de Dundee, Que.; C. T. Noble, Hatton, Ont.; C. O'Connor, Worcester, Mass.; A. J. Oliver, Cowansville, Que.; H. M. Patton, B. A., Winnipeg, Man.; J. T. Reid, Winnipeg, Man.; W. Robertson, Chesterfield, Ont.; James Ross, Halifax, N.S.; R. Ross, Quebec, Que.; W. D. Smith, Plantagenet, Ont; W. J. Telfer, Burgoyne, Ont; F. E. Thompson, Quebec, Que.; D. De J. White, Montreal, Que.; W. A. Wllson. Derby, N.B.; H. M. Williamson, Guelph, Ont.; E. H. Woodruff, B.A., St. Catherines, Ont.; F. S. Yorston, Truro, N.S.

The following gentlemen have passed their Primary Examination, which comprises the following subjects:—Anatomy, Practical Anatomy, Chemistry, Practical Chemistry, Physiology, Histology and Botany:—

G. A. Berwick, J. E. Binmore, G. A. Bowen, B. F. Boyce, F. W. A. Brown, D. A. Bruce, H. B. W. Carmichael, C. M. Carlaw, J. L. Chabot, R. J. Chipman, A. R. Day, G. H. Duncan, R. T. Glendinning, W. C. R. Graham, H. A. Grant, V. Halliday, P. J. Hayes, James Henderson, D. H. Hogg, A. F. Irwin, Thos. Jameson, Albert Johnson, F. W. Lang, A. F. Langley, A. A. Lewin, A. W. Mair, C. F. Martin, H. B. Massiah, C. J. Meade, W. F. Meikle, D. T. Mackay, J. E. McKenty, R. T. McKenzie, A. I. McKinnon, H. McNally, Lamont Paterson, E. D. Phelan, B. E. Robinson, W, Rogers, Geo. R. Shirriff, O. W. Sinclair, W. H. Smith, J. A. Stewart, T. T. Taylor, J. N. Taylor, M. M. Taplin, A. S. Wade, W. E. Walsh, W. G. Walker, H. J. Wasson, H. B. Yates.

THIRD YEAR.

The following have passed in Pharmacology and Therapeutics:—

W. W. Alexander, R. Bennie, R. A. Bowie, J. E. Brouse, W. A.

Brown, J. Busby, B. H. Calkin, C. M. Carlaw, J. Clarke, J. C. Clemesha,
A. Dewar, W. A. Farwell, R. W. Fletcher, J. A. Fulton, R. J. Gibson,
E. A. Grafton, W. F. Hamilton, J. D. Harrison, W. H. Hattie, J.
Heweston, D. B. Holden, A. Internoscia, A. F. Irwin, C. I. Kelly, E.
J. Keir, E. M. Lambert, A. Love, W. Lovering, A. I. Mader, C. G.
Main, M. McL. Martin, J. M. Moore, W. S. Morrow, A. E. A. McCann,
A. A. McCrimmon, G. F. McGauran, J. C. McGuire, J. H. McMillan,
J. A. MacPhail, J. Neill, E. A. Robertson, T. F. Robertson, O. W.
Sinclair, C. F. Smith, T. H. Smith, A. J. Sparling, J. R. Spier, C. A.
Tunstall, W. Troy, N. M. Waston, R. E. Webster, W. P. Williamson.

The following have passed in Pathology :—

W. W. Alexander, R. Bennie, R. H. Berwick, R. A. Bowie, W. A.
Brown, J. Busby, B. H. Calkin, C. M. Carlaw, J. Clarke, J. C.
Clemesha, A. Dewar, W. A. Farwell, R. W. Fletcher, R. J. Gibson, E.
A. Grafton, W. F. Hamilton, J. D. Harrison. W. H. Hattie, J.
Heweston, D. B. Holden, A. Internoscia, A. F. Irwin, C. I. Kelly, E.
J. Keir, E. M. Lambert, A. Love, W. Lovering, A. I. Mader, C. G.
Main, M. McL. Martin, J. M. Moore, W. S. Morrow, A. E. A. McCann,
A. A. McCrimmon, J. C. McGuire, J. H. McMillan, J. A. MacPhail,
J. Neill, E. A. Robertson, G. Shirriff, O. W. Sinclair, C. F. Smith, T.
H. Smith, A. J. Sparling, J. R. Spier, C. A. Tunstall, W. Troy, N. M.
Watson, R. E. Webster, W. P. Williamson.

The following have passed in Medical Jurisprudence :—

W. W. Alexander, R. Bennie, R. A. Bowie, J. E. Brouse, W. A.
Brown, J. Busby, B. H. Calkin, C. M. Carlaw, J. Clarke, J. C. Clemesha,
A. Dewar, W. A. Farwell, R. W. Fletcher, J. A. Fulton, R. J. Gibson,
E. A. Grafton, W. F. Hamilton, J. D. Harrison, W. H. Hattie, J.
Heweston, D. B. Holden, A. Internoscia, A. F. Irwin, C. I. Kelly. E.
J. Keir, E. M. Lambert, A. Love, W. Lovering, A. I. Mader, C. G.
Main, M. McL. Martin, J. M. Moore, O. Morris, W. S. Morrow, H. H.
Mackay, E. A. McCann, A. A McCrimmon, G. F. McGauran, J. C.
McGuire, J. H. McMillan, J. A. MacPhail, J. J. Neill, S. Richards, E.
A. Robertson, T. F. Robertson, G. R. Sparling, J. R. Spier, C. A.
Tunstall, W. Troy, N. M. Watson, R. E. Webster, W. P. Williamson.

FIRST YEAR.

The following have passed in Histology :—

E. D. Aylen, H. H. Barrett, H. W. Blunt, W. E. Bostwick, J. A.
Brown, J. D. Cameron, Robt. Campbell, R. W. Carroll, M. A. Cooper,
W. E. Deeks, G. F. Dewar, Ed. Duvernet, G. W. Fleming, J. A.
Fulton. C. W. Girdlestone, H. N. Goff, F. B. Gunter, Mortimer
Haight, S. W. Hewetson, G. L. Hume, A. Internoscia, W. H. Jamieson,
W. O. Lambly, J. W. Lawrence, J. T. Lewis, W. Lindsay, H. A.
Livingstone, C. H. Masten, S. R. McKenzie, A. D. McArthur, J. D.

McIntyre, R. B. MacKay, D. McLennan, K. McLennan, Wallace
McMillan, R. F. McMorine, C. L. Ogden, W. Patterson, B. E. Robinson,
R. F. Rorke, J. W. Scane, E. J. Semple, J. W. A. Seguin, G. F. Shaw,
O. W. Sainclair, W. H. Smith, G. A. Trenholme, A. S. Wade, J. L.
Walker, T. N. Walsh, Robt. Wilson, R. D. Wilson, C. A. Yearwood,
W. E. Young.

The following have passed in Batony :—

N. Anderson, E. D. Aylen, H. H. Barrett, W. E. Bostwick, J. A.
Brown, J. D. Cameron, Robt. Campbell, R. W. Carroll, M. A. Cooper,
G. F. Dewar, A. T. Dewar, Ed. DuVernet, A. S. Esty, F. M. Ferron, G.
W. Fleming, M. Haight, S. W. Hewetson, R. W. Jakes, W. H. Jamie-
son, A. Johnson, W. O. Lambly, J. W. Lawrence, J. T. Lewis, Wm.
Lindcay, H. A. Livingstone, C. H. Masten, R. Mathieson, W. C. Mills,
A. D. MacArthur, J. D. MacIntyre, R. B. MacKay, J. L. MacKenzie,
K. McLennan, Wallace McMillan, R. F. McMorine, G. W. Parker,
Wm. Patterson, E McG. Quirk, F. W. Read, D. A. Rodger, R. F.
Rorke, H. J. Robinson, J. H. Scammell, J. W. Scane, J. S. Seaton, E.
J. Semple, J. W. A. Seguin, Thos. P. Shaw, G. F. Shaw, O. W. Sinclair,
W. H. Scott, J. E. C. Tomkins, G. A. Trenholme, J. L. Walker, Robt.
Wilson, R. D. Wilson, W. E. Young, C. A. Yearwood.

The Holmes Gold Medal, for the best Examination in all
the Branches comprised in the Medical Curriculum, is awarded
to Robert Edward McKechnie, of Winnipeg, Manitoba.

The Prize for the best examination in the Final Branches,
is divided equally between Edward John Bowes, of Ottawa,
Ont., and Michael William Murray, of Beachwood Ont.

The Clemesha Prize in Clinical Therapeutics, is awarded to
Afred Henry Coleman, Belleville, Ont.

The Prize for the best examination in the Primary Branches, is divided equally between James Henderson, of Warkworth, Ont., and Thomas Jameson, of Buffalo, N. Y.

The Sutherland Gold Medal is awarded to Thomas Jameson,
Buffalo, N.Y.

The following arranged in order of merit, deserve honorable
mention :

IN THE PRIMARY BRANCHES.—J. L. Chabot, A. R. Day, H. B. W.
Massiah, C. F. Martin, H. J. Wasson, P. J. Hayes, B. F. Boyce, R. J.
Chipman, F. W. Lang.

IN THE FINAL BRANCHES.—W. D. Smith, W. E. Inksetter, F. S.
Yorston, A. F. Irwin, A. H. Coleman, John Hayes, E. J. Broderick, C.
T. Noble, W. A. Wilson, D. J. Evans.

Botany,...................................Robt. Wilson, Montreal.
Senior Anatomy,......................James Henderson, Warkworth,
Junior   "   ....J. W. Scane.

Dr. Stewart, the Registrar, then administered the usual oath to the Candidates as they stood around the dais with uplifted hands.

Dr. E. J. Bowes was then called on to deliver the Valedictory on behalf of the Graduating Class of 1890. * * *

* * * * * * * * * * · *

Whatever the measure of prosperity it may be our future lot to enjoy, we shall ever remember that it is due in no small degree to the untiring efforts of our professors to instil into our minds some of that knowledge and love of science, which has brought so much honor to themselves and to their Alma Mater. And in bidding them farewell I can pay no higher tribute to their worth, or express better wishes for the welfare of my Alma Mater, than to hope that they may long be spared to preside over her Council Boards.

To our fellow students whom we leave behind, we also extend our hearty good will. We do not purpose to inflict upon you our gratuitous and unasked for advice. We only trust that you will ever work harmoniously together for the common welfare of yourselves and your university. By so doing you will, upon reaching your final year, be able to look back upon college career with the same satisfaction with which we do to-day.

Now as we go forth into the busy world, let us pause a moment and take a last fond look at our dear old Alma Mater, for we would indeed be unworthy of the name she gives us, if passing from her portals we cast no longing, lingering look on her whose loving care has brought us to this house and made us all we are. It is needless for me to sing her praises, her reputation and renown have already spread to every quarter of the globe where the English tongue is spoken. Then her graduates by their skill have been erecting a monument to her fame. The growth of her reputation has been constant and progressive, not instantaneous, and due to the electric flash of one bright genius, who illumined her horison for a few short moments and then passed away to leave her in a deeper gloom. Her light shines with a constant and ever increasing brightness, kept aglow by the succeeding generations of her children. And whilst she has been giving her sons to other universities to build up their strength, her's is the product of her own conception, and all her professorial chairs are filled by her own graduates. When in the natural course of events, one of her honored guides passes away to seek the rest and reward of a life of ceaseless energy and priceless worth, she can always find 'one of ˌher graduates, even at considerable personal sacrifice, ever ready and willing to step into the breach, take up the work and bear her banner to the achievement of still greater renown.

Farewell, our dear old Alma Mater, you have been a kind and generous foster mother to us. You have taken us into your bosom and having nourished us with your own warm blood, you now, with your last benediction, send us forth into the world to fulfil one of the noblest duties of men.

Farewell—*ever* shall our hearts turn *to thee* with gratitude and fondest remembrance ; ever shall thy precepts be engraven upon them and rule our lives, and wheresoever we shall drift on the flood of destiny, may our every deed and motive redound to *thy* honor, *our dear old Alma Mater.*

Dr. J. C. Cameron then delivered the reply for the Faculty. (*See page* 801.)

Medical Items.

—Drs. McKechnie, Coleman, Inksetter, Smith and Vidal have been appointed Resident Medical Officers to the Montreal General Hospital for the ensuing year.

—Drs. Evans and Hamilton have been appointed Resident Medical Officers to the Montreal Maternity for the ensuing year.

—We have received the first number of the *Montreal Pharmaceutical Journal.* It is edited by Joseph Bemrose, Esq., F.L.C., the well-known chemist. We wish the new periodical every success.

THE WILLIAM F. JENKS MEMORIAL PRIZE.—The second triennial prize of $450, under the deed of trust of Mrs. William

F. Jenks, will be awarded to the author of the best essay on " The Symptomatology and Treatment of the Nervous Disorders following the Acute Infectious Diseases of Infancy and Childhood." The conditions annexed by the founder of this prize are that " the prize or award must always be for some subject connected with Obstetrics, or the Diseases of Women, or the Diseases of Children" ; and that " the trustees, under this deed for the time being, can, in their discretion, publish the successful essay, or any paper written upon any subject for which they may offer a reward, provided the income in their hands may, in their judgment, be sufficient for that purpose, and the essay or paper be considered by them worthy of publication. If published, the distribution of said essay shall be entirely under the control of said trustees. In case they do not publish the said essay or paper, it shall be the property of the College of Physicians of Philadelphia." The prize is open for competition to the whole world, but the essay must be the production of a single person. The essay, which must be written in the English language, or, if in a foreign language, accompanied by an English translation, should be sent to the College of Physicians of Philadelphia, Pennsylvania, U.S.A., before January 1, 1892, addressed to Louis Starr, M.D., chairman of the William F. Jenks Prize Committee. Each essay must be distinguished by a motto, and accompanied by a sealed envelope bearing the same motto and containing the name and address of the writer. No envelope will be opened except that which accompanies the successful essay. The committee will return the unsuccessful essays if reclaimed by their respective writers, or their agents, within one year. The committee reserves the right not to make an award if no essay submitted is considered worthy of the prize.

THE

MONTREAL MEDICAL JOURNAL.

| VOL. XVIII. | JUNE, 1890. | No. 12. |

Original Communications.

CHOLECYSTECTOMY.

BY DR. E. A. PRAEGER, NANAIMO, B.C.

E. D., æt. 68 years, a widowed lady with good family history, was first seen by me six years and a half ago, when she fractured three ribs of the left side. About five years ago was attended by me for hepatic colic, which was relieved after the passage of gallstones. Enjoyed fair health till the commencement of the year, since when she had occasional attacks of pain in the region of the gall-bladder, always attended with vomiting.

About three months ago became jaundiced, suffered from incessant vomiting, and had great pain in the right hypochondrium. She was under continual medical supervision from that time till this date (Dec. 6th, 1889), when I was summoned by telegraph to Victoria to see her in consultation. The treatment up to this time had been confined to an endeavor to check the vomiting, which had resisted almost every anti-emetic in the pharmacopœia, and had now resolved itself into free administration of cocaine and morphia and peptonised injections per rectum, nothing being given by the mouth but ice and champagne. For weeks vomiting had been incessant, the fluid ejected being sometimes of a dark bilious character, at others a thick glairy mucus. No coffee grounds, no blood.

Examination.—Patient very emaciated ; conjunctivæ and skin tinged with bile ; urine loaded with bile. Pressure over stomach caused no pain. Liver dulness normal. Two inches below the ninth costal cartilage and to the right of the external

border of the right rectus muscle there was a slight upheav[al]
the abdominal wall. Palpation revealed the existence of a [well]
defined pear-shaped tumor, giving the sensation of deep fluc[tua]
tion, which was very dull on percussion, while slight pres[sure]
caused severe pain and vomiting.

It was evident that the patient was suffering from tox[ae]
[m]ia [or] retention of bile, and that the tumor was a disten[ded]
gall-bladder. The administration of phosphate of sodium [for a]
few days was recommended, and it was further suggested [that]
if relief were not afforded within that time, the urgency of [the]
symptoms, together with the existence of a tumor, rendere[d an]
exploratory incision not only justifiable, but expedient, in o[rder]
that the gall-bladder might be dealt with surgically if f[ound]
necessary. The question of operation was mentioned to [the]
patient, whose sufferings were so acute that she readily expre[ssed]
her willingness to submit.

Jan. 14*th*, 1890.—I saw no more of the case until to-[day]
when I was again summoned by telegram, asking me to be [pre]
pared to operate. On my arrival I was told that for se[veral]
days the patient had complained of pain over the upper pa[rt of]
the abdomen : that on the previous night there was a very [great]
swelling, with redness of the integument to the right of [the]
rectus muscle, reaching as low as the umbilicus : and that no[thing]
had been vomited for some days, although vomiting had [been]
[in]cessant and uncontrollable by cocaine and morphia. This s[well]
[i]ng had been manipulated for the purpose of examination.
[b]y the time I arrived it had almost disappeared and recollec[tion]
[se]rous fluid had again taken place. There was, however, a [de]
crease of pain over the upper part of the abdomen. O[wing]
[to] the relief [?] which had taken place (*i.e.*, the disappear[ance]
[of] the tumor) the weight of opinion was unfavorable to oper[ation]
[e]specially as it was considered a case of malignant disease [of the]
stomach.

[*Jan.*] 28*th*.—There having been no amelioration of the s[ymp]
[to]ms and the patient having urgently requested operation [it was]
again resorted to. The patient had lost ground, and as I fou[nd]
[after]wards soundly in consequence of a subcutaneous injec[tion]

three-fourths of a grain of morphia, I was rather unwilling to operate, but did so at the strong request of her relatives.

Operation, 3 *p.m.*—A very small quantity of ether was required to produce anæsthesia. An incision about two inches in length was made through the abdominal wall, parallel with the outer border of the rectus, immediately over the gall-bladder, which was found enormously distended, bent on itself like a retort, and bound by adhesions to the under surface of the liver and pylorus. The cystic duct was felt for, and being also bound by adhesions, was somewhat difficult to recognize with the finger. It was found blocked with calculi, which were dislodged and pushed back into the fundus. The duct was included between two ligatures, and the gall-bladder having been carefully freed from its attachments was gradually pulled out through the incision, the abdomen being packed with sponges to guard against rupture and escape of its contents. The duct was then cut through. A couple of fingers were then passed towards the stomach, which was found adherent to the abdominal wall. The toilet having been carefully performed, the wound was closed with silkworm gut sutures and covered with borated cotton. The patient was then returned to bed, with plenty of hot-water bottles. There was very slight (if any) shock, the pulse (104) being rather stronger than before operation. 10 *p.m.*—Patient had slept more or less all the afternoon, only asking once or twice for a small piece of ice. Temperature normal ; pulse 104 ; very drowsy.

Shortly after my visit, contrary to my desire, another large dose of morphia was given subcutaneously, the patient dying at 4 A.M. without awaking.

Jan. 27th.—An autopsy was made at mid-day, eight hours after death. There had been no oozing from any of the separated adhesions and the abdominal cavity was clean and dry. The liver was of a pale yellowish-gray color. Section of the right lobe showed nothing abnormal to the naked eye, but the left appeared somewhat mottled, with patches of yellowish-white, apparently fatty. There had been some recent localized peritonitis, the anterior surface of the stomach being attached by numerous recent adhesions to the abdominal wall. On opening the stomach it was found to contain about two ounces of a dirty, yellowish-brown liquid. The mucous membrane was highly congested, and there were a few ecchymosed patches. No ulceration ; no tumor. All traces of inflammation were confined to the gastro-hepatic region. All the other abdominal organs were healthy.

Specimen.—The gall-bladder, when removed from the abdomen, measured seven inches in length, and contained from six to eight ounces of fluid, its walls being distended to their utmost capacity. Unfortunately I placed it for a few days in undiluted alcohol, which caused it to shrink considerably and its walls to appear thicker. The fluid contents (bile) passed through and mixed with the spirit. Calculi can be felt in the fundus, the blood-vessels of which are very much larger than normal, and, altogether, it shows signs of great congestion.

Remarks.—It is unfortunate that operation was so long delayed, for even had it disproved the diagnosis of distended gall-bladder, an exploratory incision, made under aseptic precautions, would have done little, if any harm. While laying claim to no personal experience in the surgery of the gall-bladder, I submit that the symptoms not only justified, but made an exploration imperative. I started with the intention of performing cholecystotomy, but abandoned this in favor of extirpation, for the following reasons : There were no adhesions between the fundus and the abdominal wall, while it was firmly bound to the liver and pylorus, and this, together with signs of a localized peritonitis, made it appear to me probable or possible that there had been a leakage of biliary fluid from some part of the neck of the gall-bladder, while its extreme flexion on itself appeared to preclude the possibility of thorough drainage ; moreover, the walls were so thin, by reason of hyper-distension, that it occurred to me it was not wise to risk suturing them to the wound. While, unfortunately, the result adds to the mortality of an operation which will probably soon cease to be regarded as a " surgical audacity," I cannot help remarking that a rather too free use of morphia was probably an important factor in the untoward termination, and that to get good results the operator should have full charge of and take the entire responsibility of the after treatment.

I desire to record my indebtedness to Staff-Surgeon Fitzgerald, R.N. (in charge of the Royal Naval Hospital, Esquimalt), and to Dr. Davis of Nanaimo, for their valuable advice and assistance.

CASES IN PRACTICE.

By EDWARD EVANS, M.D., LaCROSSE, WIS.

Case I.—VOMITING OF PREGNANCY CURED BY LOCAL TREAT-
MENT OF CERVIX.

Mrs. S., aged 27, healthy; good personal and family history; six weeks pregnant, fourth pregnancy. Vomiting for past six weeks, getting worse all the time. Appetite fair, but vomits all food; vomits during night if she sits up in bed. Treated during past six weeks without benefit by two or more physicians. There seems to be no evidence of any gastric lesion. Bowels costive. Heart, lungs and urine normal. Uterus anteverted. There is flexion of the cervix, which is large and abnormally hard, with a slight left laceration; the os red, eroded and tender. I applied Arg. Nit. (g. xl. to oz.) to os and cervix, and put in a boro-glyceride tampon. This stopped vomiting for ten hours, when she had a fright, which produced symptoms of abortion (pain and hemorrhage); these were overcome by rest and opium. After a few days, on vomiting recurring, the treatment with arg. nit. and tampon was repeated (in all four times), and in the course of ten days vomiting had ceased and she went safely to full term. During first pregnancy she vomited the whole nine months; in second, vomiting stopped by local treatment in third month; aborted in third pregnancy.

Case II.—TYPHOID FEVER RELAPSE—PNEUMONIA OF RIGHT
BASE IN PRIMARY ATTACK AND RELAPSE—RECOVERY,
FOLLOWED BY SLIGHT PARESIS.

M. F., aged 30, farmer, entered St. Francis Hospital Oct. 9th, 1889, with a history of being very sick for the past eight days, though going about part of the time, and coming in eight

pain for the past few days, caused a good deal of swelling of face and glands, and a fever going on as high as 101.5°. I gave about a drachm of chloroform. The patient was a girl 3 years old and very healthy. In a few hours after the operation she suffered from great frequency of micturition, which continued for thirty-six hours and then abated slowly. The mother noticed the urine looked dark-red, as if containing blood. It continued so for four days, when she called my attention to it, and said it had not been so previous to operation. The child apparently suffered little, complaining once of some pain in back. Had no fever, but was sleeping and eating well, and evidently much relieved by opening of abscess. Urine evidently contained much blood, acid; specific gravity 1015. Boiling and nitric acid gave quite a large deposit. Under the microscope there were numerous red blood corpuscles and a few white, but no epithelium or tube casts. The blood seemed persisting under a treatment of warm bathing, free evacuation of bowels, rest and low diet, so I gave a mixture of gallic acid and ergot, and in a few days it had entirely disappeared. (What caused the blood in urine ?)

Retrospect Department.

QUARTERLY RETROSPECT OF SURGERY.

BY FRANCIS J. SHEPHERD, M.D., C.M., M.R.C.S., ENG.

Surgeon to the Montreal General Hospital; Professor of Anatomy and Lecturer on
Operative Surgery, McGill University.

Tuberculosis of the Bladder.—This affection is by no means
so rare as is supposed, and is one of the frequent causes of these
obscure diseases of the bladder which do not yield to ordinary
treatment. Of course the difficulty of diagnosis is often great,
and other organs, as the kidney, are frequently involved, and
thus the ailment in the bladder is masked. Of late years this
disease has attracted much attention, and Guyon of Paris has
successfully treated this affection by cystotomy and cauterization
of the tubercular ulcer.

In the *N. Y. Medical Record* for May 3rd, 1890, is an interesting paper by Dr. Alex. W. Stein on " *Tuberculosis of the
Bladder.*" He states that this affection is more frequent in the
male than the female. According to Erns only one case out of
twenty-five occurred in a female. The immunity of the bladder
in the female is due no doubt to the more perfect separation of
the reproductive and urinary organs. In the male the disease
usually extends by continuity from the reproductive to the urinary
organs. All ages are affected, but is more often seen in middle
life. There is much difference of opinion as to whether the
bladder is primarily or secondarily involved. Dr. Stein says
that he believes micro-organisms can extend to the bladder from
the prostate or kidney, but he is sceptical about these organisms
extending higher—that is, from the bladder to the kidney. Socin
reports cases of tuberculosis of the urethra and prostate lasting
for years without involving the bladder.

Dr. Stein says the diagnosis of tubercular disease is often
made with extreme difficulty; if there is no obstructive disease
of the urinary outlet, no renal derangement or other exciting
cause for the vesical irritability or hæmaturia, and other organs
are affected with tubercle (the lungs, testes, etc.), then there is
strong presumptive evidence that we have a case of tubercular

cystitis.   Absence of bacilli is not convincing proof of the non-
existence of the disease.   The progress of the disease is very
slow, sometimes lasting for fifteen or twenty years, and may
often be latent, extensive disease occurring without any symptoms referable to the bladder at all.   Again, we may have
disease of the kidneys and no disease of the bladder, and yet
vesical irritability is the most prominent symptom.

As a rule, when the lesions are in the neck of the bladder,
the pain is acute and lancinating, and referred to the glans penis
at the end of micturition ; frequent and painful micturition or a
sense of discomfort attending the act are symptoms seen sooner
or later in these cases.   In some cases there may be incontinence,
in others spasms are noticed with sudden stoppage of the stream.
This may lead to retention of urine from spasmodic contraction
of the sphincter.   Tuberculosis involving the orifice of one of the
ureters may cause obstruction sufficient to produce dilatation of
the ureter and hydronephrosis of that side.   The urine is at first
acid and cloudy, the turbidity being due to mucus and pus ; it
may become ammoniacal and decidedly viscid, shreds of tissue
and blood corpuscles are seen, etc.   The ulceration may be
coated over with phosphates and give the idea of calculus.
Hæmaturia is a prominent symptom, and may be an initial symptom, before even frequent micturition.   Still, again, it may be
absent during the whole course of the disease.   The blood is
seen at the end of micturition, and is usually but a few drops ;
coagulæ are rarely passed.   It may disappear and reappear.
All the symptoms of tubercular disease of the bladder are subject to exacerbations before softening and ulceration takes place,
and bladder irritability is not a prominent symptom, but as soon
as ulceration begins, rapid destruction of the mucous surface
takes place and the symptoms become well pronounced.

For treatment, Dr. Stein says irrigation of the bladder can
only wash out the products of inflammation and thus retard the
progress of the case ; instruments irritate.   In fact there is but
little to be done in these cases except to perform perineal section
or suprapubic cystotomy, so as to give the bladder as little to do
as possible.   The results of operative interference have not been

very encouraging, the disease returning after a few months.
Guyon and Reverdin curette and cauterize the bladder, whilst
Bardenhcuer and Shatz excise the entire mucous membrane.

Prof. Guyon of Paris, at the last French Surgical Congress
(1889), (*Annals des Mal. des Voies Urin.*, Nov. 1889,) gave
the latest account of his operations performed for tubercle of the
bladder in four cases. His method is to open the bladder above
the pubes, to explore carefully, and to remove the tubercular
patches in the mucous membrane by scraping and cautery. One
patient, aged 24, operated on in July 1885, was well in August
1889, and had gained flesh and strength. Another, a male,
died two years after operation, the operation not affording relief
and leaving a vesical fistula behind ; at the autopsy both kidneys
were the seat of tuberculous disease. The third case, with
symptoms of seven months' duration, was operated on in March
1888 ; patient had disease of right kidney ; urinated as many
as many as one hundred times a night ; patient improved until
the other kidney became affected, and died in February 1889 ;
autopsy showed both kidneys tuberculous, the right completely
obliterated and destroyed, and a number of tuberculous nodules
were found in the mucous membrane of the bladder. In the
fourth case, a male aged 34, cystotomy was performed in Dec.
1884 for tubercular cystitis, and patient died March 25th, 1885 ;
the whole posterior surface of the bladder showed ulceration
and granulations. The results in these cases were not very
encouraging, except where the disease is early and primarily
affects the bladder. This condition of the bladder is not easy to
diagnose without exploratory incision.

Dr. James Bell recently had a successful case of operation for
tubercular ulcer of the bladder at the Montreal General Hospital, and several months have now passed without recurrence.
In my opinion the future of this operation is not brilliant, chiefly
because when the bladder is diseased in the large majority of
cases some other part of the genito-urinary apparatus is also
affected.

At a meeting of the Clinical Society of London, held April
25th, 1890, Mr. W. H. Battle read a paper on *Tubercular*

Ulceration of the Bladder, in which suprapubic cystotomy and scraping were done (*Lancet*, May 3rd, 1890) and recovery re. sulted. The patient was a single girl aged 20 ; she had a maternal history of phthisis. For ten months she had some increased frequency of micturition, with some pain before the act, the urine had been thick and at times had contained blood. On admission to the Royal Free Hospital she was obliged to pass urine every hour and a half, and there was a feeling of fulness and aching pain, which emptying the bladder relieved ; urine alkaline, specific gravity 1015, and contained many pus and epithelial cells. Five days after admission the urethra was dilated and an ulcerated surface of considerable extent felt at the base of the bladder and posteriorly, while on the right side, was a pouch. The surface of the ulcerated patch was soft and vascular, with a well defined mucous margin. Various solutions were used without improvement. On April 3rd, after cystoscopic examination had demonstrated that the ulceration was as extensive as at first, the parts were scraped with the finger-nail and Volkmann's spoon, and later an emulsion of iodoform was used after micturition and a couple of drachms of the emulsion left in the bladder. Other injections were also used without benefit, so on July 29th suprapubic cystotomy was performed ; the ulcerated surface was well exposed and scraped with a sharp spoon, and afterwards daubed over with a solution of zinc chloride thirty grains to the ounce. A catheter was passed into the bladder and a drainage-tube into the wound. The drainage-tube was removed August 3rd and the catheter removed on the 10th. She was about on August 31st, and discharged from hospital Sept. 20th. She was seen again April 8th, 1890, and was then in good health, having been able to work since leaving the hospital. She could retain her urine for three hours, but had to get up several times during the night.

Examination of the tissue removed at the operation showed some caseous tuberculous deposit, but no bacilli were found, nor could any be discovered in the urine. Mr. Battle thought the case one of primary disease of the bladder. The paper closed by reviewing the work of Guyon, Reverdin and others in the same field. In the discussion which followed, Mr. Heath stated that he had treated a large number of cases of ulceration of the bladder successfully in women by applying strong solutions of nitrate of silver to the raw surface *per urethram*. Mr. Harry Fenwick doubted the correctness of the diagnosis. He said there were two distinct foms of ulceration—the tubercular and scrofulous. The former often led to a fatal termination within three years ; the latter, which was solitary, remained for months and years. He thought the treatment adopted too severe and that everything necessary could have been done through the urethra. He had found a five per cent. solution of lactic acid directly applied to the ulcer followed by much benefit, and he had used the same substance as an injection in the strength of one per cent. He exhibited a table of fifty cases of vesical ulceration which he had had under treatment. Mr. R. Johnson spoke favorably of treatment by injection of iodoform emulsion as used by Mr. Berkeley Hill—(iodoform 2 parts, mucilage 4 parts, glycerine 2 parts, water 20 parts).

Prolapse of the Rectum.—Dr. J. B. Roberts of Philadelphia describes (*Annals of Surgery*, April 1890) a *New Operation for the Relief of Complete Prolapse of the Rectum*, and reports a case. The steps of the operation are as follows : A small incision is made in the middle line near the apex of the coccyx, the finger introduced, and the cellular connections behind the rectum broken down. The sphincter muscle is then divided in two places by incisions situated each about half an inch away from the posterior median line. By carrying these incisions obliquely backwards through the skin until they meet at the original incision near the tip of the coccyx, a triangular portion of tissue, having as its base about one inch of the anal sphincter, is cut out, and with scissors a long triangular piece is cut out of the posterior wall of the rectum, the apex of the triangle being situated some three inches up the gut, whilst the base corresponds with the space between the two incisions and the sphincter. Hemorrhage having been controlled, the incised walls of the rectum are brought together with chromicised catgut sutures. The divided ends of the anal sphincter are now brought together

by two catgut sutures and one wire shotted suture. The anal
aperture is thus reduced so that it is barely possible to introduce
the tip of one's finger. A drainage tube of rubber is then introduced into the space between the rectum and the coccyx and
the original incision closed by numerous shotted wire sutures
carried deeply down into the tissues.

In the case reported there was considerable suppuration,
which rather interfered with proper healing, but the patient
could go up and down stairs without any tendency to prolapse
of the rectum.

Mr. Frederick Treves contributes an interesting paper on the
" *Treatment of Prolapse of the Rectum by Excision*," with a
report of three cases in which the operation recommended by
him was carried out. (*Lancet*, Feb. 22nd, 1890.) After describing the various causes of prolapse which is especially common
in children, he says the majority of cases yields to simple measures, as rest, removal of cause of trouble, improvement of the
general health, regulation of the bowels, and the use of astringent applications. When these fail, other methods of treatment
are in vogue, as—

(1) Subcutaneous injections into the ischio-rectal fossa of
ergot, nux vomica, carbolic acid, etc.

(2) The application of nitric acid, a method entirely condemned by Mr. Treves, and which is spoken of as " little less
than barbarous," although recommended in most text-books and
frequently carried out with success.

(3) The application of the actual cautery to the mucus membrane of the prolapse or the removal of linear folds of that membrane by clamp and cautery. This method is also condemned
by Mr. Treves, who looks upon all the methods above described
as " clumsy, uncouth, uncertain, and unsafe," and therefore not
to be practised by modern surgeons. He also says that the
method of excision is simple, final, and not painful, and offers
the best claims of being a " radical cure." The operation recommended by him is performed as follows : The rectum having
been well emptied by an aperient, followed by an enema, the
patient was anæsthetized and placed in the lithotomy position.

Clover's crutch was employed and the buttocks raised. The mucous membrane within the lumen of the prolapse was seized at some height above the aperture of the bowel with tongue forceps and pulled down ; three pairs of such forceps were employed, and were applied at different points on the rectal wall. When it was evident that the whole relaxed mucous membrane was entirely drawn down, the forceps were allowed to remain attached. They served to indicate the real apex of the protrusion and to allow a hold to be taken of the part, while this weight prevented any great recesssion of the everted mucous membrane. A circular cut was now made around the base of the prolapse at the exact spot where the skin joined the mucous membrane ; the incision involved the mucous membrane only. This was next dissected off, turning the whole of it down like a cuff ; it was dissected entirely with scissors and forceps. When separation was complete the prolapse had an hour-glass shape, the waist of the hour-glass corresponding to the site of the apex of the protrusion. There was no bleeding. The external anal sphincter, hypertrophied, was now exposed, and within it the internal sphincter could be defined. The left forefinger was now introduced into the lumen of the prolapse, and it was ascertained that the prolapse consisted of mucous membrane only. This layer of mucous membrane was next divided at a level with the anus by scissors ; as each cut was made the parts were seized with pressure forceps and so all bleeding was immediately arrested. After all bleeding was controlled, the mucous membrane was attached to the skin at the margin of the anus with sutures of silkworm gut, then dressed with iodoform or wool. In his first case he was tempted to excise a portion of the external sphincter in order to lessen the size of the anus ; one inch of the muscle was removed and the divided ends brought together with catgut stitches. Mr. Treves now thinks this proceeding unnecessary, and gives rise to some pain and much tenesmus.

Operative Treatment of Cancer of the Rectum.—In the *Annals of Surgery* for March, 1890, is an interesting resumé of the present views on the operative treatment of rectal cancer and of which a short account is given below.

M. Routhier (*Bull. et Mem. de la Soc. Chirurgie de Paris*) reports a case in which he successfully removed four inches of the rectum which was the seat of an annular carcinoma. The lower border of the growth was four inches above the external sphincter. The patient was a woman aged 29. The method of operating was by the posterior or sacral method. The coccyx was removed and the lower angle of the sacrum. The rectum was easily separated from the sacrum, but the separation from the vaginal wall was more difficult; in fact, the peritoneal cul-de-sac was opened and afterwards sutured. The cancerous portion of the rectum was removed and then the two cut ends of the rectum sewn together. The wound was stuffed with iodoform gauze. The case did remarkably well. The bowels moved on the seventh day, the sphincter acting perfectly.

Statistics of excision of the rectum have been given by various men. Frank, in the *Dublin Journal of the Medical Sciences*, vol. lxxxiii, gives a mortality of 30 per cent. done by the older surgeons. Gross, in his *System of Surgery*, gives a mortality of 20 per cent. in a total of 193 cases; Ball, in 175 cases, a mortality of 16 per cent.; and Cripps puts it at 17 per cent. in 76 cases. There is much in the proper selection of cases. Czerny, out of 45 cases, considered only 25 fit subjects for operation, and of these only one died. Koenig, at the German Surgical Congress of 1888, had operated on 50 patients with a mortality of 10 per cent; 18 per cent. had no return in four years, and 10 per cent. no return in three years. Bardenheuer lowered the mortality to 5 per cent., and mentions three cases (women) which remained cured after a lapse of six, seven and eight years.

The great objection to the circular amputation is the removal of the sphincter ani. Now all operators cut the rectum across, above and below the growth, as far as possible from it. Kraske and many others slit the posterior wall of the rectum down to the sphincter before making the transverse cut below the cancer. Kraske has abandoned the complete circular suture, and in order to prevent the escape of fæces into the abdominal cavity provides an artificial anus at the line of suture. Others (Heinede and

Hochenegg) go further and suture the upper cut end of the intestine to the cutaneous borders of the sacral incision, reserving the closure of the artificial anus for a later operation. Schede, again, makes a complete suture and then establishes a temporary artificial anus in the inguinal region. All surgeons leave the sacral wound open and stuff it with iodoform gauze.

With regard to the peritoneum, Kraske proposes a deliberate opening of the peritoneum to facilitate the pulling down of the intestine. Bardenheuer strips the peritoneum from the intestine. Most operators deliberately open the peritoneum and tampon it during the rest of the operation with iodoform gauze. Some do not close the peritoneal wound and others close it only partially, leaving a drain in the opening. The abdominal cavity is closed by a few operators, the parietal peritoneum being sutured to the serous covering of the bowel.

Dr. R. Stierlin (*Brun's Beiträge zur Klin. Chirurgie*, 1889, Bd. v., Hft. 3), in an article on this subject, after giving the history and statistics of the operation, says the operation is indicated in different types of cases.

(1) In carcinoid of anal portion, the diseased tissues should be excised and the healthy mucous membrane sutured.

(2) In carcinoma extending circularly upwards from the anus, but easily detachable, Listrani's method of amputation should be practised, with, if necessary, a posterior incision of the rectum. Continence is fairly satisfactory without a pad, and hence this method is to be preferred to the sacral method of Hochenegg.

(3) For carcinoma beginning considerably above the anus and extending circularly upwards, Kraske's operation is indicated, the sphincter is saved and incision of the posterior wall avoided.

(4) For very aggravated carcinoma, the sacral method is the only one adapted.

(5) For limited tumors of the rectal wall, when near the anus, Stierlin's divided incisions will usually make them accessible. When appearing in culpse transverse, if possible, is excised, the edges united and the wound drained.

Before passing the incisions should be thoroughly and completely disinfected. That seven or eight to ten days, sutures, injections of water and harmless antiseptics by means of a tube carried well up the bowel. The bladder should be emptied immediately before operation. For primary disinfection of the wound, sublimate (1–2000) and iodoform have proven the best. The drainage must be thorough ; strips of iodoform gauze alone or an unperforated tube wrapped in the same are the best. The parts should be cleansed once or twice daily with a weak sublimate lotion. Opiates are given at first ; later, laxatives. As soon as the drain and sutures are removed, and the wound is granulating, the patient is bathed once or twice a day. The dressing consists of sublimate wool and wool cushions retained by a T bandage. The peritoneum was injured and immediately sutured without bad result. Suture of the cut ends of the gut in the operation by the sacral method is necessary. In complete circular suture it is as well to pass a large drain up the rectum beyond the sutured spot to avoid fæcal stasis. In the ordinary operation the patient should be in the lithotomy position ; in the sacral operation, on the side. Dr. Stierlin's mortality in 22 cases of radical operation was two—one from delirium tremens and one from retro-peritoneal phlegmon. As a palliative method he prefers intra-peritoneal colotomy to scraping, cauterization or linear rectotomy. With regard to the after results, six of his cases are alive after one to four years without recurrence, two are alive with recurrence, and eight have died. He considers that cases which have remained free from recurrence after three years may be regarded as definitely cured.

At the last annual meeting (1889) of the British Medical Association, held in Leeds, a most interesting discussion on *Cancer of the Rectum* took place. The discussion was opened by Mr. Jessop of Leeds. He divided the operative measures into radical and palliative. *Proctectomy* or excision of the rectum he placed among the established surgical procedures, and reported seven cases with one death. Of the six favorable cases, in three the disease was in the posterior or lateral wall of the rectum, above the sphincter, and entirely within reach of the finger ; these three patients are alive, two after 21 and 17 months, and in one there was recurrence in seven months. In a fourth case there was no return of the disease at the end of 13 months. In the two others the disease was high up, but the disease was removed without much difficulty; in one case the peritoneal cavity was opened, but no sutures were introduced, and free drainage used with good result. In these cases there has been no return in 20 and 26 weeks respectively. In the cases where no sutures were used the result was quite as good as where they were used. He washed the rectum out every eight hours for several days.

Mr. Jessop had performed colotomy (lnmbar) 103 times. He was of opinion that in cancers high up colotomy should be performed as soon as obstruction appears. The average duration of life after colotomy was 22½ months; when the operation was not performed, the average duration of life was 17 months. Complete relief of pain and distress is never obtained, but the continuous pain is lessened in severity and the almost constant desire to evacuate the bowels disappears in some and is diminished in others.

Marsh and Banks advocated a preliminary colotomy in all cases where excision of the rectum was undertaken. In colotomy Mr. Banks completely divides the colon and stitches the upper end of the gut into the wound.

Mr. H. Cripps said that excision was only applicable to a small proportion of cases (about 20 per cent.), and should not be undertaken if the upper limit of the growth is beyond the reach of the finger, or if it has extended to other organs. Of 30 cases operated on he had two deaths—one from erysipelas and one from exhaustion. The duration in the 28 cases that recovered was as follows: In six, no after history; ten, recurrence within a year; four, recurrence between the first and third years; one died without recurrence a year after operation; one no recurrence after eighteen months, and one no recurrence at end of three months; one, two years, one, three years, one, four years, and one no recurrence after nine years. Mr. Cripps operates with patient in the lithotomy position and buttocks raised. A sharp-pointed, curved bistoury is passed up the bowel and then by transfixion is made to protrude through the skin on a level with the side of the coccyx, the whole of the intervening tissues being cut through. A crescentic incision is now made, extending from the margin of the first cut to a point in the middle line in front. This cut should extend well into the fat of the ischio-rectal fossa, and, if the disease is not too low down, should go through the mucous membrane so as not to interfere with the skin at the anal margin. Dissection is now carried upwards to a point well beyond the disease, and the same is done on the opposite side. A sound in the bladder of the male will greatly assist. The bowel is then cut across and not sutured. The wound is packed for thirty-six hours, and after the second week bougies are passed regularly. Mr. Cripps reported 14 cases of lumbar and 26 cases of inguinal colotomy with only one death.

Mr. Allingham said that excision was justifiable only in those cases where there was a small annular growth freely movable, and only when this starts two inches up the rectum, and where the upper limit of the growth can be easily felt. His method of excision, which he claims can be accomplished in 15 minutes, is as follows : Lithotomy position ; left forefinger in rectum. A straight bistoury is introduced half an inch behind the rectum, keeping outside the rectum to a depth of three inches, and the cut made to the coccyx. Next the rectum is divided in the whole of its circumference between the sphincters, then with scissors the tissues on either side of the bowel are divided and a careful dissection is made along the anterior wall up to a point beyond the disease, when the rectum is cut across.

Mr. McGill had substituted colectomy for colotomy in the lumbar region. In two cases in which he did colectomy death resulted from a gangrenous condition developing as a result of retained fæces in the lower portion of the bowel. He would therefore not recommend the operation unless this upper end of the lower portion was left open in the wound.

Dr. Charles Kelsey, in a clinical lecture (*N.Y. Med. Journal*, May 3rd, 1890) describes his method of operating for cancer of the rectum. The patient is placed in the lithotomy position, with buttocks well raised. After dilating the sphincter and intro-ducing a sound into the bladder for a guide, an incision is made through the anus in the median line behind, down to the tip of the coccyx. The left index finger is now placed in the gut and a bistoury is introduced behind the growth and pushed along the cellular tissue outside the bowel until its point is fully half an inch beyond the disease. The first incision is made to extend to this depth, and is tightly packed with sponges, no time being lost in tying vessels. Next, with a pair of straight, blunt-pointed, long scissors the rectum is cut through completely by a circular incision half an inch below the growth and between it and the sphincters. Then with the finger as a guide still in the diseased bowel, the cellular tissue of the ischio-rectal fossa and the levator ani is boldly cut into, first on the right, then on the left side, until the bowel has been completely separated from its attachments on all sides, except anteriorly, and to a point at least half an inch above the disease. This takes very little time, and as fast as the incision is made it is packed tightly with sponges. The next step is a careful dissection of the rectum from its anterior attachments, and this may take some time if the disease has involved the base of the bladder and deep urethra. After the rectum is dissected anteriorly above the limit of the disease it is cut off cylindrically and removed. The sponges are now removed and the bleeding points secured. The upper end of the bowel is now sutured to the lower as closely as possible, but nothing in the way of complete apposition or suturing is attempted and the wound is intended to heal by granulation. Three deep silver wire sutures are then put in the posterior incision and left without tightening until the end of the first week, so that there may be perfect drainage. The wound is irrigated with sublimate solution, packed with charpie, and dusted with iodoform. A drainage-tube is placed on each side of the rectum. This operation can be performed in from fifteen to twenty minutes.

Radical Cure of Hernia.—Dr. D. Hayes Agnew says (*University Medical Magazine*, April, 1890) that he does not think present operators should commit themselves to present plans until both in time and in number the necessary data for the expression of an authoritative opinion have accumulated. Dr. Agnew says, with the caution gained from years of experience and observation, that "any one who has followed the literature of the different surgical processes for the radical cure of hernia, and for most of which great success has been claimed (*e.g.*, Wurtzer's operation), and then discovers that all have fallen into disuse, becomes, naturally, a little sceptical of the trustworthiness of surgical statements." At the present time he thinks the knife is out on a grand revel, and is too often used without due consideration for human life. His views as to the necessity for operative measures in cases of hernia are as follows :

(1) The radical plan should follow all cases of strangulated hernia when it is necessary to use the knife.

(2) Cases of hernia in adults which cannot be controlled by mechanical means.

(3) Children under ten years of age who have rupture are not proper subjects for operation ; such patients usually recover after wearing a truss for two or three years.

New Operations for the Radical Cure of Hernia.—Now that the radical cure of hernia has become fashionable, and is an operation frequently performed, each surgeon is devising some method which surpasses every other hitherto employed, so that the invention of a new operation for the radical cure of hernia is as common as was formerly the invention of a new pessary, and these operations are called after the inventor's name. At present we have Macewen's, Ball's, Bank's, Barker's, Frank's, McBurney's, etc. Each operation is a perfect success in the hands of the operator, but others are not so successful with them. The success of the operation is judged, not by the number of permanent cures (for usually too short a time has elapsed before the cases are reported), but by the small number of deaths due to the operation.

One of the latest operations for the radical cure of hernia is that devised by Dr. Halstead of Baltimore (*Johns-Hopkins Hosp. Bull.*, Dec. 1889), and it is as follows : The incision begins at the external abdominal ring and ends one inch or less to the inner side of the anterior (superior ?) spine of the ilium in an imaginary line connecting the anterior-superior spines of the ilia. Throughout the entire incision, everything superficial to the

... errupted, strong, silk sutur
... ... tween the skin and
... .per portion of the wou
... ... noes to the outer
... ... ernead to these sutures
... ... ne men to the inner
... ... um. The skin is
... ... very fine silk.
... ... when tied become
... ... of the skin and
... ... ivers not occupied b
... ... as wounds thi
... ... um from his
... ... disinfect the skin
... ... may e present a
... ... ng he oeration
... ... s vound truns.
... ... is een suggested
lancet Journal.
... ... Mac=won a
... ... somewhat
... ... oin
... ... vi
... ... ion.

the abdominal wall from within outwards. The same thing is done on the opposite side. When both threads are presenting through the abdominal muscular structures they are pulled up, the sac being at the same time invaginated before the finger as the threads are drawn upon ; the sac is thus turned inside out on its passage and becomes fixed as a rounded bow exactly over the internal ring. The ends of the threads are then tied firmly over the ring. Mr. Bishop says the whole pad forms, as it were, a bridge—a Roman arch—over the weak place on the abdominal wall, of which bridge the fundus forms the keystone. The article is well illustrated, and theoretically the procedure seems most excellent, but, unfortunately, the sac has not the consistency of a Roman arch, and in some cases is composed of very flimsy material indeed. However well the operation may look diagrammatically, in reality it would not, I think, come up to anticipated expectations.

At a recent meeting of the Royal Medico-Chirurgical Society of London (*Lancet*, April 12th, 1890), Mr. Barker gave the results of a study of fifty consecutive cases of operation for the radical cure of non-strangulated herniæ. There was not a single death. True suppuration of the wound only occurred in two cases. There were no cases of wound infection or shock. The ages of the patients varied from three months to seventy years. In the discussion which followed, most of the speakers advised against operation in young children, and held that if properly treated by truss the case tended to cure.

Prof. Eduard Bassini of the University of Padua reports 262 cases of radical cure of hernia (*Archiv für Klin. Chir.*, Bd. xl., Hft. 2, 1890) treated by the following operation. The incision is made through the skin and the canal slit up, the cord separated from the neck of the sac, the sac dissected out, and any adherent intestines or omentum separated. The neck of the sac is freed and ligatured and then cut off, and when the neck of the sac is large it is tied off in two pieces. The cord is then kept in the upper angle of the wound and held up, whilst the conjoined tendon is separated from the aponeurosis of the external abdominal oblique and then sutured by a continuous suture to

Poupart's ligament, the cord not being included, but is repla in its proper direction and remains superficial to this la sutures. Then, finally, the aponeurosis of the external abdom oblique is sutured over the cord, and the skin is brought toget over all. Drainage is only used when the hernia is large. the 262 cases, 12 were strangulated and 251 non-strangula both reducible and irreducible. These 251 cases occurred 216 individuals—10 females and 206 males; the youngest i 13 months and the oldest 69 years. In 196 cases the her was acquired and in 55 congenital. Of the 251 cases of n strangulated herniæ only 1 died, fifteen days after the operati and after the wound was completely healed. The cause of de was pneumonia, and the post-mortem showed that the wound l been aseptic throughout and that the pneumonia did not depe on this operation. There was no return in 108 cases in from f and a half to one year; in 33 cases from one year to six mont and from six months to one month, no return in 98 cases. 7 cases there was return, 4 cases were lost sight of, and 1 di Of these cases, in 108 complete healing took place in from n to thirteen days, in 66 from fourteen to sixteen days, and in from seventeen to thirty days. Of the 11 cases of strangulat hernia he had to excise a portion of omentum in all, and in case was the bowel gangrenous: 9 cases rapidly recovered, a 2 died—one twenty-one days after the operation, the other h hours after.

Treatment of Fractured Patella.—At a meeting of the N York Academy of Medicine, held Feb'y 10th, 1890, the ab subject was discussed, and a number of cases illustrating the sults of treatment by different methods were shown by membe

Dr. W. T. Bull read a paper on the *Results of Treatment Fracture of the Patella without Operation* (N.Y. Med. Rec March 22nd, 1890), and exhibited cases to illustrate the pap He recorded 22 cases which he had treated during the last fif years, and which he had been able to follow; 22 other ca were lost sight of. These 22 cases are represented by ninete patients, as three had fractures on both sides at different tim Six cases were refractures. Of the 16 fractures, he found :

excellent result in 14 and a bad result in 2 (87½ per cent. satisfactory). In 10 of the 14, flexion and extension of the limb was complete and strong and the ligament firm, with little or no atrophy of the thigh, so they were classified as " functionally perfect." There were 4 cases where flexion or extension was imperfectly performed, with a joint useful, according to the patient's statement, for all the purposes of his or her occupation. In 2 cases there was no power of extension at all, and the patients are compelled to wear supports or walk with a cane. In all the cases the treatment was the same, viz., plaster-of-Paris bandages after the effusion has subsided with the application beneath the splint of an adhesive plaster strip to steady the fragments, the fragments of the patella being kept in apposition by figure-of-8 turns of a bandage. The bandage is left on six weeks, then removed, and patient allowed to go about with a splint of leather to back of knee. This latter is worn for six weeks and the thigh and knee vigorously shampooed and kneaded. At the end of three months the patient can bend the limb but slightly, but power of extension has been good. In the discussion which followed, the consensus of opinion was against operative measures, and many cases of accident and some deaths were recorded as the result of wiring the patella. No doubt the results are brilliant in many cases where no complications occur, but when suppuration takes place ankylosis of the knee is a favorable termination.

Laparotomy for Appendicitis in its Quiescent Stage.—Dr. Robert Weir, in an article on the above subject (*Medical News,* March 1st, 1890), says that it cannot be considered as settled that surgery is justified in its interference by the removal of an appendix when symptoms of urgency are not present, notwithstanding the teaching of Mr. Frederick Treves. He asks that more consideration be given to this point before accepting too hastily the maxim that the " ounce of prevention" theory applies to an appendix which has given rise to sundry previous attacks of pain and perhaps dangerous tumefactions in the iliac region. He goes on to say that we are ignorant in a great measure of the simpler forms of appendical trouble, such as inflammation pure and simple, or associated after a while with stenosis of some part of its canal, and how often such a stenosis will beget trouble by accumulation of retained materials. He has been struck, when witnessing laparotomies for the ablation of the appendix in its quiescent stage, by the total absence in each case of any trace of peritoneal changes from previous attacks of pain, many of which were reported to have been severe. In most of the cases there was only stenosis with a moderate accumulation of mucus or muco-pus beyond the removed portion. He has seen fatal results follow this removal in the quiescent stage, and concludes that in any but exceptional cases (such as where the attacks of recurrent appendicitis are so frequent as to impair the patient's usefulness in life) is it justifiable to perform an operation of acknowledged risk, such as the removal of the appendix when the patient is not suffering from an attack of appendicitis.

In a discussion on the above subject at a meeting of the Practitioners Society of New York (*N.Y. Med. Record*, April 26th, 1890), Dr. W. T. Bull, after reviewing the literature on the subject, said that while he should not, in the light of present experience, encourage operations after one attack of appendicitis without urgent symptoms, he was unqualifiedly in favor of them when attacks frequently occur. Although some surgeons look upon the operation in simple uncomplicated appendicitis as one of the easiest and safest of all intra-abdominal operations, yet in his experience it was not always so, for the appendix and cæcum are often buried in adhesions and the dissection was complicated and tedious. He mentioned one case where he had performed this operation in a lady aged 63, who had attacks of appendicitis every three weeks for four months; they last only a few days and were accompanied by fever. A small ileo-cæcal tumor could be felt. On opening the peritoneum the appendix was found imbedded in a mass of plastic exudation. He decided not to dissect out the appendix, because the operation would have been prolonged, difficult and risky on account of the extensive raw surfaces which would be left behind in the peritoneal cavity, so he closed the peritoneal wound and left a drain in the wound outside the cavity. He mentioned several other similar cases. Another objection to the operation is that it is sometimes followed by serious ventral hernia. He had seen half a dozen cases during the winter, and the victims complained bitterly of their condition. With this additional uncertainty attached to the fate of the patient, and with the traditional uncertainty of the course of the disease, it is of importance that we bring every accessible fact to light that can help us to formulate a safe rule of treatment.

Dr. Peabody said the physician should decide in what cases operation was necessary. These were where the attacks frequently recurred and the danger of their recurring at a time when surgical aid could not be reached if it were demanded.

Dr. W. H. Draper said he had seen a number of cases of recurring appendicitis in which recovery had taken place without operation. He could not recall a fatal case of peritonitis from appendicitis where there had been a previous attack. In his experience the fatal cases had been in persons who had never before had an attack.

Dr. Andrew Smith recalled six cases of appendicitis with suppuration, in three of which surgeons operated and all died; while the other three not operated on recovered. Of the six, in only one case was the disease recurrent.

Dr. Geo. F. Shrady related the case of a physician who had had four attacks of appendicitis, in all of which the question of operation arose. Dr. Shrady had seen the patient in three attacks, all of which were pronounced. The fourth attack occurred in Paris, where the question of operation came up. Each attack was attended with all the severe symptoms indicating the formation of an abscess—there was dulness, tenderness, more or less rigidity, and some œdema in the neighborhood of the cæcum. In each attack the patient was willing to take the risks of operation, but in each case the symptoms gradually disappeared and he recovered. He asked Dr. Shrady, should he survive him, to examine his appendix, which was done when death occurred some time subsequently from another cause. The appendix was found perfectly normal. There was not the slightest appearance of any inflammation around it; it was not even thickened.

Dr. Partridge said there was a class of cases to which but

little attention had been paid where the appendix, when cut down upon, would be found distended, containing, perhaps, a good deal of pus, the cases giving only a history of recurrent pain, showing that a considerable time had been occupied in the production of the pathological changes, and yet very little surrounding peritoneal inflammation or adhesion would be found to have taken place. These cases, when recurrent, were highly dangerous. He concluded by saying that where there were repeated attacks of local pain pointing to appendicitis, but without induration, he would suppose the prognosis grave.

Dr. Mitchell Clark and Mr. J. Greig Smith of Bristol report (*Lancet*, May 3rd, 1890) a successful case of removal of the appendix during the quiescent period for recurrent attacks of inflammation. The patient was a girl aged 22, and had had two well-marked attacks of appendicitis. At the operation a number of adhesions were found and the appendix with great difficulty brought to the surface ; it was the size of one's thumb, thickened, red and distended. In it were found three orange pips covered with mucus and fæces; it was tied off, and, after sewing the peritoneum over the stump, returned. Mr. Greig Smith says the operation was not an easy one, and advises no one to attempt it who has not had some considerable experience in abdominal surgery and full confidence in his sense of touch. As a possible factor in the decision as to the removal during a quiescent period this question of surgical difficulty and perhaps danger must be reckoned with. A few of the cases operated upon have been easy, and then no adhesions, but a number are described as having had adhesion of the tip of the appendix to some outlying part ; in others the presence of adhesions is simply noted. Mr. Smith asks : " Is it not possible that too much weight is given to a foreign body in the appendix and too little to fixation of its apex, as a cause of irritation, catarrh, distension and rupture ?"

In an article headed *Indications for Abdominal Section and the Details of its Performance*, Mr. Lawson Tait (*N. Y. Med. Record*, May 3rd, 1890) attributes both the invention of the modern artery forceps and the introduction of the drainage-tube to Kœberlé of Strasbourg. He says the drainage-tube has reduced the mortality 10–15 per cent. He washes out the abdomen with a stream of water from a bucket, and by means of a strong current gets rid of " all rubbish from the crannies and crevices," even oozing from adhesions may be stopped by a current of water like this. The after-treatment is conducted practically by nurses. For the first twenty-four hours the patient is not allowed to swallow anything at all, except, perhaps, a little warm water. Vomiting is a serious complication after an abdominal section, but the best way to avoid vomiting is to avoid giving patients anything they can vomit. He believes that the deprivation of fluids in the stomach favors absorption of the effusion in the peritoneum. The second day he gives a few tablespoonsful of milk and soda. The third day is the critical day, and the first indication of the scondary changes is distension of the epigastrium suggestive of peritonitis. In such a case the patient is given a small saline purge and a turpentine enema, and this will enable her to pass flatus. He does not care a bit for anything save distension, and never has any trouble if it is treated at once in this way. The temperature in abdominal surgery is a matter of very secondary importance, the pulse being the great guide, and whenever it rises to 120 a minute, there is reason to be anxious. Temperature rise alone has no value as an indication of danger, but the safest guide of all is the expression of the face. An anxious expression keeps him on tenter-hooks, and a woman who will not keep quiet after an operation, but will go on chattering, is almost sure to die.

Two Hundred and Fifty Extirpations of the Thyroid Gland by Dr. Th. Kocher.—Six years ago the author reported 58 cases of extirpation of the thyroid gland, and computed the mortality of the operation as 13.9 per cent. Since then he has performed 250 operations with six deaths, a mortality of only 2.4 per cent. And if we exclude the cases in which the operation was done for malignant struma or the goitre of Basedow's disease, the mor. tality sinks to only .8 per cent. On the ground of these statistics Kocher maintains that the operation, when practised for simple goitre, is perfectly free from danger, independent of the size of the growth and the age of the patient. The author has not found it necessary to modify the technique of the operation. He warns us that in ligaturing the inferior thyroid at the point where the vertical portion of the vessel becomes horizontal, we should exercise special care to avoid wounding the recurrent nerve and the cardiac branches of the sympathetic. Of especial importance also is the most scrupulous antisepsis of the wound. To prevent the cachexia which follows complete extirpation of the thyroid gland, it is necessary to leave behind any portions of the gland still capable of performing their function. He concludes as follows : (1) Extirpation is indicated in malignant and inflamed goitres, and in diffuse hypertrophies of the thyroid gland ; it is contraindicated if healthy gland tissue is absent on the other side. (2) Enucleation is indicated in cystic goitre ; that is, goitres in which a cyst forms the main portion of the tumor, and in cases of isolated large nodular goitres which are imbedded in well-preserved gland tissue, and in cases where large nodules are present in immovable goitres, if the nodules are soft and are surrounded by a vascular zone. (3) Resection is reserved for the numerous class of cases which do not fulfil the above indications ; contraindications are malignant and immovable goitres, and those which are the seat of infectious inflammation. (4) Ligature of the thyroids is indicated in vascular goitre either as a method of treatment or as introductory to a subsequent partial extirpation or resection. Only those arteries should be tied in whose districts the changes are most marked.—(Quoted in the *Edinburgh Med. Jour.*, March, 1890.)

Hemorrhoids treated by the Clamp and Cautery.—Dr. B. Gibbs, in a paper read before the Alumni Society of Bellevue Hospital, Feb. 5th, 1890 (*N.Y. Medical Journal*, April 26th, 1890), strongly advocated this method of treatment. He has a record of over two hundred cases without a single case of hemorrhage, and he has never seen any septic complications. In five or six hours after the operation the perineal pad is removed, and if there is any soreness hot applications are applied. The patient is allowed to get out of bed to pass water as soon as the urine shows itself. After this no dressings used, and no suppositories of iodoform or others employed. A laxative is given within forty-

eight hours. He has found no pain follow this operation or retention of urine.

In the discussion which followed the reading of the paper,
Dr. Kelsey said he had formerly advocated the method by ligature, but latterly he has used the clamp and cautery with the
best results. There was less pain, no greater danger from hemorrhage, and it cured the patient in less time. Dr. Kelsey also
stated that he had formerly been a very strong advocate of the
method of injection by carbolic acid, and had reported 200 consecutive cases treated in this way without bad result, but immediately after he met with his first unfortunate case. The operation was followed by an unusually large slough, by a peri-proc-
titis or ischio-rectal abscess. The operation was not radical, and
was dangerous on account of its uncertain action. He did not
think the operation of Mr. Whitehead any better than the clamp
and cautery, and it was much more tedious.

Hospital Reports.

MONTREAL GENERAL HOSPITAL.

*Three Cases of Fracture of the 6th Cervical Vertebra, followed
by complete Paraplegia, Motor and Sensory, below the 3rd
Intercostal space, with surgical procedure in two cases
for relief of the Spinal Cord by Dr. Jas. Bell.*

(Reported by Dr. W. S. England.)

Case I.—E. P., aged 50, a French-Canadian, was brought
to the hospital, per ambulance, July 19th, 1889, having fallen
off a scaffold, a distance of thirty-five feet, striking on his feet;
thinks a falling plank struck him on the back. Personal and
family history of no importance.

Examination.—Patient is in a fair state of nutrition; assumes
the dorsal decubitus and presents the appearance of helplessness;
flexor surfaces of hands and arms dependent; elbows slightly
flexed. Respiration diaphragmatic; abdomen moves passively
with inspiration and expiration. Paralysis of body below the
arms; voluntary power of arms weakened; paralysis of flexors

and interossei ; voluntary power of extensors slight. Sensat
as to touch, pain and temperature absent below the 3rd int
costal space ; also absent over ulnar and extensor surfaces
arms ; present over radial flexor aspects. Reflexes : patell
cremasteric, abdominal and ankle clonus absent ; pupillary ref
present, pupils contracted ; no deformity of the back. Subj
tive sensations : complains of pain in the back of the ne
between shoulders, and in right elbow ; general sense of cc
ness. Urine negative ; penis passively congested ; retention
urine. *Treatment*—Palliative.

July 21st—Developed cough ; a few râles in chest.

July 22nd, a.m.—Dyspnœa ; rattling in the throat ; inte
gence still good ; loss of sensation has extended up to 2nd int
space. 7 *p.m.*—Slight delirium ; temperature 102°F.; sc
became unconscious, and died from respiratory failure.

Autopsy.—Fracture of body of 6th cervical vertebra and co
pression of about half an inch of cord ; separation of poster
ligament for about one inch ; hemorrhage into cord.

CASE II.—P. St. A., aged 40, was brought to the hospit
per ambulance, on the morning of the 25th October, 1889, h
ing fallen off a ladder on to the back of his head and ne
When first seen by the ambulance doctor, patient was quite c
scious, but paraplegic.

Examination.—Patient is a well-nourished man, in g
general health ; lies in a helpless state ; respiration wholly
phragmatic ; paralysis of body below arms ; complete paral
of flexors of arms ; paresis of extensors ; able to supinate h
to a moderate degree ; sensation lost below the 4th rib in fr
and blades of scapulæ behind, also absent over ulnar and tric
surfaces of arms, but present elsewhere ; marked tenderness
deep pressure at the lower cervical area ; bending forward
head and rotation caused pain ; reflexes absent ; pupils o
tracted ; intellect good. Complains of slight pain only an
feeling of general numbness over the body, most marked in
legs ; priaprism ; loss of desire to micturate. Pulse strong
full, 72 per minute ; temperature 102°F.; respirations 22.

Oct. 26th.—General condition unchanged. After a consultation of the staff being held, Dr. Bell decided to operate with the view of removing pressure from the spinal cord if it existed. Chloroform was administered, patient turned on his face, and occiput and back of neck shaved and cleansed. An incision about four inches long was made over the lower cervical vertebræ, reaching to the spinous processes and laminæ ; the tissues were removed by a rasparatoire. On examination, found a fracture of the left laminæ of 5th and 6th cervical vertebræ. The right laminæ were also cut by the bone forceps, and by the aid of the knife and lion forceps the membranes covering the cord were readily exposed. These appeared normal ; the spinal canal was examined above and below the opening and seemed regular and even. The dura mater was picked up and incised ; a considerable quantity of a reddish cerebro-spinal fluid escaped; the cord looked normal on its surface, no irregularity or evidence of traumatism at any part. Thought it proper to desist from further interference. Sutured membranes by a continuous fine catgut suture ; rubber drain inserted ; muscles and skin brought together by deep silk sutures ; iodoform and gauze dressing. Patient made a good recovery from the operation.

Oct. 27th.—About 8 a.m. patient took a bad turn ; dyspnœa ; brandy administered ; dry cupping over bases of lungs ; large amount of oozing of cerebro-spinal fluid. In the afternoon the patient's condition improved ; some slight expansion of chest (?).

Oct. 28th.—General condition much improved ; copious mucus râles throughout chest ; takes nourishment better ; anæsthesia over entire surface of right arm ; return of sensation in soles of feet.

Oct. 29th.—General condition not quite so good.

Oct. 29th.—This morning patient's condition remained unchanged. At 11 a.m. suddenly became much worse, and died in ten minutes.

Post-mortem examination showed a portion of the cord, about three-quarters of an inch long, opposite the 6th cervical vertebræ, soft to the touch. No dislocation of the bodies of the vertebræ, and no separation of the posterior ligament.

58

CASE III.—W. W., aged 36, was brought to the hospital, per ambulance, January 6th, 1890, suffering from several severe injuries. Patient, while white-washing a ceiling over an engine, had lost his balance and fell into the belt of a rapidly-revolving wheel, which carried him around about twenty times, inflicting a fracture of the right leg, right clavicle and pelvis, causing hæmaturia, contusions about the face, and a fracture of the cervical spine, causing paraplegia.

Examination.—Patient is a well-nourished man, in good general health; intellect clear; pulse 72, strong and full; respiration diaphragmatic; pupils contracted and react to light; patellar, abdominal, etc., reflexes absent. Loss of sensation, as to temperature, touch and pain, of the whole body below the 3rd intercostal space, also of the extensor and radial surfaces of both arms; present on the flexor surfaces. Paralysis of the body below the arms and of flexors of arms. Still possesses some voluntary power over the extensors. Is unable to help himself in the least degree. Complains of pain at the lower cervical region; marked tenderness on pressure here. On examining the spine, find a marked prominence of the spinous process of the 6th cervical vertebræ; no priapism.

Treatment.—Palliative; was unable to catheterize on account of fracture of the pelvis and laceration of the urethra.

Jan. 7th.—Consultation and decided to operate. General condition about the same as on the day of admission. Chloroform was administered, patient turned on his face, and neck and occiput shaved and cleansed. The membranes were exposed as in the former case and incised. About one inch in extent of cord substance was found very badly crushed, so ended operation by suturing membranes and bringing muscles and skin together by deep silk sutures, inserting a rubber drain, and dressing with iodoform and gauze.

Patient made a good recovery from the operation and passed a good night, although sleep was poor. He lived three days after operation without amelioration of any of the symptoms, and died comatose from respiratory failure.

Reviews and Notices of Books.

Chronic Urethritis and its Treatment. By M. BER-
KELEY HILL, M.B., F.R.C.S. With colored plates by F.
COLLINS, M.R.C.S. London: H. K. Lewis. 1890.

This little work consists of three lectures delivered at the
Royal College of Surgeons, London. These lectures were
written with the object of describing the forms of chronic urethritis as seen by reflected light, and the treatment of the
troublesome discharge termed gleet mainly by topical methods.
The healthy urethra is first described, then the morbid changes
caused by urethritis, and finally its treatment. In speaking of
" duration of contagion" in urethritis, Mr. Hill says he can offer
no definite rule for deciding this question; he says that in the
present state of our knowledge it is rash to assume that, in the
absence of gonococcus from any particular drop of discharge, the
contagion is past. He is inclined to think that when the discharge
is secreted entirely from granular patches, the crypts and ducts
of glands having ceased to furnish pus, we may consider the discharge to be no longer specific in character or capable of communicating disease to others. A narrow meatus is a frequent
cause for the continuation of a gleet, which disappears on enlarging this opening; other causes are stricture (single or multiple),
patches of inflammation, and granular areas. The commonest
cause is stricture, even though in many cases it means merely a
lessening of the natural distensibility of the urethra. These
strictures are most frequently met with between the third and
fourth inch from the meatus. In all cases, the average duration
of treatment before cure was effected was two and a half months.
Treatment is described in detail by soluble bougies and instillations of nitrate of silver by Guyon's catheter and syringe. When
nitrate of silver instillations were used, cure was made more
rapid by a preliminary stretching of the urethra with large bougies. In the third lecture, prostatitis and tubercle of the prostate
are described. In prostatitis, the most advantageous local remedy
is found to be the repeated application of strong astringent solu-

tions to the membrano-prostatic portion of the urethra, combin
with a thorough dilatation of the urethra with sounds gradua
increasing to No. 30 French.   Mr. Hill is of opinion that gon
rhœa is indirectly an exciting cause of tubercle in the geni
organs.   In tubercular ulcers of the prostate he has found t
thorough washing out of the bladder to clean out the pus a
urine from the parts and then the injection of quinine gr. ii-
of which solution about two ounces should be left in the bladd
a good plan.   In chronic cystitis he gets the best results by
jecting an emulsion of iodoform (iodoform 2 parts, mucilag
parts, glycerine 2 parts, water 20 parts).   The book is ful
interest to all urethral surgeons, and should be carefully stud
The arrangement of the matter is not as orderly and conveni
as it might be, but the matter itself is unquestionably good, a
the result of a ripe and wide experience.   The colored illus
tions, which are beautifully executed, add much to the valu
this work, and will be of great service to all who examine
urethra by reflected light—a method of examination at o
scientific and accurate.

Essentials of Diseases of the Skin, including Syphilodermata. By HENRY W. STELWAGON, M PhD.   Philadelphia: W. B. Saunders.   1890.

This small book adds another to that innumerable grou
compends written for students of medicine with the objec
compressing all necessary information on various subjects int
small a space as possible.   This method of studying medical
jects we have before condemned, and think it tends to r
students less thorough and to encourage the idle.   However
subject of skin diseases is rather outside a medical curriculum
students generally acquire but a smattering during their co
so if by any means this small amount of knowledge can b
creased we must not object, even if compends have to be i
use of.   The subject-matter is arranged in the form of ques
and answers, and certainly the answers are very concise, a
rate, and to the point, and will be useful for those who have
little time to consult the larger works on skin diseases.   T

are numerous illustrations throughout the work, which add to its value. Students will find it a handy pocket volume for use in clinics on skin diseases.

Diseases of Women and Abdominal Surgery. By Lawson Tait, F.R.C.S., Edin. and Eng., LL.D., Professor of Gynæcology, Queen's College, Birmingham ; Surgeon to the Birmingham and Midland Hospital for Women, &c., &c. Vol. I. Philadelphia : Lea Brothers & Co.

The advent of Mr. Tait's book is regarded with great interest by the whole profession. It is entirely characteristic of its distinguished author. To Mr. Tait, more than any man living, modern gynæcology owes its remarkable position. Amongst the concluding words of the author's preface are the following : " My chief object is to offer the results of my own experiences in as condensed a form as possible." The book is a clinical digest of the author's enormous experience, and is, therefore, in certain directions, because of that experience, of a value that can only be appreciated by one who has seen him at work.

The first part of the book is devoted to what may be called the minor diseases of women. In the chapter on physical examination, Mr. Tait makes some of his characteristic strong statements. These will not be universally accepted. However true they may be of gynæcologists of large experience, they cannot apply to the many whose opportunities have been moderate in extent, and who, though still learners, must do a large amount of the work in this department of medicine. Thus, for a pelvic examination, Mr. Tait says the position of the patient on the left side is the best for both vaginal (digital) and bimanual. We venture to say that few observers of experience of the dorsal position will subscribe to this statement. We, however, quite agree with him in his denunciation of the use of instruments, to the neglect of the far more instructive, careful use of the educated finger and opposite hand. So, not many who have thoroughly acquired the Sims' method of examination will agree with him when he says that by far the best speculum for almost every purpose is the glass-barrelled Fergusson's speculum.

In the chapter on the diseases of the uterus, Mr. Tait mere
mentions Emmet's operation for torn cervix, and then only
denounce it. "Nothing more useless than Emmet's operat
has ever been introduced into surgical practice." Surely
does not speak from experience. In speaking of chronic cervi
metritis and endometritis no mention is made of the value
iodine or systematic tamponade. In the treatment of cancer
the uterus, Mr. Tait has little to say in favor of any surg
treatment, and is entirely opposed to total extirpation. In
treatment of displacements of the uterus, he does not appr
of shortening the round ligaments.

The chapter on uterine myoma is, as might have been expect
most interesting and satisfactory. Contrary to the opinion of ma
Mr. Tait reiterates his belief, many times already expres
that myoma is often a fatal disease. It is therefore, accord
to him, to be dealt with promptly. He gives a table of :
cases of removal of the appendages, with four deaths. He, h
ever, classes separately pyosalpinx and hydrosalpinx occur
with myoma, as a much more serious condition. For the
rapidly-growing myoma, extirpation is the only procedure
considers advisable.

The chapter on chronic, inflammatory. and other diseas
the uterine appendages is full of interest, but we have not s
to say more than that the author is evidently as strong an
cate as ever for prompt operation for their removal.

The last chapter of this first volume, consisting of a hun
pages, is devoted to ectopic gestation and pelvic hæmatocel
the author's many brilliant contributions to gynæcologica
gery, none is so remarkable as his work in the treatment o
condition, and his unique experience commands attention to
word he says on the subject.

Such, in brief, is the scope and character of the first vol
We await with impatience the appearance of the second.
work of the well-known publishers is entirely satisfactory.

Insomnia and its Therapeutics. By A. W. MacFarlane, M.D., Fellow of the Royal College of Physicians, Edinburgh, Examiner in Medical Jurisprudence in the University of Glasgow, &c. London : H. K. Lewis, 136 Gower street.

Dr. MacFarlane's work is one of great value to the practitioner, for of all troublesome conditions that he is called upon to treat few are so annoying and persistent as sleeplessness. The difficulties that present themselves in unravelling the mysteries that give rise to insomnia are very great, and frequently tax the patience and acumen of the ablest and most experienced physician. The author of this work has done a great service in bringing together the scattered information that we have in all that relates directly and indirectly to sleeplessness.

We have, first, an introductory chapter on the physiology of sleep, followed by one on the conditions which influence sleep and sleeplessness. Then, in order, is taken up the affections of the different systems which conduce to insomnia. First of all, we have the great group of nervous affections ; over work, shock, depressing emotions, neurasthenia, hypochondriasis, the organic and the toxic affections. The gastro-intestinal, renal, respiratory and circulatory disturbances which tend to bring on insomnia are fully treated in this connection.

One of the best chapters in the book is that devoted to gouty insomnia. The insomnia of fever is also dealt with.

The work, on the whole, is one that will well repay diligent perusal, and no practitioner can read it without feeling that the author has done his work well.

Spinal Concussion. Surgically Considered as a Cause of Spinal Injury, and Neurologically restricted to a certain Symptom Group, for which is suggested the designation Erichsen's Disease, as one form of the Traumatic Neuroses. By S. V. Clevenger, M.D., late Pathologist to County Insane Asylum, Chicago. With thirty wood engravings. Philadelphia and London : F. A. Davis. 1889.

This work not only deals with concussion of the spine, but also with a great many other subjects, as medical electricity, medical

politics, medical education, the anatomy and physiolrgy of
sympathetic system, etc., etc. It is difficult to see what c
nection there is between such subjects. The work on the wl
represents a great amount of diligent research and study, ;
will no doubt be a very useful work of reference in cerl
medico-legal cases. We would advise the author, if ever a sec
edition is called for, to eliminate all such subjects as do not bel
to " concussion of the spine." The amount of padding is 1
gether too great. It is unfortunate for both the author and
hypothesis that there is so much of it.

Essay on Medical Pneumatology. A Physiolog
Clinical and Therapeutic Investigation of the Gases.
J. N. DEMARQUAY, Surgeon to the Municipal Hosp
Paris. Translated by SAMUEL S. WALLIAN, A.M., M
Illustrated. Philadelphia and London : F. A. Davis. 1£

This work is devoted mainly to the consideration of the p
macology and therapeutics of oxygen. Under the latter h
we have a very full account of what has been written on
value of oxygen both in medicine and surgery. In our opin
the most valuable part of the work is the translator's n
comments and additions.

Handbook of Materia Medica, Pharmacy and The
peutics. Including the Physiological Action of Dr
the Special Therapeutics of Disease, Official and Ex
poraneous Pharmacy, and Minute Directions for Pres
tion Writing. By SAMUEL O. L. POTTER, M.A., M
Professor of the Theory and Practice of Medicine ii
Cooper Medical College of San Francisco. Second edi
Revised and enlarged. Philadelphia : P. Blakiston, S
Co. 1890.

The second edition of Dr. Potter's Handbook is in many
pects a considerable improvement on the first. It is now o
the most useful of the many textbooks on this subject.
section on pharmacy and the act of prescription writing is
and ably prepared, and would itself well repay any practiti

who is not thoroughly conversant with this necessary part of
his professional work. A considerable part of the work is devoted to special therapeutics. This is in a great measure an
elaborate index to the more important diseases and their treatment. The publishers have performed their part of the work
with great credit.

Annual of the Universal Medical Sciences. A Yearly
Report of the Progress of the General Sanitary Sciences
throughout the World. Edited by CHARLES E. SAJOUS,
M.D., Lecturer on Laryngology and Rhinology in Jefferson
Medical College, Philadelphia; and 70 Associate Editors,
assisted by over 200 Associate Editors, Collaborators and
Correspondents. Illustrated with chromo-lithographs, engravings and maps. Five volumes. F. A. Davis, Philadelphia, New York and London. 1889.

The five volumes of this excellent work more than sustains
the reputation gained by the issue of the previous year. We
have here a judicious and critical review of all the important
medical papers and publications issued in different parts of the
world for the past year.

Electricity in the Diseases of Women. By BETTON
MASSEY, M.D. Second edition. F. A. Davis, publisher,
Philadelphia and London. 1890.

This well known author on electricity has written a most useful little work on the subject. It is very similar to other works
which have gone before it, and we can recommend it to all who
are interested in the treatment of diseases of women by electricity.

May's Diseases of Women. Second edition. Revised
by LEONARD S. RAW, M.D. Philadelphia : Lea Bros. &
Co. 1890.

This little work, intended for senior students and practitioners,
has some very excellent qualifications, but in some instances is
very much behind the present practice of teaching. In regard

to sutures, the author speaks of using wire where silkworm gut is in more recent favor ; also, he advises the use of many silver sutures in the operation of primary perineorrhaphy, where one is all that is necessary. The author leaves out altogether the mechanism of the pessary in treating retroversion, and does not mention the very important direction to always return the uterus to its forward position before the pessary can be applied. This is a very grave omission, as it would result in a serious abuse of the pessary by the inexperienced. The book, however, will have its usefulness, and can be read with pleasure.

The Doctor in Canada. His Whereabouts and the Laws which Govern Him. A Ready Book of Reference. By ROBERT WYNYARD POWELL, M.D., Ottawa.

Dr. Powell has performed a very useful piece of work in giving to the profession the work in question. It deals with all subjects of special interest to the medical practitioner in Canada. We have first the various acts which are in force in the different Provinces, the Public Health Acts. We have next detailed information on the different teaching and licensing bodies. Then follow accounts of the hospitals, asylums, etc., of the country. The book should be in the hands of every practitioner in Canada.

Society Proceedings.

HAMILTON MEDICAL AND SURGICAL SOCIETY.

Stated Meeting, May 20th, 1890.

DR. CAVILLER IN THE CHAIR.

DR. A. B. OSBOHNE read a paper entitled,

SPECTACLES AS THERAPEUTIC AGENTS.

If " the proof of the pudding is in the eating," then the value of any therapeutic measure consists in its successful application. The results—remote and direct—of strain upon certain portions of the ocular mechanism are being rapidly ascertained and are becoming recognized by the profession. So far reaching are the effects of ocular strain that an examination of the eye is considered incomplete unless the state of the refraction and motor apparatus is fully noted, and many chronic inflammatory affections of the eyes become much more amenable to treatment when the ciliary strain is removed by glasses.

The constant occurrence of certain symptoms in cases of hypermetropia and astigmatism, as well as the equally constant relief to these symptoms afforded by wearing glasses, point at once to a strain of the ciliary muscle as the prime factor in their production.

Headache is one of the commonest manifestations of ciliary strain ; in fact, refractive errors are so productive of this disorder that every case of chronic or recurring headache should be tested for glasses. The headache may occur in almost any form, but is most frequently frontal, accompanied by a sensation of weariness and a desire to close the eyes. It is rarely present upon first awakening in the morning, but commences during the day or in the evening after the eyes have been in use for some time. Among school children who are compelled to study at night these headaches are specially frequent ; a good night's rest usually removes the trouble completely, but only to return at the end of another day's work. The sufferer may be quite unaware of any defect of the eyes, as there are frequently no symptoms pointing directly to them and the vision may be excel-

A large percentage of squints are the outcome of ciliary strain, and many oculists can cite cases where, having seen the patient before the squint had become a confirmed habit, it disappeared completely under the use of atropine and correcting glasses. Similarly a simple surgical correction without the assistance of spectacles is too frequently a complete failure. So well known has this fact become that surgeons do not operate upon squints without first testing the vision and ordering the requisite glasses.

Chronic affections of the lids, as blepharitis and recurring styes, may be kept up by ciliary strain; these cases recover rapidly when glasses are worn. This is also true of a chronic form of conjunctivitis affecting principally the palpebral conjunctiva. The writer has found a considerable proportion of his cases of chalazion associated with hypermetropia and astigmatism, and the correction of these defects has materially lessened the irritation. Photophobia, lachrymation, and an apparent hyperæsthesia of the retina may all be produced by strain of the refractive mechanism.

The hypertrophy of the ciliary muscle resulting from the continuous strain necessary in hypermetropia and astigmatism is an important factor in the production of glaucoma.

Lastly, the asthenopia produced by some forms of ocular strain is familiar to all; it disappears rapidly after proper glasses are worn.

The large number of children wearing spectacles in the present day is frequently adduced as evidence of the deterioration of the species. It would be more correct to call this an index of the advance of science, inasmuch as we are now able to relieve diseases by means of glasses which our predecessors were barely able to diagnose, much less treat.

From what has been said it will be seen that spectacles occupy a prominent place among our therapeutic agents, not only in relieving visual defects and in the treatment of some painful reflex symptoms, but also in diminishing the danger to eyes later in life from such serious diseases as cataract and glaucoma.

DR. LAFFERTY then read the notes of a case of

TABES DORSALIS.

J. M., a laborer, aged 51, married ; has served in the British army for eleven years. With the exception of smallpox thirty-two years ago, has had no sickness of any kind. Drank very hard until about twelve years ago. During this latter period he had been a total abstainer. Family history good ; parents both lived to 80. Never contracted any venereal disease ; in fact, never required any medical attention until about four years ago, when he experienced some difficulty in micturating. The urine contained a considerable quantity of white substance, milky in appearance. Had retention, and was relieved by means of a catheter. This deposit has gradually increased in quantity ever since, being almost constantly present. About this time pains began to be felt in the sacral and gluteal regions, darting and shooting down both legs to the heels. Little notice was taken of it, believing it to be sciatica, until in May 1887, three years ago, there was a decided weakness in his lower extremities. The pain was more frequent and severe, and shortly after, while walking with a friend at night, fell down on the sidewalk and had to be assisted home by his companion. In August of this same year (1887) I was summoned to attend him ; found the patient in bed, complaining of pain in both limbs, especially in the calves. While lying on his back with his legs crossed, when endeavoring to change their position by lifting the top one, there would be a disposition for the lower one to move first. Has considerable difficulty in walking, and in the dark stumbles from side to side. If walking during the day, cannot look back without first stopping ; that is, he cannot look back over his shoulder and still keep moving forward. Has a tendency to fall under these circumstances. Eyesight good, pupils equal ; no arcus senilis ; conjunctival normal. No evidence of paralysis ; has good power of muscles. Can stand steadily when eyes are open, but when asked to close them begins to sway backwards and forwards and is quite unsteady. With closed eyes can place right index finger on tip of nose without any hesitation ; the left is slower in movement, and does not find the nose so conveniently.

Walks with a staggering gait, bringing the heel down with the toes. Diminished sensation in both extremities. Tendon reflex *nil ;* bowels very constipated ; appetite diminished and variable. Describes a feeling of numbness most noticeable in right leg and foot, and a sense of constriction about the body as if a rope was tied around him above the hips. Urine somewhat increased in quantity ; very slight trace of albumen, no sugar ; sp. gr. 1022, turbid and alkaline. After micturating a light, creamy deposit was frequently passed. Sexual powers normal. Pulse 65. Weighs 160 lbs.

Diagnosis—Tabes dorsalis, non-syphilitic. Ordered rest in bed, a liberal dose of castor oil as bowels had not been moved for four days, and 'fluid ext. Calabar bean ♏ ii four times a day.

Aug. 21st.—Bowels moved thoroughly ; feels much more comfortable.

Sept. 2nd.—Allowed up ; pains slight ; appetite good ; sleeps well. Takes pulv. glycyrrhizæ co. every alternate day.

Oct. 15th.—Retention, relieved by catheter. Complains of a fatigued feeling generally ; marked numbness in both legs ; pain increased ; has to use a cane to steady himself when walking at night. Ordered pil. argentum nitrate ¼ gr. three times a day in addition to previous prescription.

Nov. 20th.—No improvement. Thinking that owing to his military career and previous intemperate habits there might possibly be a specific cause, pot. iodid. was given in gradually increased doses. This drug produced gastric disturbance and was intolerable at times, hence discontinued it after a trial of a few weeks and substituted fld. ext. Calabar bean ♏ ii, with four minims of acid phos. dil. four i.d.

Aug. 30th, 1888.—Galvanism has been systematically used for the last two months. The pains are somewhat relieved by its use. Walks very slowly, assisted by a cane ; dare not venture out at night alone. Occasional doses of morphia have to be administered to relieve pain. Greater loss of sensation in lower extremities ; numbness extends higher up the waist. Complains of tightness from the ribs down. Slight numbness in right arm. Sensation in soles of feet when walking as though stepping on spongy material. On pinching the neck the pupils

do not respond by dilating as is seen in normal subjects. Power
of co-ordination much lessened ; in fact, the conditions present
a year ago are now greatly exaggerated. Prescribed syr. trip.
phos. 3i ter in die.

May, 1889.—Is so much disabled as to be unable to go out.
Goes around the house with a crutch under each arm. Pains
in the lumbar region and down both legs very troublesome. Says
stiffness and tightness has become worse. Sensation leaving
right arm and shoulder ; can remove the hair from his arm without
out feeling it. Left arm normal. Is now given Sayre's apparatus, which is attached to the ceiling. By means of this he is
to be raised off his feet once a day and allowed to hang five
minutes each time. When raised, he described the sensation as
if being pulled apart ; could feel the spine, as it were, separating.
Found almost immediate benefit, pain and stiffness being relieved.
Bowels began to move without purgatives, and four weeks after
walked from the street car into my office, the only assistant being
a heavy cane.

Aug., 1889.—Went to Toronto on a visit for a month, using
Sayre continually, taking syr. trip. phos., and still improving.

Dec., 1889.—The pain, stiffness, etc., has again returned,
although he has persevered with the treatment recommended.
Is forced to use the crutches once more. Has lost all sexual
desire and power. Urine is now clear and normal. Muscles do
not respond to a very strong faradic current. Sensation in legs
almost entirely gone ; can strike them with a heavy stick without feeling it, as he puts it, " they are just like a board." Loss
of sensation extends over upper right half of body, limited by
clavicle and scapula above and the median line before and behind.

April, 1890.—General condition much the same as in December last. Sayre's apparatus is of no benefit to him now further
than some temporary relief for an hour or so. Has taken nothing
in the way of drugs for the last three months, except an occasional half grain of morphia as may be found necessary.

THE ANNUAL MEETING OF THE ASSOCIATION OF AMERICAN PHYSICIANS.

Held at Washington, D.C., May 13, 14 and 15, 1890.

The proceedings of the Association, so far as its scientific work was concerned, opened with a paper by Dr. J. E. Reeves of Chattanooga, Tenn., upon *Some Points in the Natural History of Typhoid Fever*, in which he considered the character, course, and complications of the disease from its inception through to convalescence.

In the discussion, DR. J. C. WILSON of Philadelphia spoke of his belief in the great value of Brandt's method of using the cold bath whenever the temperature rises to a point over 101.5°, and briefly detailed the favorable results obtained by him in the treatment of thirty cases of the disease in the wards of the German Hospital in Philadelphia. In the majority of these no medicine was given, in a few a little calomel being occasionally used to evacuate the bowels at the beginning of the attack, and in every instance the results were extraordinarily good.

DR. ALFRED L. LOOMIS of New York stated that he failed to recognise the distinct forms of typhoid fever characterized by Dr. Reeves as mild, intermediate, and malignant, and expressed surprise at the statement of the author that he had seen five recoveries in typhoid fever after perforation of the bowel had occurred. He himself had never seen a recovery where perforation really took place ; although he had observed cases in which peritonitis of a localized or diffuse character had complicated typhoid fever, not due to perforation, and resulting in recovery. Dr. Loomis believed that cardiac softening is a very common complication of typhoid fever, and asserted that if a loud systolic murmur is heard at the apex the prognosis is unfavorable, as it shows that softening has occurred, and that thrombosis or sudden dilatation has taken place, the latter resulting from some sudden movement straining the softened viscus. He thought that getting up too soon probably caused the symptoms of a weak, dilated heart following typhoid fever. Dr. Loomis then proceeded to state that he had recently seen in New York a form

59

of nervous trouble consequent upon typhoid fever which, as far as he was aware, had been described nowhere except in a paper by Dr. V. P. Gibney, in which the author had detailed several instances of what he was pleased to call "typhoid spine." This condition is marked by great pain and tenderness over the spinous processes of the vertebræ, and has been confused by some physicians with lumbago and other similar conditions. Eventually the cases which had consulted Dr. Loomis were cured by the use of the hot iron and a particular jacket devised by Dr. Gibney.

DRS. S. WEIR MITCHELL and ABRAHAM JACOBI objected very strongly to the idea that typhoid spine was in any way a new or distinct sequelæ of typhoid fever, both agreeing that it was simply a spondylitis.

DR. H. A. JOHNSON of Chicago stated that he had seen a case of what he believed to be recovery after perforation of the intestine in typhoid fever, and detailed the symptoms which gave rise to this belief.

DR. WM. PEPPER of Philadelphia agreed with the opinions of Dr. Mitchell and Dr. Jacobi, and expressed the thought that the immunity from typhoid fever in Chattanooga, as stated by Dr. Reeves, was very extraordinary, and must be largely dependent upon some peculiar condition of the soil. He also insisted upon the great value of the use of nitrate of silver internally in typhoid fever throughout the attack as a means of avoiding complications and lessening its severity.

The paper of DR. N. BRIDGES of Chicago on *Appendicitis* (see page 937) was discussed by several of the physicians present.

DR. ATKINSON of Baltimore stated that in his opinion the surgeon is often called too late, and yet, on the other hand, a large proportion of the cases get well if left alone ; leaving us in a position of indecision as to what course is to be pursued.

DR. R. FITZ of Boston believed that there were many cases of mild catarrh of the appendix that never come to the care of the physician, and gave the conclusions derived by him from 72 cases which he had personally seen. He thought that the 500 cases previously collected by him and reported some four years ago had been somewhat misleading in respect to the results derived from them. His opinion at present is that there are half as many females affected as males, and he added that while 11 per cent. in his statistics had recurring attacks, 44 per cent. in his personal experience had recurring attacks. Dr. Fitz also made the interesting statement that recurring attacks take place with equal frequency, whether the cases be treated medically or surgically, unless the appendix be removed, the general average of recovery being 74 per cent. He believed that the mortality of medical treatment is only 11 per cent., while that of surgical treatment is 40 per cent., but it is to be remembered that the high percentage of surgical treatment rests largely upon the serious and advanced condition of the disease before the surgeon is called in or given the opportunity to operate. He also thought that two simple rules could readily be formulated—namely, that where the symptoms were very urgent, or where a tumor was present, the surgeon should operate, but that in cases of slow recurrence without urgent symptoms medical treatment is to be resorted to, as surgical treatment is difficult owing to the changes produced in the relative positions of the parts caused by previous attacks.

Dr. Jacobi of New York objected to the term " turn the case over to the surgeon," saying that in his opinion physicians should be able to perform four surgical operations—namely, intubation, tracheotomy, herniotomy, and abdominal section for appendicitis. He did not think that localized peritonitis in the right groin should be operated upon during its stage of activity, but punctured if necessary and operated upon in the course of a week or two, after the severity of the inflammation had passed, provided that it was considered necessary to use the knife.

Dr. Pepper, on the other hand, did not believe that any physician should operate upon such a case, and thought it required all the skill of the thoroughly trained surgeon to undertake such a procedure, the physician always sharing his responsibility with a surgeon.

Dr. J. H. Musser spoke of tuberculosis as a cause of appendicitis, having seen three such cases.

The paper of DR. LUSK on *Antisepsis during Labor* was d
cussed by Drs. Welch, Pepper and Roosevelt, who all express
their interest in the conclusions reached by the essayist, a
agreed with him as to the inadvisability of the vaginal touch
most cases.   The fact that the hands of the accoucheur cot
not be considered sterile, although they might be aseptic, ev
if a very strong solution of bichloride of mercury was used, v
pointed out by Dr. Welch.

DR. DANA read a paper upon *Seizures Accompanied
Shock and Coma*, which was discussed by Drs. Lyman, E
and Loomis. Dr. Loomis spoke of the difficulty of differentiati
embolism, apoplexy, and thrombosis in diagnosis. In many ca
he has found supposed apoplexy to be in reality cerebral thro
bosis with softening. The patient in embolism, however, ge
rally does not lose consciousness, and he thought that bef
fifty years of age such attacks are always due to extravasati
and after fifty to thrombosis and softening. In his opinion, t
uræmic coma cannot be diagnosed by the condition of the pu
Dr. Jacobi stated that in his experience the œdema of uræ
coma is often unilateral, not bilateral, and that its diagno
cannot rest upon any such diffusion of the puffiness.

The paper of DR. S. WEIR MITCHELL, as referee, upon *L
orders of Sleep*, was unusually interesting, and dealt with
psychical, motor and sensory disturbances of the præ-dormiti
and post-dormitium, including sensory, motor, and emotio
overflows or explosions, as well as the condition of the subje
of waking numbness, and post-somnic paresis and paralysis.
Mitchell also dwelt on the curious nervous disorders known
night neuralgias, night choreas, and failures of respiration
sleep.

DR. FOLSOM, the co-referee, considered the physiology
sleep, the causes and conditions of insomnia, the influence
habit, and the various diseases and poisons which produce
He also spoke of the vaso-motor conditions associated with c
orders of sleep, and discussed quite fully the treatment of th
by measures directed to the improvement of hygienic surrou
ings of the patient and by the use of certain drugs. He belie

that drugs are to be generally avoided as far as possible, but chloral, hyoscin, methylal, and sulphonal are the best remedies to be resorted to if drugs are necessary. Dr. Pepper added that a person might train himself to sleep and to put aside all mental effort, arranging the body in such a manner as to let it rest entirely upon the skeleton, thereby affording the muscular system total relaxation and rest. As the superior oblique and external rectus muscles of the eye are generally severely strained by prolonged eye-work, and ache, he advised rotation of the eye-balls upward during the endeavor to obtain sleep, in such a way as to relieve these muscles from all exertion. Dr. H. M. Lyman of Chicago said that he believed that many cases of insomnia were due to rheumatism, and recommended the use of milk of sulphur and bitartrate of potassium in the proportion of one to five parts. Dr. G. L. Peabody of New York related a case where full doses of soda and rhubarb cured insomnia which had resisted all other remedies. Dr. M. Allen Starr of New York expressed great confidence in sulphonal as a hypnotic, and believed it to be valuable, particularly if food is taken just before instead of just after its administration.

In closing the discussion, Dr. Mitchell remarked that many cases of insomnia, though depending upon gastric or other trouble, failed to recover from the disease causing the insomnia unless sleep was induced by the use of drugs. He also recommended the administration of sufficiently large doses of hypnotics to make the production of sleep sure of occurrence, as the use of smaller doses, if they fail, produces a condition of doubt in the patient's mind as to his ability to sleep, or the power of remedies to make him sleep, which is unfortunate and interferes with successful results. He advocated the administration of thirty or more grains of bromide at once, or that one-hundredth of a grain of hyoscin should take its place. Finally, if these both fail, he depended upon sulphonal.

DR. C. L. DANA of New York followed with a paper upon a study of the *Sensory Disturbances in Hysteria*, which showed careful study of the entire subject, and was received with great interest.

The paper of DR. WHARTON SINKLER of Philadelphia u *Migraine* dealt very largely with its causes, its unusual vi phenomena, and particularly with its treatment. He rec mended phenacetin, antipyrine, eucalyptus, and caffein in la doses as the best means of treatment.

A very interesting demonstration was that of DR. HARI ERNST of Boston, who showed to the Society the body of a rab which was one of three to which he had given, by means o hypodermic needle, in the abdominal region, five or six drop milk derived from the udder of a tuberculous cow. All abdominal viscera were thickly studded with miliary tubercl but the lungs were not affected. Dr. Ernst naturally believ this to be a very strong evidence of the communicability of tub culosis by means of milk to human beings, and asserted that was sure that the rabbit which had died was not affected tuberculosis arising independently of his injection of the mi as rabbits which did not receive the milk were healthy at t date. He then proceeded to discuss briefly and to place record certain studies carried out by Dr. Stephen Martin Boston, concerning the *contagium vivum* of cowpox and vacci material. Dr. Martin had been able to make cultures throu five generations of this material, and had inoculated childr with matter derived from the fifth generation with success, sin these children, when vaccinated with lymph which had be found active in other children, failed to develop the typi vesicles. He stated that Dr. Martin was continuing his inve gations, and would report further upon them at future meetii of the Association.

DR. D. W. PRENTISS of Washington showed a man with extraordinarily slow pulse, the pulse-beat at the time of the hibition being but 30 per minute, but had been as low as 11, respirations being 32. He also presented a boy suffering fr rheumatic purpura, in whom so large an amount of blood h been poured out beneath the skin on the anterior belly wall to produce a slough. In the discussion of this last case I Atkinson of Baltimore stated that he had seen somewhat simi cases, and knew of instances where similar sloughs had occurre

Dr. Tyson of Philadelphia also mentioned one such occurrence in his experience. Dr. Jacobi expressed the belief that all these cases were dependent upon changes in the bloodvessel walls, and that in those instances where the blood had undergone a change the leakage which resulted was due to alterations in the bloodvessels resulting from the hæmic alterations.

DR. W. H. WELCH of Baltimore then reported a case of *Acute Diphtheritic Colitis with Peri-pancreatic Fat-necrosis.* The patient, 53 years old, had been a hard drinker. Three days before death he became delirious and was admitted to hospital. Temperature elevated—when first observed, 101.5°F.; on day of death, 105.4°F. Pulse 120 to 132, compressible. Spleen not enlarged. Abdomen tympanitic, tender on pressure, especially in epigastrium. Urine slightly albuminous. Tongue clean and moist. No diarrhœa until a few hours before death, when he had an offensive liquid stool. Urine and fæces passed involuntarily. Patient became unconscious and died two days after admission to hospital. At the autopsy, which was made a short time after death, were found numerous foci of so-called fat-necroses in the transverse meso-colon and in the adipose tissue around the pancreas, with beginning sequestration of the pancreas. Liver intensely fatty. Contents of bile-ducts and of gall-bladder viscid, clear, with only slight yellowish tint. Renal epithelium fatty. Ecchymoses, small ulcers, superficial necroses and diphtheritic exudation in large intestine. The foci of fat-necroses, as well as the liver, bile and spleen, contained in large number a single species of bacteria, which was isolated and studied in pure culture. The organisms are bacilli, belonging to the group of colon bacilli, and probably identical with the bacterium coli commuue. Cultures and microscopical specimens from this case were exhibited,

He also reported a case in which symptoms suggesting intestinal obstruction existed. Exploratory laparotomy was performed. Numerous foci of fat-necrosis were found in the omentum and mesentery and a swelling in the region of the pancreas, but no intestinal obstruction existed. Portions of the omentum containing necrotic foci were excised and were examined microscopically by the writer. The patient recovered.

Following this report, DR. REGINALD FITZ of Boston described a *Case of Acute Pancreatitis*, which illustrated the suppurative in contrast with the hæmorhagic and gangrenous varieties of the disease. Microscopical preparations were shown and the recent literature on the subject was reviewed.

DR. E. O. SHAKESPEARE of Philadelphia then read a paper entitled *What Can and Should be Done to Limit the Prevalence of Tuberculosis in Man?* In this essay the speaker advanced the following propositions :

1. The bacillus tuberculosis is the sole active or exciting cause of the disease, which is infectious or contagious and non-hereditary.

2. Whilst on the one hand the discovery of the bacillus has advanced our methods of treatment but little, on the other hand it has revealed most important principles upon which to base efficient means of preventing the spread of the disease.

3. In view of the admitted inefficiency of all present modes of treatment of actual cases of tuberculosis, effective prophylactic measures are infinitely more important to the general public, and should also be to the physician, than the most skilful therapeutic measures.

4. Since analysis of the fullest records bearing upon the relation of family history to the causation of tuberculosis can possibly account, through hereditary predisposition, for little more than one-fourth of the cases, the most perfect measures conceivable for the lessening of that influence cannot be ratiocally compared in importance to those which are essentially based upon the destruction of an infective poison, which is virulent enough to produce the disease, not alone in the comparatively few who may be born with hereditary predisposition, but also to cause tuberculosis in the majority who succumb, notwithstanding the absence of an hereditary weakness.

The following general principles underlie an efficient system of prevention of tuberculosis :

1. From the standpoint of the already diseased, effective and preventive measures should look to the rapid destruction of the tubercle bacilli in the excretions and secretions, and by as little association of the well with the sick as possible.

2. From the standpoint of those liable to become infected, nothing which may contain the living tubercle bacillus should be permitted to enter the digestive apparatus. Rigid inspection of meat and milk is a necssity.

3. Tuberculous subjects should not be admitted to hospital wards in which those with other diseases, especially of the lungs, are confined. In general hospitals, consumptives should be assigned to special consumptive wards.

4. Special hospitals for the treatment of consumption should be established.

DR. F. P. KINNICUTT followed with a paper upon *Methods of Diagnosis in Diseases of the Stomach.*

DR. F. C. SHATTUCK also read a paper upon the same subject.

The meeting closed with *A Report of Two Cases of Acromegaly*, by DR. J. E. GRAHAM of Toronto.—(*Medical News.*)

Selections.

INFLAMMATIONS OF THE APPENDIX AND CÆCUM AND THE DUTY OF THE PHYSICIAN REGARDING THEM.

BY NORMAN BRIDGE, A.M., M.D., CHICAGO.

[*From the Medical News.*]

To anyone who reads the recent literature of this subject it will be apparent that it has received its chief study of late, not at the hands of general medical practitioners, who have the greatest opportunities for observing cases of these inflammations, but at the hands of surgeons, men who make surgery a specialty, and who see few cases in their incipiency of inflammation of the abdominal organs. The character and effects of these inflammations have been revealed to a large degree by post-mortem examinations, but it was left for modern surgery with its antiseptic methods to illuminate the subject of the treatment of many of their results as well as their character and tendencies. In proportion to the number of cases falling under the observation and management of surgeons the results in many ways have been profitable and encouraging. The surgeons have reached certain conclusions as to the character of these inflammations and what ought to be done for them, some of which are rather sweeping, and which encounter doubt and opposition on the part of many practitioners who give little or no attention to surgery. If the results attained by surgery were put with the observations of large numbers of cases never requiring surgical interference, and which are never seen by workers in the field of surgery, we should have the safest guide for diagnosis and treatment.

It is certain that these diseases are frequently not recognized and are often mistreated, and that the notions of doctors generally regarding them need to be radically revised. An obstacle to the exact understanding of the whole subject is the reluctance practitioners manifest to reporting their unfortunate results and bad diagnoses.

One prevalent misconception regarding these inflammations is is of their actual and relative frequency. Primary inflammation of the cæcum is rare, while that of the appendix is very common. Of all organs of the abdomen in males the appendix is most prone to dangerous inflammation. In females this tendency is exceeded by the pelvic organs only. Of 300 autopsies at random Toft reports that 36 per cent. revealed evidence of disease of the appendix. Such evidence doubtless consisted of adhesions of the organ to adjacent parts, and of various changes in its structure and condition which can be caused only by inflammation of some degree or character. Often these appearances are found in cases not known to have ever had abdominal inflammation. Four-fifths of all cases collected by Fitz were in males, showing a marked predisposition difficult to explain. While of all cases of appendicitis without extension only 20 per cent. were in females, 26 per cent. of cases of perityphlitis were of that sex. This does not prove, perhaps, that women are more prone to perityphlitis from inflammation of the appendix than men, but the increased percentage may be explained by the possibly greater tendency in them to pure cæcitis from foreign bodies— aggravated by constipation—since irritation within the cæcum sometimes leads to perforation and perityphlitis.

Dr. Ludvig Hektoen of Chicago, a careful observer, has noted the condition of the appendix in 280 post-mortem examinations, and found that in 42 cases (15 per cent.) there were evidences, in adhesions or otherwise, of peri-appendicitis from which the patient had recovered. Cases of existing inflammation were not counted. So in Chicago, among people who find their way into the County Hospital, fifteen in every hundred have had inflammation of the peritoneal surface of the appendix or the connective tissues posterior to it or both, and have recovered. ·These figures are not inconsistent with the records of Toft, since he observed all diseases of the appendix both inside and out, while Hektoen only recorded cases showing inflammation of the outside of the appendix, and which had recovered.

While primary inflammation of the cæcum is unusual, its secondary involvement from appendicitis and resulting perityphlitis or circumscribed peritonitis is doubtless common.

It must be extremely unusual for the cæcum to be primarily attacked, except when irritated by foreign bodies from within. Even in such cases it is rare for perforation to occur, this process usually beginning from without, when a perityphlitic abscess opens into the cæcum.

The vast majority of cases of so-called typhlitis and perityphlitis begin as appendicitis; the tissues of and about the cæcum become inflamed secondarily and usually as a result of perforation of the appendix. These two pathological conditions are often confounded; probably in most instances perityphlitis is the term to use. It is not the inflammation of the cæcum that is usually a menace to life, but that of the cellular tissue and peritoneum which so often leads to induration and to abscess with its manifold dangers of spontaneous opening in perilous directions.

Probably failure of free evacuation of the appendix is the first step in the causation of its commonest inflammation. The moment its contents are unduly retained harmful decomposition begins, deposits of lime salts occur upon retained fæcal matter, if such is present, and enteroliths are formed which press too hard on the swollen and tense mucous membrane, which finally yields in the weakest spot, and an ulcer is present. Only occa-

...ally are similar consequences produced by foreign b...
the appendix. In a considerable proportion of cases th...
...occurs without the irritation of a hard body of any kind
ulcer deepens b... persistence of its causes till it touc
internal surface... the covering peritoneum, or the cellul...
if within the mesentery; then trifling peritonitis or cell
both occur... ...ing in a few days if the causative proce...
If, however the ulcer deepens it perforates the app...
...its contents is extruded, when peritonitis or p
...idly ensues. In some instances the perit...
...localised and plastic exudation bars the irrita...
...from the general peritoneal cavity, and intra-p...
...forms; in others a general peritonitis occurs, and
...in a few days.

...the perforation is within the mesentery a cellular i...
...results, and we have the common perityphlitis—as
...ually independent of more or less peritonitis—and i...
...roportion of cases such induration as may be easil...
...rated, and within this, pus.

Most cases in males of so-called " inflammation of the
...are simply instances of inflammation of the appendix or
...ith or without the involvement of the connective tiss...
...them, or the peritoneum, or both. It is equally true t...
...ases of peritonitis in men and boys, and not a few i...
...also, are due solely to perforation and infection conse...
these diseases. Until discovered after death this cause
...rally not suspected. I venture the assertion that most...
...after peritonitis in the male sex reveal this etiology—and
...are made in only a meagre minority of such cases.

A case in point came under my observation in con...
about two years ago:

" Mr. S., a large, robust man, 45 years of age, had
apparent perfect health for many years. After att...
banquet he stood for half an hour, dressed in thin cl...
without an overcoat, in a cold and windy doorway waiti...
carriage. The next day he felt uncomfortable; later,...
pain and slight tenderness in the abdomen; the next d...

and some vomiting. A consultation a day or two later discovered simply the evidences of mild general peritonitis; there was neither much fever, pain, tenderness nor prostration, and the tenderness was localized in the lower zone of the abdomen, and to the same degree on either side. There was moderate tympanites, but no dulness on percussion. He was somewhat under the influence of opiates. He continued in much the same condition for nearly a week, when the symptoms suddenly became worse, collapse soon appeared, and death in a few hours. The autopsy revealed a fresh general peritonitis, a peritonitis of longer standing localized about the appendix, the intestines glued together by thick, plastic deposits, a pocket of pus, with fæcal matter, by the side of the appendix, and the latter perforated at its junction with the cæcum. The steps in the case were appendicitis, ulceration, perforation, extrusion of fæcal particles, localized peritonitis and abscess, extension of the poison and the process to the general peritoneal cavity, general peritonitis and death."

Many cases of supposed intestinal obstruction, such as intus-susception and volvulus, with some evidence of inflammation, are instances of peritonitis from perforation of the appendix, or of abscess due to previous inflammation of the appendix and its results. The fallacious theory that is often held is that an obstruction has occurred, which in a few hours has developed inflammation. A case in my own hospital service well illustrates this error:

" A youth of less than 20 years walked into the hospital from a cab at the curbstone, complaining of pain in the abdomen. He said he had been sick for several days with this pain to such a degree that he could not lie down, but must sit in bed bent forward. His friends said it had been impossible at times to keep him in bed, his suffering was so great. The sickness had, it was declared, come on suddenly, and he had repeatedly vomited. After his arrival he vomited yellowish fluid having a stercoraceous odor. He had considerable fever, a pulse of 130, a tense abdomen, and a look of desperate sickness. A consultation with my surgical colleague, Dr. Graham, resulted in the conclusion that the case was probably one of obstruction followed by peri-

tonitis.   Certain to die speedily without surgical relief, h
given the chance of laparotomy.   Nothing but peritoniti
discovered.   This was afterward found to have resulted fi
perforation of the appendix."

It is probable that abscess rarely occurs until after perfor:
which may be regarded as the direct cause of it.   Inflamm
of small surfaces of the peritoneum with adhesions, how
often supervene, as well as probably some degree of cellula
flammation, without perforation.

The mortality from appendicitis, considering the frequen
the disease, cannot be regarded as great.   The mortality i
those cases eventuating in perforation of the appendix, howe
is great, since this is the condition that leads to induration
extra-peritoneal abscess, and to acute severe local peritonitis
intra-peritoneal abscess, or to general peritonitis.   The gen
peritonitis means almost sure death, and the abscess, wher
it is and however well it may appear to be surrounded by
tecting plastic deposits, is a constant menace to life, as al
dantly shown by its spontaneous opening into the abdon
cavity, the venous canals, the bladder, and the chest cavit
well as externally and into the intestinal canal.

In view of these considerations, it is of the highest mo
that we should be able, if possible, to distinguish the mild
the grave cases.   One-fourth at least of all post-mortems
recoveries from previously existing inflammation, or other dis
of the appendix, and probably 15 per cent. show recoveries
peri-appendicitis.   The duty and aim of the doctor must
determine, clinically, if possible, the cases that form this
class and commit them strictly to medical treatment, whi
insists on surgery for those that lead to death directly, or
hazardous results of abscess.   Can this determination be
with certainty ?

The diagnosis of perityphlitis is usually easy.   Localized
sometimes masked early by pain elsewhere, often in the e
trium, and by vomiting ; more especially, localized tende:
soon some evidence, both by palpation and percussion, of
faction in the cæcal region ; possibly pain in this region o

ing the thigh, and with some fever—all perhaps following or attending diarrhœa—are ordinarily sufficient. Percussion dulness is often present over the tumor, though tympanites sometimes masks it completely, but palpation discovers an induration even of small size if it is done carefully and in comparison with the opposite side. The diagnosis of acute appendicitis before the advent of perityphlitis is more difficult, from the absence of any tumor and the deep location in the abdomen of the tenderness. The appendix sometimes hangs down into the true pelvis and far from the anterior wall of the abdomen. An appendicitis may be ushered in by vomiting and pain in the epigastrium, which may evoke such complaint as to mask the pain in the cæcal region. In only a little over one-half of all cases of acute inflammation in the cæcal region is the pain mostly in that locality, while in nearly one-third the pain is attributed to the abdomen generally. Sometimes there is a misleading sensation of induration to touch due to the tension of the abdominal muscles over the tender point, a condition that wholly disappears under anæsthesia. For purposes of diagnosis the hypodermic needle is permissible only when it is absolutely certain that it may be passed into the centre of the induration without entering the general peritoneal cavity. It is unsafe to use it in a supposed intraperitoneal abscess. The absence of fluctuation over an induration is no proof of the absence of pus ; pus is present in all large and in most small indurations of a few days' standing. In a few cases (it must be very few) digital exploration of the rectum will discover indurated tissue below the cæcal region.

A large proportion of first attacks, and probably many subsequent attacks, of acute appendicitis will doubtless recover without abscess, and with slight cellulitis or local peritonitis and adhesions, under proper treatment ; namely, quiescence in bed, hot applications, anodynes, light diet, and a rigid avoidance of all influences that can provoke general intestinal peristalsis. It can hardly be questioned that a majority of such cases recover even without these wholesomely safe measures of treatment and hygiene. Many cases of chronic appendicitis utterly fail to improve much under any treatment, albeit treatment doubtless often prevents such from passing on to ulceration.

When to go beyond medical treatment of these diseases ᵢ
insist on operation probably cannot be determined by any ab
lute rule. Each case must be dealt with by itself to some degr
since cases differ widely ; but there are certain general princip
that ought to guide us, in view of which we cannot shirk our fi
responsibility.

Reliance on medical treatment is justifiable in acute inflamm
tion in the cæcal region (i.e., appendicitis, perityphlitis, or typl
litis) of moderate severity, in the absence of strong evidence ᴏ
perforation, abscess, peritonitis, or marked tender induratio
lasting two or three days without some sign of decrease, and ᴏ
high temperature either continuous or recurring, rapid wea
pulse, or rapid anxious respiration. But we can never kno
when a catastrophe is to occur, even in an apparently mild ca
such as is here characterized. A few cases falling in this cat
gory will suffer sudden perforation, general peritonitis, and deat
but nearly all of them, failing of prompt recovery, will, if pᵉ
foration occurs, have sharply localized peritonitis or perityphlit
and probably abscess that will be easily discovered, and ᴡ
demand surgical treatment. That, in a high percentage of
large number of post-mortem examinations made on all sorts
cases, there should have been found evidence of previous,
covered appendicitis would seem to justify the position here tal

Reliance on medical treatment is also justifiable in suba
and chronic inflammation where the constitutional symptoms
mild, pain and tenderness slight, and the induration small
not increasing. Such cases frequently suffer occasional ᵉ
exacerbations of short duration, which do not positively ind
the need of an operation, unless each recurrence increase
size of the tumor or its sensitiveness to pressure, or dev
other proof that it is an abscess. To say that every perceᵖ
induration at the site of the cæcum should receive the min
tions of surgery is not justifiable ; and probably numerous ᵢ
might be reported of operation on small indurations withou
covering pus. One such is here presented :

" Mr. A. B. entered my hospital service complaining of ᵉ
pain and tenderness in the right iliac region, and giving a hi

of several attacks of acute inflammation within a year. In each attack there was moderate fever, and in the beginning frequent diarrhœa. A small induration over the lower part of the cæcum was distinctly made out ; it was slightly tender to pressure, and forward movement of the right thigh was embarrassed. This case was transferred to my surgical colleague, Dr. Parkes, in the belief that an operation should be made. He performed laparotomy, and found some thickened omentum, numerous adhesions, some of which he separated, but neither abscess nor appendicitis. The wound healed promptly."

The two outlines given above include the vast majority of all cases, and if the premises are correct, then these cases are most properly committed to strictly medical treatment, and the only proper treatment is the conservative course already described.

But surgical interference is demanded in certain cases of inflammation in the region under consideration, whether they happen to be called typhlitis, appendicitis, perityphlitis, or by some other name, and the weight of first responsibility is on the physician more than the surgeon.

1. Surgery is imperative in cases of acute inflammation in the cæcal region, with rather protracted high temperature, and with distinct induration, sensitive to pressure, that does not show positive evidence of subsidence within two days, or three or four days from the beginning. This rule becomes more urgent if the induration continues to increase in size and sensitiveness after two days, or if symptoms of general peritonitis occur, or rapid, weak pulse, or rapid respiration. The vast majority of such cases if left to themselves eventuate in abscess in less than a week, and many before that time lead to mortal peritonitis. Some require operation in less than two days from the beginning of the attack, and most of them have perforation of the appendix as early as the beginning of the symptoms.

I am aware that a few cases here characterized do not require operation and would recover without it, but the number is so small compared to those in the greatest peril, to which it is a crime not to offer the benefit of surgery, and the danger of an antiseptic operation is so slight that they constitute no impeachment of the rule.

60

2. Operation is required in cases of undoubted severe acute inflammation in the region of the appendix, even though no particular induration is demonstrable, and in cases of acute localized peritonitis having its origin certainly at the appendix and causing marked constitutional symptoms. In the one situation there is almost certainly such violent inflammation of the appendix as seriously to threaten perforation, with all its dire possibilities; in the other, perforation has occurred and an abscess is probably forming. In the one case there should be laparotomy and extirpation of the appendix; in the other, laparotomy, extirpation of the appendix, if possible, and treatment of the abscess. Probably these two classes cannot be distinguished from each other; many of the symptoms of the one belong to the other. Practically, it is hardly important that they should be distinguished, as both abundantly justify surgical interference; the patients are in vastly less jeopardy with the operation, when carefully made, than without it.

3. Surgery is especially promptly required in that small class of acute cases in which a large, sensitive induration develops rapidly, with high fever and general evidence of severe constitutional disturbance. Here extensive deposit and large abscess are almost certain to be present, and the danger of early rupture into the peritoneal cavity is considerable, hence the necessity of prompt action.

4. Surgical aid is demanded in all cases which have advanced to the subacute or chronic stage with distinct induration of considerable size, or with any induration that steadily increases in size for many days, since in most such cases pus is present. These are the cases where sometimes weeks and months after the acute stage a tumor of variable size is found in the iliac region, slightly tender, dull on percussion, and attended by a slight stiffness in walking dependent on pain in flexing the right thigh. Usually in such cases there are frequent exacerbations of moderate suffering in the affected region, often with slight fever, and disabling the patient for a day or two. Unless the tumor is very small pus is almost invariably found in its midst, the quantity varying from a few drachms to many ounces. The

patient cannot be safe so long as an abscess is present in the
neighborhood of the cæcum, but the danger is in proportion to
the size of the abscess. Some portion of the cæcum must generally form a part of the abscess wall, hence the liability of rupture into this canal and into the peritoneal cavity. In a case
seen by the writer in consultation with Dr. J. B. Murphy, a
perityphlitic abscess had undoubtedly existed for a year, since
the date of a previous illness in which there were dull pain and
fever for several weeks. The abscess ruptured into the abdominal cavity while the patient was scrubbing a floor; peritonitis
rapidly supervened; a circumscribed large peritoneal abscess
formed, which was opened by Dr. Murphy, and a quart of pus
evacuated. This case also exemplifies the large induration developing rapidly already referred to. The apparently small
difference between cases sure to die without operation and those
likely to recover without it, as well as the difficulty in finding
the line of duty in management, is shown in the two cases that
follow:

" D. F. G., aged 14 years, robust and active, went hunting
on April 30, 1881, and became very tired. The whole of the
next day he felt fatigued.

May 2nd.—Felt a little better, but had a mild diarrhœa;
next day more diarrhœa, pain, and slight tenderness on pressure
in the cæcal region. *4th*—I was called and found the diarrhœa
better, but still some pain and tenderness at the point mentioned;
pulse was 100 and temperature 101°F. *5th*—Patient was improved; slight tumefaction in the cæcal region; pulse 100 and
temperature 101.7°F. *6th*—No pain; tenderness less; pulse
100, temperature 99°F. *7th*—Temperature 99°F. There had
been no increase in respiration rate, and the patient felt convalescent. The next day at 11 p.m. a piercing pain was felt in the
lower abdomen at the right side, lasting only a few minutes.
Some tenderness was found soon afterward, but no tympanites;
the pulse was 100 and small, temperature 98.5°F.; respiration
20. Collapse came on in six hours, pulse was 150, temperature
98.5°F., and death in four hours more. It was found, post
mortem, that perforation of the appendix had led to an intra

peritoneal abscess containing an ounce of pus ; that the plast
wall of this abscess had given way at its superior point, a fu
minating general peritonitis being instantly lighted up. Th
rupture was at the distal end of the appendix, which was gai
grenous."

" G. B., aged 30, salesman, strong and active, had had occ
sional attacks of pain in the abdomen lasting for a few hour
He was seized last February, in the morning, with severe pa
in the lower abdomen, and went home and to bed. By evenin
his temperature was 104.5°F. ; then he discovered that the pai
which had continued to some degree all through the day, w
most intense in the right iliac region. His bowels were movi
by an enema. I saw him first at this time and found tumefa
tion and dulness in the cæcal region with the slightest possib
tenderness ; next day and the day after, the evidence of tum
was greater than at this time, the tenderness being reduce
The second day of attendance the temperature was over 103°]
the third day 102°, and the day following 99°, from which tii
convalescence was rapid, and he was out in a week from t
onset. The pulse was at no time much above 100, and t
respiration was not accelerated ; there was no diarrhœa and t
patient was tranquil in mind."

It will be seen that the temperature rapidly fell after the thi
day of the sickness ; with its fall the evidence of tumor rapic
disappeared. In this case tumefaction and dulness on percuss
were marked in the cæcal region, and entirely disppeared w
recovery, and there was never any notable tenderness. In 1
case of D. F. G., clinical evidence of tumor was slight, but d
ing the first week there was constantly more or less tenderne
a symptom we now know as some indication for surgical relie

5. Surgery is justifiable in all cases of undoubted chro
appendicitis with occasional exacerbations even if no indurat
is present. In all such cases we cannot doubt that the pati
is in constant danger of perforation of the appendix and mor
peritonitis or perityphlitis—a danger greater than that involv
in an antiseptically done laparotomy and extirpation of the lit
organ entire.

If the diagnosis was positive in every case there could be no objection to this proposition, for it covers only cases with some persistent cause of the inflammation, and not those with a temporary cause, and a single seizure with no special tendency to a recurrence. The persistent cause is usually something within the appendix that makes pressure and irritation, and back of that some constriction of the appendicular opening or some fault of its valve ; the cases of one mild attack and quiescence afterward are those in which there is no incarceration of irritating matter of any sort, and where the exit from the canal is free.

Fitz says catarrhal appendicitis is probably not recognizable. The diagnosis of such cases is beset with difficulties, and probably many of them cannot be diagnosed, but some may be, and these should not fail to receive the benefit of surgery simply because they may not appear for the moment to be formidable. The diagnosis must often be made by exclusion, and is easier in males than females, since in the latter the pelvic organs are apt to produce symptoms resembling those of appendicitis. The following case is illustrative :

" A lady of 28 years, vigorous and robust, had experienced from time to time since girlhood slight pain in the right groin and thigh, often aggravated by exercise. Occasionally there was accompanying but less pain in the left groin and thigh. Last summer she had what appeared to be a dysenteric attack, passed bloody stools, had much pain in the abdomen, especially on the right side, and fever. She recovered and resumed her active life, which required her to be much upon her feet. Soon pain in the abdomen recurred, then came slight fever, anorexia, occasional vomiting and constipation, tenderness over the hypogastrium, and pain in the thigh. At the end of six weeks she entered my hospital service and was carefully examined, my gynæcological colleague, Dr. Merriman, assisting. Then she was in bed, unable to move without pain in the abdomen, and suffering considerably in the thighs, hypogastrium, and right inguinal region. The abdomen was tender over its right side, from the border of the ribs to Poupart's ligament, but no tumefaction or dulness was discoverable. An examination of the pelvic organs

revealed nothing pathological, nor could any induration be fe
through the vagina or rectum. She had a daily rise of temper
ture to 100° or 101°F. The thighs were kept flexed much
the time, and pain in the psoas region occurred on flexing tl
right thigh against resistance ; a daily enema was requirec
the appetite was poor, and the sleep much disturbed by pai
She soon began to improve, and in a month or six weeks cou
turn in bed with only slight discomfort ; her appetite was bette
the pain less, and the temperature much of the time norma
The tenderness in the abdomen, however, persisted and becar
more marked over the cæcal region ; and one or two tentati
efforts at sitting up were followed by rise of temperature ai
return of pain lasting two days or more. It now seemed th
the history and course of the case had excluded every oth
pathological condition but some chronic inflammation at the loc
tion of the cæcum and appendix, and that the time for surgic
exploration had arrived, and my colleagues, Drs. Parkes ai
Merriman, examined her at my request and agreed that :
operation was justifiable. Laparotomy was made by Dr. Park·
and the appendix was found enlarged in its diameter, hard a
tense. projecting forward in an erect position, and deeply cc
gested. No other pathological condition was discovered in t
abdomen. The appendix was extirpated and found to conta
three small enteroliths, and a quantity of thick, tenacious mucι
its walls were thickened. On laying it open longitudinally
assumed instantly a rolled form in the reverse direction—ap
rently the peritoneum contracted and the thickened muc·
membrane and muscular tissue became extended. The pati·
made a good recovery from the operation and her sympto
have disappeared."

There was in this case no evidence of beginning ulceratior
the appendix, and so no immediate danger of a perforation, l
the tension of the organ was so great as to prove the existei
of an almost complete closure of its opening, and must have
to ulceration sooner or later. Moreover, the patient apparen
would have been a permanent invalid without the operation.

Anæsthetics in Natural Labor.—Obstetric anæsthesia is quite different from surgical anæsthesia, the latter being indicated for all obstetrical operations. Obstetric anæsthesia may be general or local. For the former are used ether, chloroform, chloral, and a variety of mixtures, including the bromide of ethyl and the protoxide of nitrogen. Chloral can hardly be considered as a general anæsthetic in the same sense as ether and chloroform· An injection of three or four grammes of chloral in solution given during the period of dilatation, and repeated, perhaps, in four or five hours, will often prove of the greatest benefit and comfort to the patient, regulating the pains, moderating the suffering of the patient, and abbreviating the duration of labor. In the latter part of labor chloral is less useful than chloroform, this substance being now almost universally used in parturition. When it is employed only in the first stage of anæesthesia no particular influence is exerted upon the contractions. If it is pushed to the second stage the contractions are retarded, but soon resume their normal rhythm. In the third stage of chloroform anæsthesia the contractions are diminished, or may cease altogether. This is a stage of danger, for not only the uterus but the heart and other muscular organs may be paralyzed. The fœtus experiences very little of the effect of the chloroform. The author's experience is thus summed up :

1. Chloroform given in small doses produces a condition of physical and moral calm in the patient.

2. If the inhalations are prolonged for a considerable time, the result will usually be an attenuation of the uterine pain. The perceptions of the patient become less keen and the uterine contractions are slower.

3. If the period of complete anæsthesia is reached with analgesia, there is surgical and not obstetrical anæsthesia.

4. In some cases chloroform excites instead of calming, and in such cases its use should be discontinued.

5. In some cases chloroform has unquestionably diminished the retractability of the uterus, and has thus been the cause of more or less severe hemorrhage after labor.

6. Chloroform has no action upon the fœtus.

7. Chloroform given during the period of expulsion has a l
decided effect upon the contractions of the abdominal musc
and the resistance of the perineum than is generally suppos
The sensation of pain at that period is not entirely abolish
the contractions are frequent.

Chloroform is especially indicated :

1. In primiparæ who are nervous and excitable, and in wh
the pain may even cause delirium ; also in those with whom t
labor is greatly prolonged, thus becoming a source of danger.

2. In all cases in which there is spasm, contraction, or rigidi
of the neck or body of the uterus. Contra-indications are t
absence of severe suffering, the existence of placenta prævi
general prostration, disease of the circulatory or respirato
organs, cerebral disease, alcoholism, etc.

During the period of dilatation chloroform is most require
but only to the exteut of obstetric anæsthesia, as a rule.
sometimes gives rise to nausea, vomiting, headache, and vario
nervous trouoles. Hemorrhage is not likely to result unless t
anæsthesia is profound. Chloroform cannot cause convulsion
on the contrary, it is one of the best means for relieving the
It may also be useful in warding off puerperal mania from tho
patients in whom the intense pain of parturition might lead
such a result. Dutertre has found reports of forty cases
sudden death during labor attributable to chloroform, but of t
number thirteen should be eliminated as irrelevant. Of
others, some had cardiac or pulmonary disease, some suffe
from alcoholism, and in others the narcosis was too profound.
first condition in the use of chloroform is that it be chemica
pure ; death from respiratory syncope may follow the use of
impure article. Small quantities should be given, the pati
being in the horizontal position, and there should be an inter
between successive inhalations.

Subcutaneous injections of antipyrine, 25 centigrammes a
dose, have been used in a number of cases to produce obstet
anæsthesia. Other mixtures have been suggested, in most
which ether, chloroform, or chloral is an element. The autl
expresses his views upon the subject as follows :

1. Nothing can be applied to relieve the pain caused by the distension of the lower segment of the uterus which causes the pain felt during the contractions.

2. Applications of cocaine may give relief if they reach the nerve-endings of the supravaginal and infravaginal portions of the cervix and the nerves of the vagina. Thus the pain of dilatation may be modified.

3. For the pain produced by compression of the nerve trunks of the pelvis no local application will avail.

4. The pain in the vulva and vaginal mucous membrane during expulsion may be somewhat modified by local applications.

As to the value of hypnotism in parturition it must have a limited range. Of thirteen cases in which it was tried, it was successful in only four, the patients all being of a hysterical temperament.—(*Dr. A. F. Currier ; N. Y. Med. Journal.*)

THE

Montreal Medical Journal.

VOL. XVIII.	JUNE, 1890.	No.

ASYLUM MANAGEMENT.

It has now been authoritatively ascertained that nearly hundred persons—mostly women—lost their lives in the dr ful holocaust at the Longue Pointe Asylum. In additio these, a large, but uncertain, number of the patients have s died in consequence of the exposure, hardships, and incre mental excitement following the fire. It was, indeed, an a ling and a heartrending calamity, and it is sincerely to be h that the Government of this Province will take steps to en as far as human foresight can, against any possibility of a tition in the future of such a wholesale sacrifice of human It is a foregone conclusion that no radical change will be in the method of caring for the insane in this Province. method is the old everywhere-else discarded plan of farming the lunatics—a plan, the fundamental defects of which been exposed and condemned by all alienists of modern tim a plan which, with especial reference to this very Asylum, shown by Dr. Tuke years ago to lie at the very root of the c abuses and the mouldy mediævalism which pervaded all it partments. The opposite method, the direct care of the ir by the Government, which appoints the superintendents, b the asylums, and controls all their operations—is that commends itself to every intelligent man who gives the m a moment's consideration ; and is the method employed ir other Provinces where the management of the asylums has highly spoken of by all experts who have visited them. T can be no comparison between the two systems. It is us for anyone at the present day to attempt a defence of the farming system, but in spite of that, we are obliged to say as we have already said, that no change in the direction of the modern treatment of our lunatics is to be hoped for. The nuns will get a new contract and will go on in the old way. The whole community was stirred by the simple narration of the facts gathered by Dr. Tuke at his inspection of the establishmont. Some people, more sanguine than those who know the Province better, believed that this event was bound to lay the foundation of a new era. But public interest in the matter soon began to flag; no sturdy philanthropists appeared to keep the matter under discussion and by frequent repetition prevent a too-easily satisfied public from relapsing into its former apathy. Thus, after a few months, new topics of interest took the place of that of asylum-management, and everything has been going on as before. Then came the great fire and its dreadful loss of life. The newspapers point out that the duty of the Government is to re-consider the entire question, and especially to take over the direct care and management of their helpless wards. That duty is as clear as day; but, will they do it? As already stated, all information goes to show that that duty will not be performed—but that in this matter we shall remain, as heretofore, a standing reproach and a shame.

CHANGES IN McGILL.

The old friends of Dr. Fenwick will regret to learn that, owing to impaired health, he has been obliged to resign his professorship in McGill University. As Demonstrator of Anatomy, as Professor of Clinical Surgery, and now for many years as Professor of Surgery, Dr. Fenwick has done admirable teaching work, has well maintained the high reputation of his department bequeathed to him by Dr. Geo. Campbell, and has taken a large part in moulding the present generation of Canadian practitioners. His keen interest in matters of surgical progress has never abated, and his great operative skill yet remains to him. He has won a well-merited rest from the laborious work of teaching,

and will, in future, have more time to devote to his *client*
We trust that, with the renewed vigor secured by a lessen
of his labors, Prof. Fenwick may yet live for many years
continue his much appreciated work in the interest of his patie
and the public. We are glad to know that the Governors of
University, in view of his long and great services to the Colle
have raised him to the position of Professor Emeritus, so t
the Faculty still will have the benefit of his presence and
wise counsels.

The vacancy thus created has been filled by the appointm
of Prof. T. G. Roddick to be Professor of Surgery. Dr. Rodd
will, however, retain his chair of Clinical Surgery in addit
and will continue to take an active part in hospital work du
the winter sessions. We are certain that this appointment
meet with enthusiastic acceptance from the Canadian med
public.

In future, Dr. James Bell, who for some years has had
perience in the teaching of practical surgery with the ju
class, will assume the majority of the lecture and clinique
with the senior class. He has been appointed to the positi
Lecturer on Clinical Surgery. Dr. Bell's already large ex
ence in general surgery, the care and skill he has shown :
operator, and his zeal as an investigator, ensure his doing
work in the important department which he now assumes.

THE FATAL AFTER-ACTION OF CHLOROFO1

Recently attention has been directed to a fatal action of c
form coming on some hours or even days after its administr
Ostertag, in a paper published in the *Deut. Med. Zeitun*
cords the result of a series of experiments he performed o
bits, dogs and cats. By keeping the animals under chlor
for several hours, he almost invariably found that fatty de
rative changes were induced in different organs. The
heart and kidneys were found to be the most frequent s
these changes. That similar changes are possible in man is
probable. The subject is one which has received but little :
tion. That chloroform may bring about a fatal issue days

its administration from a destructive action on the cellular elements of the blood is a well recognized fact. Such a condition has, we believe, come under our observation. The case was one where chloroform had been given for several hours ; the patient became cyanotic and icteroid, and died within twenty-two hours. The practical lesson to be derived from these observations is, that prolonged chloroform anæsthesia has its special dangers and should be avoided.

TOXIC ALBUMINURIA.

It is well known that albuminuria can be experimentally induced by certain drugs. Digitalis, for instance, will, in animals, as surely give rise to albuminuria, as the compression of the renal artery or vein and the mode of action is similar in the two cases. Digitalis acts by practically inducing compression of the renal arterioles. Strychnine has been proved to have a similar action to digitalis. Both of these agents induce albuminuria through their influence on the circulation.

We have a second class of drugs which bring about albuminuria by a direct action on the secreting texture of the kidneys. Cantharides, lead, mercury and chlorate of potassium act in this way.

It has recently been pointed out that albuminuria is not infrequent in those afflicted with the morphia habit. In a communication to the Société Méd. des Hop., Huchard advances the view that this accident is due to the action of the drug in lowering the blood tension. He narrates a case fatal with uræmic symptoms. It is important that the urine in all cases of the abuse of morphia should be examined, for the presence of albumen in it would certainly be an important guide to judicious treatment.

—An interesting ceremony took place recently in the surgical theatre of the General Hospital at Munich. The occasion was the celebration of the return to work of Prof. Nussbaum after a long and dangerous illness. The festal reception given him by his assistants and students, and the enthusiasm with which he

was greeted, showed the profound respect and affection whi
entertained for this great surgeon. He expressed his grati
for their kindly welcome, and felt thankful to the Almighty
he was once more spared to go out and in among them.

—The malaria plasmodia are now being universally recogi
throughout Europe. Within the last few months L. Pfeifi
Wiesbaden, R. Paltauf of Vienna, V. Jaksch of Gratz, and F
of Berlin, have had opportunity to investigate cases of mal
and have all, without exception, recognized the correctne
Laveran's description.

Personal.

—H. S. Birkett, M.D., has been appointed Laryngolog
the Montreal Dispensary.

—Archie W. Campbell, M.D., has started practice as a
cialist in laryngology in this city.

—T. Johnson-Alloway, M.D., has been appointed Assi
Gynæcologist to the Montreal General Hospital.

—T. A. Rodger, M.D., surgeon to the Grand Trunk Rail
has been appointed Assistant Surgeon to the Montreal Gei
Hospital.

—Dr. Burgess, the recently appointed superintendent of
Protestant Hospital for the Insane in this city, has arrived,
will in a few days be able to receive patients. Dr. Burgi
a welcome addition to the professional men of Montreal.

Medical Items.

—A monument to the memory of Dr. Mesmer, from w
mesmerism derives its name, was lately unveiled at Dresde

—Dr. H. C. Wood of Philadelphia has been appointe
deliver one of the public addresses at the International Mec
Congress in Berlin.

—A committee has been formed at the Sarbonne for encouraging foreigners to study at the University of Paris. M. Pasteur is president. It is proposed to give special facilities to foreign students immediately upon their arrival in Paris.

TYPHOID FEVER.—A. Wiltschour of St. Petersburg, examined, in 28 cases, the stools of typhoid patients. He never found the specific bacilli earlier than the tenth day, after which date it was almost constantly present in the proportion of 1 to 25 or 30 of the other bacteria. Out of 35 cases where the blood was examined microscopically and by cultivation methods the characteristic bacillus was found once on the eighth day.

—During the past few years the subject of hygiene has received marked attention from the German Government. In nearly all the leading universities there are now hygienic institutes, thoroughly equipped in every way to afford to students excellent opportunities of acquiring a sound knowledge of this important subject. Last month the new Hygienic Institute in the University of Halle was opened by an address from Professor Benk. The Institute has a lecture-room which can accommodate sixty students, and also special chemical, physical and bacteriological laboratories. It is hoped that before long McGill University will possess a hygienic institute which will rival in completeness that of the German universities.

—J. B. Lippincott Company announce, in press, an important work on " Regional Anatomy in its relation to Medicine and Surgery," by George McClellan, M.D., Lecturer on Descriptive and Regional Anatomy at the Philadelphia School of Anatomy, etc., etc. With about one hundred full-page fac-simile illustrations reproduced from photographs taken by the author of his own dissections, expressly designed and prepared for this work, and colored by him after nature. To be complete in two volumes of about 250 pages each ; large quarto. The object of the work is to convey a practical knowledge of regional anatomy of the entire body ; the text to embrace, besides a clear description of the part in systematic order, the most recent and reliable infor-

mation regarding anatomy in its medical and surgical rela
The illustrations are intended to verify the text and to
before the reader the parts under consideration in as reali
manner as possible. Vol. I. will be ready for publication
December 9th, and the second volume is expected to a
shortly thereafter. The work will be sold by subscription

ONTARIO MEDICAL ASSOCIATION.—The following are
officers of this Association for the ensuing year:—

President—Dr. W. H. Moorehouse, London.

Vice-Presidents—Dr. Charles Sheard, Toronto ; Dr.
Gibson, Belleville ; Dr. Powell, Ottawa ; Dr. Wishart, Lo

General Secretary—Dr. J. Gibb Wishart, Toronto.

Assistant Secretary—Dr. W. P. Caven.

Treasurer—Dr. E. J. Barrick, Toronto.

Committee on Credentials—Dr. Shaw, Hamilton ; Dr. L
Acton.

Committee on Public Health—Dr. W. J. Charlton, We
Dr. Farley, Belleville.

Committee on Legislation—Hon. M. Sullivan, King
Dr. Waugh, London.

Committee on Publication—Dr. J. L. Davison, Toronto
A. Primrose, Toronto.

Committee on By-laws—Dr. Griffin, Hamilton ; Dr. C
Toronto.

Committee on Ethics—Dr. A. R. Harvie, Orillia ; Dr.
W. Ross, Toronto.

The following were elected honorary members: Dr.
Emmet, New York ; Dr. E. M. Moore, Rochester ; Dr. J
Workman, Toronto ; and Dr. William Mickle, London, E

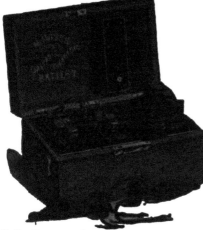

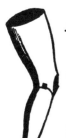
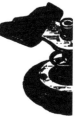

In corresponding with advertisers please mention Montreal Medical Journal.

'THIS IS AN AGE OF APOLLINARIS WATER."

Walter Besant.

Apollinaris

"THE QUEEN OF TABLE WATERS

The filling at the Apollinaris Spring (Rhenish Prussia) amounted to

11,894,000 **BOTTLES IN** **1887,**

12,720,000 **BOTTLES IN** **1888**

AND

15,822,000 **BOTTLES IN** **1889.**

" *The annual consumption of this favorite beverage affords a striking proof of the widespread demand which exists for table water of absolute purity, and it is satisfactory to find that, wherever one travels, in either hemisphere, it is to be met with; it is ubiquitous, and should be known as the cosmopolitan table water. ' Quod ab omnibus, quod ubique.' "—* BRITISH MEDICAL JOURNAL.

SOLE EXPORTERS:

THE APOLLINARIS COMPANY, LIMITED,

19 REGENT STREET, LONDON, S.W.

FROM IMPERFECT NUTRITION.

LACTOPEPTINE precisely represents in composition the natural digestive juices of the Stomach, Pancreas and Salivary Glands, and will therefore, readily dissolve all foods necessary to the recuperation of the human organism.

LACTOPEPTINE, Elixir.

We call special attention to our Elixir, which we have recently greatly improved, establishing as a fact that the compound forming Lactopeptine can, by employing a proper menstruum, be entirely incorporated and suspended in fluid form.

Each fluid ounce contains 35 grains of Lactopeptine.

Dose.—One to two teaspoonfuls after each meal.

SPECIAL NOTICE TO THE MEDICAL PROFESSION

Whenever satisfactory results are not obtained from the administration of **LACTOPEPTINE**, we will consider it a favor if such facts are reported to us, for there can be no doubt that substitution of Papain, or some of the cheap imitations of Lactopeptine has been practiced, whenever the therapeutic activity of Lactopeptine is so uniformly recommended in its indications.

You address to or our new Medical Almanac, containing valuable

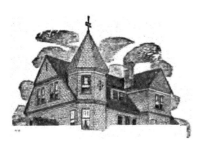

In corresponding with advertisers please mention Montreal Medical Journal.

M^CGILL UNIVERSITY, MONTREA

FACULTY OF MEDICINE.

FIFTY-SIXTH SESSION, 1889–90.

FACULTY:

SIR WILLIAM DAWSON, LL.D., F.R.S., Principal and Professor of Natural Hist
ROBERT CRAIK, M.D., Dean of the Faculty.

Emeritus Professors.

W. WRIGHT, M.D., L.R.C.S. | DUNCAN C. McCALLUM, M.D., M.R.

Professors.

ROBERT CRAIK, M.D., Professor of Hygiene.

G. E. FENWICK, M.D., Prof. of Surgery.

G. P. GIRDWOOD, M.D., M.R.C.S., Eng., Professor of Chemistry.

GEORGE ROSS, A.M., M.D., Professor of Medicine.

THOS. G. RODDICK, M.D., Professor of Clinical Surgery.

WILLIAM GARDNER, M.D., Professor of Gynæcology.

F. J. SHEPHERD, M.D., M.R.C.S., Eng., Professor of Anatomy.

F. BULLER, M.D., M.R.C.S., Eng., Professor of Ophthalmology.

JAMES STEWART, M.D., L.R.C.P.R. fessor of Materia Medica and Therape and Registrar to Faculty.

GEORGE WILKINS, M.D., M.R.C.S., Professor of Medical Jurisprudence Lecturer on Histology.

D. P. PENHALLOW, B.Sc., Profes Botany.

RICHARD L. MACDONNELL, B.A., M.R.C.S., Eng., Professor of Cl Medicine.

WESLEY MILLS, M.A., M.D., L.R. Lond., Professor of Physiology.

J. CHALMERS CAMERON, M.D., M. L., Prof. Midwifery & Diseases of In

Demonstrators, Instructors, &c.

R. F. RUTTAN, B.A., M.D., Lecturer on Chemistry.

WM. SUTHERLAND, M.D., L.R.C.P., Lond. Assistant Demonstrator of Anatomy.

GEO. W. MAJOR, B.A., M.D., Instructor in Laryngology.

A. D. BLACKADER, B.A., M.D., M.R.C.S., Eng., Instructor in Diseases of Children.

WYATT G. JOHNSTON, M.D., D strator of Pathology.

JAMES BELL, M.D., Assistant to th fessor of Clinical Surgery.

T. JOHNSON ALLOWAY, M.D., Inst in Gynæcology.

F. G. FINLEY, M.D., Assistant D strator of Anatomy.

H. S. BIRKETT, Assistant Demons of Anatomy.

The Collegiate Courses of this School are a Winter Session, extending the 1st of October to the end of March, and a Summer Session from the e the first week in April to end of the first week in July.

The fifty-seventh session will commence on the 1st of October, and will be tinued until the end of the following March; this will be followed by a Su Session, commencing about the middle of April and ending the first wee July.

Founded in 1824, and organized as a Faculty of McGill University in this School has enjoyed, in an unusual degree, the confidence of the Profe throughout Canada and the neighboring States.

One of the distinctive features in the teaching of this School, and the o which its prosperity is largely due, is the prominence given to Clinical Ins tion. Based on the Edinburgh model, it is chiefly Bed-side, and the Stu personally investigates the cases under the supervision of special Profess Clinical Medicine and Surgery.

The Primary subjects are now all taught practically as well as theoreti For the department of Anatomy, besides a commodious and well-li dissecting-room, there is a special anatomical museum and a bone The other branches are also provided with large laboratories for v courses. There is a Physiological Laboratory, well stocked with apparatus; a Histological Laboratory, supplied with thirty-five microscopes; a Pharmacological Laboratory, in which experiments will be performed demonstrating the action of drugs, &c.; a large Chemical Laboratory, capable of accommodating 76 students at work at a time.

Besides these, there is a Pathological Laboratory, well adapted for its special work, where accommodation is provided for students and practitioners wishing to do special work in Morbid Anatomy and Bacteriology.

About a year ago, at a great expense, extensive additions were made to the building and the old one entirely remodelled, so that besides the Laboratories, there are two large lecture-rooms capable of seating 300 students each, also a demonstrating-room for a smaller number. There is also a Library of over 10,000 volumes, and a museum, as well as Reading-rooms for the students.

In the recent improvements that were made, the comfort of the students was also kept in view.

Matriculation.

Students from Ontario and Quebec are advised to pass the Matriculation Examination of the Medical Councils of their respective Provinces before entering upon their studies. Students from the United States and Maritime Provinces, unless they can produce a certificate of having passed a recognized Matriculation Examination, must present themselves for the Examination of the University, on the first Friday of October, or the last Friday of March.

Hospitals.

The Montreal General Hospital has an average number of 150 patients in the wards, the majority of whom are affected with diseases of an acute character. The shipping and large manufactories contribute a great many examples of accidents and surgical cases. In the Out-Door Department there is a daily attendance of between 75 and 100 patients, which affords excellent instruction in minor surgery, routine medical practice, venereal diseases, and the diseases of children. Clinical clerkships and dresserships can be obtained on application to the members of the Hospital staff.

University Dispensary.

This was established four years ago for the purpose of affording to senior students practical instruction in Diseases of Women, and has proved very successful. Three other special departments have been added—viz., Diseases of Children, Diseases of the Skin, and Diseases of the Nervous System.

Clinics.

The Clinical teaching is conducted in the wards and theatre of the General Hospital, daily, throughout the session. Ample opportunities are afforded to the Student to investigate the cases, medical and surgical.

Requirements for Degree.

Every candidate must be 21 years of age, have studied medicine during *four* six months' Winter Sessions, and *one* three months' Summer Session, one Session being at this School, and must pass the necessary examinations.

FEES, arranged according to years, are as follows:—

First Year, $69; Second Year, $91; Third Year, $97; Fourth Year, $65; Hospital Ticket (6 months), $8; Lying-in Hospital (6 months), $8; Graduation, $30.

All Fees are payable strictly in advance.

For further information, or Annual Announcement, apply to

JAMES STEWART, M.D., Registrar,
Medical Faculty, McGill College

MEDICAL DEPARTMENT
OF THE
UNIVERSITY OF VERMO[
BURLINGTON, VERMONT, U.S.A.,
WILL BEGIN
On the Last Thursday of February, 1890, and continue Twenty W

FACULTY OF MEDICINE.

MATTHEW H. BUCKHAM, D.D., - - - - PRESIDENT.

JOHN ORDRONAUX, M.D., LL.D., Emeritus Professor of Medical Jurispruder

J. W. WRIGHT, A.M., M.D., NEW YORK CITY, Emeritus Professor of Princip Practice of Surgery.

A. F. A. KING, A.M., M.D., WASHINGTON, D.C., Professor of Obstetrics and I of Women.

A. P. GRINNELL, M.D., BURLINGTON, VT., Dean of the Faculty, Professor Theory and Practice of Medicine.

R. A. WITTHAUS, A.M., M.D., NEW YORK CITY, Prof. of Chemistry and Tox

J. HENRY JACKSON, A.M., M.D., BARRE, VT., Professor of Physiology and] copic Anatomy.

WM. B. TOWLES, M.D., UNIVERSITY OF VIRGINIA, Professor of General and | Anatomy.

J. H. WOODWARD, B.C., IM.D., BURLINGTON. .VT., Professor of Materia . and Therapeutics.

A. M. PHELPS, M.D., NEW YORK CITY, Professor of Surgery.

PROFESSORS OF SPECIAL SUBJECTS.

ROBERT W. TAYLOR, M.D., NEW YORK CITY, Professor of Diseases of th and Venereal Diseases.

STEPHEN M. ROBERTS, A.M., M.D., NEW YORK CITY, Professor of Dises Children.

ADRIAN THEODORE WOODWARD, M.D., BRANDON, VT., Professor of S Diseases of Women.

EDWARD D. FISHER, NEW YORK CITY, Professor of Diseases of the Mii Nervous System.

J. H. WOODWARD, M.D., BURLINGTON, VT., Professor of Diseases of the Eye al

WILDER A. BURNAP, A.M., BURLINGTON, VT., Professor of Medical Jurispre

——————————, M.D., RUTLAND, VT., Professor of Sanitary Science.

GEORGE B. HOPE, M.D., NEW YORK CITY, Professor of Diseases of the Throa

CHARLES B. KELSEY, M.D., NEW YORK, Professor of Diseases of the Rectum

HENRY C. TINKHAM, M.D., BURLINGTON, VT., Demonstrator of Anatomy.

The Lectures on special subjects, by gentlemen recognized as authorities in the ticular departments, will be delivered during the regular session without extra fee.

New College Building.—Owing to the generosity of Mr. John P. How: Burlington, Vt., a new College Building has been erected, with all modern improve capable of seating about four hundred students.

Hospital Advantages.—The MARY FLETCHER HOSPITAL, with its comm amphitheatre, is open for clinical instruction during the session. The Medical and S Clinics of the College will be held in the amphitheatre attached to the Hospital.

The PRELIMINARY TERM, consisting of a Course of Lectures and Recitations various branches of Medicine and Surgery, will begin on the First Thursday of Nov each year, and continue until March 1st. Fee, $30.00.

The REGULAR WINTER SESSION will commence on the last Thursday of Fel 1890, and continue twenty weeks. This Course will consist of from five to six Lectures in the various departments of Medicine and Surgery.

FEES FOR THE REGULAR SESSION:

Matriculation Fee, payable each Term ....$

Fees for the full Course of Lectures by all the Professors..............

Perpetual Ticket 1

Examination Fee, not returnable ....

Students who have already attended two full courses of lectures in other regular s are admitted on paying the matriculation fee and $40. Students who have attended o course in some regular established medical school and one full course in this College : mitted to a third course on paying the Matriculation Fee and $25. Graduates of this are admitted without fee. Graduates of other regular schools, and Theological Studen admitted by paying the Matriculation Fee.

For further particulars and circular, address the Dean.

PROF. A. P. GRINNELL, M.D., BURLING

THE MONTREAL MEDICAL JOURNAL.

EDITORS :

GEORGE ROSS, A.M., M.D. | T. G. RODDICK, M.D. | JAS. STEWART, M.D.

SUBSCRIPTION, $2.00 Per Annum. Payable in Advance.

HALF RATE TO MEDICAL STUDENTS.

ADVERTISING SCALE OF PRICES :

One Page (8vo. Demy)—12 Months $60—6 Months				-	-	-	-	-	-	$35
Half " "	"	35	"	-	-	-	-	-	-	20
Quarter Page "	"	20	"	-	-	-	-	-	-	12
Eighth " "	"	12	"	-	-	-	-	-	-	7

☞ Monthly, two monthly or three monthly Advertisements payable in advance ; half-yearly and yearly Advertisements payable quarterly in advance. Any omission of insertion during contract to be made up by extra insertion at end of term. Business communications to be addressed to the Publisher,

Address, THE MONTREAL MEDICAL JOURNAL CO.,

P.O. Box 386,   MONTREAL.

Subscriptions received by

J. H. CHAPMAN, SURGICAL SUPPLY DEPOT,

2294 St. Catherine Street, MONTREAL.

A
CLASSIFICATION OF ADVERTISEMENTS

In Corresponding with Advertisers please ment "Montreal Medical Journal."

NEW YORK
Post-Graduate Medical School and Hospital.

Incorporated by Special Act of the Legislature of the State of New York.

FOR PRACTITIONERS OF MEDICINE EXCLUSIVELY.

EIGHTH YEAR — SESSIONS OF 1889-'90.

FACULTY.

D. B. ST. JOHN ROOSA, M.D., LL.D.,
Professor of Diseases of the Eye and Ear; Surgeon to the Manhattan Eye and Ear Hospital; President of the Faculty.

CHARLES L. DANA, M.D ,
Professor of Diseases of the Mind and Nervous System; Professor of Physiology Woman's Medical College, Physician to Bellevue Hospital.

ANDREW H SMITH, M D.,
Professor of Clinical Medicine and Therapeutics; Physician to the Presbyterian Hospital; Consulting Physician to the Orthopædic Hospital.

WILLIAM OLIVER MOORE, M D ,
Professor of Diseases of the Eye and Ear; Professor of Diseases of the Eye and Ear, University of Vermont, and Woman's Medical College, New York.

BACHE McE. EMMET, M.D.
Professor of Diseases of Women; Assistant Surgeon to the New York State Woman's Hospital.

EDWARD KERSHNER, M.D., U.S N.,
Professor of Naval, Military, and State Hygiene.

AMBROSE L. RANNEY, M.D.,
Professor of the Anatomy and Physiology of the Nervous System ; Professor of Diseases of the Mind and the Nervous System, University of Vermont.

WILLIAM HENRY PORTER, M D ,
Professor of Clinical Medicine and Pathology ; Curator of the Presbyterian Hospital.

J. H. NILSEN, M.D.,
Professor of Diseases of Women

STEPHEN SMITH BURT, M.D.,
Professor of Clinical Medicine and Physical Diagnosis , Physician to the Out-Door Department, Bellevue Hospital.

SENECA D. POWELL, M D.,
Professor of Clinical Surgery, Surgeon to St. Elizabeth's Hospital

C A. VON RAMDOHR, M D.,
Professor of Obstetrics , Physician to the German Poliklinik.

HORACE T. HANKS, M.D ,
Professor of Diseases of Women; Assistant-Surgeon to the New York State Woman's Hospital

LEWIS S PILCHER, M.D.,
Professor of Clinical Surgery, Surgeon to the Methodist Episcopal Hospital, Brooklyn.

HENRY J. GARRIGUES, M.D.,
Professor of Obstetrics , Surgeon to the Maternity and German Hospitals.

CLARENCE C. RICE, M.D.,
Professor of Diseases of the Throat and Nose; Consulting Surgeon to the Out-Door Department, Bellevue Hospital, Secretary of the Faculty

CHARLES CARROLL LEE, M.D.,
Professor of Diseases of Women; Surgeon to the New York State Woman's Hospital; Consulting Surgeon to Charity Hospital.

GRAEME M HAMMOND, M.D.,
Professor of Diseases of the Mind and Nervous System.

GEORGE B. FOWLER, M.D.,
Professor of Clinical Medicine and Medical Chemistry; Physician to Bellevue Hospital; Visiting Physician N Y. Infant Asylum

ROBERT ABBE, M.D.,
Professor of Clinical Surgery; Surgeon to St. Luke's Hospital.

A M. PHELPS. M.D.,
Professor of Orthopædic Surgery; Professor of Orthopædic Surgery, University of Vermont; Instructor in Orthopedic Surgery in the University of the City of New York.

HENRY D. CHAPIN, M.D ,
Professor of Diseases of Children; Visiting Physician Out-door Department Bellevue Hospital

A. D ROCKWELL, M.D,
Professor of Electro-Therapeutics.

L. BOLTON BANGS, M.D.,
Professor of Venereal and Genito-Urinary Diseases; Surgeon to St. Luke's Hospital.

O. B. DOUGLAS, M.D.,
Professor of Diseases of the Nose and Throat; Surgeon to the Manhattan Eye and Ear Infirmary.

PETER A. CALLAN, M.D.,
Professor of Diseases of the Eye; Surgeon to the New York Eye and Ear Infirmary.

JOSEPH O'DWYER, M.D.,
Professor of Diseases of Children

R W. TAYLOR, M'D.
Professor of diseases of the Skin.

J. B. EMERSON, M.D.,
Professor of diseases of the Eye and Ear.

FREDERICK BAGOE, PH. B.
Professor of Pharmacology

J. H RIPLEY, M.D.,
Professor of Diseases of Children.

FRANK FERGUSON, M.D.
Professor of Pathology, Pathologist to the New York Hospital.

CHARLES B. KELSEY, M D ,
Professor of Rectal Diseases.

REYNOLD W. WILCOX, M.D.,
Professor of Clinical Medicine.

CHARLES H. KNIGHT, M D ,
Professor of Laryngology and Rhinology.

This school was founded by members of the Post-Graduate Faculty of the University of the City of New York, and was the first institution in the United States to present a systematic system of clinical instruction for graduates in medicine.

All the lectures are clinical. It is a place of instruction where the practitioner, by actually handling the cases under the guidance of the professors and instructors, may learn the use of instruments for examination and treatment, and observe the effects of remedies. Its facilities are unrivaled. Each hospital to which the teachers are attached forms a part of the field of instruction. The general schedule is so arranged that there is no conflict in the hours of attendance of the professors. The clinics begin at 9 A.M., and continue until 9 P.M. each day. The Hospital of the School contains eighty-five beds—a new building having been lately added to the premises already occupied. This Hospital has been in active operation for five years, and furnishes most important clinical cases for study. It is open nine months of the year. The Babies' Wards are open the whole year.

☞ Sessions continue throughout the year. Physicians may join the classes at any time. For Catalogue and further information, address

CLARENCE C. RICE, M.D., Secretary of the Faculty,
226 East 20th Street, NEW YORK CITY.

C

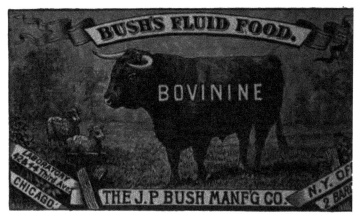

"NUTRITION IS THE PHYSICAL BASIS OF L

This axiom, formulated by the lamented Fothergill, conveys a v meaning to the intelligent physician. If a food can be obtained con all the elements necessary for the nourishment and support of the bo which can also be readily assimilated under every condition of dise immense advantage is obtained in controlling symptoms and restoring tissues. Mal-nutrition and mal-assimilation are potent factors in train of critical ailments. Bush's Fluid Food BOVININE combine concentrated form all the extractive or albuminous properties of un beef, together with its stimulating salts.

Dr. Geo. D. Hays, of New York Post-Graduate School, in an exh essay on Artificial Alimentation, thus alludes to BOVININE: "Of t parations of raw food extracts one has a clinically proved value. It in nitrogenous substances and phosphates. It is readily digested a sorbed, and can be relied upon for the entire sustenance of the bo considerable period."

The blood corpuscles, which carry such a wealth of vitalizing pow found in BOVININE intact, as revealed by the microscope in co thousands.

B. N. Towle, M.D., of Boston, in a notable paper on Raw Foods, read the American Medical Association at Washington, D.C., May 6th, 18S refers to BOVININE: "I have given it continually to patients for with signal comfort, especially in complicated cases of dyspepsia a by epigastric uneasiness from inervation, and in nervous debility standing. Raw food is equally adapted to acute lingering diseases."

In stomach and intestinal troubles of childhood proceeding fro gestion, its administration is followed by marked benefits, while bo infants thrive wonderfully upon it, five to fifteen drops being adde feeding. A decided change for the better is often seen in weakly i twenty-four hours. BOVININE is palatable to the most fastidious t

Samples to physicians on application.

CAREFULLY PREPARED BY
The J. P. Bush Manufacturing Comp
2 BARCLAY STREET, NEW YORK CITY.

LABORATORY, 42 & 44 THIRD AVENUE, CHICAGO.

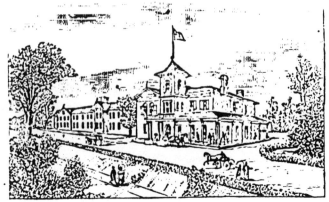

*A Private Asylum for the Care and Treatment of the Insane,
Inebriates, and the Opium Habit.*

DIRECTORS.

J. W. LANGMUIR, Esq., Ex-Inspector of Asylums, Etc., for Ontario, *President.*
E. A. MEREDITH, Esq., LL.D., Ex-Chairman of the Board of Inspectors of Asylums for
Canada, *Vice-President.*
F. W. JARVIS, Esq., Sheriff of the County of York.
ROBERT JAFFRAY, Esq., Vice-President of the Land Security Company, Toronto.
JAMES A. HEDLEY, Esq., Editor *Monetary Times*, Toronto.

MEDICAL SUPERINTENDENT.

DR. STEPHEN LETT, Assistant Medical Superintendent for 13 years of the London and
Toronto Lunatic Asylums.

CONSULTING PHYSICIAN.

JOSEPH WORKMAN, Esq., M.D., Medical Superintendent for 23 years of the Provincial
Lunatic Asylum, Toronto.

This admirably appointed and salubriously situated Retreat, whilst possessing all the
advantages of a larger institution, enjoys the privacy and quietness of a gentleman's residence.

The number of patients being limited, each case comes under the direct personal care
and attention of the Medical Superintendent.

There are a few vacancies for both male and female patients.

Application for admission should be made to the Medical Superintendent, either personally or by letter, giving a short outline of the history and symptoms of the proposed patient,
whereupon the requisite blank forms will be furnished with full instructions as to their
execution.

Habit Cases and Inebriates are received upon their voluntary application according to a
prescribed form.

For terms and other information, address

DR. STEPHEN LETT, Homewood Retreat, GUELPH, Ont

MONTREAL TRUSS FACTORY.

J. HUDSON,

692 CRAIG STREET, - - MONTREAL,

MANUFACTURER OF

All Kinds of Deformity Apparatus.

**TRUSSES,   SUPPORTERS,   BRACES,
CRUTCHES,   ARTIFICIAL LIMBS,   Etc.**

Seeley's celebrated Hard Rubber Trusses and the Celluloid Company's
Trusses, of all sizes and shapes, in stock.

PARTURITIOI

Aletris Cordial [Rio] given in Teaspoonful
every hour or two AFTER PARTURITION, is the
agent to prevent after-pains and hemorrhage. I
DIRECT tonic action on the uterus, it expels blood-
closes the uterine sinuses, causes the womb to con
and prevents subinvolution. In severe cases, it ca
combined with ergot in the proportion of one oun
fluid Ext. Ergot to three ounces Aletris Cordial
is the experience of eminent practitioners, in all
where ergot is indicated, that its action is rendered r
more efficacious by combining it with Aletris Cordi
the proportions above stated.

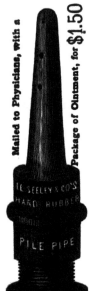

WYETH'S

Beef, Iron and Wir

Extract of Beef, Citrate of Iron a Sherry Wine.

In this preparation are combined the stimulant properties of W the nutriment of BEEF with the tonic powers of IRON, the effect of w the blood is so justly valued. For many cases in which there is

Pallor, Weakness, Palpitation of the Heart,

with much nervous disturbance, as, for example, where there has bee loss of blood, or during the recovery from wasting fevers, this article found especially adapted. The peculiar feature of this combination is

Combines Nutriment with Stimulus.

Prompt results will follow its use in cases of sudden exhaustion, from either acute or chronic diseases, and will prove a

Valuable Restorative for all Convalescents.

As a Nutritive Tonic it would be indicated in the treatment of ir nutrition, impoverishment of the blood, and in all of the various f general debility. Each tablespoonful contains the essence of one o Beef, with two grains of Citrate of Iron, dissolved in Sherry Wine.

IMPORTANT.

MARCH 1st,

We have been advised by Physicians and Druggists of Imitat our BEEF, IRON AND WINE, so similar in appearance (the bo style of label being an exact copy, with *verbatim* wording), that would be deceived, rendering it necessary for the purchaser to see t NAME is on the LABEL to avoid being imposed upon.

The reputation of this combination has been created by that manufacture, and we feel that Physicians should give our article the ence, as they can depend upon the quality of the material, as well intelligent manipulation in its preparation ; while a great deal that i and claimed to be equal to ours, is disagreeable to the taste, offer stomach, and must disappoint the prescriber.

JOHN WYETH & B